**Therapeutic Nanocarriers in Cancer Treatment:
Challenges and Future Perspective**

Editors: Neeraj Mishra, Ashish Garg and Neeraj Upmanyu

ISBN (Online): 978-981-5080-50-6

ISBN (Print): 978-981-5080-51-3

ISBN (Paperback): 978-981-5080-52-0

First published in 2023.

Therapeutic Nanocarrie
Cancer Treatment: Chall
and Future Perspecti

Edited by

Neeraj Mishra
Amity Institute of Pharmacy
Amity University Madhya Pradesh
Gwalior (M.P.)
India

Ashish Garg
Department of P. G. Studies and Research in C
and Pharmacy, Rani Durgavati Universit
Jabalpur (M.P.)
India

&

Neeraj Upmanyu
Sagar Institute of Research & Technology-Phar
Pro Vice-Chancellor, Sage University
Bhopal
India

need for a court order if at any point you breach any terms of this License Agreement. In no event will any delay or failure by Bentham Science Publishers in enforcing your compliance with this License Agreement constitute a waiver of any of its rights.

3. You acknowledge that you have read this License Agreement, and agree to be bound by its terms and conditions. To the extent that any other terms and conditions presented on any website of Bentham Science Publishers conflict with, or are inconsistent with, the terms and conditions set out in this License Agreement, you acknowledge that the terms and conditions set out in this License Agreement shall prevail.

Bentham Science Publishers Pte. Ltd.
80 Robinson Road #02-00
Singapore 068898
Singapore
Email: subscriptions@benthamscience.net

BENTHAM
SCIENCE

CONTENTS

FOREWORD

Research in nanomedicine is a fast-emerging topic of study with broad application potential throughout the whole healthcare sector. They include a wide range of technologies, ranging from particles to networks and nanostructures and theragnostic applications. A selection of the most recent and representative breakthroughs in nanomedicine, which have been carried out in the context of a wide range of different cancer varieties, are presented in this book. This book is primarily concerned with the use of nanomedicine and nanotechnology in the treatment of different types of cancer. There will be an introduction to a variety of nano-carriers, specifically nanoparticulate systems, NLCs, and carbon nanostructures, polymer nanocomposites. There will also be an introduction to a variety of methodological techniques for the treatment and targeting of a number of cancer groups, such as lung, cervical, breast, and ovarian cancer, head and neck cancer, prostate cancer, and others. It emphasizes some of the most important aspects related to synthesis strategies for a wide range of nanostructures, and it offers readers to research on the creation of surface-modified nano-systems for cancer detection and treatment. The chapters include a wide variety of advanced data from existing and ongoing clinical research, as well as major regulatory considerations and issues. This reference book will be of great use to oncologists, health care professionals, research scientists, physicians, pathologists, biologists, biochemistry specialists, chemists, pharmacists, and people interested in cancer biology and nanomedicine and renowned professionals who are engaged in ground-breaking research.

Amit K. Goyal
Department of Pharmacy, School of Chemical Sciences and Pharmacy
Central University of Rajasthan
Rajasthan, India

Kamal Dua
Australian Research Centre in Complementary and
Integrative Medicine of Technology Sydney
Ultimo, 2007 New South Wales
Australia

Subheet K. Jain
Department of Pharmacy, Guru Nanak Dev University
Amritsar (Punjab)
India

Sanyog Jain
National Institute of Pharmaceutical Education and Research (NIPER) S.A.S.
Nagar Sector 67, S.A.S.
Nagar (Mohali)-160062, Punjab, India

PREFACE

Nano-carriers are an innovative and promising alternative technology for cancer treatment, which show many advantages over conventional cancer therapies. It provides new opportunities for early detection, improved treatment, and diagnosis of cancer. Currently, available cancer treatments include radiation therapy, targeted therapy, surgery, chemotherapy, radiation therapy, immunotherapy, and some existing symptomatic treatments. The present challenges faced for the treatment of cancer are mainly due to the heterogenicity of some cancers, drug resistance, late diagnosis, few treatment advances for early-stage cancer, non-selectivity of drugs towards cancer cells leading to side effects and many more, which are still in the dark. The development of such ligand decorated nano- carriers modifies the anticancer drug accumulation and distribution, thus producing the best possible therapeutic effects to the cancerous cells that will finally reduce the dose and dosing frequency of the anticancer drug. Nano-drug delivery by various drug delivery systems has emerged as a commanding technology for the treatment of various cancers. Nanotechnology provides new rays of hope for the effective treatment of different types of cancer. Nanotechnology-based drug delivery carriers (NCs), such as nanoparticles, liposomes, dendrimers, polyplexes, solid lipid nano-carriers and many more, offer treatment strategies due to their ability to target cancer cells. Nano-carriers are used for targeted drug delivery of medicaments to the desired site along with their surface modification which has shown their significance in the management of cancer. The book contains thirteen chapters, including an introduction to cancer biology, nanotechnology for cancer treatment: an introduction, potential approaches for delivery of surface decorated nano-carriers in the management of carcinoma, the importance of surface-modified nano-carriers in the management of cancer, Importance of nano-carriers in prostate cancer, Future prospects and challenges in toxicology related to nanoparticles, Nano-carriers and its role in the treatment of breast cancer, the importance of surface-modified nano-carriers in the management of cervical cancer, the importance of nano-carriers in colon cancer, nano-carriers in treatment of head and neck cancer, accounts on nano-carrier system for diagnosis purpose, cancer drug products containing nanomaterials: key regulatory issues and future prospects and challenges in treatment of cancer. Each chapter discusses an introduction to the cancer biology role of nanotechnology, potential approaches for delivery of surface decorated nano-carriers in the management of carcinoma, and cancer drug products containing nanomaterials: key regulatory issues and future prospects and challenges in the treatment of cancer. We hope the book shall be a useful compilation for undergraduate, postgraduate, and doctoral students and researchers working in cancer and drug delivery research, research and development, and national research institutes. We hope to receive feedback, suggestions, and inputs from researchers and students that will help improve the next edition of the book.

ACKNOWLEDGMENTS

I am thankful to my Honorable Vice Chancellor Lt. Gen. V. K. Sharma, AVSM (Retd.), and Pro-Vice Chancellor Prof. (Dr.) M. P. Kaushik, Amity University Madhya Pradesh, Gwalior, India, for his continuous encouragement. I am very also grateful to Dr. S. Mohana Lakshmi, Director, Amity Institute of Pharmacy, Amity University Madhya Pradesh, Gwalior, for his support during the writing of this book. Finally, I would like to express my wholehearted appreciation to the faculty members and students of Amity Institute of Pharmacy, Amity University, Madhya Pradesh, Gwalior.

Neeraj Mishra
Amity Institute of Pharmacy,
Amity University of Madhya Pradesh
Gwalior (M.P.)
India

Ashish Garg
Department of P. G. Studies and Research in Chemistry and Pharmacy
Rani Durgavati University
Jabalpur (M.P.)
India

Neeraj Upmanyu
Sagar Institute of Research & Technology-Pharmacy &
Pro Vice-Chancellor, Sage University
Bhopal
India

List of Contributors

A. Tiwari	Department of Pharmacy, Shri G. S. Institute of Technology and Science, Indore, India
Aakanchha Jain	National Institute of Pharmaceutical Education and Research (NIPER) –Ahmedabad, Palaj, Gandhinagar, Gujarat, India Bhagyoday Tirth Pharmacy College, Sagar, M.P., India
Aakriti Garg	School of Pharmaceutical Sciences, Apeejay Stya University, Gurgaon, India
Ajay Sharma	Department of Pharmacognosy, Delhi Pharmaceutical Sciences and Research University, Pushp Vihar Sector 3, MB Road, New Delhi-110017, India
Amrita Kumari Panda	Department of Biotechnology, Sant Gahira Guru University, Ambikapur, Chhattisgarh, India
Anchal Pathak	National Institute of Pharmaceutical Education and Research, Raebareli, India
Anoop Kumar	Department of Pharmacology, Delhi Pharmaceutical Sciences & Research University (DPSRU), New Delhi, India
Arghya Kusum Dhar	School of Pharmacy, Neotia University, Sarisa, D.H. Road, 24 Pgs (South) West Bengal 743368, India
Ashish Garg	Department of P.G. Studies and Research in Chemistry and Pharmacy, Rani Durgavati University, Jabalpur, M.P.482001, India
Ashok kumar Datusalia	Department of Pharmacology and Toxicology, National Institute of Pharmaceutical Education and Research (NIPER), Raebareli, Lucknow, India
Awesh k Yadav	National Institute of Pharmaceutical Education and Research, Raebareli, India
Azmi Khan	Department of Pharmaceutics, Delhi Pharmaceutical Sciences and Research University, Pushp Vihar Sector 3, MB Road, New Delhi-110017, India
B. Patil	Department of Pharmacy, Shri G. S. Institute of Technology and Science, Indore, India
Dolly Jain	Oriental University, Indore, M.P., India
Farhan Mazahir	National Institute of Pharmaceutical Education and Research, Raebareli, India
Firdos Khan	Department of Pharmacology, BM College of Pharmaceutical Education and Research, Indore, MP – 452020, India
Hari Krishnareddy Rachamalla	Department of Biochemistry and Molecular Biology, Mayo Clinic, 500 San Pablo Road, Jacksonville, FL-32224, USA
Jinu Mathew	Department of P.G. Studies and Research in Chemistry and Pharmacy, Rani Durgavati University, Jabalpur, M.P.482001, India
Madhu Gupta	Department of Pharmaceutics, Delhi Pharmaceutical Sciences and Research University, Pushp Vihar Sector 3, MB Road, New Delhi-110017, India
Manisha thakur	Department of Pharmacology and Toxicology, National Institute of Pharmaceutical Education and Research (NIPER), Raebareli, Lucknow, India
Meghna A. Singh	Department of Pharmaceutics, Delhi Pharmaceutical Sciences and Research University, Pushp Vihar Sector 3, MB Road, New Delhi-110017, India

N. Upmanyu	School of Pharmacy and Research, Peoples University, Bhopal, India Sagar Institute of Research & Technology-Pharmacy, Bhopal, India
Nagma Parveen	Department of Zoology, Kumaun University, Nainital, Uttarakhand, India
Neeraj Mishra	Amity Institute of Pharmacy, Amity University, Gwalior, 474005, MP, India
Neha Srivastava	Faculty of Pharmaceutical Sciences, PCTE Group of Institutes, Ludhiana (Punjab), India School of Pharmaceutical Science, Lovely Professional University, Phagwara (Punjab), India
P. Jangied	Department of Pharmacy, Shri G. S. Institute of Technology and Science, Indore, India
Pallav Namdeo	Department of P.G. Studies and Research in Chemistry and Pharmacy, Rani Durgavati University, Jabalpur, M.P.482001, India
Prakash Pandey	RKDF College of Pharmacy, Sarvepalli Radhakrishnan University, Bhopal, M.P., India
Rajeev K. Singla	Institutes for Systems Genetics, Frontiers Science Center for Disease-related Molecular Network, West China Hospital, Sichuan University,, Chengdu, 610041, Sichuan, China Global Research and Publishing Foundation, New Delhi, India
Richa Jain	People's University, CSRD, Bhopal, M.P., India
Rupesh K. Gautam	Department of Pharmacology, MM School of Pharmacy, Maharishi Markandeshwar University,Ambala-Chandigarh Highway, Sadopur- Ambala-134007 (Haryana), India
S.P. Pandey	Department of Pharmacy, Shri G. S. Institute of Technology and Science, Indore, India
Santanu Kaity	Mylan Laboratories Limited, R&D Center, Bollaram (V), Hyderabad, India
Santosh Kumar Behera	National Institute of Pharmaceutical Education and Research (NIPER) –Ahmedabad, Palaj, Gandhinagar, Gujarat, India
Satpal Singh Bisht	Department of Zoology, Kumaun University, Nainital, Uttarakhand, India
Shiv Kumar Prajapati	Department of Pharmacy, Ram-Esh Institute of Vocational and Technical Education, Greater Noida, UP, India
Shvetank Bhatt	Amity Institute of Pharmacy, Amity University, Gwalior, Madhya Pradesh (AUMP), Gwalior, 474005, India
Sidhartha S. Kar	Institute of Pharmacy & Technology, Salipur, Cuttack, Odisha, India
Sumel Ashique	Department of Pharmaceutic, Bharat Institute of Technology (BIT), School of Pharmacy), Meerut- 250103, UP, India
Sweta Garg	Shri Ram Institute of Pharmacy, Jabalpur, M.P., India
T. Shukla	Institute of Pharmaceutical Sciences, SAGE University, Indore, India
Tarani P. Shrivastava	Department of Pharmacology, Delhi Pharmaceutical Sciences and Research University, Pushp Vihar Sector 3, MB Road, New Delhi-110017, India
Tripathi A.	Sagar Institute of Research & Technology-Pharmacy, Sage University, Bhopal, India

Ujala Gupta	National Institute of Pharmaceutical Education and Research, Raebareli, India
Vaibhav Kumar S. Gawali	Department of Internal Medicine/Nephrology, College of Medicine, University of Cincinnati,, OH, USA
Vijay Mishra	School of Pharmaceutical Science, Lovely Professional University, Phagwara (Punjab), India
Vijay Sagar Madamsetty	Department of Biochemistry and Molecular Biology, Mayo Clinic, Jacksonville, Florida 32224, USA
Vinod Gauttam	IES Institute of Pharmacy, IES University, Bhopal 462044, India
Yachana Mishra	Department of Zoology, School of Bioengineering and Biosciences, Lovely Professional University, Phagwara (Punjab), India

CHAPTER 1

Cancer Biology

Aakanchha Jain[1,2,*], **Shiv Kumar Prajapati**[3], **Dolly Jain**[4], **Richa Jain**[5], **Amrita Kumari Panda**[6], **Nagma Parveen**[7], **Satpal Singh Bisht**[7] and **Santosh Kumar Behera**[1]

[1] *National Institute of Pharmaceutical Education and Research (NIPER) – Ahmedabad, Palaj, Gandhinagar, Gujarat, India*

[2] *Bhagyoday Tirth Pharmacy College, Sagar, M.P., India*

[3] *Department of Pharmacy, Ram-Esh Institute of Vocational and Technical Education, Greater Noida, UP, India*

[4] *Oriental University, Indore, M.P., India*

[5] *People's University, CSRD, Bhopal, M.P., India*

[6] *Department of Biotechnology, Sant Gahira Guru University, Ambikapur, Chhattisgarh, India*

[7] *Department of Zoology, Kumaun University, Nainital, Uttarakhand, India*

Abstract: As stated by Globocan, there were around 82 lakh cancer-related deaths and 141 lakh new cancer diagnoses worldwide in 2012. Normal genes that are expressed improperly or exhibit aberrant expression may cause neoplasia, often known as cancer. Oncogenes are mutated forms of normal cellular genes that contribute to the development of cancer. Typically, oncogenes govern cell development and differentiation. Proapoptotic genes initiate cell death and decrease the number of cells. Antioncogens, or tumour suppressor genes, regulate cell division negatively. Tumours are caused by genes that directly or indirectly control cellular proliferation or inhibition, or that govern apoptosis or any sort of cell death. As a target for the development of novel cancer treatments, tumour cell metabolism has gained substantial attention. Identification of cancer has always been a crucial aspect of diagnosis and therapy. Markers for cancer are one of the most effective approaches for recognising, diagnosing, treating, monitoring progressions, and evaluating chemical resistance. A biomarker is "a distinctive biochemical, genetic, or molecular characteristic or material that signals a particular biological state or treatment." Tumour biomarkers are often seen in moderation in the absence of a tumour. The activation of CDKs (protein kinases) aids in the progression of cells from one phase of the cell cycle to the next. Various isoforms of CDK/cyclin complexes are capable of binding with a regulating cyclin protein. Aloisine is a potent inhibitor of CDK1, CDK 2, and CDK 5, and it has been observed that GSK3 (Glycogen synthase kinase 3) terminates cell division. Antimicrotubule medicines cause the mitotic Chk to halt the cell cycle by inhibiting

* **Corresponding author Aakanchha Jain:** National Institute of Pharmaceutical Education and Research (NIPER) –Ahmedabad, Palaj, Gandhinagar, Gujarat, India; Tel: 9407525548;
E-mails: jainaakanchha83@gmail.com; aakanchha.jain@niperahm.ac.in

microtubules. The presence of cancer cells results in enhanced cell proliferation and expansion. They can result in an absence of apoptosis and excessive cell proliferation. DNA damage or significant cellular stress might result in cell death. In cancer cells, proapoptosis is often missing or inhibited. iPSCs and cancer cells have comparable transcriptome profiles, including surface antigen markers identified by the immune system. MSCs producing IFN- accelerate the killing of tumour cells, augment NK cell activity, and decrease angiogenesis. This chapter provides an introduction of the fundamentals of cancer biology, including its characteristics, metabolic processes, and biomarkers.

Keywords: Biomarkers, Cancer biology and tumour vasculature, Cell Cycle, Genes, Metastasis.

INTRODUCTION

Cancer is a leading cause of death worldwide, and its treatment has been hampered to a large extent by the current COVID-19 pandemic situation due to hospital closures, overcrowded healthcare settings, and so on. Cancer occurrence differs between ethnic groups due to alterations in risk factor exposures and obstructions to high-throughput cancer prevention and early stage detection tools. On This entry was published in August 1, 2010 [1]. The use of targeted drugs in cancer treatment decreases the side effects of conventional chemotherapy and also induces the death of cancer cells with high efficiency. The targeted drugs are mainly categorised into two categories: (i) the first type, which inhibits angiogenesis; and (ii) the second type, which inhibits tumour growth by interfering with the signal transduction pathway. Many new drugs and strategies have been designed and got approval to be used in cancer therapy due to their ability to target various cell cycle checkpoints and protein kinases and their potency to force cancer cells to exit from the cell cycle. Cancer cells divide uninterruptedly due to various DNA mutations and increased cyclin-dependent kinases (CDK) activity, which makes CDKs a striking target for cancer treatment. Palbociclib, abemaciclib and ribociclib were three recently FDA approved drugs for treatment of breast cancer [2].

These drugs target CDK4/6 and force the cancer cells to exit the cell cycle and also induce apoptosis in cancer cells. Adavosertib is another approved drug in phase-II clinical trials that targets Wee1 kinase, which regulates the mitotic entry checkpoints by ensuring DNA damage repair before G2/M progression. Targeting Wee1 has also been proven as a potential strategy in the treatment of thyroid cancer [3].

Vinca alkaloid is one of the effective chemotherapy drugs that interrupt mitotic spindle formation and target the mitotic checkpoint to stop cells in mitosis.

Each cell has a unique biomarker signature that signifies the functions of genes and the pathological and metabolic status of that cell. The process of carcinogenesis is primarily developed due to mutations, mainly in tumour suppressor genes, oncogenes, and DNA repair genes. These gene mutations act as genetic biomarkers for cancer diagnostics and therapeutics. In addition to these mutations that down or up-regulated gene expressions, altered metabolites, DNA methylation, and modified chromatin condensation drive carcinogenesis. The identification of such types of biomarkers acts as an important cancer diagnostic and detection tool. The occurrence of circulating tumour cells (CTCs) in the bloodstream is a very dominant biomarker in oncology. The increased number of CTCs indicates the progression of disease, whereas the CTCs' decreased number indicates the efficacy of treatment method. Cancer cells secrete many proteins into the extracellular fluid that can act as serum biomarkers. Some important cancer antigens include prostate specific antigen (PSA) for prostate cancer, Alpha-foetoprotein for hepatocellular carcinomas, Cancer antigen 125 for ovarian and fallopian tube cancer, BRCA-1 and BRCA-2 for breast cancer, TGF for malignant tumours, and thyroglobulin for papillary and follicular thyroid cancer. This chapter gives an overview of the basic cancer biology, its hallmarks, metabolic transformations, cancer biomarkers that are used to diagnose cancer and a summary of the different targeted cancer treatments, with a focus on stem cell targeted therapy.

CANCER INCIDENCE AND ETIOLOGY

The word cancer is derived from the "Greek word Karkinos meaning crab having the supply of thick veins around itself". Cancer is the most devastating diseases that affects a large population throughout the world. It can be said as the uncontrolled division of abnormal cells leading to swelling without any sign of inflammation or the abrupt generation of an abnormal cell in the body with or without any sign of inflammation or the abrupt generation of cells in the body with or without blood supply. It may be characterised by the accumulation of detrimental variation in the genome by single and multiple mutations in the genome over several years of life.

Recognition of cancer has been a major issue at all times for the diagnosis and treatment. Manually identifying a malignant growth from a biopsy picture seen through a microscope is subjective and depends on the person's skill and other factors, such as the lack of clear and exact quantitative measurements to classify the biopsies as normal or tumorous [4].

The computerised detection of tumorous cells from microscopic biopsy images assists in eliminating worries and achieving improved outcomes. The advancement in medical technology has increased the possibility of getting cured of threatening diseases like cancer. Rather, curing the cancer is easy at its early stage if it is well diagnosed. The cancer can be benign or malignant, and the selection of treatment approach is simply based on the stage of cancer or can be said to be based on its malignancy level. Various techniques which are being used for the imaging of cancer cells are: Computer Tomography (CT) scan, Magnetic Resonance Imaging (MRI), Positron Emission Tomography (PET), ultrasound, and X-ray, along with many other pathological (urine/blood) examinations.

Histopathology

Histopathology is the investigation of illnesses of the tissues and includes inspecting tissues and, additionally, cells under a confocal microscope. For the accurate detection of cancer, histopathologists make tissue diagnoses and help clinicians plan patients' care. In the histopathology, the histology slides are prepared, which is perhaps the foundation for this procedure. Ultimately, these prepared slides are examined under a microscope. The preparation of slides is completed in five steps: fixing, processing, embedding, sectioning, and last but by no means least, staining. Eventually, these readied slides are inspected under a microscope. The planning of slides finishes in five stages. These are: fixing, handling, inserting, separating, and last, but in no way, shape, or form least, staining. Tissue sectioning is significant on the grounds that suitably thin slices facilitate easy and clearer electron microscopy or light microscopy monitoring. The desired thickness of the section depends on tissue type and the depth of analysis. Sectioning is done using a microtome. If the sections are in frozen forms, then the instrument is clubbed with cryostats. The cells/tissues are dyed (one or more stains) to easily detect them under a microscope. The staining exposes the cellular component. On the other hand, counterstains give the details of colour, visibility, and contrast. Various staining components, such as Melanin stains and Haemotoxylin stains, give the nucleus a blue color, whereas Eosin stains other parts, such as connective tissue and cytoplasm, pink or color [5]. Microscopic methods of biopsies are generally less invasive and are supposedly good for screening of disease; they can even detect cancerous cells and cell constellations [6, 7].

Cancerous and non-cancerous cells can be differentiated by observing abnormalities in the sample on the basis of their colour, size, shape, and cytoplasm amount. High resolution microscopic biopsy renders credible information to distinguish normal and cancerous tissues [8].

The regular highlights utilised for the discovery and analysis of malignant growth from the biopsy pictures incorporate the dimension of cells, cores of cells, and cellular distribution. The concise portrayals of these highlights are given in further sections [9].

The size and shape of the normal tissues and cells are generally normal and regular in shape, while the tumorous cells may be shorter or larger and irregular in shape. Typically, the size and state of the malignant cell core are frequently not typical, decentralized, bigger and hazier than those of ordinary ones, and size fluctuates significantly. Another element of the core of a malignancy cell is that in the wake of being stained with specific colors, the dangerous cell looks more obscure under a magnifying instrument. The core of a malignant growth cell is bigger and hazier on the grounds that it contains a lot of DNA. The better arrangement and cell distribution are the properties of normal cells. In carcinogenic cells, the quantity of healthy cells is less in number.

CANCER GENETICS

Cancer genetics is the logical control that scrutinises the qualities and pathways that drive malignancy development. Malignancy genetics utilize a few methodologies, including the investigation of the genomes of diseased patients' tumours. Genes carry the instructions to make proteins for the functioning of a cell. The alteration in genes causes cells to prevent usual growth controls and results in the development of cancer. The changes in gene expression may enhance the output of a protein that helps cells grow. The human body is comprised of billions of tissue specific cells which are developing, separating/ differentiating, and dying every day. Every stage is exceptionally constrained via the progression of genes that are actuated or deactivated according to the need. Cells take delivery of definite biochemical signals after various stimuli, which may be internal or external. Any distraction may occur, which may cause an imbalance. Furthermore, this early precariousness convinces a succeeding course of events that are expected to cause malignancy. The signs may originate from adjoining cells, steroidal and polypeptide exposures, various environmental variables like patients lifestyle (deskbound or activity based), pH of blood, dietary habits *etc*. Acidic medium is best suited for the growth of cancerous cells. As the signs are received, they reach to the nucleus of receptor cells and the basic changes are made in light of such signs, which articulate or actuate specific genes and quiet others [10]. When a cell undergoes many cell divisions and loses its self-control, clones of cells are formed that cross the safety regulations of the cell. This leads to high proliferation, angiogenesis (new blood vessel growth), metastasis, and resistance to normal cell death, making them highly immortal [11, 12]. This process is passable to generations when in germ cells but not when in somatic cells.

The human body works on the principal of genes, or genetics. There are some normal genes which function normally and there are obviously some abnormal genes which function abnormally, which may cause cancer. On the other hand, if normal genes are expressed abnormally or they show abnormal expression, they may lead to neoplasia, *i.e.*, cancer. Normal genes may convert in to abnormal genes during division or may be during inheritance. Mutation is another common method by which these normal genes can be converted into abnormal genes. Mutation, sudden inheritable changes may occur and can be caused by a varying number of factors.

Normal cells or normal genes undergo mutation and are called as mutated genes and the cells called mutated cells. These mutated cells may undergo such changes, which may cause them to divide rapidly, and such process is called clonal expansion. Clonal means similar type of cells are formed at an expanding rate, which ultimately leads to the tumour, or termed as neoplasia.

The factors which may lead to mutation of genes or cells are commonly known as carcinogens because these are the factors which cause the mutation and lead to conversion of normal genes to mutated genes, therefore making them carcinogens. Carcinogens may chemicals, radiological or virus. The cells divide from exposure to carcinogenic substances (chemicals in tobacco smoke), and radiation (ultraviolet rays). Somatic changes are genetic changes that persuade after conception. Some DNA changes may occur if it affects only one unit (nucleotide) and may be or may not be replaced by another nucleotide. Rearrangements, deletions, or duplications of long strands of DNA are also some abnormal changes. The addition or deletion of chemical marks "epigenetic modifications" on DNA can affect the gene's "expression"- that is, whether and how much messenger RNA is produced. In general, cancer cells possess added genetic changes than those in normal cells. As the cancer persists to grow, some auxiliary changes, which causes differentiation at molecular levels, continue to occur. Even within the same region of tumour, cells may have different genetic changes [13].

Many genetic and epigenetic changes in genes accumulate to play a vital role in regulating cell proliferation in cancer cells. The genes which directly or indirectly affect cellular proliferation or inhibition or regulate apoptosis or any type of cell death or cause damage in auto DNA repair are the ones which generate tumour [14]. The four key genetic regulators of cancer are protooncogenes, antioncogenes, apoptosis-regulating genes, and DNA repair genes. Even slight modification in their structure can cause tumour germination and development. Any mutation or any change during inheritance or cell division that leads to a change in these genes may lead to cancer because of the inability to function normally.

Protooncogene

An oncogene is a mutated form of a normal cellular gene-called a proto-oncogene-that contributes to the development of a cancer. Proto-oncogenes typically regulate cell growth and cell differentiation. In this case, *proto* means original and *onco* means dividing. These are originally dividing genes which may be physiologically functional and causes physiological division at a normal rate and within normal limits. When these genes are affected by any of these causes causes, the gene converted into oncogenes, and this division is uncontrolled and rapid, and not required, which may lead to tumour formation. Oncogenes are dominant over protooncogenes. Most proto-oncogenes encode enzymes. The oncogenic forms of these enzymes have a higher level of activity, either because of an altered affinity for substrate or a loss of regulation. The mutations that convert proto-oncogenes to oncogenic alleles are known for activating mutations [15, 16].

Antioncogenes

In contrast to oncogenes, the antioncogenes, or tumour suppressor genes act as negative regulators of cell division.

In the case of cancer cells, suppressor genes could be defined as "police" genes that keep a close watch and detect cells that might be manifesting abnormal behaviour because some of their oncogenes or pathological genes are activated, causing the "bad" cells to die and be eliminated.

These are against the division of the cells *i.e.*, they suppress the cell growth. Physiologically it is needed that protooncogenes undergo division, but they need to be controlled by some regulatory phenomenon. Here comes the role of antioncogenes because they are against the division. So their expression may lead to suppression of growth, which is important and keeps a check on the non-required growth and hence the cancer. When they undergo mutation or rather mutated inactivation, they are unavailable to keep a check on the growth and therefore, they are unable to suppress the growth. They assess the protooncogenes and may lead to continuous division *i.e.*, progression of the growth and ultimately tumour mass [16].

Apoptosis Regulator Gene

Apoptosis is a programmed cell death, or what we can say pre-decided suicide. If a cell is undergoing any injury or if the cells themselves recognise that they are not able to function normally, there is no need for it to survive. So the cells undergo programmed cell death on their own *i.e.*, apoptosis. There are two types of genes involved in this process. The first are antiapoptotic genes and the second are proapoptotic gene. Antiapoptotic genes are against the apoptosis, which is against the cell death, so these cells promote cell division and hence cancer. While the proapoptotic genes are initiator of cell death. These reduces the cells number and therefore keep a check on the normal functioning of cells [14].

DNA Repair Gene

Dysregulations in DNA damage or DNA repair steps play an important role in tumour advancement, leading to higher gene un-stability, increased rates of mutation, and enhanced tumour heterogenecity. Chromatin remodelling, double strand break repair and redox homeostasis are the three basic modes which causes change in cell metabolic activities and largely influence DNA damage or DNA repair [17, 18].

TUMOUR VASCULATURE

The disproportion of angiogenic regulators develops tumour vasculature with entirely different properties than the normal tissues. Various approaches are being used to target tumour vasculature for their treatment. The tumour vasculature helps in survival of tumour and facilitates its growth. For this, it is vital that tumour cells ought to be at a specific distance from the perfused vein where they will get the oxygen and different supplements to multiply and endure. Thus, the tumour tends to become more angiogenic. Four mechanisms are involved in the vascularization: (i) co-option, (ii) intussusception, (iii) sprouting (angiogenesis), and (iv) vasculogenesis [19]. The tumour cells manage to have increased blood supply by the phenomenon of angiogenesis, not only in small venules and capillaries but also in large vein supplies in the affected area of host cell. The network of capillaries develops in the direction of tumour and anastomose and the process of angiogenesis continues in the periphery of tumour, leading to increase in their size. The venous vessels of host cells are amended and modernized before they proceed to be integrated with those of the tumour cells. However, the arterial vessels remain unchanged before interacting with tumour cells. Tumour cappilaries grow strangely, dilate, become convoluted, and retain their capillary-like framework. The blood vessels that supply of host cells get dilated, thinner in diameter and shredded. The tortuous vessels may result in fluctuation of perfusion. On increasing the tumour size, the interstitial pressure increases and small vessels get blocked permanently, leading to the blood immobility and the development of necrosis near the tumour centre [20].

HALLMARKS TO CANCER

Cancer/tumour biomarkers (CB) or cancer hallmarks are biomolecules produced by cancerous cells in response to a tumour. These biomarkers were first used in medicine about 170 years ago; after Bence Jones identified a novel protein with unique temperature clotting properties in the urine samples of patients with multiple myeloma [21]. Biomarkers may help with the molecular concept of cancer because each single cell does have its own molecular signature and recognisable features like levels or actions of a range of proteins, genes, or supplementary molecular characters. Genetic alterations in cancerous cells, such as point mutations, gene reconfiguration/amplifications, and the associated unregulated cell division and multiplication, are displayed by the generation of biological markers in the majority of cancer patients. As a result, they may be used as cancer biomarkers and treatment response predictors [21]. A biomarker can be defined as "a unique biochemical, genetic, or molecular feature or substance that indicates a specific biological condition or procedure" [22]. As per the National Cancer Institute, it is a biomolecule present in blood and other body fluids, or tissues that is an indication of a regular or irregular procedure, or of a disease or disorder such as cancer. A biomarker is a trait that can be measured accurately and used to characterise a normal or anomalous biological condition [23, 24] in a life form by analysing biological molecules such as DNA, RNA, protein, and peptide [25].

There are three mechanisms that could explain the increase in CB levels in every biological fluid. The first process is gene amplification or overexpression of the target gene, or an increase in epigenetic alterations (which regulate gene expression). The release of protein substrates by the cells or the loss of membrane proteins is indeed the second mechanism of acceleration that can be used on serum biomarkers. A serum biomarker such as alpha-fetoprotein (AFP) can be an example. The third approach involves cell invasion and angiogenesis, which is shown by prostate-specific antigen (PSA). Usually, the prostatic epithelium makes it, but a crooked basement membrane in the prostatic cell and lymph undergoes angiogenesis [21], causing the PSA level to rise.

To validate the use of such therapeutic or intervening therapies, cancer biomarkers are increasingly linked to deregulations of molecular pathways and /or cancer pathogenesis [25]. To differentiate between normal and pathogenic processes, various onco-markers can be used. A perfect or ideal biomarker is one that comes from cancer cells, which is undetectable in normal and benign tissues but can be detected in biological specimens using basic methods (biological fluids). It needs to be responsive, precise, and cost-effective [26].(Fig. **1**), illustrates the criteria for selecting a diagnostic biomarker where the parameters should be carefully considered.

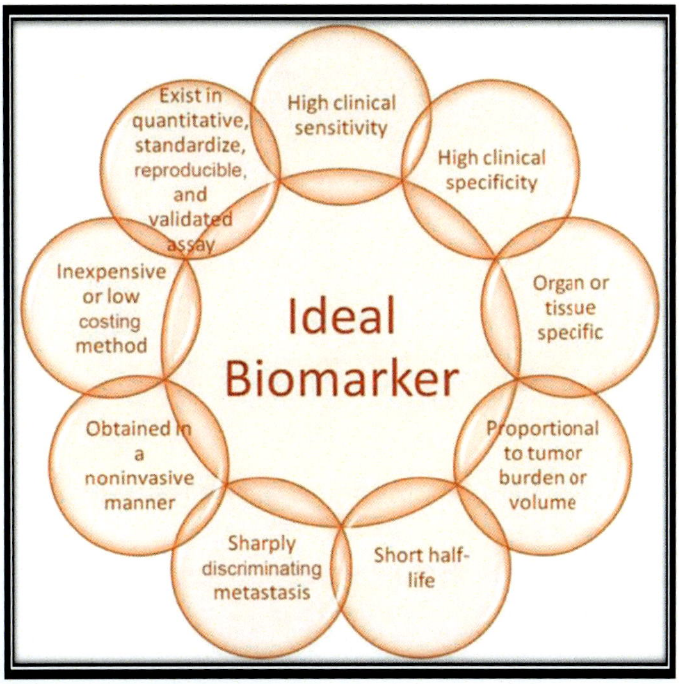

Fig. (1). Physiognomies of an idyllic Biomarker.

BIOMARKERS FOR CANCER: WHAT ARE THEY AND HOW DO THEY HELP?

Based on their applications, cancers biomarkers are divided into three categories: predictive, prognostic and diagnostic. Predictive biomarkers, like HER2 activation, which correlates with trastuzumab reaction in breast cancer, are used to predict the impact of specific treatment approaches. Prognostic biomarkers, at the other hand, are not specifically related to or cause particular treatment strategies but rather serve to warn clinicians about the likelihood of treatment outcome like cancer recurrence or disease progression. The 21-gene reappearance rate was predictive of reiteration and overall survival in node-negative, tamoxifen-treated breast cancer patients. A diagnostic biomarker is a test that determines whether or not a person has a particular disease [25].

Genetic (point mutations, repeat number variations, matrix RNA expression), epigenetic (DNA methylation pattern variations), proteomic (structure and protein expression profile variations), and metabolic biomarkers (Fig. **2**) are the four types of cancer biomarkers [26]. DNA, RNA, miRNA, and protein markers are the main types of molecular markers [27].

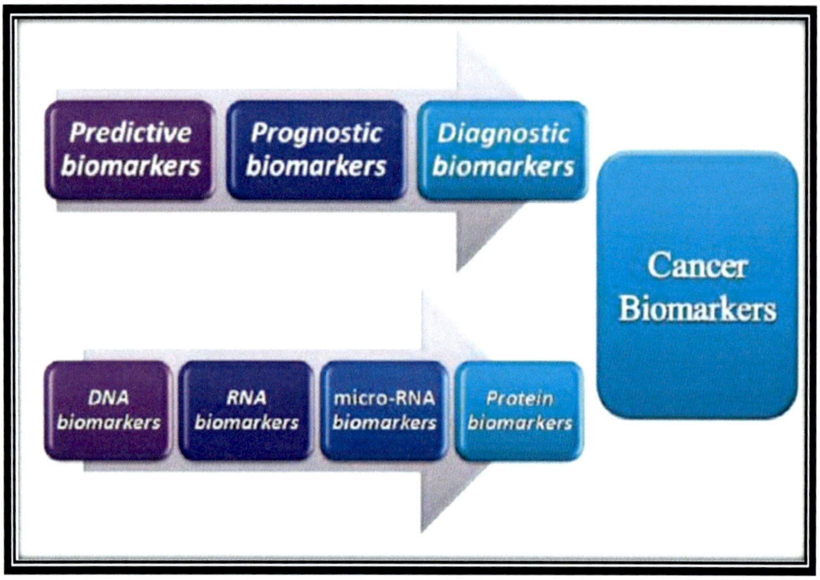

Fig. (2). Various Biomarkers based on Biomolecule and their Uses.

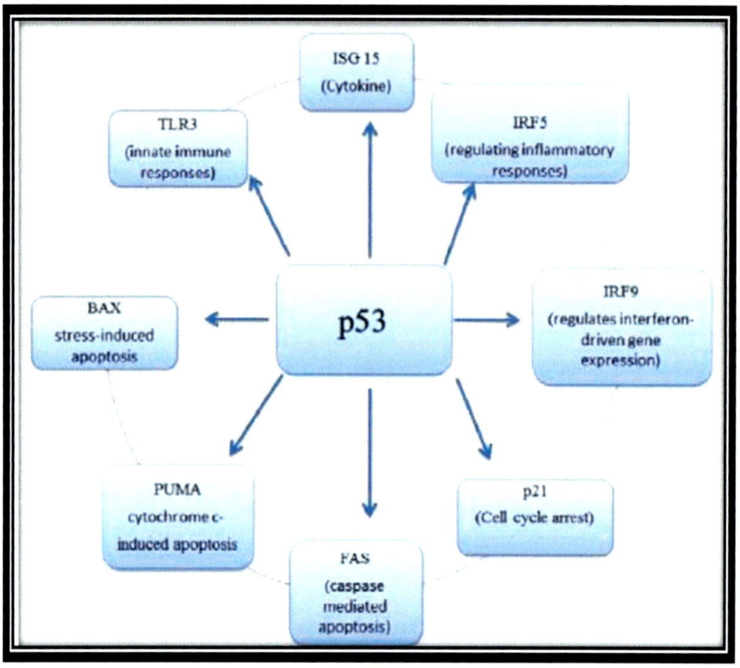

Fig. (3). Targets of p53.

1. **DNA Markers:** There are noticeable epigenetic shifts like DNA methylation, which have a major impact on expression of genes. Recent research has shown

that abnormal DNA methylation occurs frequently and quickly in human carcinogenesis [21, 27] [Kamel and Al-Amodi, 2016; Ghafouri-Fard et al., 2014]. Chromosome 9 loss is a very distinct shift observed most often in Ta/T1 bladder cancers and on fewer occasions in muscle invasive bladder cancers (MIBC). On chromosome 9, LOH (Loss of heterozygosity) has been linked to cancer production instead of initiation. It's also useful for keeping track of patients suffered from superficial bladder cancer who have received Bacillus Calmette-Guerin (BCG) immunotherapy, particularly if cytology investigations are ambiguous. BCL2, CDKN2A, and NID2 are a few examples, as well as CDH1, APC, GSTP1, ARF, MGMT, RARb2, CDKN2A, TIMP3, and RASSF1A genes found in urine [27].

2. **RNA Markers:** The expression levels of Aurora-A kinase in bladder cancer tend to be substantially greater than in non-tumour tissues. The presence of a vital marker for urothelial carcinoma in urine cytology samples has been suggested. Urothelial carcinoma-associated 1 (UCA1) is a unique non-coding RNA gene that has been found to be significantly up-regulated in TCC [27].

3. **MicroRNA (miRNA) Markers:** Intracellular regulators of gene activity, miRNAs, are 18-24 nucleotide long RNA molecules that work by degrading RNA or inhibiting translation. In cancer, modified alterations of miRNA expression can be used as new biomarkers for earlier monitoring and recognition of therapeutic responses. This panel of miRNAs can diagnose bladder cancer with 94 percent sensitivity, 51 percent specificity, and 86 percent concordance, where the group of miRNAs includes miR-135b, microRNA-15b, and microRNA-1224-3p.

4. **Protein Markers:** BTA, d-Dimer, FAS, hyaluronidase (HA), carcinoembryonic antigen (CEA),, interleukins such as IL-1, IL-6, IL-8, and vascular endothelial growth factor (VEGF) are the few protein biomarkers that have demonstrated major differences in NMIBC and MIBC [27].

Some Other Important Cancer Biomarkers

Benjamin and de Lima [28] list the following breast cancer biomarkers: the BRCA1 (type 1) and BRCA2 (type 2) genes; tenascin-C (TN-C); oestrogen receptor (ER); DNA methyltransferase (DNA-MTase); apurinic/apyrimidinic endonuclease 1 (APE1); matrix metallopeptidase 9 (MMP-9), murine double minute 2 (MDM 2), (NFk-B), and mucin-like carcinoma-associated antigen (MCA). Just like breast cancer biomarkers, there are some markers which help in the diagnosis and therapeutics of bladder cancer. For example, complement factor H associated protein in urine, NMP22, Ki67 (an independent prognostic marker), Mcm5 protein, BCL2, CDKN2A and NID2, Aurora-A in tissue samples, p16INK-

4a in urinary bladder lavages, APC, GSTP1, CDH1, CDKN2A, ARF, RARb2, TIMP3, MGMT, and RASSF1A gene products in urine, *etc* [27, 29].

Lung cancer is the most common cancer and the leading cause of cancer-related deaths worldwide, accounting for approximately 18 lakh new cases and 16 lakh deaths in 2012.Lung cancer patients have a five-year rate of survival of around 13-15%. So, early and accurate diagnosis is very important in this case, too. EPCAM (epithelial cell adhesion molecule), CYFRA 21-1 (cytokeratins), ProGRP (pro-gastrin-releasing peptide), AGER, CEACAM (carcinoembryonic antigen), C10orf116, PRX,ADD2, SYNM,LAMB3, SPTA1, HBE1,ANK1, HBG1, TNXB,CA1, HBA1, MMRN2, COL6A6, CAV1, HBB, SDPR, C1orf198, APOA2,CLIC2, EHD2, NDUFB7, LAMA3, LBN, PRKCDBP, are some important protein biomarkers, useful in lung cancer detection [26].

METABOLIC TRANSFORMATION IN CANCER

Tumour cell metabolism has attracted considerable focus as an area for the progression of newer cancer drugs for their therapeutic usage. The transformed metabolism is regarded as pivotal in the transformation of normal cells into cancerous cells. The intermediated metabolic transformation are crucial for controlling different events of malignancy, including bioenergetic, invasiveness, and related proliferative activities including migration. As the cell alters its activity, its metabolism should be transformed to supply catabolic, synthetic, or bioenergetic necessities to change the activity of cells. The malignant calibre of the neoplastic cell is constrained to change in its metabolism *i.e.*, "metabolic transformation" to deliver the bioenergetic, synthetic, and catabolic requirements of malignancy. When there is no metabolic transformation, the cancerous cells will not become malignant [30]. In cancer, malignant cells attain metabolic variations to retort diverse extrinsic and intrinsic indications of cell. Certain variations initialise the progression of transformation, while some of them encourage malignant cell growth and render them prone to inhibitors of major pathways. "Cancer metabolism" and "metabolic reprogramming" are often preferred to represent a pooled pathways noticed in immensely multiplying cancerous cells or tumour [31]. Initially, the growth of tumour requires various nutrients and biosynthesis, with supplementary metabolic need emerging in locally infiltrating cancer. In the later stages, tumour necessitates newer pathways for their progression.

The metabolic alteration comprises of turning on metabolic possessions for anabolic purposes, endorsing the formation of intermediates of biosynthesis pathways and precursors for new cell growth and proliferation. The cancer cells uptake nutrients and other metabolic requirements and are more transformed than normal cells. The notable metabolic activity in cancer cells involves glycolysis (aerobic), macromolecular synthesis, redox homeostasis, macromolecular synthesis; these endorse the necessities of exponential growth and proliferation. All these pathways are controlled by oncogenic signalling and transcription network within cell. Understanding of these pathways may assist in fixing metabolic dependencies and will be a transcendent therapeutic pathway to target various cancers. Non-cancerous cells transform into oncogenic cells through the transformation of normal cells involving seamlessly immutable metabolic switch for the activation of glucose transport and use in further suppression of mitochondrial respiration [32]. If the respiratory mechanism is normal, glycolysis will be controlled by substitute metabolic pathways to achieve energy equilibrium [33]. Glutamine is a crucial bioenergetic and anabolic substrate for numerous types of cancer cells. Tumours tends to undergo aerobic glycolysis and they depend on glutamine as a source for proper running of Tricarboxylic acid (TCA) cycle. Glutamine also acts as an intermediate herald for other biosynthetic cycles in conjunction with the TCA cycle. The dual role of acetyl-CoA, primarily generation of energy (catabolism) and as intermediate in anabolism, are vital for existence of tumour cells. It is well known that the metabolic alteration in glucose renders excess energy to help in growth in tumour. So, the hang-up of the glycolysis process and other biosynthetic pathways will reduce cell proliferation and tumour growth [34].

Cell Cycle–Targeted Cancer Therapies

The cell cycle is an event that permits each cell to duplicate genetic material that is further equally distributed to daughter cells. In the somatic cell, the G1 and the G2 phases acts as cycling intervals between Synthesis phase (S phase) where DNA is synthesised and mitosis phase (M phase) where cell division occurs. The activity of checkpoints at the S/ G2/ M phases is demolished by the inactivation of tumour suppressor gene and the mutated oncogene can raise the reliance of cancer cell on CDK of G1 phase and can even increase replication stress leading to DNA damage in the S phase [35]. Generally normal cells delay the progression of cell cycle to fix the damages. Shortcomings in cell cycle capture the pathways that develop in cancer cells and possibly make them vulnerable to die when DNA is damaged [36]. The tactic of targeting in cancer is supposed to lessen the dose related toxicities which impact the normal body cells and have higher accuracy than the conventional agents to hit tumour cells [35]. The loss in activity of CHK1 causes DNA damage in p53 deficient cells.

Major constraints of the cell cycle includes CDKs, whose activation helps cells move from one stage to the next stage of the cell cycle and the division is monitored at cell cycle checkpoints (Chk). Thus, these CDKs, have been identified as cancer targets [37]. CDKs are able to bind with a regulatory cyclin protein, various isoforms of CDK/cyclin complexes thereby regulating gradual progression via the cell cycle [38]. The CDK-focused drug also targets the proliferating section of cell but without causing the genotoxicity. CDK targeted drugs causes minimum toxicity and are well tolerated [39]. A, B, D, and E cyclin activate CDKs, whereas CDKIs (CDK inhibitors) down regulated them [40]. The two major checkpoints of cell cycle are incentivized in response to DNA damage, and this leads to synthesis of pre-DNA and post-DNA during G1 and G2 stages, respectively. The cell cycle checkpoint kinase CHK1 and CHK2 are important signal transducers. The CDC 25 family of phosphatases performs the function of dephosphorylation and activation of CDKs [41, 42]. Targeted therapy is designed for the treatment of the majority of cancer. After the initial efficiency of pan-CDK "flavopiridol" and CDK inhibitors "roscovitine" by Meijer and Raymond [43] various other studies have been conducted on new chemical entities and have shown improved preclinical efficacy. Various pyrazolopyrimidinones have been reported to act as inhibitors to CDK 1, 2, and 4 [44]. Bis(aminopyrimidine), have shown inhibition of CDK 1, CDK 2, and CDK 5. The molecule strongly inhibits CDK 1 and CDK 2, while it shows non-competitive inhibition of CDK4 at micromolar concentrations. Aloisine, being a powerful inhibitor of CDK 1, CDK 2, and CDK 5. Glycogen synthase kinase 3 (GSK 3) has been reported to terminate cell division by acting on both G1 and G2 phases. While aloisine A was extremely selective for these over CDK4 (more than 1000-fold) and 20 other kinases. A selectivity study of aloisine executed on 26 kinases confirmed its selectivity for cyclin B/ CDK 1 [45].

CDK4 kinase regulates the shift of G1-to-S phase within the cell cycle. Palbociclib was the first inhibitor of CDK 4 to be approved [46]. Based on CDK 4/6 inhibitory action, the USFDA approved the use of ribociclib, abemaciclib, and palbociclib for the treatment of oestrogen receptor positive breast cancer [47, 48]. It has been reported that selective CDK 4/6 inhibition causes a reduction in toxicity with promising anticancer efficacy in variety of tumour types [49]. Abemaciclib inhibits CDK 4/6 by inducing G1 phase arrest and reducing the RB1 phosphorylation in melanoma xenografts and colon-rectal cancers [50, 51]. Ribociclib at nanomolecular concentration inhibits the growth of neuroblastoma and liposarcoma cell lines by inhibiting CDK 4/6, resulting in G1 arrest and a marked reduction in tumour burden [52, 53]. The abovementioned agents bind within the ATP-binding pocket of CDK 4 and CDK 6, causing obstruction in kinase activity with higher discernment for CDK 4 and CDK 6, compared with CDK1 and CDK2 (Fig. **4**). The arrest of G1 phase was seen due to an inhibitory effect on CDK 4/6 with IC50 values less than 40 nM [49, 54]. Flavopiridol and bryostatin are the novel CDL inhibitors (CDKi). Flavopiridol has shown its potential to induce cell cycle arrest when tested on several cell lines by directly inhibiting CDK 1 (cyclin B1-Cdc2 kinase), CDK 2, 4, and 6 [55]. Bryostatin is a cell-cycle inhibitor that inactivates CDK 2 and inhibits tumour cell growth by inducing p21^Kip1^ [56] and downregulating cyclin B1. Bryostatin-1 activates protein kinase C through translocating it from the cell membrane, cytoskeleton, or nucleus [57]. Seliciclib inhibits (*R*-roscovitine) and various kinases, including CDK 2, CDK 7, and CDK 9, resulting in cell apoptosis [58]. Some other inhibitors of CDK 2 to target them include SNS-032 and imidazopyridines that are in early phases of development [59].

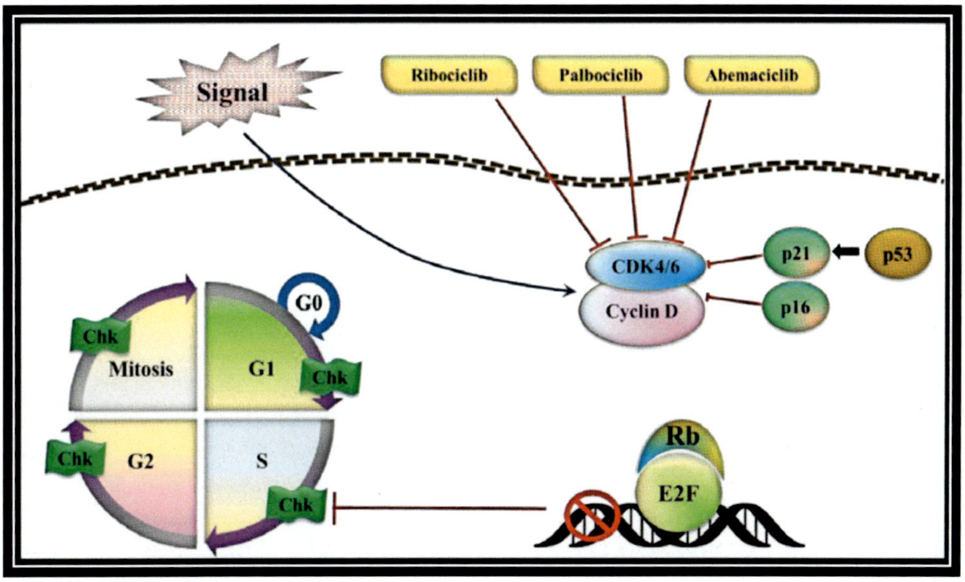

Fig. (4). The cell cycle and the functions of CDK6/ 4 restraint.

Another target is Chk. It responds to improper replication and other internal or external stimuli, causing DNA damage and disrupting the cell cycle. They work continuously until the stress is corrected or resolved fully. For example, G1 phase arrest and anti-proliferative signals are induced by Chks before being entered into S phase. Similarly, S phase arrest and G2 phase arrest are evoked by stress influencing replication fork if DNA is damaged or during unlinking of chromosomes, respectively. Currently, approaches for the targeting of Chk are being developed to enhance the efficacy and selectivity of chemotherapeutic agents. The ionising radiation acts on both G1 and G2 phase Chks and breaks down the dual stranded DNA. Some genotoxins, such as inhibitors of Topo II and alkylating agents, can induce G2 phase Chk, whereas, anti-microtubule drugs induce the mitotic Chk, causing the cell cycle to be arrested [60, 61]. The first G-2 Chk inhibitors include caffeine and its derivative pentoxifylline, 2-aminopurine,

6-dimethylaminopurine, staurosporine and its derivative 7-hydroxy staurosporin (UCN-01) [62]. Some studies have shown CDK10-13 inhibitors are structurally related to UCN-01 aglycone, which has been reported to inhibit CDK 4 [63]. p53-lacking cells rely on initiation of the checkpoint kinase Chk 1 pathway for cell cycle arrest in the G2 phase and repair of DNA after DNA damage [64]. This pathway is also known as the "survival pathway for cancer cells". UCN-01 inhibits both Chk1, 2 kinases. This leads to the cell exiting the G-2 phase before DNA repair and finally causing apoptosis [65]. Isogranulatimide is another Chk inhibitor that acts on G2 phase. It is comprised of a indole/ maleimide/ imidazole skeleton identified in a phenotypic cell-based screen, It also inhibits protein kinase Cβ and structurally resembles UCN-01. The UCN-01 in the cell cycle enhances chemosensitivity by holding down the expression of crucial events. It is a selective inhibitor of protein kinase C (PKC) and repeals the S/G2 phases of Chk via a Cdc2-dependent pathway and also dephosphorylates retinoblastoma gene product [66].

Gemcitabine is used for various types of cancer and has very short half-life [67]. Gemcitabine damages DNA by inducing the cell cycle arrest in G2 phase or S phase by inhibiting Chk1. Arrest of the cycle allows time for DNA repair before the cell advances to the next phase. Like other DNA-harming products, gemcitabine initiates cell cycle halt in the S or G2 stage in a way controlled by Chk1 [68]. Damage to DNA turns on the checkpoint, and this is when a Chk1 inhibitor will stop the cell cycle from moving forward [69, 70]. In a study, the Chk1 inhibitor "MK-8776" administered 18 hours after 40 mg/kg of gemcitabine showed the marker γH2AX (DNA damage marker). Thus, the combination therapy showed the efficacy of MK-8776 in killing the cells arrested in S phase [71]. Paclitaxel has the ability to kill the cancer cells by causing p53 mutation and targeting p53 pathways. It specifically provokes arrest in the G2/M phase of the cell cycle and then stops apoptosis [72, 73].

APOPTOSIS AND CANCER

Apoptosis is the controlled death of cells that is needed for the growth and survival of living organisms. It is a consecutively controlled suicide programme in which cells release enzymes that destroy their own nuclear and various protein components of the nucleus and cytoplasm [74]. If apoptosis did not occur, there would be no way to control cell growth and tissue homeostasis would be lost. Cancer cells lead to increased cell proliferation and growth. They also lead to a loss of apoptosis along with too much cell growth.

Apoptosis is distinguished by a sequence of distinctive morphological features, like cell shrinkage, release of mitochondrial cytochrome C, fission into membrane-bound apoptotic vesicles, and ultimately rapid phagocytosis by adjacent cells [75, 76]. Two signalling mechanisms exist for the activation of apoptosis, an intrinsic and an extrinsic. The mitochondrial or intrinsic pathway is regulated by a group of proteins concerned with the Bcl-2 family [77]. There are two main types of Bcl-2 proteins: "(i) pro-apoptotic proteins (*e.g.* Bad, Bak, Bax, Bcl-Xs, Bid, Bik, Bim and Hrk), and (ii) anti-apoptotic proteins (*e.g.* Bcl-2, Bcl-W, Bcl-XL, Bfl-1, and Mcl-1)" [78].

As said previously, cell death is triggered by DNA damage or severe cell stress following activation of proapoptotic protein. This ultimately results in pro-apoptosis. This pro-apoptosis is usually absent or halted in cancer cells [79]. Re-establishing the inborn expert apoptotic pathway after it has been inactivated may advance tumour cell demise. The death receptor or "Extrinsic pathway" is activated in response to diverse external signals such as Apo2L/ TRAIL and when death ligands bind to a death receptor. The well-known death receptors are TNF receptor (TNFR1) and a protein called Fas (CD95). The ligands for these are TNF and Fas ligand (FasL), respectively [80]. This pathway can possibly initiate the demise of tumour cells separately from the intrinsic pathway. Both pathways ultimately stimulate a set of enzymes called caspases. Caspase 8 is an initiator caspase which instigates apoptosis by splitting other downstream or executioner caspases [79], which move out the mass proteolysis that leads to apoptosis. The caspases interact with inhibitors of apoptosis protein (IAP) or the Bcl-2 family of proteins, which independently have either pro or anti-apoptotic properties. There are several ways a malignant cell can attain apoptosis resistance. Typically, there are a few mechanisms that are involved in evasion of apoptosis: (i) impaired balance of pro-apoptotic and anti-apoptotic proteins; (ii) decreased caspase function, and (iii) deformed death receptor signalling [81]. (Fig. **5**) describe the mechanisms of apoptosis and carcinogenesis

STEM CELLS TARGETED CANCER THERAPY

Cancer is one among the primary causes of death worldwide, out of which India has 9% of overall deaths [82]. A better understanding of cancer biology allows the researchers to design better therapeutic strategies. Depending upon the type of cancer, the treatment methods vary, but the primary methods include surgery (to remove localised solid tumours), fractionated radiotherapy (kill tumours), chemotherapy (halt tumour growth by the use of toxic drugs) and immunotherapy (use of monoclonal antibodies) [83]. These therapeutic methods have many disadvantages, such as nonspecific-target effects, tumour recurrence, immune responses, and drug tolerance ability. Metastatic cancer cells cannot be removed by traditional therapies, and recurrence is particularly possible. Therefore, researchers are trying to develop novel therapies with minimum toxicity to adjacent normal cells. Stem cell therapy has brought a hopeful choice and improves the therapeutic ability due to better targeting of tumourogenic cells, thereby decreasing nonspecific-target events. Many stem cell-based therapies are under preclinical and clinical trials, that reflect great potential and huddles for cancer treatment [84]. In these parts of this chapter, you'll learn about the different types of stem cells, how they work to treat cancer, and what's new in this therapy.

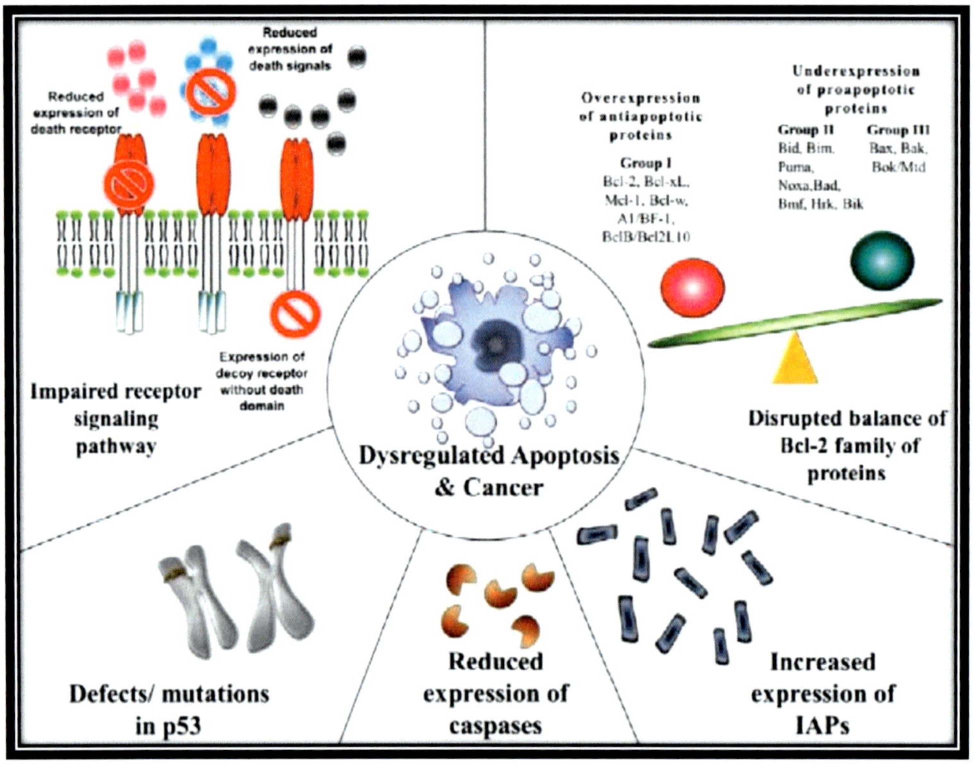

Fig. (5). Mechanisms involved in evasion of apoptosis and carcinogenesis.

Pluripotent Stem Cells (PSCs) in Cancer Treatment

Adult somatic cells transformed into induced pluripotent stem cells (iPSCs) by introducing four transcription factors that convert their epigenetic state to that of embryonic pluripotent stem cells [85]. iPSCs and cancer cells share similar transcriptomic signatures, including immune-system-recognized surface antigen markers [86, 87]. These iPSCs are important sources for anti-cancer vaccine production [88] and the induction of "Natural Killer" (NK) cells [89]. Kooreman et al. [90] compared the expression profiles of human iPSC clones with embryonic stem cells and cancer tissues through RNA sequencing and observed that human iPSCs express tumour-related, tumour-specific antigens and revealed overlap of gene expression profiles among iPSCs and various cancer types.

Adult Stem Cells in Cancer Treatment

Mesenchymal stem cells (MSCs) differentiate to a diversity of cell types such as adipocytes, osteocytes, and chondrocytes, and play a significant role in tissue repair and regeneration. MSCs are used to deliver therapeutic agents to treat various cancers [91]. In most human malignancies, abnormal expression of tumour suppressor genes, oncogenes, and onco-microRNAs is a common feature. Many studies reported that MSCs-derived exosomes can be loaded by variety of miRNAs and used to suppress tumour growth for example exosomes produced from MSCs inhibit breast cancer cell angiogenesis *in-vitro* through controlling the mTOR/HIF-1/VEGF signalling pathways [92]. Scientists proved that MSCs with apoptotic genes target tumour more effectively for example the interferon-γ expression in MSCs successfully kill glioma cells [93]. In a mouse prostate cancer lung metastasis model, MSCs expressing IFN- promote tumour cell death, increase NK cell activity, and inhibit angiogenesis [94]. MSCs are striking cancer therapy vehicles, earlier research provides evidence that genetically modified MSCs affect tumour development kinetics by delivering high doses of therapeutic anticancer proteins directly into the tumour mass [93, 95]. In a pre-established mouse model with metastasis of breast, melanoma, and hepatoma cancers, engineered MSCs that produce IL-12 prevented metastasis into the internal organs and boosted tumour cell death [96]. MSCs that were modified to express IL-12 were also examined in glioma models in mice [97].

Cancer Stem Cells (CSCs) in Cancer Treatment

CSCs are tumour-initiating cells that result from epigenetic alterations in normal stem cells or progenitor cell fusion. Identification of CSCs can be done on the basis of cellular surface markers. For example, CD44 can be used as a hallmark for CSC identification in various types of cancers like breast, lung, prostate, pancreatic, hepatocellular, and squamous cell carcinoma. CSCs, which are located inside tumour tissues, aid in the progression, metastasis, and recurrence of cancer [98]. CSCs may hold the key to diagnosing and treating a variety of solid cancers. CSCs are more resistant to radiotherapy due to various extrinsic factors (growth factors, acidic pH, cytokines, shortage of oxygen and nutrient shortage) and intrinsic factors (DNA repair capacity, stimulated cell cycle checkpoints and depleted proteasome activity). Therefore, radiation therapy must be replaced by other therapeutic methods [99]. The current cancer treatment methods are not at all effective at targeting CSCs, so they cannot remove progressive tumours.

Immunotherapy methods have a great potential to target CSCs. Duan et al. [100] proposed a synergistic nano-system immunotherapy method that uses photothermal agent polydopamine and immunomodulator CpG oligode oxynucleotides to boost immune response through dendritic cell maturation and T lymphocyte activation.

TUMOUR SUPPRESSOR GENES IN CANCER

Cellular stress circumstances such as DNA impairment, oncogene activation, and so forth activate tumour-suppressor genes that regulate stress responses, *e.g.* cell cycle arrest at check points and programmed cell death. Loss of function or decrease in function of these genes, in addition to other genetic mutations, facilitates cancer development [101 - 103].

p53

The p53 transcription factor is a master regulatory transcription factor expressed in response to several cellular stress conditions such as DNA damage and regulates a variety of cellular mechanisms such as cell cycle arrest, apoptosis, and senescence by targeting numerous genes. (Fig. **3**) [104]. p53 encoding gene TP53 mutations are linked with many sporadic human cancers [105]. Many of the TP53 mutations cause single amino acid substitutions in the p53 protein's DNA-binding domain, and mutp53 loses its capacity to trigger p53 target genes. MDM2 and CHIP (E3 ubiquitin ligases) enhance proteasome-mediated degradation of mutp53 proteins, making them unstable [106]. The activity of ubiquitin ligases is inhibited in cancer tissues due to mutp53's continuous interaction with chaperones Hsp70, Hsp90 and further Hsp40/DNAJA1 co-chaperones that support cancer cell survival [107]. Mutp53 sustains glucose uptake in tumour cells by inducing glucose transporter GLUT1 membrane translocation and also inhibits autophagy-dependent proteolysis caused by glucose deprivation [108]. Mutp53 also induces aerobic glycolysis and oxidative phosphorylation by inhibiting AMP-activated protein kinase [109] in tumour tissue. As the incidence of TP53 mutation is high in various human tumours, strategies that target blocking of mutp53 can have a massive impact on cancer therapeutics. Anticancer medications focusing on the mutp53 target are still in the initial stages of progress; the lone molecule, APR-246 (PRIMA-1Met), which restores mutp53 function to a wild type-tumour suppressor role, has been effectively tested in phase I/II clinical trials [110]. The pro-drug APR-246 is converted to methylene quinuclidinone that covalently binds to the –SH groups of cys-124 and 277 in the mutp53 main domain and finally causes p53 reactivation. When APR-246 is given, p53 refolds back into its normal shape and p53-targeting pathways are activated [111].

Retinoblastoma (Rb)

The tumour suppressor retinoblastoma (RB) is a principal cell cycle regulator and is functionally deactivated in most human cancers. This transcriptional regulator interacts with transcription factors of the E2F family and chromatin remodelers that cause many gene repressions that are significant for cell cycle progression. The functions of RB include telomere maintenance, DNA repair, chromosome cohesion and condensation, and gene silencing of repetitive DNA regions [112]. Retinoblastoma protein is made up of three parts: p105 (product of gene RB1), p107 (from gene RBL1) and p130 protein (gene RBL2) [113]. Mutations either in the RB1 gene or genes involved in its pathway are the main causes of a variety of human cancers due to cyclin and CDKs overexpression [114].

PTEN (Phosphatase and Tensin Homologue)

Phosphatase and tensin homolog (PTEN) is a protein and lipid phosphatase that acts on the AKT/ phosphatidylinositol-3-kinase (PI3K) signalling pathway as a negative regulator [115]. PTEN removes phosphate from 3′ position of phosphatidylinositol-3, 4, 5-triphosphate (PIP3) and converts it back to PIP2, causing PIP3 synthesis to decrease [116]. Decreased production of PIP3 indirectly affects AKT-mediated signalling pathways. AKT phosphorylates MDM2 and MDMX, which stabilises MDM2-MDMX complexes which maintain the p53 level low in the cells [117]. The better understanding of PTEN-regulated metabolism leads to the development of future cancer targeted therapies that aim at PTEN-regulated signalling cascades. Nowadays many strategies developed to reactivate PTEN, including CRISPR-Cas mediated gene editing for correction of PTEN somatic mutations and to restore PTEN tumour suppressor activities for cancer therapy [118].

CONCLUSION

Recent developments in the realm of molecular biotechnology have provided medical researchers with new pathways to explore when developing targeted medications and therapeutic approaches for the treatment of cancer. The research into cancer biomarkers, the locating of signalling pathways, and the development of novel targeted medications have all contributed to the beginning of a new age in the treatment of cancer. The discovery of cell surface indicators that are connected with cancer stem cells enables researchers to target CSCs more effectively and also properly, which is a significant step toward removing progressing tumours, which is one of the most difficult aspects of treating cancer. Methods of immunotherapy in which antigens derived from tumour cells are utilised to create cytotoxic lymphocytes, which then kill cancer stem cells (CSC). The latest information that scientists have gained about cancer hallmarks may give them with a better answer to the problem of developing innovative cancer therapy strategies.

CONSENT FOR PUBLICATION

Not applicable.

CONFLICT OF INTEREST

The authors declare no conflict of interest, financial or otherwise.

ACKNOWLEDGEMENT

The authors, Aakanchha Jain and Santosh K. Behera are thankful to former Director, NIPER-A for providing necessary literature searching facilities.

REFERENCES

[1] Siegel RL, Miller KD, Fuchs HE, Jemal A. Cancer Statistics, 2021. CA Cancer J Clin 2021; 71(1): 7-33.
[http://dx.doi.org/10.3322/caac.21654] [PMID: 33433946]

[2] Braal CL, Jongbloed EM, Wilting SM, Mathijssen RHJ, Koolen SLW, Jager A. Inhibiting CDK4/6 in breast cancer with palbociclib, ribociclib, and abemaciclib: similarities and differences. Drugs 2021; 81(3): 317-31.
[http://dx.doi.org/10.1007/s40265-020-01461-2] [PMID: 33369721]

[3] Lu YL, Huang YT, Wu MH, Chou TC, J Wong R, Lin SF. Efficacy of adavosertib therapy against anaplastic thyroid cancer. Endocr Relat Cancer 2021; 28(5): 311-24.
[http://dx.doi.org/10.1530/ERC-21-0001] [PMID: 33769310]

[4] Rahane W, Dalvi H, Magar Y, Kalane A, Jondhale S. Lung cancer detection using image processing and machine learning healthcare. 2018 International Conference on Current Trends towards Converging Technologies (ICCTCT). 1-5.
[http://dx.doi.org/10.1109/ICCTCT.2018.8551008]

[5] Brian Wu. MD Candidate, Keck School of Medicine, Los Angeles, USA. Hamilton, New Zealand: Dermatologist 2015. https://dermnetnz.org/topics/histology-stains/

[6] Gurcan MN, Boucheron LE, Can A, Madabhushi A, Rajpoot NM, Yener B. Histopathological image analysis: a review. IEEE Rev Biomed Eng 2009; 2: 147-71.
[http://dx.doi.org/10.1109/RBME.2009.2034865] [PMID: 20671804]

[7] Allam M, Cai S, Coskun AF. Multiplex bioimaging of single-cell spatial profiles for precision cancer diagnostics and therapeutics. NPJ Precis Oncol 2020; 4(1): 11.
[http://dx.doi.org/10.1038/s41698-020-0114-1] [PMID: 32377572]

[8] Liao S, Law MWK, Chung ACS. Dominant local binary patterns for texture classification. IEEE Trans Image Process 2009; 18(5): 1107-18.
[http://dx.doi.org/10.1109/TIP.2009.2015682] [PMID: 19342342]

[9] Kumar R, Srivastava R, Srivastava S. Detection and classification of cancer from microscopic biopsy images using clinically significant and biologically interpretable features. J Med Eng 2015; 2015: 1-14.
[http://dx.doi.org/10.1155/2015/457906] [PMID: 27006938]

[10] https://lagenetica.info/en/genetics-present-and-future/genetics-and-cancer

[11] Rapizzi E, Ercolino T, Fucci R, *et al.* Succinate dehydrogenase subunit B mutations modify human neuroblastoma cell metabolism and proliferation. Horm Cancer 2014; 5(3): 174-84. [http://dx.doi.org/10.1007/s12672-014-0172-3] [PMID: 24595825]

[12] Garrigue P, Bodin-Hullin A, Balasse L, *et al.* The evolving role of succinate in tumor metabolism: an 18F-FDG–based study. J Nucl Med 2017; 58(11): 1749-55. [http://dx.doi.org/10.2967/jnumed.117.192674] [PMID: 28619735]

[13] https://www.cancer.gov/about-cancer/causes-prevention/genetics#identifying-genetic-chang-s-in-cancer

[14] Arumugam J, Jeddy N, Ramamurthy A, Thangavelu R. The expression of Bcl-2 in oral squamous cell carcinoma—A review. J Orofac Sci 2017; 9(2): 71. [http://dx.doi.org/10.4103/jofs.jofs_88_16]

[15] Bozzone DM. Cancer Genetics (The Biology of Cancer). Garland Science Press 2007.

[16] Bunz F. Principles of cancer genetics. New York, NY, USA: Springer Dordrecht 2008; p. 14. [http://dx.doi.org/10.1007/978-1-4020-6784-6]

[17] Ronen A, Glickman BW. Human DNA repair genes. Environ Mol Mutagen 2001; 37(3): 241-83. [http://dx.doi.org/10.1002/em.1033] [PMID: 11317342]

[18] Turgeon MO, Perry NJS, Poulogiannis G. DNA damage, repair, and cancer metabolism. Front Oncol 2018; 8: 15. [http://dx.doi.org/10.3389/fonc.2018.00015] [PMID: 29459886]

[19] Jain RK, Martin JD, Chauhan VP, Duda DG. Tumor microenvironment: vascular and extravascular compartment. In: Niederhuber JE, Armitage JO, Kastan MB, Doroshow JH, Tepper JE (Eds.) Abeloff's Clinical Oncology; 6th edition. 2020; Elsevier: pp. 108-126.e7.

[20] Siemann DW. The unique characteristics of tumor vasculature and preclinical evidence for its selective disruption by Tumor-Vascular Disrupting Agents. Cancer Treat Rev 2011; 37(1): 63-74. [http://dx.doi.org/10.1016/j.ctrv.2010.05.001] [PMID: 20570444]

[21] Kamel HFM, Al-Amodi HSB. Cancer Biomarkers. In: Wang M, Witzmann FA (Eds.). Role of Biomarkers in Medicine. London: IntechOpen; 2016. [http://dx.doi.org/10.5772/62421]

[22] Getzenberg RH. Cancer Biomarkers Cancer: Prevention, Early Detection, Treatment and Recovery. 2nd ed., John Wiley & Sons, Inc. 2019.

[23] Mishra A, Verma M. Cancer biomarkers: are we ready for the prime time? Cancers (Basel) 2010; 2(1): 190-208. [http://dx.doi.org/10.3390/cancers2010190] [PMID: 24281040]

[24] Henry NL, Hayes DF. Cancer biomarkers. Mol Oncol 2012; 6(2): 140-6. [http://dx.doi.org/10.1016/j.molonc.2012.01.010] [PMID: 22356776]

[25] Goossens N, Nakagawa S, Sun X, Hoshida Y. Cancer biomarker discovery and validation. Transl Cancer Res 2015; 4(3): 256-69. [PMID: 26213686]

[26] Zamay T, Zamay G, Kolovskaya O, *et al.* Current and Prospective Protein Biomarkers of Lung Cancer. Cancers (Basel) 2017; 9(12): 155. [http://dx.doi.org/10.3390/cancers9110155] [PMID: 29137182]

[27] Ghafouri-Fard S, Nekoohesh L, Motevaseli E. Bladder cancer biomarkers: review and update. Asian Pac J Cancer Prev 2014; 15(6): 2395-403. [http://dx.doi.org/10.7314/APJCP.2014.15.6.2395] [PMID: 24761840]

[28] Benjamin SR, de Lima F. Current and Prospective of Breast Cancer Biomarkers. Biomarkers. In: Sedykh S (Ed.). Molecular Biotechnology [Internet]. London: IntechOpen; 2020 [cited 2023 Jan 04].

Available from: https://www.intechopen.com/chapters/71368.
[http://dx.doi.org/10.5772/intechopen.91151]

[29] Proctor I, Stoeber K, Williams GH. Biomarkers in bladder cancer. Histopathology 2010; 57(1): 1-13. [http://dx.doi.org/10.1111/j.1365-2559.2010.03592.x] [PMID: 20579130]

[30] Costello LC, Franklin RB. The genetic/metabolic transformation concept of carcinogenesis. Cancer Metastasis Rev 2012; 31(1-2): 123-30. [http://dx.doi.org/10.1007/s10555-011-9334-8] [PMID: 22109079]

[31] Faubert B, Solmonson A, DeBerardinis RJ. Metabolic reprogramming and cancer progression. Science 2020; 368(6487): eaaw5473. [http://dx.doi.org/10.1126/science.aaw5473] [PMID: 32273439]

[32] Koppenol WH, Bounds PL, Dang CV. Otto Warburg's contributions to current concepts of cancer metabolism. Nat Rev Cancer 2011; 11(5): 325-37. [http://dx.doi.org/10.1038/nrc3038] [PMID: 21508971]

[33] Pfeiffer T, Schuster S, Bonhoeffer S. Cooperation and competition in the evolution of ATP-producing pathways. Science 2001; 292(5516): 504-7. [http://dx.doi.org/10.1126/science.1058079] [PMID: 11283355]

[34] Jang M, Kim SS, Lee J. Cancer cell metabolism: implications for therapeutic targets. Exp Mol Med 2013; 45(10): e45. [http://dx.doi.org/10.1038/emm.2013.85] [PMID: 24091747]

[35] Sherr CJ, Bartek J. Cell Cycle–Targeted Cancer Therapies. Annu Rev Cancer Biol 2017; 1(1): 41-57. [http://dx.doi.org/10.1146/annurev-cancerbio-040716-075628]

[36] Taylor WR, Grabovich A. Targeting the cell cycle to kill cancer cells.Pharmacology. Academic Press 2009; pp. 429-53. [http://dx.doi.org/10.1016/B978-0-12-369521-5.00017-8]

[37] Feng M, Jiang W, Kim BYS, Zhang CC, Fu YX, Weissman IL. Phagocytosis checkpoints as new targets for cancer immunotherapy. Nat Rev Cancer 2019; 19(10): 568-86. [http://dx.doi.org/10.1038/s41568-019-0183-z] [PMID: 31462760]

[38] Malumbres M, Barbacid M. Cell cycle, CDKs and cancer: a changing paradigm. Nat Rev Cancer 2009; 9(3): 153-66. [http://dx.doi.org/10.1038/nrc2602] [PMID: 19238148]

[39] Lapenna S, Giordano A. Cell cycle kinases as therapeutic targets for cancer. Nat Rev Drug Discov 2009; 8(7): 547-66. [http://dx.doi.org/10.1038/nrd2907] [PMID: 19568282]

[40] Schwartz GK, Shah MA. Targeting the cell cycle: a new approach to cancer therapy. J Clin Oncol 2005; 23(36): 9408-21. [http://dx.doi.org/10.1200/JCO.2005.01.5594] [PMID: 16361640]

[41] Collins I, Garrett M. Targeting the cell division cycle in cancer: CDK and cell cycle checkpoint kinase inhibitors. Curr Opin Pharmacol 2005; 5(4): 366-73. [http://dx.doi.org/10.1016/j.coph.2005.04.009] [PMID: 15964238]

[42] Bartek J, Lukas J. Chk1 and Chk2 kinases in checkpoint control and cancer. Cancer Cell 2003; 3(5): 421-9. [http://dx.doi.org/10.1016/S1535-6108(03)00110-7] [PMID: 12781359]

[43] Meijer L, Raymond E. From Starfish Oocytes to Clinical Trials. Roscovitine and other purines as kinase inhibitors. From starfish oocytes to clinical trials. Acc Chem Res 2003; 36(6): 417-25. [http://dx.doi.org/10.1021/ar0201198] [PMID: 12809528]

[44] Markwalder JA, Arnone MR, Benfield PA, *et al.* Synthesis and biological evaluation of 1-aryl-4-5-dihydro-1H-pyrazolo[3,4-d]pyrimidin-4-one inhibitors of cyclin-dependent kinases. J Med Chem

2004; 47(24): 5894-911.
[http://dx.doi.org/10.1021/jm020455u] [PMID: 15537345]

[45] Mettey Y, Gompel M, Thomas V, *et al.* Aloisines, a new family of CDK/GSK-3 inhibitors. SAR study, crystal structure in complex with CDK2, enzyme selectivity, and cellular effects. J Med Chem 2003; 46(2): 222-36.
[http://dx.doi.org/10.1021/jm020319p] [PMID: 12519061]

[46] Schwartz G. The Development of CDK4 Inhibitors for Cancer Therapy. Ann Oncol 2015; 26: ii7.
[http://dx.doi.org/10.1093/annonc/mdv083.2]

[47] Yuan K, Wang X, Dong H, Min W, Hao H, Yang P. Selective inhibition of CDK4/6: A safe and effective strategy for developing anticancer drugs. Acta Pharm Sin B 2021; 11(1): 30-54.
[http://dx.doi.org/10.1016/j.apsb.2020.05.001] [PMID: 33532179]

[48] Goel S, DeCristo MJ, McAllister SS, Zhao JJ. CDK4/6 inhibition in cancer: beyond cell cycle arrest. Trends Cell Biol 2018; 28(11): 911-25.
[http://dx.doi.org/10.1016/j.tcb.2018.07.002] [PMID: 30061045]

[49] O'Leary B, Finn RS, Turner NC. Treating cancer with selective CDK4/6 inhibitors. Nat Rev Clin Oncol 2016; 13(7): 417-30.
[http://dx.doi.org/10.1038/nrclinonc.2016.26] [PMID: 27030077]

[50] Tate SC, Cai S, Ajamie RT, *et al.* Semi-mechanistic pharmacokinetic/pharmacodynamic modeling of the antitumor activity of LY2835219, a new cyclin-dependent kinase 4/6 inhibitor, in mice bearing human tumor xenografts. Clin Cancer Res 2014; 20(14): 3763-74.
[http://dx.doi.org/10.1158/1078-0432.CCR-13-2846] [PMID: 24850847]

[51] Gelbert LM, Cai S, Lin X, *et al.* Preclinical characterization of the CDK4/6 inhibitor LY2835219: in-vivo cell cycle-dependent/independent anti-tumor activities alone/in combination with gemcitabine. Invest New Drugs 2014; 32(5): 825-37.
[http://dx.doi.org/10.1007/s10637-014-0120-7] [PMID: 24919854]

[52] Rader J, Russell MR, Hart LS, *et al.* Dual CDK4/CDK6 inhibition induces cell-cycle arrest and senescence in neuroblastoma. Clin Cancer Res 2013; 19(22): 6173-82.
[http://dx.doi.org/10.1158/1078-0432.CCR-13-1675] [PMID: 24045179]

[53] Zhang YX, Sicinska E, Czaplinski JT, *et al.* Antiproliferative effects of CDK4/6 inhibition in CDK4-amplified human liposarcoma in vitro and in vivo. Mol Cancer Ther 2014; 13(9): 2184-93.
[http://dx.doi.org/10.1158/1535-7163.MCT-14-0387] [PMID: 25028469]

[54] Hamilton E, Infante JR. Targeting CDK4/6 in patients with cancer. Cancer Treat Rev 2016; 45: 129-38.
[http://dx.doi.org/10.1016/j.ctrv.2016.03.002] [PMID: 27017286]

[55] Carlson BA, Pearlstein RA, Naik RG, Sedlacek HH, Sausville EA, Worland PJ. Inhibition of CDK2, CDK4 and CDK7 by flavopiridol and structural analogs. Proc Am Assoc Cancer Res 1996; 37: 424.

[56] El-Rayes BF, Gadgeel S, Shields AF, Manza S, Lorusso P, Philip PA. Phase I study of bryostatin 1 and gemcitabine. Clin Cancer Res 2006; 12(23): 7059-62.
[http://dx.doi.org/10.1158/1078-0432.CCR-06-1419] [PMID: 17145828]

[57] Isakov N, Galron D, Mustelin T, Pettit GR, Altman A. Inhibition of phorbol ester-induced T cell proliferation by bryostatin is associated with rapid degradation of protein kinase C. J Immunol 1993; 150(4): 1195-204.
[PMID: 8432975]

[58] Le Tourneau C, Faivre S, Laurence V, *et al.* Phase I evaluation of seliciclib (R-roscovitine), a novel oral cyclin-dependent kinase inhibitor, in patients with advanced malignancies. Eur J Cancer 2010; 46(18): 3243-50.
[http://dx.doi.org/10.1016/j.ejca.2010.08.001] [PMID: 20822897]

[59] Mikhail S, Albanese C, Pishvaian MJ. Cyclin-dependent kinase inhibitors and the treatment of

gastrointestinal cancers. Am J Pathol 2015; 185(5): 1185-97.
[http://dx.doi.org/10.1016/j.ajpath.2015.01.008] [PMID: 25747534]

[60] Kuntz K, O'Connell MJ. The G2 DNA damage checkpoint: Could this ancient regulator be the Achilles heel of cancer? Cancer Biol Ther 2009; 8(15): 1433-9.
[http://dx.doi.org/10.4161/cbt.8.15.9081] [PMID: 19574738]

[61] Gabrielli B, Brooks K, Pavey S. Defective cell cycle checkpoints as targets for anti-cancer therapies 2012; 3: 9.
[http://dx.doi.org/10.3389/fphar.2012.00009]

[62] Anderson HJ, Andersen RJ, Roberge M. Inhibitors of the G2 DNA damage checkpoint and their potential for cancer therapy. Prog Cell Cycle Res 2003; 5: 423-30.
[PMID: 14593736]

[63] Jain A, Jain R, Jain S, Khatik R, Veer Kohli D. Minicapsules encapsulating nanoparticles for targeting, apoptosis induction and treatment of colon cancer. Artif Cells Nanomed Biotechnol 2019; 47(1): 1085-93.
[http://dx.doi.org/10.1080/21691401.2019.1593848] [PMID: 30942626]

[64] Busby EC, Leistritz DF, Abraham RT, Karnitz LM, Sarkaria JN. The radiosensitizing agent 7-hydroxystaurosporine (UCN-01) inhibits the DNA damage checkpoint kinase hChk1. Cancer Res 2000; 60(8): 2108-12.
[PMID: 10786669]

[65] Kortmansky J, Shah MA, Kaubisch A, *et al.* Phase I trial of the cyclin-dependent kinase inhibitor and protein kinase C inhibitor 7-hydroxystaurosporine in combination with Fluorouracil in patients with advanced solid tumors. J Clin Oncol 2005; 23(9): 1875-84.
[http://dx.doi.org/10.1200/JCO.2005.03.116] [PMID: 15699481]

[66] Shah MA, Schwartz GK. Cell cycle-mediated drug resistance: an emerging concept in cancer therapy. Clin Cancer Res 2001; 7(8): 2168-81.
[PMID: 11489790]

[67] Prajapati SK, Malaiya A, Kesharwani P, Soni D, Jain A. Biomedical applications and toxicities of carbon nanotubes. Drug Chem Toxicol 2020; 1-6.
[PMID: 31908176]

[68] Thompson R, Eastman A. The cancer therapeutic potential of Chk1 inhibitors: how mechanistic studies impact on clinical trial design. Br J Clin Pharmacol 2013; 76(3): 358-69.
[http://dx.doi.org/10.1111/bcp.12139] [PMID: 23593991]

[69] Kohn EA, Ruth ND, Brown MK, Livingstone M, Eastman A. Abrogation of the S phase DNA damage checkpoint results in S phase progression or premature mitosis depending on the concentration of UCN-01 and the kinetics of Cdc25C activation. J Biol Chem 2002; 277: 26553-64.
[http://dx.doi.org/10.1074/jbc.M202040200] [PMID: 11953432]

[70] Montano R, Chung I, Garner KM, Parry D, Eastman A. Preclinical development of the novel Chk1 inhibitor SCH900776 in combination with DNA-damaging agents and antimetabolites. Mol Cancer Ther 2012; 11(2): 427-38.
[http://dx.doi.org/10.1158/1535-7163.MCT-11-0406] [PMID: 22203733]

[71] Montano R, Khan N, Hou H, *et al.* Cell cycle perturbation induced by gemcitabine in human tumor cells in cell culture, xenografts and bladder cancer patients: implications for clinical trial designs combining gemcitabine with a Chk1 inhibitor. Oncotarget 2017; 8(40): 67754-68.
[http://dx.doi.org/10.18632/oncotarget.18834] [PMID: 28978069]

[72] Wahl AF, Donaldson KL, Faircnild C, *et al.* Loss of normal p53 function confers sensitization to Taxol by increasing G2/M arrest and apoptosis. Nat Med 1996; 2(1): 72-9.
[http://dx.doi.org/10.1038/nm0196-72] [PMID: 8564846]

[73] Wang TH, Wang HS, Soong YK. Paclitaxel-induced cell death. Cancer 2000; 88(11): 2619-28.

[http://dx.doi.org/10.1002/1097-0142(20000601)88:11<2619::AID-CNCR26>3.0.CO;2-J] [PMID: 10861441]

[74] Sankari SL, Masthan KMK, Babu NA, Bhattacharjee T, Elumalai M. Apoptosis in cancer--an update. Asian Pac J Cancer Prev 2012; 13(10): 4873-8.
[http://dx.doi.org/10.7314/APJCP.2012.13.10.4873] [PMID: 23244073]

[75] Saraste A, Pulkki K. Morphologic and biochemical hallmarks of apoptosis. Cardiovasc Res 2000; 45(3): 528-37.
[http://dx.doi.org/10.1016/S0008-6363(99)00384-3] [PMID: 10728374]

[76] Li XM, Luo XG, Wang N, *et al.* The extract of Hypericum ascyron L. induces bacterial cell death through apoptosis pathway. J Ethnopharmacol 2015; 166: 205-10.
[http://dx.doi.org/10.1016/j.jep.2015.03.034] [PMID: 25796407]

[77] Lowe SW, Lin AW. Apoptosis in cancer. Carcinogenesis 2000; 21(3): 485-95.
[http://dx.doi.org/10.1093/carcin/21.3.485] [PMID: 10688869]

[78] Reed JC. Bcl-2 family proteins: regulators of apoptosis and chemoresistance in hematologic malignancies. Semin Hematol 1997; 34(4) (Suppl. 5): 9-19.
[PMID: 9408956]

[79] Karp G. Cell and molecular biology: Concepts and experiments. John New Jersey: Wiley and Sons 2008; 653-657: 5.

[80] Hengartner MO. Apoptosis. Cell 2001; 104(3): 325-8.
[http://dx.doi.org/10.1016/S0092-8674(01)00219-7] [PMID: 11239389]

[81] Wong RSY. Apoptosis in cancer: from pathogenesis to treatment. J Exp Clin Cancer Res 2011; 30(1): 87.
[http://dx.doi.org/10.1186/1756-9966-30-87] [PMID: 21943236]

[82] WHO. World Health Statistics 2019: Monitoring Health for the SDGs. Geneva, Switzerland: World Health Organization 2018.

[83] Vanneman M, Dranoff G. Combining immunotherapy and targeted therapies in cancer treatment. Nat Rev Cancer 2012; 12(4): 237-51.
[http://dx.doi.org/10.1038/nrc3237] [PMID: 22437869]

[84] Gomes JPA, Assoni AF, Pelatti M, Coatti G, Okamoto OK, Zatz M. Deepening a simple question: Can MSCs be used to treat cancer? Anticancer Res 2017; 37(9): 4747-58.
[PMID: 28870893]

[85] Takahashi K, Yamanaka S. Induction of pluripotent stem cells from mouse embryonic and adult fibroblast cultures by defined factors. Cell 2006; 126(4): 663-76.
[http://dx.doi.org/10.1016/j.cell.2006.07.024] [PMID: 16904174]

[86] de Almeida PE, Meyer EH, Kooreman NG, *et al.* Transplanted terminally differentiated induced pluripotent stem cells are accepted by immune mechanisms similar to self-tolerance. Nat Commun 2014; 5(1): 3903.
[http://dx.doi.org/10.1038/ncomms4903] [PMID: 24875164]

[87] Ghosh Z, Huang M, Hu S, Wilson KD, Dey D, Wu JC. Dissecting the oncogenic potential of human embryonic and induced pluripotent stem cell derivatives. Cancer Res 2011; 71: 5030-9.
[http://dx.doi.org/10.1158/0008-5472.CAN-10-4402] [PMID: 21646469]

[88] Ouyang X, Telli ML, Wu JC. Induced pluripotent stem cell-based cancer vaccines. Front Immunol 2019; 10: 1510.
[http://dx.doi.org/10.3389/fimmu.2019.01510] [PMID: 31338094]

[89] Knorr DA, Ni Z, Hermanson D, *et al.* Clinical-scale derivation of natural killer cells from human pluripotent stem cells for cancer therapy. Stem Cells Transl Med 2013; 2(4): 274-83.
[http://dx.doi.org/10.5966/sctm.2012-0084] [PMID: 23515118]

[90] Kooreman NG, Kim Y, de Almeida PE, *et al.* Autologous iPSC-based vaccines elicit anti-tumor responses in vivo. Cell Stem Cell 2018; 22(4): 501-513.e7. [http://dx.doi.org/10.1016/j.stem.2018.01.016] [PMID: 29456158]

[91] Lin W, Huang L, Li Y, *et al.* Mesenchymal stem cells and cancer: clinical challenges and opportunities. BioMed Res Int 2019; 2019: 1-12. [http://dx.doi.org/10.1155/2019/2820853] [PMID: 31205939]

[92] Pakravan K, Babashah S, Sadeghizadeh M, *et al.* MicroRNA-100 shuttled by mesenchymal stem cell-derived exosomes suppresses in vitro angiogenesis through modulating the mTOR/HIF-1α/VEGF signaling axis in breast cancer cells. Cell Oncol (Dordr) 2017; 40(5): 457-70. [http://dx.doi.org/10.1007/s13402-017-0335-7] [PMID: 28741069]

[93] Nakamizo A, Marini F, Amano T, *et al.* Human bone marrow-derived mesenchymal stem cells in the treatment of gliomas. Cancer Res 2005; 65(8): 3307-18. [http://dx.doi.org/10.1158/0008-5472.CAN-04-1874] [PMID: 15833864]

[94] Ren C, Kumar S, Chanda D, *et al.* Cancer gene therapy using mesenchymal stem cells expressing interferon-β in a mouse prostate cancer lung metastasis model. Gene Ther 2008; 15(21): 1446-53. [http://dx.doi.org/10.1038/gt.2008.101] [PMID: 18596829]

[95] Pereboeva L, Curiel DT. Cellular vehicles for cancer gene therapy: current status and future potential. BioDrugs 2004; 18(6): 361-85. [http://dx.doi.org/10.2165/00063030-200418060-00003] [PMID: 15571421]

[96] Chen X, Lin X, Zhao J, *et al.* A tumor-selective biotherapy with prolonged impact on established metastases based on cytokine gene-engineered MSCs. Mol Ther 2008; 16(4): 749-56. [http://dx.doi.org/10.1038/mt.2008.3] [PMID: 18362930]

[97] Nakamura K, Ito Y, Kawano Y, *et al.* Antitumor effect of genetically engineered mesenchymal stem cells in a rat glioma model. Gene Ther 2004; 11(14): 1155-64. [http://dx.doi.org/10.1038/sj.gt.3302276] [PMID: 15141157]

[98] Chang JC. Cancer stem cells: Role in tumor growth, recurrence, metastasis, and treatment resistance. Medicine (Baltimore) 2016; 95: S20-S25.

[99] Atashzar MR, Baharlou R, Karami J, *et al.* Cancer stem cells: A review from origin to therapeutic implications. J Cell Physiol 2020; 235(2): 790-803. [http://dx.doi.org/10.1002/jcp.29044] [PMID: 31286518]

[100] Duan Y, Yang H, Gao J, *et al.* Immune Modulator and Low-Temperature PTT-Induced Synergistic Immunotherapy for Cancer Treatment. ACS Appl Bio Mater 2021; 4(2): 1524-35. [http://dx.doi.org/10.1021/acsabm.0c01397] [PMID: 35014502]

[101] Chaffer CL, Weinberg RA. How does multistep tumorigenesis really proceed? Cancer Discov 2015; 5(1): 22-4. [http://dx.doi.org/10.1158/2159-8290.CD-14-0788] [PMID: 25583800]

[102] Weinberg RA. Coming full circle-from endless complexity to simplicity and back again. Cell 2014; 157(1): 267-71. [http://dx.doi.org/10.1016/j.cell.2014.03.004] [PMID: 24679541]

[103] Hanahan D, Weinberg RA. Hallmarks of cancer: the next generation. Cell 2011; 144(5): 646-74. [http://dx.doi.org/10.1016/j.cell.2011.02.013] [PMID: 21376230]

[104] Bursac S, Brdovcak MC, Donati G, Volarevic S. Activation of the tumour suppressor p53 upon impairment of ribosome biogenesis. Biochim Biophys Acta 1842; 2014: 817-30.

[105] Kandoth C, McLellan MD, Vandin F, *et al.* Mutational landscape and significance across 12 major cancer types. Nature 2013; 502(7471): 333-9. [http://dx.doi.org/10.1038/nature12634] [PMID: 24132290]

[106] Li D, Marchenko ND, Schulz R, *et al.* Functional inactivation of endogenous MDM2 and CHIP by

HSP90 causes aberrant stabilization of mutant p53 in human cancer cells. Mol Cancer Res 2011; 9(5): 577-88.
[http://dx.doi.org/10.1158/1541-7786.MCR-10-0534] [PMID: 21478269]

[107] Schulz-Heddergott R, Moll U. Gain-of-function (GOF) mutant p53 as actionable therapeutic target. Cancers (Basel) 2018; 10(6): 188-203.
[http://dx.doi.org/10.3390/cancers10060188] [PMID: 29875343]

[108] Rodriguez OC, Choudhury S, Kolukula V, *et al.* Dietary downregulation of mutant p53 levels via glucose restriction. Cell Cycle 2012; 11(23): 4436-46.
[http://dx.doi.org/10.4161/cc.22778] [PMID: 23151455]

[109] Mantovani F, Collavin L, Del Sal G. Mutant p53 as a guardian of the cancer cell. Cell Death Differ 2019; 26(2): 199-212.
[http://dx.doi.org/10.1038/s41418-018-0246-9] [PMID: 30538286]

[110] Bykov VJN, Wiman KG. Mutant p53 reactivation by small molecules makes its way to the clinic. FEBS Lett 2014; 588(16): 2622-7.
[http://dx.doi.org/10.1016/j.febslet.2014.04.017] [PMID: 24768524]

[111] Magri J, Gasparetto A, Conti L, *et al.* Tumor-Associated Antigen xCT and Mutant-p53 as Molecular Targets for New Combinatorial Antitumor Strategies. Cells 2021; 10(1): 108.
[http://dx.doi.org/10.3390/cells10010108] [PMID: 33430127]

[112] Vélez-Cruz R, Johnson D. The Retinoblastoma (RB) Tumor Suppressor: Pushing Back against Genome Instability on Multiple Fronts. Int J Mol Sci 2017; 18(8): 1776.
[http://dx.doi.org/10.3390/ijms18081776] [PMID: 28812991]

[113] Dick FA, Rubin SM. Molecular mechanisms underlying RB protein function. Nat Rev Mol Cell Biol 2013; 14(5): 297-306.
[http://dx.doi.org/10.1038/nrm3567] [PMID: 23594950]

[114] Sherr CJ, McCormick F. The RB and p53 pathways in cancer. Cancer Cell 2002; 2(2): 103-12.
[http://dx.doi.org/10.1016/S1535-6108(02)00102-2] [PMID: 12204530]

[115] Downes CP, Ross S, Maccario H, Perera N, Davidson L, Leslie NR. Stimulation of PI 3-kinase signaling via inhibition of the tumor suppressor phosphatase, PTEN. Adv Enzyme Regul 2007; 47(1): 184-94.
[http://dx.doi.org/10.1016/j.advenzreg.2006.12.018] [PMID: 17343901]

[116] Vivanco I, Sawyers CL. The phosphatidylinositol 3-Kinase–AKT pathway in human cancer. Nat Rev Cancer 2002; 2(7): 489-501.
[http://dx.doi.org/10.1038/nrc839] [PMID: 12094235]

[117] Chen CY, Chen J, He L, Stiles BL. PTEN: tumor suppressor and metabolic regulator. Front Endocrinol (Lausanne) 2018; 9: 338.
[http://dx.doi.org/10.3389/fendo.2018.00338] [PMID: 30038596]

[118] Lee YR, Chen M, Pandolfi PP. The functions and regulation of the PTEN tumour suppressor: new modes and prospects. Nat Rev Mol Cell Biol 2018; 19(9): 547-62.
[http://dx.doi.org/10.1038/s41580-018-0015-0] [PMID: 29858604]

CHAPTER 2

Nanotechnology for Cancer Treatment: An Introduction

Farhan Mazahir[1], **Anchal Pathak**[1], **Ujala Gupta**[1] and **Awesh K. Yadav**[1,*]

[1] *National Institute of Pharmaceutical Education and Research, Raebareli, India*

Abstract: Cancer is the leading cause of death worldwide. The treatment of cancer remains a challenge for medical professionals. Although various options, like chemotherapy, radiation, and surgery, are available to manage cancer, their use could be limited due to serious adverse effects. Therefore, advancements are highly essential to treat cancer properly. Nanotechnology provides new rays of hope for the effective treatment of cancer. Nanotechnology-based drug delivery carriers (NCs), such as nanoparticles, liposomes, dendrimers, polyplexes, and many more, offer treatment strategies due to their ability to target cancer cells. As these NCs target cancer cells, the exposure of other tissues to the drug is very less. Hence, these NCs exhibit fewer side effects in comparison with standard anti-cancer drugs. Here, we try to summarize a precise introduction of different NCs and their role in cancer therapy.

Keywords: Cancer, EPR, Inorganic Nanocarriers, Nanotechnology/ Nanomedicines.

INTRODUCTION

Cancer has been considered a leading cause of death worldwide. Also, the treatment of such horrible diseases seems very challenging till now. Chemotherapy (alone and in combination with radiotherapy) and surgery are considered first-line therapy for solid tumors. But, classical chemo-therapeutics suffer from terrible side effects. Thus, formulating anti-cancer molecules into Nanoparticles (NPs) /Nanocarriers (NCs)/Nanomedicines (NMDC) has become an attractive and important technique (Fig. **1**). Moreover, NPs or NCs increase the quality of the therapeutic index of cytotoxic agents. Thousands of research articles and approved nanomedicine have been witnessed in the last three decades. These NPs target the tumor *via* the enhanced permeability and retention (EPR) effect. The EPR effect is a peculiar characteristic of solid tumors. Due to the leaky and abnormal architecture of blood vessels around the tumor mass, the EPR effect

* **Corresponding author Awesh K. Yadav:** National Institute of Pharmaceutical Education and Research, Raebareli, India; Tel: +91-8989154900; E-mail: aweshyadav@gmail.com

Neeraj Mishra, Ashish Garg and Neeraj Upmanyu (Eds.)

predominates, as shown in Fig. (**2**). The EPR effect was first described by Matsumura and Maeda in 1986. Doxil™, Marqibo™, Abraxane™, onivyde™, and Daunoxome™ in the U.S., Genexol-PM™ in Korea, SMANCS™ in japan, and Mepact™ and Myocet™ in Europe, are good examples of NMDC and currently being used in the clinical management of different cancers. Vyexos™ (Liposomal formulation encapsulated with daunorubicin and cytabarine) has received approval from the FDA for the management of cancer. Vyexos™ increased the improved overall survival for 9.56 months in the patients with high-risk acute myeloid leukemia, while the patients who received daunorubicin and cytarabine had an increased survival only of 5.95 months [1 - 3]. A draft (docket no. FDA-2010-D-0530) was prepared by the FDA to provide the guidelines for the industry to regulate nanotechnology-based products, which states that materials that fall on the scale of nano range, *i.e.*, 1 nanometer (nm) to 100 nm, in any dimension and can exhibit either different biological or chemical or physical effects in comparison with large scale, materials. The word "product" means products, ingredients, materials, medical devices, biological products, dietary supplements, and food products, *i.e.*, food for animals, tobacco, and cosmetic products. Moreover, if the change in any dimension can increase potency, bioavailability, or reduce the potency and toxicity of drug products, highly protective packaging material foods improve the detection of pathogens and better delivery of nutrients or functional ingredients in the food [4]. Moreover, NPs offer effortless purification, easy sterilization, a chance to target the drug, release over a long time, and the best use of the EPR effect [5, 6]. NPs could be exploited for the controlled release and tumor targeting application due to multiple ligand coupling [7]. This chapter is dedicated to nanotechnology and its applications for the clinical management of various cancers. So, we tried our best to present the recent advancements and role of NMDC/NPs/NCs to treat illnesses like cancer.

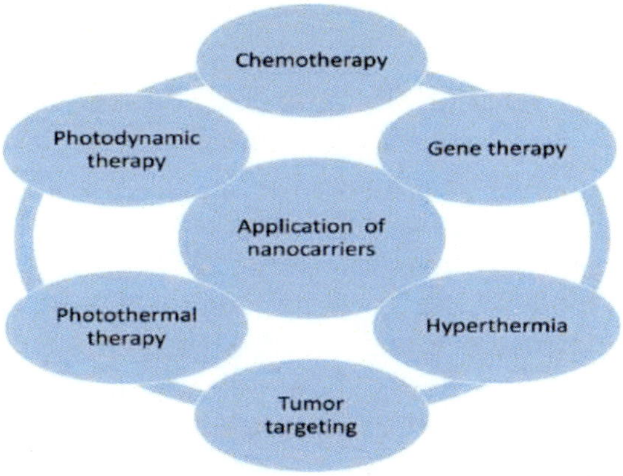

Fig. (1). Illustration of the role of nanotechnology in the management of cancer.

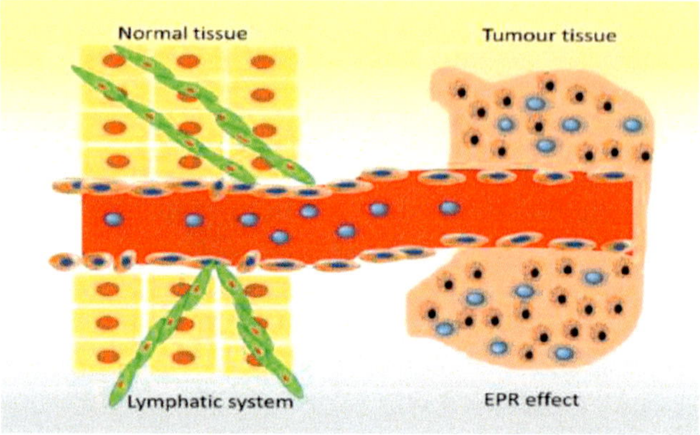

Fig. (2). Schematic illustration of EPR effect.

POLYMERIC NCS

Over the recent decades, numerous highly effective polymeric NMDCs have been delivered to improve the potential of therapeutic agents. The Polymeric NPs, due to their nano size, can access leaky vasculature of tumors and their surface could be modified easily for targeted delivery. Polymers can offer the feasibility to synthesize particles with different shapes, porosity, and size. Interestingly, the desirable release profile of active ingredients could be achieved *via* the change in molecular weight of the polymer. Synthetic polymers (Polycaprolactone (PCL), poly(lactic-co-glycolic acid) (PLGA), *etc*., and natural polymers (Chitosan and many more), have been used successfully for the production of NMDC. In this section, we present precise and recent glimpses of polymeric NPs and their usefulness in the treatment of cancer [8].

Polymeric NCs: Polycaprolactone (PCL) NCs

PCL has received approval from FDA (Food and Drug Administration) for biomedical applications. Due to its excellent bio-degradation in biological conditions, the delivery of drugs over a long time could be possible. A continuous nanoscale encapsulation of 5-Fluorouracil (5-FU) and Paclitaxel into the PCL has been reported by Iqbal *et al.*, that the process accomplished with the help of core-shealth technology using dimethyl formamide (DMF). The dimension of PCL-based nanofibers was found in the 22-90 nm range. Also, an inverse relationship between pH and drug release rate was observed. Moreover, the addition of PVA during the nanofibre formation clearly showed the presence of nanocrystals on the surface of nanofibres. These 5-FU encapsulated nanofibres were tested against PC-3 cells for their therapeutic usefulness. The *in-vitro* data suggested that only 33.8% of cells were found to be alive when treated with a 5 μm concentration of nanofibres in comparison with free drug, *i.e.*, 43% survived cells [9]. The NPs containing curcumin, prepared from enzyme responsive PCL based triblock co-polymers, functionalized with (ACP)-GPLGIAGQr9-(ACP) peptide, were found to be internalized *via* macropinocytosis and displayed a targeted drug delivery profile. The peptide GPLGIAGQr9 was designed in such a way that it could be degraded with MMP-2. But, GPLGIAGQr9 was used to enhance cellular uptake of triblock co-polymer NP. Also, PEG is known for *in-vivo* prolonging the retention effect. Furthermore, cellular toxicity and uptake were assessed in non-small cell lung cancer (NSCLC) A549 and L929 mouse embryonic fibroblasts cells. The strong fluorescence behavior of curcumin helped to analyze the *in-vivo* distribution. Moreover, triblock co-polymer NPs were found to be effective against *in-vivo* lung cancer treatment [10]. Polycaprolactone NPs functionalized with folic acid, PEG-modified, and comprised of ditelluride and doxorubicin (DOX) embedded, were assessed against *in-vitro* and *in-vivo* breast tumor (4T1 cells-based models). The *in-vitro* drug release suggested the detection of 76.71% of DOX in the presence of Glutathione (GSH), indicating the redox-sensitive behavior. Also, the internalization was found to be folic acid-mediated endocytosis. Based on the *in-vitro* and *in-vivo* results, such redox-sensitive and folic acid functionalized could be the choice for the treatment of breast cancer [11]. Another, amphiphilic triblock co-polymer consisting of PCL-PEG-PCL was used to fabricate the 86.71% DOX loaded 'flower-like NPs of 130.08 nm dimension having 0.200 PDI, which were tried against ovary cancer for evaluation of its therapeutic purpose. The *ex-vivo* study suggested that DOX-embedded amphiphilic triblock co-polymer NPs demonstrated excellent targeting, and accumulation at the site of *in-vivo* tumors by exploiting the EPR mechanism. Hence, DOX-loaded NPs composed of amphiphilic triblock co-polymer could be a choice for cancer therapy [12]. Sorafenib loaded and d-α-tocopherol polyethylene glycol 1000 succinate conjugated polycaprolactone (TPGS-b-PCL) NPs synthesized by modified precipitation were evaluated against hepatocellular carcinoma in HepG2 hepatoma cells and an HCC xenograft mouse model. The flow cytometry, western blotting, and MTT assay revealed the tumor-suppressing effect in HepG2 hepatoma cells and an HCC xenograft model. Also, no adverse effects were observed in the sorafenib-loaded NPs. The data suggested that TPGS-b-PCL NPs could be a trial for the management of hepatocellular carcinoma [13]. Also, in different studies, the combinatorial effect (chemo-photothermal) of cholic acid functionalized, conjugated with AS1411 aptamers-polydopamine and DOX embedded (PCL-ran-PLA) NPs, were evaluated. Due to their fabulous bio-properties, uncomplicated preparation process, significant drug concentration at the tumor site, lesser side effects, and enough tumor elimination properties, multimodal NPs for biomedical purposes could be useful for the elimination of cancer [14].

Polymeric NCs: Poly (Lactic-Co-Glycolic Acid) (PLGA) NPs

5-boronopicolinic acid (BA) functionalized and camptothecin-carrying PLGA nanoparticles were used for the treatment of tumors with overexpression of sialic acid. PLGA NPs functionalized *via* electrostatic interaction between the nanoparticles and BA. The BA functionalized PLGA NPs in a 1:20 molar ratio demonstrated higher cellular uptake and excellent *in-vivo* tumor efficacy in 4–5 weeks-old female BALB/c mice (20 ± 3 g) tumor model [15]. Bioinspired co-delivery of small interfering RNA (siRNA), targeting E7 and Paclitaxel, was used against HeLa Cancer. These bioinspired NPs demonstrated all the essential physicochemical characteristics for NPs-mediated drug delivery. Moreover, the desirable *in-vivo* distribution derived the 3-fold higher accumulation in the HeLa-bearing mouse models [16]. CD-340 functionalized (a type of Human epidermal growth factor receptor 2 (HER 2)) and DOX embedded PLGA NPs were tested for their *in-vitro* and *in-vivo* efficacy against various breast cancer cells. Moreover, confocal microscopy, flow cytometry, and gel electrophoresis were used to confirm the conjugation of the ligand. Also, the highest level of caspase was found in SKBR-3 in comparison with MDA-MB-23 and MCF-7. Also, the release of DOX from the functionalized particles was found for 96 hrs [17]. Interestingly, Paclitaxel-carrying NPs demonstrated significant tumor penetrating ability, while injected with iRGD, a tumor penetrating peptide. Paclitaxel-carrying PLGA NPs arrested the cell cycle at the G2/M phase. Moreover, migration and invasion of the tumor were diminished. Hence, the NPs could be the choice for the cell or tissue-specific delivery of the anti-tumor drug by co-administration of penetrating agents [18]. CXCL12 anchored PLGA/Pluronic F127 NPs were used to mitigate the migration of cells. The role of CXCL12/CXCL4 has been established in the metastasis of tumor cells. Also, CXCL4 has been targeted with different peptides and or CXCL12-derived peptides. Intriguingly, CXCL12 anchored NPs did not provoke an immune reaction and displayed significant compatibility. The CXCL12 anchored NPs did not initiate cell invasion but rather inhibited the migration of THP-1 cells. However, the internalization of NPs increased by the expression of CXCR4 in culture medium/FBS [19]. A dual-targeting approach has also been utilized for the novel *in-vitro* treatment for the human primary malignant glioblastoma (U87MG) cell line. To achieve dual drug targeting, both hyaluronic acid and RGD peptide were used to modify the PLGA NPs. RGD peptide has an affinity toward Integrin ($\alpha_2\beta_3$), a kind of protein used to over-express in different cancers. This dual drug approach displayed a lesser IC_{50} value against U87MG. Also, better uptake was observed in the case of RGD peptide-anchored PLGA NPs [20]. In another experiment, the inhibition of glucose transport to the tumor cell was used to mitigate the growth of tumor cells with the help of glucose-functionalized PLGA and chitosan NPs. The level of expression of GLUT-1 and GLUT-4 after the treatment with glucose-functionalized NPs was evaluated. The expression of GLUT-1 mRNA was found to be 45% less after the 72 hrs treatment. More than 80% of glucose-decorated NPs were found to be stable at 40°C and different pH 5.4 to 7.4. Both, glucose-modified PLGA and chitosan NPs were found to be effective in inhibiting the survival rate of HT-29 cells up to 54% [21]. Leutolin encapsulated and HER2 modified PLGA NPs were validated for their *in-vitro* therapeutic efficacy against gastric cancer SGC-7901 cells. Luteolin was found to be induced early and late apoptotic events in the gastric cancer cells. In the case of HER2-modified PLGA NPs, the level of FOXO 1 (forkhead box protein O1) mRNA was found to be altered by 6.75 fold, indicating the inhibition of growth of SGC-7901 cells has direct linked with the increased expression of FOXO 1. But, the high expression of FOXO 1 protein was found in the cells treated with luteolin encapsulated HER2 tethered PLGA NPs [22]. Oxaliplatin containing folic acid-coated PLGA NPs proved their maximized efficacy against the xenograft model of colorectal cancer. Oxaliplatin is third-generation platinum and has a place in the therapeutic regime for colorectal cancer. PLGA NPs were designed to minimize the side effects, metastasis, and resistance to the drug and to enhance apoptosis. The xenograft model of colorectal cancer was developed by injecting CT-26 cells into the right flank of male Balb/c mice. The weight of the tumor in the treated group was found to be decreased in comparison with the saline-treated group ($p<0.0001$) [23]. A co-polymer of PEG-PLGA was used to prepare the rapamycin (RAP) encapsulated PLGA NPs. PEG-PLGA NPs (118.8 nm) were used to accumulate in the tumor area through enhanced permeability and retention effect. Rapamycin (RAP) is known to inhibit the mTOR signaling pathway. The RAP has been found to exert anti-proliferation, anti-inflammation, and anti-migration. Also, RAP is popular for its autophagy-inducing property. The release behavior of RAP from PEG-PLGA NPs was detected for 96 hrs and followed the non-fickian diffusion mechanism. Also, prepared NPs formulation showed desirable pharmacokinetic behavior indicating its importance and could be a better option for the treatment of cancer [24]. Near-infrared radiation is being used as a stimulus to modulate the drug release at the desired site, an excellent stimulus for PTT (photo-thermal therapy). PTT has gained big attention due to minimal hurt to the peripheral tissue. Also, due to metastasis, drug resistance tendency, and other factors, monotherapy for the treatment of cancer is not effective. So, the combination of chemotherapy with other treatment modalities is more effective. Hence the combination of PTT and chemotherapy displayed huge potential. Guo *et al.* developed PLGA-based NPs containing superparamagnetic iron oxide (SPIO), perfluorohexane, paclitaxel, and herceptin antibody attached to the surface of constructed drug delivery system. Perfluorohexane forms gas bubbles and assists in the imaging developed by sonography, herceptin targets HER2 receptor, and paclitaxel (well known for its anti-tumor effects). SPIO could convert the NIR into thermal energy. PLGA is used for its easy surface modification, biodegradability, and longer circulation time. Hence the design of NCs was designed in a manner so that they could target HER2-expressed breast cancer cells *i.e.* SKBR3 [25]. Nano carriers comprising PLGA and pH-responsive N-acetyl histidine modified D-α-tocopheryl polyethylene glycol succinate was developed, and used for the co-encapsulation of DOX and indocyanine green. DOX is a popular anti-tumor agent and indocyanine was incorporated as a photothermal agent. The protonation of N-acetyl histidine modified D-α-tocopheryl polyethylene glycol succinate was observed at acidic pH and assisted in the cellular uptake. Upon intravenous injection, these protonated nanocarriers were found to be deposited around TRAMP-C1 solid tumor-bearing mice. Extravasation and tumor permeation was found to be prominent through vessel/tumor tissue ablation. This may help in the mitigation of tumor growth [26]. Co-encapsulation of SPIO NPs and DOX in PLGA-based nanoparticles and modified with AS1411 aptamer (Apt) for the treatment of murine C26 colon carcinoma cells was proposed. This constructed nanoscale platform displayed 130 nm size with a narrow size range. These SPIO, DOX encapsulated, AS1411 aptamer modified, and nucleolin targeted NPs successfully demonstrated excellent and effective tumor inhibition, and demonstrated prolonged animal survival of C26 colon carcinoma xenografts models [27]. Unique core/shell-structure comprised of PLGA NPs, hematoporphyrin monomethyl ether (HMME), folate, and melanin nanoparticles were fabricated. The core was comprised of melanin NPs to obtain the photoacoustic image. HMME, a derivative of porphyrin sonosensitizer, has a high and selective uptake by cancer cells in comparison with other porphyrin-related agents, as well as the corresponding more pronounced cytotoxic effect when combined with ultrasonic irradiation. Especially, HMME has been extensively used in the diagnosis and treatment of various tumors, including bladder cancer, brain glioma, and lung cancer. These nanoplatforms were found to be effective to enhance the light stability of HMME and sonodynamic imaging of melanin NPs. A high *in-vitro* and *in-vivo* anti-tumor activity was found to be selective due to the generation of reactive oxygen species. So, based on tumor inhibition activity, it could be concluded that NPs could be useful to inhibit tumor growth *via* selective generation of ROS at the tumor site [28]. A hybrid nano-composite based on PLGA, DOX, and gold NPs (Au NPs) was prepared as core/shell NPs. Angiopep 2 was successfully conjugated to Au by sulfur bond. So, this type of prepared drug delivery system could be an example of combined therapy *i.e.* thermal and cancer therapy. Also, the release of DOX from the system exhibited dependency on the NIR. Besides the thermal ablation property, the X-ray imaging property was also observed. Furthermore, such a synthesized nano carrier platform could be an example of targeted, photothermal, X-ray imaging, and targeted delivery of DOX [29]. In another multipurpose PLGA-based NPs were designed to be useful for MRI imaging, thermal ablation of the tumor, and selective delivery of DOX. Mn^{+2} is allowed to coordinate with DOX and entrapped inside the NPs. The Mn^{+2} demonstrated its thermal property and was also found to be suitable for magnetic resonance imaging. Hence, imaging ability and more tumor inhibition in comparison with alone DOX, make such a system attractive for the therapy for the management of cancer [30].

Polymeric NCs: Polyplexes

Polyplexes belong to the non-viral vectors that are being used as a carrier to deliver the gene for therapeutic purposes. The formation of polyplexes may occur due to electrostatic interaction between negatively charged oligonucleotide/s and cationic carriers such as polypeptides, cationic lipids, polyethyleneimine (PEI), or dendrimer. Interestingly, due to high positive charge density, PEI attracts the attention of researchers to synthesize polyplex. The negatively charged phosphate groups present in DNA interact with cationic PEI. Thus, it forms polyplex and may exhibit amazing endosmotic inaction [31]. Especially, the polymer having high molecular weight encompasses highly efficient intracellular delivery and transfection with genes [32]. Faria *et al.* developed polyplex of different sizes (<373 nm) based on PEI and a p53 encoding plasmid DNA and also carrying methotrexate (MTX) (PEI-p53-MTX) and evaluated for their therapeutic activity against fibroblast and HeLa cells. These *in-vitro* studies related to the therapeutic efficacy of PEI-p53-MTX indicated folate receptor-mediated endocytosis, significant accumulation inside the cancerous cells, and optimum transfection. Hence, these types of tri-functional polyplex-based NCs could favor further research for translational medicine for the treatment fo terminal diseases like cancer [31]. Also, in a different set of the research experiment, the polyplexes were formed with the help of PEI (having low molecular weight) with a ketal-containing linker and further coated with hyaluronic acid (HA) to protect the positive charge from the physiological environment. HA prevents the adsorption of various negatively charged serum proteins after systemic administration of polyplexes. Moreover, the HA coating may assist to target CD44 receptor-mediated targeting of different CD44 positive cancerous tissue. Also, HA-coated polyplexes may demonstrate better *in-vitro* and *in-vivo* transfection efficiency. Hence the inconsistencies related to safety and efficiency could be overcome through this unique approach [32]. T-shaped polyplexes comprised of cationic lipids and oligonucleotides were developed for the co-delivery of siRNA (anti-tumor) and miRNA. To deliver the polyplexes to the T24 bladder cancerous cells through the epidermal growth factor receptor, maleimide-polyethylene glycol-GE11 (Mal-PEG-GE11) was introduced. GE11 is used as a targeting ligand. Thus, resultant polyplexes were found to have size ranges of 120-150 nm. Furthermore, cysteines were added to the end of maleimide-PEG-GE11. However, treatment of T24 cells and MDA-MB-231 having Mal-GE11 in a ratio equivalent to 0.8 moles diminished growth and migration, altering the cell cycle, and increasing the sensitivity towards DOX. Also, delivery of EG5 siRNA through cationic lipid-oligonucleotide to the Huh7 cells demonstrated antitumoral activity and diminished growth at the G2/M phase [33]. Another study demonstrated that PEG grafted and prostate-specific membrane antigens (PSMA) conjugated PEI (PEI-PEG-PSMA) based polyplexes were used to deliver DOX and shRNAs against Bcl-xL. The combination therapy of shRNA and DOX-induced intrinsic apoptosis in LNCap (PSMA overexpressed prostate cancer cell lines). PEI-PEG-PSMA polyplex exhibited 17 times less IC_{50} value in comparison with a mixture of shRNA and drug or lipofectamine and drug [34].

Polymeric NCs: Dendrimers (DDMs)

DDMs are precisely defined as monodispersed, homogeneous, radially symmetrical, and hyperbranched NCs. These hyperbranched dendrimers were first reported by Fritz Vogtle in 1978 and Donald Tomalia and co-workers in 1980. Also, George R. Newkome, independently reported these hyperbranched molecules in 1980 [35]. Hundreds of published scientific reports indicate the importance of DDMs for cancer therapy. In this section, we try to present a few recent works demonstrating the usefulness of DDMs as a carrier for antitumor drug delivery. Poly(amidoamine) DDMs functionalized with EpDT3 aptamer and grafted with PEG was used to deliver pMEG3 to castration-resistant prostate cancer (CRPC) cells. The EpDT3 aptamer is a ligand for EpCAM. EpCAM is a type of glycoprotein and is found to be overexpressed on the surface of malignant epithelial tumor cells. EpCAM is found to play a crucial role in the development of resistance of prostate cancer to chemotherapy and radiation *via* actuating the PI3/Akt/mTOR pathway. lncRNA *MEG3* arrests the proliferation of CRPC cells and upregulates the expression of p53 in CRPC cells. The p53 is a housekeeping gene and checks the excessive growth of cells. Both *in-vitro* and *in-vivo* studies suggested that functionalization with EpDT3 promoted endocytosis and exerted its effects against CRPC. Thus, proving its efficacy to deliver genes, efficiently [36]. Histidine-modified and transferrin-anchored PAMAM-based DDMs in the form of NCs, having disulfide bonds, were used to deliver the DOX to the acidic and redox-responsive microenvironment of tumors. The concentration of GSH, the most abundant thiol species, was found to be four times higher in tumor cells. Interestingly, histidine was found to have a positive charge at pH below 6, *i.e.*, pH of the endosome. Thus, promotes the "Proton Sponge" effect. Transferrin was used for the active targeting of tumor cells as shown in Fig. (**3**). The internalization in HepG2 has been achieved *via* clathrin-mediated endocytosis. Also, pH and redox-sensitive PAMAM DDMs reduced the cardiac toxicity associated with DOX. Thus, pH and redox-sensitive PAMAM DDM could be the right choice for the treatment of cancer and to reduce the side effects associated with cytotoxic agents [37]. Poly (propylene imine) (PPI) based and maltose tethered glycosylated DDM (PPI DDM) to deliver the cytarabine to the resistant tumor and evaluated for its therapeutic benefit against leukemia. Cytarabine, a nucleoside analog, displays its anti-cancer activity while it undergoes bio-transform into bio-active triphosphate form inside the cancerous cells. But, cytarabine suffers intracellular accumulation and limited therapeutic efficacy due to the resistance of the tumor to cytarabine. Moreover, the cationic charge present on the PPI DDM is found to be responsible for interacting with the negative charge present on the triphosphate forms. More apoptotic activity was observed rather than free cytarabine and its free bioactive triphosphate form when evaluated against 1301 cells (leukemia cells) [38]. PPI DDM engineered with dextran has been assessed for the site-specific delivery of DOX. Also, modification with dextran has shown less hemolytic activity and increased cytotoxicity in comparison with free drugs. *In-vitro*, cellular uptake studies confirmed the significantly high uptake in A549 cells. The macromolecular nature of dextran-modified PPI DDM selectively targeted the tumor mass due to leaky angiogenesis. Also, improved *in-vivo* pharmacokinetic profile and better tissue distribution suggested its role as a vector for selective delivery of cytotoxic agents [39].

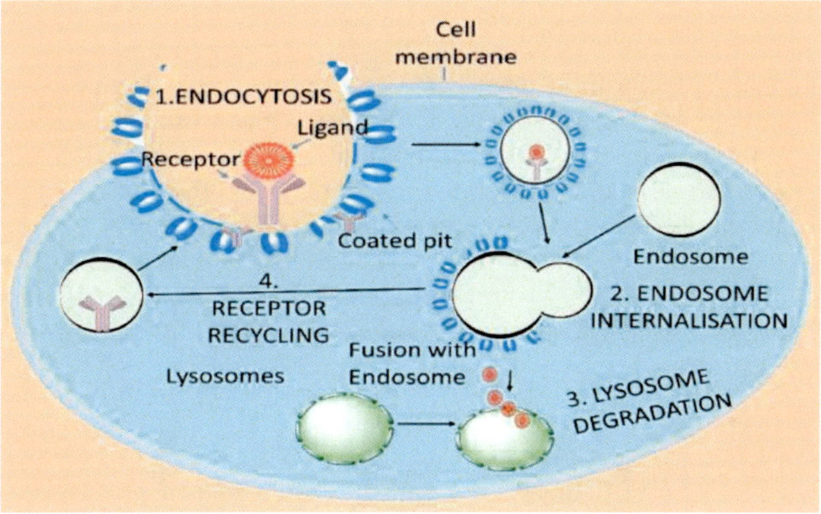

Fig. (3). The concept of active targeting and events during receptor-mediated endocytosis.

Polymeric NCs: Chitosan (CHN) NPs

CHN is found to be composed of units of D-glucosamine and N-acetyl-d-glucosamine. Additionally, it possesses two hydroxyl groups and one amino group in the repeating glycosidic unit. The presence of an amino group has been used for the functionalization and modification of CHN. CHN is bio-compatible, bio-degradable, and non-immunogenic. Chitosan NPs can encapsulate polypeptides, oligosaccharides, and various anti-cancer drugs. Moreover, CHN NPs can be administered *via* oral, ocular, intranasal, or intra-venous routes [40]. Trimethyl and Thiolated CHN NPs engineered with TAT peptides and hyaluronic acid (HA) was used for the co-delivery of signal transducer and activator of transcription-3 (STAT3) and (Small interfering Ribonucleic Acids (siRNA) to silent programmed cell death 1 (PD-L1). STAT3. STAT3 regulates proliferation, differentiation, inflammation, and angiogenesis of tumor cells. PD-L1 has an intrinsic property to modulate the phenotype of cancer stem cells, epithelial-mesenchymal transition, metastasis, and insensitivity to the treatment. The role of PD-L1 blockade in the management of cancers like Bladder, breast, lung, renal cell carcinoma, and melanoma has been acknowledged. Various studies suggested that the double inhibitions of STAT3 and PD-L1 with co-delivery of STAT3 and PD-L1 siRNA *via* CHN NPs modified with TAT and HA could be a novel strategy to suppress the growth of the tumor. Also, the CHN NPs could be used to deliver the oligonucleotide to treat cancer [41]. In another work, Nikhoo *et al.* used carboxymethyl dextran trimethyl (CMDT) CHN NPs to deliver the BV6 and STAT3 siRNA to mitigate the progress of cancerous cells. BV6 is a SMAC mimic and induces the death of various cancer cells. SMAC mimic molecules have an antagonist effect against IAP proteins (proteins that inhibits apoptosis). Co-delivery of BV6 and STAT3 siRNA in the form of encapsulation into CMDT CHN NPs synergistically induced *in-vitro* programmed cell death in melanoma, colorectal, and breast cancer cells. Moreover, proliferation, angiogenesis, migration, colony formation and anti-apoptotic effect were inhibited. Thus, indicating the usefulness and accelerated investigation in the animal models [42]. Also, transmembrane TNF (tumor necrosis factor) α-coated CHN NPs displayed significant and potential anti-proliferative activity against MCF-7 cells in comparison with MDA-MB-231 and HeLa cells. TNF-α is a cytokine and holds anti-proliferative action. Moreover, TNF-α coated CHN NPs exhibited dose-dependent cell death [43].

MICELLES (MCS)

MCs have a size of less than 100 nm and possess a special propensity to skirt clearance by the MPS (mononuclear phagocyte system). Polymeric MCs demonstrated high stability as compared to surfactant-based MCs, and were effective in solubilizing a considerable amount of hydrophobic drug into their core. Due to their hydrophobic core and hydrophilic shell, they revealed longer *in-vivo* circulation time and preferential accumulation in cancerous tissue [44]. Teniposide carrying self-assembled and monodisperse MCs, by using monomethoxy-poly (ethylene glycol)-poly (Ɛ-caprolactone-co-d, l-lactide) (MPEG-PCLA), was prepared without the addition of a surfactant or any additives. These MPEG-PCLA-based MCs exhibited the slow and uninterrupted *in-vitro* release of teniposide and displayed improved terminal life ($t_{1/2}$) and area under the curve of teniposide in comparison with commercially available formulation, *i.e.*, VM-26. Also, these self-assembled MCs displayed *in-vitro* enhanced cellular uptake by MCF-7 cells. Moreover, intravenous administration of MPEG-PCLA MCs mitigated the growth of breast cancer in contrast to VM-26 [45]. Cross-linked, polypeptide and reducible MCs based on the conjugation of lipoic acid and peptide 6 (cytosol and inter-cellular localization peptide) embedded were designed and prepared for the co-delivery of docetaxel (DTX) and siATG7 to arrest the growth of breast cancer. The encapsulation of siATG7 silenced the ATG7 gene, thus enhancing the apoptotic effect of DTX and exhibiting synergistic effects for the effective management of breast cancer. Interestingly, Cy5, an indicator, confirmed the accumulation in breast cancer and demonstrated the target efficiency of breast cancer. The combination of DTX and siATG7 into MCs displayed a minimum 1.84 fold higher *in-vivo* inhibition of breast tumor rather than DTX-loaded micelles [46]. In a comparative study, the tumor suppressor efficacy of MCs based on two different modified polymers, *i.e.*, monomethoxy poly(ethylene glycol)-poly(Ɛ-caprolactone) (mPEG-PCL) and monomethoxy poly(ethylene glycol)-poly(d, l-lactic acid) (mPEG-PLA) were prepared and assessed for their therapeutic efficacy. The micelles of both mPEG-PCL and mPEG-PLA, with the incorporation of DTX proved their usefulness for the therapy of cancer than free DTX. Although, DTX embedded mPEG-PCL showed remarkable and higher concentration in both plasma and cancerous tissue. Genotoxicity and acute toxicity studies confirmed that DTX-mPEG-PCL had minimal damage to DNA than MCs of mPEG-PLA [47].

MICELLES (MCS): NIOSOMES

Niosomes could be derived from amphiphilic and non-ionic surfactants. Both, hydrophobic and hydrophilic cargo could be encapsulated with significant and remarkable and offers coast-effective loading of therapeutics. They are non-immunogenic. Niosomes carrying essential oil extracted from *Trachyspermum copticum* have been evaluated by Trinh and co-workers and proved their therapeutic importance due to their cytotoxic activity against HepG2 (Hepatocellular carcinoma) cell lines [48]. Niosomes prepared using the reverse-phase evaporation method, comprised of span 60, cholesterol, and PEG 6600, encapsulating 76% gingerol, were evaluated against T47D breast cancer cell lines. Results showed that the presence of PEGylated niosomes showed a lower IC 50 value in comparison with gingerol [49].

NANOSTRUCTURED LIPID CARRIERS (NLCS)

NLCs could be prepared by mixing liquid lipids (LL) and solid lipids (SL). These NLCs may belong to the amorphous solid matrix. NLCs exist in the form of the amorphous solid matrix at room and body temperatures. The presence of LL in the NLCs has an important role. LL imparts certain specific features and defines the differences between NLCs and Solid lipid NPs (SLNPs). LL creates an amorphous lattice with significant deformities. Thus, higher loading of therapeutic agents can be loaded in comparison with SLNPs (crystalline state) [50, 51]. Interestingly, the NLCs displayed better localization and the accumulation of a significant amount of drug in the lung after modification with surfactants. The increased concentration of drug in the lungs was found due to inhibition of P-gp efflux. P-gp plays a crucial role in the development of drug-resistant cancer. Thus, NLCs may provide an important research area to search for effective NCs for the better management of lung cancer [52, 53].

INORGANIC NCS (INCS)

The delivery of gold, silver, and iron metal oxides to cancerous tissue, attracted enormous attention and is considered to be superior to organic nanocarriers in several aspects. Besides size, shape, and target accumulation-dependent properties, modified metallic NPs offer properties of photoluminescence, surface plasmon resonance, and super-paramagnetism, which can be utilized for imaging, sensing, photodynamic therapy, and photothermal therapy [54]. Furthermore, these features can be modified by adjustment in the composition, shape, and size of inorganic NCs, and also external stimuli like magnetic fields, temperature or light can be utilized to develop smart nanomaterials [55].

Inorganic NCs (INCs): Iron-Based NCs

The mechanism behind the synthesis of iron-based NCs formation relies on the reduction of Fe^{2+}/ Fe^{3+} ions into crystallized nanoparticles of Fe, which may be surrounded by stabilizing layer whose properties are characterized by Fe oxide composition compromising size between 5-380 nm and surface charge dependent upon nature of stabilizing layer. Iron-oxide NCs (Fe_2O_3 NCs) have shown significant anti-cancerous activities against several cancer cells like colon, cervical, neuroblastoma, leukemia, ovarian, and breast cancer cells due to their extraordinary superparamagnetic and magnetic healing characteristics, which permit their accumulation at a specific site [56]. Fabrication of nanosystems *via* conjugation of Fe_2O_3 NCs with drugs is known to have efficient magnetic thermotherapy characteristics, *in-vivo* magnetic resonance imaging, and magnetically targeted functionalization with combined delivery of drugs. Also, surface modification of Fe_2O_3 NCs *via* aptamers, transferrin, aptamers, folate, and hyaluronic acid further enhances the efficacy of the drug delivery system [57]. Also, iron oxide nanosystems are used to maintain Hb levels in cancer patients and are utilized as an important adjunct in erythropoietin agents [58]. Nanocomposites were prepared using magnetic Fe-oxide, coated with silica by hydrothermal method for the delivery of DOX for liver cancer therapy and MRI imaging to induce enhanced cell necrosis. It showed no considerable toxicities within HepG2 and Huh 7 liver cancer cell line [59]. In the current studies, iron oxide nanosystems are being utilized for magnetic hyperthermia for the treatment of cancer due to their lower systemic toxicity and enhanced targeting capability. Hedayatnasab et. al, synthesized Fe_2O_3 NCs coated with polycaprolactone polymer shell and stabilized *via* controlled micellar conformation and observed potent cytotoxicity on HepG2 by inducing hyperthermia achieved *via* polymer coated NCs in the presence of alternating magnetic field exposure [60]. A different study by Stankovic *et al.*, combined magnetic nanosystem-mediated hyperthermia with radionuclide therapy to suppress tumors. They utilized superparamagnetic Fe_2O_3 NCs to achieve proper hyperthermic conditions, and over the surface, ^{131}I-radiolabeled CC49 antibody was attached, which further provided localized retention and specificity. The results showed significant suppression of tumor growth without toxicity [61]. Theranostic systems are emerging tool for cancer treatment and control, which comprises the simple synergistic system of the therapeutic agent and diagnostic features into a single system that provides accurate diagnosis coupled with efficient therapy. Ribeiro *et al.* prepared magnetic hydroxyapatite NCs by doping hydroxyapatite nanoparticles chemically with 10% iron (III) ions which were further evaluated in terms of biological responses and *in-vitro* toxicity utilizing human triple-negative breast cancer cell lines. These iron (III) doped hydroxyapatite NCs not only generated highly contrast effects on MRI, and induction of mitochondrial and cell membrane damage but also proved to be extremely toxic against cancerous cells (A549 and HeLa cell lines) [62]. In recent studies, Rajkumar *et al.*, synthesized mPEG and folic acid-coated Fe_3O_4@Au NPs to deliver DOX to cancerous tissue that can be utilized for MR/CT imaging and photothermal therapy. The nanosystem loaded with DOX showed pH-dependent dependent drug release. Further, conjugation of NPs with targeting ligand indicated enhanced cellular uptake and cytotoxicity against Hela cell lines [63]. Further, Shu *et al.*, prepared sialic acid modified, polydopamine anchored and DOX embedded superparamagnetic iron oxide nanoconstruct with Fe^{3+} ion, novel theranostic NCs for MRI-guided chemo-photothermal therapy that has been utilized to target hepatic tumor sites effectively [64]. Khaniyabadi *et al.*, designed and created a promising bimodal nano-agent in which trastuzumab (targeting ligand) was conjugated with Porphyrin-superparamagnetic iron oxide (MRI contrasting agent) for MRI and photothermal therapy in HER2 positive breast cancer cells [65].

Inorganic NCs (INCs):Au - Based NCs

Au-based drug therapy for rheumatoid arthritis was recently approved by USFDA for rheumatoid arthritis, thus inferring its biocompatibility. Au- based nanosystems confer superiority in-terms of physiological stability, surface functionalization, and adjustable surface plasmon resonance phenomenon, thus promising candidates for various biological applications involving diagnostic, bioimaging, and therapeutics [66]. Au-NCs optical properties have been utilized to enhance localized temperature in the targeted site to induce a hyperthermic response. Au NCs target specifically deep tissue at targeted sites to avoid side effects and allow the NIR radiation absorption for efficient cancer therapy [67]. Magnetic nanohybrid system synthesized by Dharwesh *et al.*, where functionalization of magnetic nanoparticles with gold shown to exhibit radiosensitization effect which displayed enhanced cancerous cell death and shown intensive arrest of cancer cell division thus causing high cancer cell apoptosis [68]. In another study by Cheng *et al.*, an advanced microwave-triggered heat-shocked protein coupled with a gold nano cage as a "Photothermal therapy" (PTT) agent and further functionalized with the anti-HSP monoclonal antibody, showed improved targeting ability and significant anti-tumor activity [69]. In another recent study, Ahmed *et al.*, fabricated nano-gold by utilizing bio-enzyme (β galactosidase), which further showed significant cytotoxicity against liver (Hep 3B), cancer cells, breast (MCF-7), and human cervical (HeLa) [70]. Various gold nanosystems utilized for cancer targeting have been enlisted in Table **1**.

Table 1. Au nano-delivery vehicles for cancerous cell targeting.

S. No.	Type of Gold NCs	Morphology	Modifying/ Therapeutic Agent	Cell Lines/ Targets	Effects	References
1	Gold nanogels	-	DOX and 6-mercaptopurine	Human breast adenocarcinoma cell line	Enhanced apoptosis of tumor cells during subG0/G1 phase and efficient drug release	[70]
2	Gold nanospheres	13 nm- 50 nm spheres	CpG oligonucleotides	RAW - blue macrophage cell line	Efficient immuno-stimulatory activity	[71]
3	Gold nanoparticle - attached with CGKRK conjugate	17 – 80 nm	PD - L1 siRNA and STAT3siRNA	Melanoma	Increased expression levels of CD8 and CD4	[72]

(Table 1) cont.....

S. No.	Type of Gold NCs	Morphology	Modifying/ Therapeutic Agent	Cell Lines/ Targets	Effects	References
4	Gold-leaf	20 nm and 39 nm	Folate and cysteamine	HT 29 cancer cells	Detection and targeting of the overexpressed Folate Receptor	[73]
5	Gold nano-bipyramids	785 nm	Indocyanine Green (ICG), PLA	Murine melanoma B16-F10	Photothermal and Photodynamic activities	[74]
6	Nano-conjugate (AuNP-PEG-RGD)	40–45 nm	RGD peptide and glucose oxidase	MCF-7 cells	Reduced MDR development and re-activation of MDR breast cancer cells to be sensitive to drugs.	[75]
7	Gold nano-architectures	Fruit-like diameter of 112.1 ± 21.0 nm	Cisplatin prodrug-modified poly(L-Lysine)	SCC-25 and UPCI:SCC-154 cell lines	Ultrasmall-in-nano design for combined anti-tumor therapeutic applications, such as photodynamic therapy-PTT and chemo-radiotherapy	[76]
8	Au@XL-MSN-CpG/PEG	1–2 nm	XL-MSN	CT26 colon carcinoma cell line (ATCC)	Efficient drug delivery	[77]
9	Gold nanorod@ metal-organic frameworks	Length~ 53.8 ± 2.1 nm Width~ 25.2 ± 1.7 nm	Lipoic acid and PEG-(SH) polymer	4T1 cells	Damaging the cancer cells and tumor growth inhibition	[78]

Inorganic NCs (INCs): Gadolinium (Gd) Based NCs

Gadolinium (^{157}Gd)-based nanosystems, due to their higher X-ray attenuation coefficient, have been utilized for imaging modalities, *i.e.*, CT imaging, optical imaging, *etc.* Surface-decorated Gd hybrid-based nanocomposites loaded with anticancer drugs were proposed for imaging probes and as photosensitizers for cancer imaging [79, 80]. Similarly, Maghsoudinia *et al.* fabricated gadolinium-loaded nanodroplets *via* nano-emulsion methods and functionalized them with folic acid as a dual-modal magnetic resonance/ ultrasound contrasting agent which delivers complementary reports for therapeutic monitoring and early cancer diagnosis. The cytotoxicity studies on mouse hepatocellular carcinoma (Hepa1-6) and mouse fibroblast (L929) showed biocompatibility of nanodroplets and *in-vivo* studies showed no significant induction in organ toxicity and insignificant hemolytic activity in human RBCs [81]. Another strategy for the management of cancer demonstrated by Yun *et al.* showed that Gd-DTPA complexes (as a contrasting agent) (CA) decorated with chitosan/gelatin shell provided a unique technique to release CA by switching off (prohibited release)/switching on (burst release) fashion in response to different pH environment. The contrasting systems showed enhanced sensitivity and selectivity with varying environmental conditions [82]. Usman *et al.* developed a theranostic nanohybrid delivery system using Gadolinium- Zn/Al layered double hydroxide (LDH) as a nanocarrier. In this nanohybrid system, chlorogenic acid (CA) was used as a therapeutic agent and Gd as a diagnostic contrast agent. The surface of the nanohybrid system was coated with gold NPs for improved contrast of the MRI image. Cell viability studies against liver cancer cell lines (HepG2) displayed significant cytotoxicity [83]. The delivery systems of Gd-based nanocarrier in the MRI, cancer therapy, and NCT (Neutron capture therapy) are exemplified in Table **2**.

Table 2. Gd nano-delivery vehicles for cancerous cell targeting.

S. No.	Type of Gd NCs	Morphology	Modifying Agents	Cell Lines	Application	References
1	Gadolinium oxide (Gd_2O_3) NPs	8.3 ± 0.5 nm	PEG and L-Cys	RAW264.7 cells.	Cytocompatibility and specific cancer cells targetting and activation of dual-mode MR imaging of lung metastasis cancer model	[83]
2	Fe2O3/Gd2O3 nanopeanut theranostic system and platinum(IV) prodrug	Peanut shape with a length of ~150 nm and width of ~40 nm	Transferrin-labeled amino polyethylene glycol (Tf-PE--NH_2)	PC-3 cells	Diagnostic capability for tumor identification and MRI-guided dual-modal cancer therapy.	[84]
3	Dendrimer-DOX loaded Gd/Cobalt@Iron oxide- Nanoseed	25-30 nm	Glucosamine ligand	PC3 cells	Chemo-photothermal therapy of resectable breast and prostate cancers	[85]
4	Gd-labeled branched glycopolymer-PTX conjugate and Cathepsin B-responsive nano theranostics	95.17 nm	Glycylphenylalanylleucylglycine (Gly-Phe-Leu-Gly, GFLG) tetra-peptide linker wand fluorescent probe pheophorbide a (Ppa)	4T1 cell line	Biocompatibility, enhanced tumor targeting ability, and anti-tumor efficacy	[86]
5	Fe_3O_4 NPs coated with Gd ions	72 nm	Polycyclodextrin (PCD) layer	MCF 10A and 4T1	Improved cancer theranostics	[87]

MESOPOROUS SILICA-BASED NPS (MSNPS)

MSNs are another potential candidate whose nanostructures are utilized for tumor detection and cancer treatment due to their biocompatibility and ultra-high surface. Recently, NPs diagnostic system based on Si was approved by USFDA and named "Cornell dots" for clinical trial Phase I, which is considered a significant step toward clinical viability of MSNCs [88, 89]. Surface modifications and conjugation of MSNPs with targeting ligands such as mannose, folic acid, and transferrin are developed for tumor targeting and photodynamic therapy in cancer treatment.

MSNPs and Tumor Targeting

MSNPs are suitable to carry both soluble and insoluble anticancer drugs for ensuring a high level of targeting to the cancer cells. In a novel study by Mozafarinia *et al.*, for targeting breast cancer, MSNs with the amine-functionalized surface, Trastuzumab anchored, and DOX were evaluated. After further surface modification with fluorescein dye, fluorescence images were obtained, which revealed the significant attachment of surface-modified MSNs to the plasma membrane of breast cancer cell lines (HER2 overexpressed in SKBR3). Also, a quantum chemical study at the B3lyp/6–311++g** level of theory revealed the pH-dependent release of DOX [90].

MSNPs Based NPs in Photothermal Therapy (PTT)

MSNPs are utilized for photothermal-chemotherapy by Guo *et al.*, Encapsulation of DOX into mesoporous Si, which was allowed to grow on reduced graphene oxide through supramolecular interaction and further bound with A44F octadecanoic acid-modified PEG (C_{18}PEG) for improved stability, solubility and to release the loaded drug in the inter-cellular acidic surrounding [91]. Also, Hu et. al., developed modified mesoporous silica with bovine serum albumin (BSA)-mediated Cu sulfide nanosystem carrying DOX. In the developed targeted drug delivery nanosystem, BSA is used to respond to redox reaction *via* glutathione to ensure DOX release through MSN pore exposure, and CuS converts light energy into heat for PTT. Incubation with cancer cells showed a diminished survival rate of up to 49%, thus improving the efficiency to treat cancer [92]. Despite the wide range of reports available for the use of nanomaterials in PDT (Photodynamic therapy)/PTT, compliance achievement is still questionable.

MSNs in Gene Therapy

Gene therapy utilizes DNA, antisense oligonucleotide, and siRNA for alteration of gene expression responsible for cancer therapy. However, the major issue involves gene penetration at the intracellular site. MSNPs, due to their good high gene payload and biocompatibility, have attracted attention, recently. In a recent study, shape-controlled carboxy-functionalized magnetic-MSN was produced, and further surface modified with PEG-g-PLL that confers positive charge for absorption of TK plasmid and the integrated MRI-guided, hyperthermia-augmented suicide gene treatment for hepatocellular carcinoma simultaneously into a single system. It was observed that rod-like MSNs exhibited faster prodrug release behavior, higher loading capacity, and stronger magnetically improved gene delivery with magnetic hyperthermia properties [93]. In a different study, Sun *et al.*, prepared MSNPs, enclosing a core-shelled hierarchical mesoporous system of organ silicate system that exhibited effective downregulation of P-glycoprotein efflux to enhance cellular and nuclear localization of DOX and siRNA. The nanosystem has shown targeted, effective knockdown of a gene associated with drug resistance and enhanced sensitivity of drug-resisted cancer cells to DOX [94]. Some of the recently developed NCs have been mentioned in Table **3**.

Table 3. Mesoporous silica nanosystem/nano-delivery vehicles for cancerous cell targeting.

S. No.	Nanosystem	Morphology	Therapeutic agent	Cell lines	Application	References
1	Monodispersed Zn-containing MSNs	54.6 ± 8.9 nm	DOX	MDA-MB-231 and MCF-7 (ER+)	Biodegradable system releasing therapeutic ion inside cells.	[94]
2	H_2O_2-operated nano- valves on ferrocene modified MSNs and PNIPAM as shell	100–150 nm	DOX	Hela cells	Temperature and H_2O_2-dependent drug release	[95]
3	Large-pore mesoporous silica microspheres	3-20 nm	Pro-apoptotic NCL antagonist agent (N6L)	PANC-1 cells	Controlled drug release rate, 60% inhibition of cell survival	[96]
4	Prostate-specific membrane antigen (PSA)-targeted manganese oxide–MSNs	46–52 nm	-	LNCap and HSF cells	Prostate cancer detection, MRI	[97]

(Table 3) cont.....

S. No.	Nanosystem	Morphology	Therapeutic agent	Cell lines	Application	References
5	MSNs with folic acid	194 nm	Tetrandrine (Tet)	Hela and A549 cells	High cytotoxicity, cell-targeted uptake capacity	[98]

OTHER CARRIERS FOR PTT

Ag-based NCs

Silver NCs (AgNCs) are broadly used metallic drug delivery systems for anticancer drugs due to their unique physiochemical, biological, and optical characteristics. Recently novel chemotherapeutic drugs, extracted from the leaf of Zingiber officinale were formulated *via* spherical Ag NCs in the average size of 18.93 nm for pancreatic cancer cells. It showed very low cell viability, dose-dependent efficacy against human pancreatic cancer, and antioxidant potential [99, 100]. Recently, Ag nanosystems of different sizes (5 nm, 10 nm, 15 nm, and 30 nm) were prepared for the evaluation of proapoptotic and antiproliferative effects of capecitabine on human breast cancer cells (MCF-7) using XTT and Annexin V. It was observed that NCs with 10 nm size shown the least toxic effect and enhanced early and late apoptotic cells on MCF-7 cell lines [101]. The effect of paclitaxel bonded Ag nanosystem was studied in different cancerous cell lines, *i.e.*, Saos-2, MDA-MB-231, MCF-7, 4T1, and non-cancerous HUVEC cells. Enhanced sensitivity of Saos cells towards Ag nanosystems was monitored, while no toxicity was observed on non-cancerous HUVEC cells. The viability of cancer cells was seen to be reduced significantly [102]. Bioactive components of medicinal plant extracts have the potential to be utilized as anticancer agents as well as fabrication of metallic nanosystems to enhance the metal properties and minimize the side effect of cancer cells [103]. Table **4** enlists biologically obtained therapeutic agents that have been delivered *via* Ag NCs to exhibit cancerous activity.

Table 4. AgNCs synthesized utilizing green chemistry to exhibit anticancer.

S.No.	NCs	Biological material	Morphology	Cell lines	Application	References
1	Bioactive AgNCs	Phenolic bioactive component of *C. serrulata*	29.28nm, Spherical	A549	Potential cytotoxicity for cancerous cells	[103]

(Table 4) cont.....

S.No.	NCs	Biological material	Morphology	Cell lines	Application	References
2	Silver NCs	Aqueous Pollen extract of *Phoenix dactylifera* (Male Date Palm) flowers	27 nm	MCF-7	Apoptotic cell death *via* modulation of gene expression of the anti-apoptotic and pro-apoptotic proteins	[104]
3	Colloidal nanosilver	Aqueous extract of Eucalyptus Camaldulensis leaves	12-23 nm	Caco-2 cells	High cytotoxicity to cancerous cells	[105]
4	Silver nanoparticle	Extract *Punica granatum* fruit peel (polysaccharide (PSP001)	30 nm, spherical	A549	Caspase-mediated programmed cell death for lungs cancer	[106]
5	Silver nanosystem	Aqueous Aspergillus niger Cell-free filtrate	20-25nm, spherical	HT29	Caspase-3 activation and Apoptotic cell death *via* ROS generation for	[107]

Copper Sulfide-based NCs

Copper sulfide-based nanosystem serves as a versatile platform for photothermal therapy, gene therapy, and multimodal imaging therapy that includes MRI, photoacoustic, or fluorescence for cancer due to its low toxicity, biocompatibility, and low price [108, 109]. In the fields of photo-thermal and photodynamic therapies, Wang *et al.*, fabricated Graphene oxide-loaded CuS quantum dots, which showed effective cytotoxicity against MCF-7 cell line *via* NIR irradiation and highly effective for PTT for breast cancer [110]. In different studies, polydopamine was utilized as a bio-template for CuS nanocomposite synthesis with excellent photothermal properties and high stability. Also, the integration of MRI and PTT was exhibited to be a more effective treatment approach (Table **5**) [111].

Table 5. CuS-based nano-delivery vehicles for cancerous cell.

S. No.	NCs	Modifying agent	Morphology	Cell line	Application	References
1	Alanine capped CuS Quantum dots	Alanine	100 nm Flower/irregular/ Rod-Shaped,	HeLa cells	Anticancer therapy	[112]
2	CuS-NP	-	390-336nm Sphere, cube	MCF-7 cells	Phototherapy of Cancerous cells	[113]

(Table 5) cont.....

S. No.	NCs	Modifying agent	Morphology	Cell line	Application	References
3	CuS–MnS2(Manganese sulfide) nano-flowers	-	400 nm Nanoflower	A2780 cells	Multifunctional theranostic MRI/ Phototherapy	[114]
4	CuS nanodot	PEG	2-5nm, Rhombohedral	4 T1 cells	PA imaging and Fenton catalyst-based tumor therapy	[115]
5	CuS-DOX@ Graphene Quantum Dots (GQD)	Graphene Quantum Dots	121nm Spherical	MDA-MB-231 cells	Dual Photo and Chemotherapy	[116]
6	CuS-NP	Hepatitis B virus-like particles	33.2 nm Spherical	U87MG cells	Phototherapy	[117]

However, PDT therapy is only effective for early tumors and won't be sufficient in the case of recurrence. In that case, chemo-phototherapy is a recently developed potent treatment approach that utilizes photosensitizers for photothermal effects and anti-neoplastic agents for chemotherapy. Recently, a dual-purpose CuS nanosystem was developed that utilizes polymer peptide DSPE-PEG-LANNPs and docetaxel (therapeutic agent). The radiation with near-IR light absorption and enhanced uptake of nanosystem resulted in enhanced cytotoxic activity, photothermal ablation, efficient drug release, and potential ROS generation, thus resulting in the efficient delivery of dexamethasone and hyperthermia resulting in chemo-phototherapeutic therapy [112].

Table 6. List of nanotechnology-based approved medicine for the management of cancer.

S. No.	Name	Manufacturer	Type	Active Constituent(s)	Indication(s)	Approved (Year)	References
1	Abraxane	Celgene	Albumin Nanoparticles	Paclitaxel	Metastatic breast cancer (secondary), and Pancreatic cancer (Primary)	FDA (2005) EMA (2008)	[118, 119]
2	Patisiran	Alnylam Pharmaceuticals	Lipid nanoparticles	RNAi	Transthyretin mediated amyloidosis	FDA (2018)	[120]
3	NBTXR3 Hensify	Nanobiotix	Nanoparticles	Hafnium oxide	Soft Tissue Sarcoma	CE MARK (2019)	[121]
4	Doxil Caelyx	Janssen	PEGylated Liposomes	Doxorubicin	Breast, Ovarian, Prostate, Solid Tumour	FDA 1995 EMA 1996	[118]

(Table 6) cont.....

S. No.	Name	Manufacturer	Type	Active Constituent(s)	Indication(s)	Approved (Year)	References
5	VYXEOS	Jazz Pharmaceuticals	Liposomes	Cytabarine Doxorubicin	Acute myeloid leukemia	FDA (2017)	[122]
6	DaunoXo-me	Galen	PEGylated Liposomes	Daunorubicin	HIV-associated primary Kaposi sarcoma	FDA (1996)	[123]
7	MEPACT	Millennium	Non-PEGylated Liposomes	Mifamurtide	Osteosarcoma	EMA 2009	[124]
8	Marqibo	Spectrum	Non-PEGylated Liposomes	Vincristine	Philadelphia chromosome-negative acute lymphoblast-ic leukemia (tertiary)	FDA (2012)	[125]
9	Onivyde	Merimeck	PEGylated Liposomes	Irinotecan	Metastatic Pancreatic Cancer	FDA (2015)	[126]

CONCLUSION

Based on the information presented above in this chapter, it could be concluded that nanotechnology has a vast role in the diagnosis, treatment, and diminishing of the growth of cancers. Nanotechnology provides long-term release of therapeutic agents in a predetermined controlled way. Also, they can travel across the leaky tumor vasculature and penetrate the cancerous mass under physiological conditions. Thus, no healthy tissues are exposed to cytotoxic drugs.

CONSENT FOR PUBLICATION

Not applicable.

CONFLICT OF INTEREST

The authors declare no conflict of interest, financial or otherwise.

ACKNOWLEDGEMENTS

The authors are thankful to the National Institute of Pharmaceutical Education and Research, Raebareli (NIPER-R), Department of Pharmaceuticals, Ministry of Chemicals and Fertilizers, Govt. of India, for providing support in every possible form. Also, the communication number is **"220"** for the submission of this chapter provided by the NIPER-R.

REFERENCES

[1] Shi Y, van der Meel R, Chen X, Lammers T. The EPR effect and beyond: Strategies to improve tumor targeting and cancer nanomedicine treatment efficacy 2020; 10: 7921-4.

[2] Golombek SK, May JN, Theek B, *et al.* Tumor targeting via EPR: Strategies to enhance patient responses 2018; 130: 17-38.

[3] Rosenblum D, Joshi N, Tao W, Karp JM, Peer D. Progress and challenges towards targeted delivery of cancer therapeutics. Nature Communications. Nature Publishing Group 2018; Vol. 9: pp. 1-12. www.nature.com/naturecommunications Internet

[4] FDA. https://www.fda.gov/regulatory-information/search-fda-guidance documents/considering-whether-fda-regulated-product-involves-application-nanotechnology

[5] Yadav AK, Mishra P, Mishra AK, Mishra P, Jain S, Agrawal GP. Development and characterization of hyaluronic acid-anchored PLGA nanoparticulate carriers of DOX. Nanomedicine Nanotechnology. Biol Med 2007; 3(4): 246-57. https://pubmed.ncbi.nlm.nih.gov/18068091/ [Internet]. [PMID: 18068091]

[6] Yadav AK, Mishra P, Jain S, Mishra P, Mishra AK, Agrawal GP. Preparation and characterization of HA–PEG–PCL intelligent core–corona nanoparticles for delivery of doxorubicin. J Drug Target 2008; 16(6): 464-78. https://pubmed.ncbi.nlm.nih.gov/18604659/ [http://dx.doi.org/10.1080/10611860802095494] [PMID: 18604659]

[7] Yadav AK, Agarwal A, Rai G, *et al.* Development and characterization of hyaluronic acid decorated PLGA nanoparticles for delivery of 5-fluorouracil. Drug Deliv 2010; 17(8): 561-72. https://www.tandfonline.com/action/journalInformation?journalCode=idrd20 [http://dx.doi.org/10.3109/10717544.2010.500635] [PMID: 20738221]

[8] Ahuja R, Panwar N, Meena J, Singh M, Sarkar DP, Panda AK. Natural products and polymeric NCs for cancer treatment: a review. Environmental Chemistry Letters. Springer Science and Business Media Deutschland GmbH 2020; Vol. 18: pp. 2021-30. https://link.springer.com/article/10.1007/s10311-020-01056-z Internet

[9] Iqbal S, Rashid MH, Arbab AS, Khan M. Encapsulation of anticancer drugs (5-Fluorouracil and Paclitaxel) into polycaprolactone (PCL) nanofibers and in vivo testing for sustained and targeted therapy 2017; 13(4): 355-66.

[10] Guo F, Wu J, Wu W, *et al.* PEGylated self-assembled enzyme-responsive nanoparticles for effective targeted therapy against lung tumors. J Nanobiotechnology 2018; 16(1): 57. [http://dx.doi.org/10.1186/s12951-018-0384-8] [PMID: 30012166]

[11] Pang Z, Zhou J, Sun C. Ditelluride-bridged PEG-PCL copolymer as folic acid-targeted and redox-responsive nanoparticles for enhanced cancer therapy. Front Chem 2020; 8: 156. https://pubmed.ncbi.nlm.nih.gov/32181244/ [http://dx.doi.org/10.3389/fchem.2020.00156] [PMID: 32181244]

[12] Tang X, Lyu Y, Xie D, Li A, Liang Y, Zheng D. Therapeutic effect of sorafenib-loaded TPGS-b-PCL nanoparticles on liver cancer. J Biomed Nanotechnol 2018; 14(2): 396-403. https: //pubmed.ncbi.nlm.nih.gov/31352936/ [http://dx.doi.org/10.1166/jbn.2018.2529] [PMID: 31352936]

[13] Zhang L, Chen Z, Wang H, *et al.* Preparation and evaluation of PCL–PEG–PCL polymeric nanoparticles for doxorubicin delivery against breast cancer. RSC Advances 2016; 6(60): 54727-37. https://pubs.rsc.org/en/content/articlehtml/2016/ra/c6ra04687h [Internet]. [http://dx.doi.org/10.1039/C6RA04687H]

[14] Kong N, Deng M, Sun XN, Chen YD, Sui XB. Polydopamine-functionalized CA-(PCL-ran-PLA) nanoparticles for target delivery of docetaxel and chemo-photothermal therapy of breast cancer. Front Pharmacol 2018; 9(FEB): 125.www.frontiersin.org [http://dx.doi.org/10.3389/fphar.2018.00125] [PMID: 29527167]

[15] Hao X, Gai W, Wang L, *et al.* 5-Boronopicolinic acid-functionalized polymeric nanoparticles for targeting drug delivery and enhanced tumor therapy. Mater Sci Eng C 2021; 119: 111553. https://pubmed.ncbi.nlm.nih.gov/33321617/

[http://dx.doi.org/10.1016/j.msec.2020.111553] [PMID: 33321617]

[16] Xu C, Liu W, Hu Y, Li W, Di W. Bioinspired tumor-homing nanoplatform for co-delivery of paclitaxel and siRNA-E7 to HPV-related cervical malignancies for synergistic therapy 2020; 10(7): 3325-39.

[17] Mondal L, Mukherjee B, Das K, *et al.* CD-340 functionalized doxorubicin-loaded nanoparticle induces apoptosis and reduces tumor volume along with drug-related cardiotoxicity in mice. Int J Nanomedicine 2019; 14: 8073-94.
[http://dx.doi.org/10.2147/IJN.S220740] [PMID: 31632019]

[18] Zhong Y, Su T, Shi Q, Feng Y, Tao Z, Huang Q, *et al.* Co-administration of irgd enhances tumor-targeted delivery and anti-tumor effects of paclitaxel-loaded plga nanoparticles for colorectal cancer treatment 2019; 14: 8543-60.
[http://dx.doi.org/10.2147/IJN.S219820]

[19] Pisani A, Donno R, Gennari A, *et al.* Cxcl12-plga/pluronic nanoparticle internalization abrogates cxcr4-mediated cell migration. Nanomaterials (Basel) 2020; 10(11): 2304.www.mdpi.com/journal/nanomaterials
[http://dx.doi.org/10.3390/nano10112304] [PMID: 33233846]

[20] Asati S. Development and characterization of RGD embellished drug-conjugate loaded NPs for dual targeting of tumor cells. Asian J Pharm Pharmacol 2019; 5(5): 948-58.
[http://dx.doi.org/10.31024/ajpp.2019.5.5.14]

[21] Abolhasani A, Biria D, Abolhasani H, Zarrabi A, Komeili T. Investigation of the role of glucose decorated chitosan and PLGA nanoparticles as blocking agents to glucose transporters of tumor cells 2019; 14: 9535-46.
[http://dx.doi.org/10.2147/IJN.S228652]

[22] Ding J, Li D, Li Q, *et al.* Luteolin-loading of Her-2-poly (lactic-co-glycolic acid) nanoparticles and proliferative inhibition of gastric cancer cells *via* targeted regulation of forkhead box protein O1. J Cancer Res Ther 2020; 16(2): 263-8. https://pubmed.ncbi.nlm.nih.gov/32474511/
[http://dx.doi.org/10.4103/jcrt.JCRT_438_18] [PMID: 32474511]

[23] Oliveira ALC d. Maximizing the potency of oxaliplatin coated nanoparticles with folic acid for modulating tumor progression in colorectal cancer 2021; 120. https://pubmed.ncbi.nlm.nih.gov/33545840/

[24] Cheraga N, Sun NC, Huang XX, Ye Z, Xiao QR, Huang NP. Optimized rapamycin-loaded PEGylated PLGA nanoparticles: Preparation, characterization and pharmacokinetics study. J Drug Deliv Sci Technol 2021; 61: 102144.
[http://dx.doi.org/10.1016/j.jddst.2020.102144]

[25] Guo Y, Wang XY, Chen YL, *et al.* A light-controllable specific drug delivery nanoplatform for targeted bimodal imaging-guided photothermal/chemo synergistic cancer therapy. Acta Biomater 2018; 80: 308-26. https://pubmed.ncbi.nlm.nih.gov/30240955/
[http://dx.doi.org/10.1016/j.actbio.2018.09.024] [PMID: 30240955]

[26] Hung CC, Huang WC, Lin YW, *et al.* Active tumor permeation and uptake of surface charge-switchable theranostic nanoparticles for imaging-guided photothermal/chemo combinatorial therapy. Theranostics 2016; 6(3): 302-17.
[http://dx.doi.org/10.7150/thno.13686] [PMID: 26909107]

[27] Mosafer J, Abnous K, Tafaghodi M, Mokhtarzadeh A, Ramezani M. In vitro and in vivo evaluation of anti-nucleolin-targeted magnetic PLGA nanoparticles loaded with doxorubicin as a theranostic agent for enhanced targeted cancer imaging and therapy. Eur J Pharm Biopharm 2017; 113: 60-74. https://pubmed.ncbi.nlm.nih.gov/28012991/
[http://dx.doi.org/10.1016/j.ejpb.2016.12.009] [PMID: 28012991]

[28] Huang J, Liu F, Han X, *et al.* Nanosonosensitizers for highly efficient sonodynamic cancer theranostics 2018; 6178-94.

[http://dx.doi.org/10.7150/thno.29569]

[29] Hao Y, Zhang B, Zheng C, *et al.* 2015; The tumor-targeting core-shell structured DTX-loaded PLGA@Au nanoparticles for chemo-photothermal therapy and X-ray imaging 220: 545-55. https://pubmed.ncbi.nlm.nih.gov/26590021/

[30] Xi J, Da L, Yang C, *et al.* Mn^{2+}-coordinated PDA@DOX/PLGA nanoparticles as a smart theranostic agent for synergistic chemo-photothermal tumor therapy. Int J Nanomedicine 2017; 12: 3331-45. [http://dx.doi.org/10.2147/IJN.S132270] [PMID: 28479854]

[31] Faria R, Sousa Â, Neves AR, Queiroz JA, Costa D. Methotrexate-plasmid DNA polyplexes for cancer therapy: Characterization, cancer cell targeting ability and tuned in vitro transfection. J Mol Liq 2019; 292: 111391. [http://dx.doi.org/10.1016/j.molliq.2019.111391]

[32] He H, Bai Y, Wang J, *et al.* Reversibly cross-linked polyplexes enable cancer-targeted gene delivery *via* self-promoted DNA release and self-diminished toxicity. Biomacromolecules 2015; 16(4): 1390-400. https://pubs.acs.org/doi/abs/10.1021/acs.biomac.5b00180 [http://dx.doi.org/10.1021/acs.biomac.5b00180] [PMID: 25756930]

[33] Müller K, Klein PM, Heissig P, Roidl A, Wagner E. EGF receptor targeted lipo-oligocation polyplexes for antitumoral siRNA and miRNA delivery. Nanotechnology 2016; 27(46): 464001. https://iopscience.iop.org/article/10.1088/0957-4484/27/46/464001 [http://dx.doi.org/10.1088/0957-4484/27/46/464001] [PMID: 27736810]

[34] Kim E, Jung Y, Choi H, *et al.* Prostate cancer cell death produced by the co-delivery of Bcl-xL shRNA and doxorubicin using an aptamer-conjugated polyplex. Biomaterials 2010; 31(16): 4592-9. https://pubmed.ncbi.nlm.nih.gov/20206379/ [http://dx.doi.org/10.1016/j.biomaterials.2010.02.030] [PMID: 20206379]

[35] Abbasi E, Aval SF, Akbarzadeh A, Milani M, Nasrabadi HT, Joo SW, *et al.* Dendrimers: Synthesis, applications, and properties. Nanoscale Research Letters. Springer New York LLC 2014; Vol. 9: pp. 1-10.http://www.nanoscalereslett.com/content/9/1/247 Internet

[36] Tai Z, Ma J, Ding J, *et al.* Aptamer-functionalized dendrimer delivery of plasmid-encoding lncrna meg3 enhances gene therapy in castration-resistant prostate cancer. Int J Nanomedicine 2020; 15: 10305-20. [http://dx.doi.org/10.2147/IJN.S282107] [PMID: 33376323]

[37] Hu Q, Wang Y, Xu L, Chen D, Cheng L. Transferrin conjugated ph-and redox-responsive poly(Amidoamine) dendrimer conjugate as an efficient drug delivery carrier for cancer therapy. Int J Nanomedicine 2020; 15: 2751-64. [http://dx.doi.org/10.2147/IJN.S238536] [PMID: 32368053]

[38] Szulc A, Pulaski L, Appelhans D, Voit B, Klajnert-Maculewicz B. Sugar-modified poly(propylene imine) dendrimers as drug delivery agents for cytarabine to overcome drug resistance. Int J Pharm 2016; 513(1-2): 572-83. https://pubmed.ncbi.nlm.nih.gov/27667754/ [http://dx.doi.org/10.1016/j.ijpharm.2016.09.063] [PMID: 27667754]

[39] Agarwal A, Gupta U, Asthana A, Jain NK. Dextran conjugated dendritic nanoconstructs as potential vectors for anti-cancer agent. Biomaterials 2009; 30(21): 3588-96. https://pubmed.ncbi.nlm.nih.gov/19344947/ [http://dx.doi.org/10.1016/j.biomaterials.2009.03.016] [PMID: 19344947]

[40] Rostami E. Progresses in targeted drug delivery systems using chitosan nanoparticles in cancer therapy: A mini-review 2020; 101813. [http://dx.doi.org/10.1016/j.jddst.2020.101813]

[41] Bastaki S, Aravindhan S, Ahmadpour Saheb N, *et al.* Codelivery of STAT3 and PD-L1 siRNA by hyaluronate-TAT trimethyl/thiolated chitosan nanoparticles suppresses cancer progression in tumor-bearing mice. Life Sci 2021; 266: 118847. https://pubmed.ncbi.nlm.nih.gov/33309720/ [http://dx.doi.org/10.1016/j.lfs.2020.118847] [PMID: 33309720]

[42] Nikkhoo A, Rostami N, Farhadi S, *et al.* Codelivery of STAT3 siRNA and BV6 by carboxymethyl dextran trimethyl chitosan nanoparticles suppresses cancer cell progression. Int J Pharm 2020; 581: 119236.
[http://dx.doi.org/10.1016/j.ijpharm.2020.119236] [PMID: 32240809]

[43] Bhattacharyya S, Ghosh SS. Transmembrane TNFα-Expressed Macrophage Membrane-Coated Chitosan Nanoparticles as Cancer Therapeutics. ACS Omega 2020; 5(3): 1572-80.
[http://dx.doi.org/10.1021/acsomega.9b03531] [PMID: 32010831]

[44] Jones MC, Leroux JC. Polymeric micelles – a new generation of colloidal drug carriers. Eur J Pharm Biopharm 1999; 48(2): 101-11.
[http://dx.doi.org/10.1016/S0939-6411(99)00039-9] [PMID: 10469928]

[45] Chu B, Shi S, Li X, *et al.* Preparation and evaluation of teniposide-loaded polymeric micelles for breast cancer therapy. Int J Pharm 2016; 513(1-2): 118-29.
[http://dx.doi.org/10.1016/j.ijpharm.2016.09.005] [PMID: 27596115]

[46] Gong C, Hu C, Gu F, *et al.* Co-delivery of autophagy inhibitor ATG7 siRNA and docetaxel for breast cancer treatment. J Control Release 2017; 266: 272-86. https://pubmed.ncbi.nlm.nih.gov/28987884/
[http://dx.doi.org/10.1016/j.jconrel.2017.09.042] [PMID: 28987884]

[47] Tan L, Ma B, QianZhao , *et al.* Toxicity evaluation and anti-tumor study of docetaxel loaded mPEG-polyester micelles for breast cancer therapy. J Biomed Nanotechnol 2017; 13(4): 393-408.
[http://dx.doi.org/10.1166/jbn.2017.2356] [PMID: 29384603]

[48] Trinh LH, Takzare A, Ghafoor DD, *et al.* Trachyspermum copticum essential oil incorporated niosome for cancer treatment. J Drug Deliv Sci Technol 2019; 52: 818-24.
[http://dx.doi.org/10.1016/j.jddst.2019.05.046]

[49] Behroozeh A, Mazloumi Tabrizi M, Kazemi SM, *et al.* Evaluation the anti-cancer effect of PEGylated Nano-niosomal Gingerol, on breast cancer cell lines (T47D), *in-vitro*. Asian Pac J Cancer Prev 2018; 19(3): 645-8. https://pubmed.ncbi.nlm.nih.gov/29580033/ [Internet].
[PMID: 29580033]

[50] Müller RH, Radtke M, Wissing SA. Nanostructured lipid matrices for improved microencapsulation of drugs. Int J Pharm 2002; 242(1-2): 121-8. https://pubmed.ncbi.nlm.nih.gov/12176234/
[http://dx.doi.org/10.1016/S0378-5173(02)00180-1] [PMID: 12176234]

[51] Haider M, Abdin SM, Kamal L, Orive G. Nanostructured lipid carriers for delivery of chemotherapeutics: A review 2020; 12 https://pubmed.ncbi.nlm.nih.gov/32210127/

[52] Kaur P, Garg T, Rath G, Murthy RSR, Goyal AK. Development, optimization and evaluation of surfactant-based pulmonary nanolipid carrier system of paclitaxel for the management of drug resistance lung cancer using Box-Behnken design. Drug Deliv 2014; 23(6): 1-14.
[http://dx.doi.org/10.3109/10717544.2014.993486] [PMID: 25544602]

[53] Sharma N, Bhandari S, Deshmukh R, Yadav AK, Mishra N. Development and characterization of embelin-loaded nanolipid carriers for brain targeting. Artif Cells Nanomed Biotechnol 2017; 45(3): 409-13. https://www.tandfonline.com/action/journalInformation?journalCode=ianb20
[http://dx.doi.org/10.3109/21691401.2016.1160407] [PMID: 27012597]

[54] Yang K, Zhang S, He J, Nie Z. Polymers and inorganic nanoparticles: A winning combination towards assembled nanostructures for cancer imaging and therapy. Nano Today 2021; 36: 101046.
[http://dx.doi.org/10.1016/j.nantod.2020.101046]

[55] Henriksen-Lacey M, Carregal-Romero S, Liz-Marzán LM. Current challenges toward *in vivo* cellular validation of inorganic nanoparticles. Bioconjug Chem 2017; 28(1): 212-21.
[http://dx.doi.org/10.1021/acs.bioconjchem.6b00514] [PMID: 27709892]

[56] Barani M, Bilal M, Sabir F, Rahdar A, Kyzas GZ. 2021; Nanotechnology in ovarian cancer: Diagnosis and treatment 266: 118914.
[http://dx.doi.org/10.1016/j.lfs.2020.118914]

[57] Zhi D, Yang T, Yang J, Fu S, Zhang S. Targeting strategies for superparamagnetic iron oxide nanoparticles in cancer therapy. Acta Biomater 2020; 102: 13-34. [http://dx.doi.org/10.1016/j.actbio.2019.11.027] [PMID: 31759124]

[58] Mdlovu NV, Lin KS, Mavuso FA, Weng MT. Preparation, characterization, and in-vitro studies of doxorubicin-encapsulated silica coated iron oxide nanocomposites on liver cancer cells. J Taiwan Inst Chem Eng 2020; 117: 190-7. [Internet]. [http://dx.doi.org/10.1016/j.jtice.2020.11.037]

[59] Hedayatnasab Z, Dabbagh A, Abnisa F, Wan Daud WMA, Wan A. Polycaprolactone-coated superparamagnetic iron oxide nanoparticles for in vitro magnetic hyperthermia therapy of cancer. Eur Polym J 2020; 133: 109789. [Internet]. [http://dx.doi.org/10.1016/j.eurpolymj.2020.109789]

[60] Mihailovi J, Mirkovi M, Radovi M, *et al.* Aminosilanized fl ower-structured superparamagnetic iron oxide nanoparticles coupled to 131 I-labeled CC49 antibody for combined radionuclide and hyperthermia therapy of cancer 2020; 587.

[61] Ribeiro TP, Monteiro FJ, Laranjeira MS. Duality of iron (III) doped nano hydroxyapatite in triple negative breast cancer monitoring and as a drug-free therapeutic agent 2019; 0-1. [http://dx.doi.org/10.1016/j.ceramint.2020.03.231]

[62] Rajkumar S, Prabaharan M. Multi-functional core-shell Fe_3O_4@Au nanoparticles for cancer diagnosis and therapy. Colloids Surf B Biointerfaces 2019; 174: 252-9. [http://dx.doi.org/10.1016/j.colsurfb.2018.11.004] [PMID: 30469046]

[63] Shu G, Chen M, Song J, *et al.* Sialic acid-engineered mesoporous polydopamine nanoparticles loaded with SPIO and Fe^{3+} as a novel theranostic agent for T1/T2 dual-mode MRI-guided combined chemo-photothermal treatment of hepatic cancer. Bioact Mater 2021; 6(5): 1423-35. [http://dx.doi.org/10.1016/j.bioactmat.2020.10.020] [PMID: 33210034]

[64] Khaniabadi PM, Shahbazi-Gahrouei D, Aziz AA, *et al.* Trastuzumab conjugated porphyrin-superparamagnetic iron oxide nanoparticle: A potential PTT-MRI bimodal agent for herceptin positive breast cancer. Photodiagn Photodyn Ther 2020; 31: 101896. [http://dx.doi.org/10.1016/j.pdpdt.2020.101896] [PMID: 32585402]

[65] Li X, Kono K. Functional dendrimer-gold nanoparticle hybrids for biomedical applications. Polym Int 2018; 67(7): 840-52. [http://dx.doi.org/10.1002/pi.5583]

[66] Ali MRK, Farghali HAM, Wu Y, *et al.* Gold nanorod-assisted photothermal therapy decreases bleeding during breast cancer surgery in dogs and cats 2019. [http://dx.doi.org/10.3390/cancers11060851]

[67] Darwesh R, Aboushoushah SF, Almarhabi S, Aldahlawi AM, Elbialy NS. TurboBeads magnetic nanoparticles functionalized with gold as a promising nano-radiosensitizer for potential breast cancer radiotherapy: In vitro study. Inorg Chem Commun 2021; 123: 108348. [http://dx.doi.org/10.1016/j.inoche.2020.108348]

[68] Cheng Y, Bao D, Chen X, *et al.* Microwave-triggered/HSP-targeted gold nano-system for triple-negative breast cancer photothermal therapy 2021; 593: 120162. [http://dx.doi.org/10.1016/j.ijpharm.2020.120162]

[69] Ahmed F, Faisal SM, Ahmed A, Husain Q. Beta galactosidase mediated bio-enzymatically synthesized nano-gold with aggrandized cytotoxic potential against pathogenic bacteria and cancer cells. J Photochem Photobiol B Biol 2020; 29: 111923. [http://dx.doi.org/10.1016/j.jphotobiol.2020.111923]

[70] Ghorbani M, Hamishehkar H. A novel multi stimuli-responsive PEGylated hybrid gold/nanogels for co-delivery of doxorubicin and 6-mercaptopurine. Mater Sci Eng C 2018; 92: 599-611. [http://dx.doi.org/10.1016/j.msec.2018.07.019] [PMID: 30184786]

[71] Yue J, Pallares RM, Cole LE, *et al.* Smaller CpG-Conjugated Gold Nanoconstructs Achieve Higher Targeting Specificity of Immune Activation. ACS Appl Mater Interfaces 2018; 10(26): 21920-6. [http://dx.doi.org/10.1021/acsami.8b06633] [PMID: 29873227]

[72] Gulla SK, Kotcherlakota R, Nimushakavi S, *et al.* Au-CGKRK Nanoconjugates for Combating Cancer through T-Cell-Driven Therapeutic RNA Interference. ACS Omega 2018; 3(8): 8663-76. [http://dx.doi.org/10.1021/acsomega.8b01051] [PMID: 31458997]

[73] Soleymani J, Hasanzadeh M, Somi MH, Jouyban A. Differentiation and targeting of HT 29 cancer cells based on folate bioreceptor using cysteamine functionalized gold nano-leaf 2020; 107: 110320. [http://dx.doi.org/10.1016/j.msec.2019.110320]

[74] Campu A, Focsan M, Lerouge F, *et al.* ICG-loaded gold nano-bipyramids with NIR activatable dual PTT-PDT therapeutic potential in melanoma cells. Colloids Surf B Biointerfaces 2020; 194: 111213. [http://dx.doi.org/10.1016/j.colsurfb.2020.111213] [PMID: 32622254]

[75] Zhang J, Liang L, Li Z, *et al.* Multi-functionalized Nano-conjugate for combating multidrug resistant breast Cancer via starvation-assisted chemotherapy. Mater Sci Eng C 2020; 116(May): 111127. [http://dx.doi.org/10.1016/j.msec.2020.111127] [PMID: 32806277]

[76] Mapanao AK, Santi M, Voliani V. Combined chemo-photothermal treatment of three-dimensional head and neck squamous cell carcinomas by gold nano-architectures. J Colloid Interface Sci 2021; 582(Pt B): 1003-11. [http://dx.doi.org/10.1016/j.jcis.2020.08.059] [PMID: 32927167]

[77] Ong C, Cha BG, Kim J. Mesoporous silica nanoparticles doped with gold nanoparticles for combined cancer immunotherapy and photothermal therapy. ACS Appl Bio Mater 2019; 2(8): 3630-8. [http://dx.doi.org/10.1021/acsabm.9b00483] [PMID: 35030750]

[78] Zeng JY, Zhang MK, Peng MY, Gong D, Zhang XZ. Porphyrinic Metal-Organic Frameworks Coated Gold Nanorods as a Versatile Nanoplatform for Combined Photodynamic/Photothermal /Chemotherapy of Tumor. Adv Funct Mater 2018; 28(8): 1705451. [http://dx.doi.org/10.1002/adfm.201705451]

[79] Zeng Y, Li H, Li Z, *et al.* Engineered gadolinium-based nanomaterials as cancer imaging agents. Appl Mater Today 2020; 20: 100686. [http://dx.doi.org/10.1016/j.apmt.2020.100686]

[80] Maghsoudinia F, Tavakoli MB, Samani RK, *et al.* Folic acid-functionalized gadolinium-loaded phase transition nanodroplets for dual-modal ultrasound/magnetic resonance imaging of hepatocellular carcinoma. Talanta 2021; 228: 122245. https://linkinghub.elsevier.com /retrieve/pii /S0039914021001661 [http://dx.doi.org/10.1016/j.talanta.2021.122245] [PMID: 33773745]

[81] Yun SY, Seo D, Kim HJ, *et al.* Inorganic-Polymer Core-Shell with Gadolinium Complex for Switching on/off CT/MRI Dual Detection System of Cancer Cells upon pH Change. J Ind Eng Chem 2021; 95: 28-36. [http://dx.doi.org/10.1016/j.jiec.2020.12.002]

[82] Usman MS, Hussein MZ, Kura AU, Fakurazi S, Masarudin MJ, Ahmad Saad FF. Chlorogenic acid intercalated Gadolinium–Zinc/Aluminium layered double hydroxide and gold nanohybrid for MR imaging and drug delivery. Mater Chem Phys 2020; 240: 122232. [http://dx.doi.org/10.1016/j.matchemphys.2019.122232]

[83] Sui Y, Li Y, Li Y, Jin H, Zheng Y, Huang W, *et al.* Tumor-specific design of PEGylated gadolinium-based nanoscale particles: Facile synthesis, characterization, and improved magnetic resonance imaging of metastasis lung cancer 2020; 202: 111669. [http://dx.doi.org/10.1016/j.jphotobiol.2019.111669]

[84] Zhang G, Zhang L, Si Y, Li Q, Xiao J, Wang B, *et al.* Oxygen-enriched Fe3O4/Gd2O3 nanopeanuts for tumor-targeting MRI and ROS-triggered dual-modal cancer therapy through platinum (IV)

prodrugs delivery 2020; 388: 124269.
[http://dx.doi.org/10.1016/j.cej.2020.124269]

[85] Patharkar A, Raval N, Kalyane D, *et al.* Glucosamine-conjugated nanoseeds for chemo-magneto hyperthermia therapy of cancer. J Drug Deliv Sci Technol 2021; 61: 102295.
[http://dx.doi.org/10.1016/j.jddst.2020.102295]

[86] Cai H, Xiang Y, Zeng Y, Li Z, Zheng X, Luo Q, *et al.* Cathepsin B-responsive and gadolinium-labeled branched glycopolymer-PTX conjugate-derived nanotheranostics for cancer treatment. Acta Pharm Sin B 2021; 11(2): 544-559.
[PMID: 33643830]

[87] Mansouri H, Gholibegloo E, Mortezazadeh T, *et al.* A biocompatible theranostic nanoplatform based on magnetic gadolinium-chelated polycyclodextrin: *in vitro* and *in vivo* studies. Carbohydr Polym 2021; 254: 117262.
[http://dx.doi.org/10.1016/j.carbpol.2020.117262] [PMID: 33357850]

[88] Barkat A, Beg S, Panda SKS, Alharbi K, Rahman M, Ahmed FJ. Functionalized mesoporous silica nanoparticles in anticancer therapeutics. Semin Cancer Biol 2021; 69: 365-75.
[PMID: 31442571]

[89] Mozafarinia M, Karimi S, Farrokhnia M, Esfandiari J. *In vitro* breast cancer targeting using Trastuzumab-conjugated mesoporous silica nanoparticles: Towards the new strategy for decreasing size and high drug loading capacity for drug delivery purposes in MSN synthesis. Microporous Mesoporous Mater 2021; 316: 110950.
[http://dx.doi.org/10.1016/j.micromeso.2021.110950]

[90] Guo D, Yang H, Zhang Y, Chen L. Constructing mesoporous silica-grown reduced graphene oxide nanoparticles for photothermal-chemotherapy. Microporous Mesoporous Mater 2019; 288(May): 109608. [Internet].
[http://dx.doi.org/10.1016/j.micromeso.2019.109608]

[91] He R-X, Wang Q, Li B, Jia J, Lu W-J, Shuang S-M. HE RX. Construction of protein-mediated copper sulfide bonded mesoporous silica nanoparticles vector for chemo-photothermal synergistic therapy of cancer. Chin J Anal Chem 2020; 48(2): 197-205. [Internet].
[http://dx.doi.org/10.1016/S1872-2040(19)61216-8]

[92] Wang Z, Chang Z, Lu M, *et al.* Shape-controlled magnetic mesoporous silica nanoparticles for magnetically-mediated suicide gene therapy of hepatocellular carcinoma. Biomaterials 2018; 154: 147-57.
[http://dx.doi.org/10.1016/j.biomaterials.2017.10.047] [PMID: 29128843]

[93] Sun L, Wang D, Chen Y, *et al.* Core-shell hierarchical mesostructured silica nanoparticles for gene/chemo-synergetic stepwise therapy of multidrug-resistant cancer. Biomaterials 2017; 133: 219-28.
[http://dx.doi.org/10.1016/j.biomaterials.2017.04.028] [PMID: 28441616]

[94] Chen S, Greasley SL, Ong ZY, *et al.* Biodegradable zinc-containing mesoporous silica nanoparticles for cancer therapy. Mater Today Adv 2020; 6: 100066.
[http://dx.doi.org/10.1016/j.mtadv.2020.100066]

[95] Guo F, Li G, Zhou H, Ma S, Guo L, Liu X. Temperature and H_2O_2-operated nano-valves on mesoporous silica nanoparticles for controlled drug release and kinetics. Colloids Surf B Biointerfaces 2020; 187: 110643.
[http://dx.doi.org/10.1016/j.colsurfb.2019.110643] [PMID: 31744758]

[96] Belbekhouche S, Poostforooshan J, Shaban M, *et al.* Fabrication of large pore mesoporous silica microspheres by salt-assisted spray-drying method for enhanced antibacterial activity and pancreatic cancer treatment. Int J Pharm 2020; 590: 119930.
[http://dx.doi.org/10.1016/j.ijpharm.2020.119930] [PMID: 33010394]

[97] Du D, Fu HJ, Ren W, Li X-L, Guo L-H. PSA targeted dual-modality manganese oxide–mesoporous

silica nanoparticles for prostate cancer imaging. Biomed Pharmacother 2020; 121: 109614. [http://dx.doi.org/10.1016/j.biopha.2019.109614]

[98] Li Y, Wang S, Song FX, *et al.* A pH-sensitive drug delivery system based on folic acid-targeted HBP-modified mesoporous silica nanoparticles for cancer therapy. Colloids Surf A Physicochem Eng Asp 2020; 590(January): 124470. [Internet]. [http://dx.doi.org/10.1016/j.colsurfa.2020.124470]

[99] Wang Y, Chinnathambi A, Nasif O, Alharbi SA. Green synthesis and chemical characterization of a novel anti-human pancreatic cancer supplement by silver nanoparticles containing Zingiber officinale leaf aqueous extract. Arab J Chem 2021; 14(4): 103081. https://linkinghub.elsevier.com/retrieve/pii/S1878535221000964 [Internet]. [http://dx.doi.org/10.1016/j.arabjc.2021.103081]

[100] Hepokur C, Kariper İA, Mısır S, *et al.* Silver nanoparticle/capecitabine for breast cancer cell treatment 2019; 61.

[101] Danışman-Kalındemirtaş F, Karİper İA, Hepokur C, Erdem-Kuruca S. Selective cytotoxicity of paclitaxel bonded silver nanoparticle on different cancer cells. J Drug Deliv Sci Technol 2021; 61: 102265. [http://dx.doi.org/10.1016/j.jddst.2020.102265]

[102] Vaid P, Raizada P, Saini AK, Saini R V. Biogenic silver, gold and copper nanoparticles - A sustainable green chemistry approach for cancer therapy 2020; 16: 100247. [http://dx.doi.org/10.1016/j.scp.2020.100247]

[103] Palaniappan P, Sathishkumar G, Sankar R. Fabrication of nano-silver particles using Cymodocea serrulata and its cytotoxicity effect against human lung cancer A549 cells line. Spectrochim Acta A Mol Biomol Spectrosc 2015; 138: 885-90. [http://dx.doi.org/10.1016/j.saa.2014.10.072] [PMID: 25467657]

[104] Banu H, Renuka N, Faheem SM, *et al.* Gold and Silver Nanoparticles Biomimetically Synthesized Using Date Palm Pollen Extract-Induce Apoptosis and Regulate p53 and Bcl-2 Expression in Human Breast Adenocarcinoma Cells. Biol Trace Elem Res 2018; 186(1): 122-34. [http://dx.doi.org/10.1007/s12011-018-1287-0] [PMID: 29552710]

[105] Zein R, Alghoraibi I, Soukkarieh C, Salman A, Alahmad A. In-vitro anticancer activity against Caco-2 cell line of colloidal nano silver synthesized using aqueous extract of *Eucalyptus Camaldulensis* leaves. Heliyon 2020; 6(8): e04594. [http://dx.doi.org/10.1016/j.heliyon.2020.e04594] [PMID: 32885066]

[106] Padinjarathil H, Joseph MM, Unnikrishnan BS, *et al.* Galactomannan endowed biogenic silver nanoparticles exposed enhanced cancer cytotoxicity with excellent biocompatibility. Int J Biol Macromol 2018; 118(Pt A): 1174-82. [http://dx.doi.org/10.1016/j.ijbiomac.2018.06.194] [PMID: 30001604]

[107] Chengzheng W, Jiazhi W, Shuangjiang C, *et al.* Biogenic Synthesis, Characterization and Evaluation of Silver Nanoparticles from Aspergillus niger JX556221 Against Human Colon Cancer Cell Line HT-29. J Nanosci Nanotechnol 2018; 18(5): 3673-81. [PMID: 29442882]

[108] Nikam AN, Pandey A, Fernandes G, *et al.* Copper sulphide based heterogeneous nanoplatforms for multimodal therapy and imaging of cancer: Recent advances and toxicological perspectives. Coord Chem Rev 2020; 419: 213356. [Internet]. [http://dx.doi.org/10.1016/j.ccr.2020.213356]

[109] Wang L, Yan J. Superficial synthesis of photoactive copper sulfide quantum dots loaded nano-graphene oxide sheets combined with near infrared (NIR) laser for enhanced photothermal therapy on breast cancer in nursing care management. J Photochem Photobiol B 2019; 192: 68-73. [http://dx.doi.org/10.1016/j.jphotobiol.2018.12.024]

[110] Xiong Y, Sun F, Zhang Y, *et al.* Polydopamine-mediated bio-inspired synthesis of copper sulfide

nanoparticles for T1-weighted magnetic resonance imaging guided photothermal cancer therapy. Colloids Surf B Biointerfaces 2019; 173: 607-15.
[http://dx.doi.org/10.1016/j.colsurfb.2018.10.023]

[111] Poudel K, Thapa RK, Gautam M, *et al.* Multifaceted NIR-responsive polymer-peptide-enveloped drug-loaded copper sulfide nanoplatform for chemo-phototherapy against highly tumorigenic prostate cancer. Nanomedicine 2019; 21: 102042.

[112] Mofokeng TP, Moloto MJ, Shumbula PM, Tetyana P. Synthesis, characterization and cytotoxicity of alanine-capped CuS nanoparticles using human cervical carcinoma HeLa cells. Anal Biochem 2019; 580: 36-41.
[http://dx.doi.org/10.1016/j.ab.2019.06.008] [PMID: 31185196]

[113] Wang L, Ma X, Cai K, Li X. Morphological effect of copper sulfide nanoparticles on their near infrared laser activated photothermal and photodynamic performance. Mater Res Express 2019; 6(10): 105406.
[http://dx.doi.org/10.1088/2053-1591/ab3a01]

[114] Chen W, Wang X, Zhao B, *et al.* CuS–MnS2 nano-flowers for magnetic resonance imaging guided photothermal/photodynamic therapy of ovarian cancer through necroptosis 2019; 12983-9.

[115] Hu R, Fang Y, Huo M, *et al.* Ultrasmall Cu2-xS nanodots as photothermal-enhanced Fenton nanocatalysts for synergistic tumor therapy at NIR-II biowindow. Biomaterials 2019; 206: 101-14.
[http://dx.doi.org/10.1016/j.biomaterials.2019.03.014]

[116] Zheng S, Jin Z, Han C, *et al.* Graphene quantum dots-decorated hollow copper sulfide nanoparticles for controlled intracellular drug release and enhanced photothermal-chemotherapy. J Mater Sci 2020; 55(3): 1184-97.
[http://dx.doi.org/10.1007/s10853-019-04062-x]

[117] Jia Q, Li D, Zhang Q, *et al.* Biomineralization synthesis of HBc-CuS nanoparticles for near-infrared light-guided photothermal therapy. J Mater Sci 2019; 54(20): 13255-64. [Internet].
[http://dx.doi.org/10.1007/s10853-019-03613-6]

[118] Anselmo AC, Mitragotri S. Nanoparticles in the clinic: An update. Bioeng Transl Med 2019; 4(3): e10143.
[http://dx.doi.org/10.1002/btm2.10143] [PMID: 31572799]

[119] FDA approves first treatment for certain types of poor-prognosis acute myeloid leukemia fda.gov/news-events/press-announcements/fda-approves-first-treatment-certain-types-poor -prognosi--acute-myeloid-leukemia

[120] Wood H. FDA approves patisiran to treat hereditary transthyretin amyloidosis. Nat Rev Neurol 2018; 14(10): 570.
[http://dx.doi.org/10.1038/s41582-018-0065-0] [PMID: 30158559]

[121] Nanobiotix Announces First Ever Radioenhancer to Receive European Market Approval. https://www.globenewswire.com/news-release/2019/04/04/1797273/0/en/Nanobiotix Announces-First-Ever-Radioenhancer-to-Receive-European-Market-Approval.html

[122] European medicine agency. Vyxeos liposomal (previously known as Vyxeos) ema.europa.eu/en/medicines/human/EPAR/vyxeos-liposomal

[123] Sevastre AS, Horescu C, Carina Baloi S, *et al.* Benefits of nanomedicine for therapeutic intervention in malignant diseases. Coatings 2019; 9(10): 628.
[http://dx.doi.org/10.3390/coatings9100628]

[124] Mepact. https://www.ema.europa.eu/en/medicines/human/EPAR/mepact

[125] Anselmo AC, Mitragotri S. Nanoparticles in the clinic. Bioeng Transl Med 2016; 1(1): 10-29. [http://dx.doi.org/10.1002/btm2.10003] [PMID: 29313004]

[126] Aetna™. Irinotecan Liposome Injection (Onivyde) aetna.com/cpb/medical/data/900_999/0902.html

CHAPTER 3

Potential Approaches for Delivery of Surface Decorated Nano-carriers in the Management of Carcinoma

B. Patil[1], A. Tiwari[1], S.P. Pandey[1], T. Shukla[2,*] and **N. Upmanyu[3,4]**

[1] *Department of Pharmacy, Shri G.S Institute of Technology and Science, Indore, India*

[2] *Institute of Pharmaceutical Sciences, SAGE University, Indore, India*

[3] *School of Pharmacy and Research, Peoples University, Bhopal, India*

[4] *Sagar Institute of Research & Technology-Pharmacy, Bhopal, India*

Abstract: Cancer is one of the leading causes of death worldwide, affecting the entire world irrespective of demographic and economic variations. In the last few decades, development concerning cancer diagnosis and treatment has witnessed significant advancement but still lags far behind in terms of targeted delivery to the targeted site without much adverse effect. Changes in the structure and pathophysiology of cancer tissue, like leaky vasculature, pH, temperature, over-expression of certain receptors, *etc*., are being utilized for the development of different approaches of targeted drug delivery to such tissues avoiding the adverse effects associated with cancer chemotherapy. The utilization of enhanced permeability retention (EPR) and surface modification of the nano-sized formulation with different ligands, such as proteins, aptamers, antibodies, *etc*., are some common ways used for the above.

The current chapter includes the different nano-carriers used for targeted drug delivery of medicaments to the affected site along with their surface modification which has shown their significance in the management of cancer.

Keywords: Cancer management, Ligands, Nano-carriers, Surface modification.

INTRODUCTION

Cancer

Cancer is accounted to be the second leading cause of death worldwide and may be defined by uncontrolled cell multiplication and the absence of cell death, which

* **Corresponding author T. Shukla:** Institute of Pharmaceutical Sciences, SAGE University, Indore, India; Tel: 9098288338; E-mail: drtriptishukla17@gmail.com

Neeraj Mishra, Ashish Garg and Neeraj Upmanyu (Eds.)

results in an abnormal cell mass, or tumor except for blood cancer [1]. When tumor cells are contained, they are called benign; however, if they spread to the surrounding tissues, they are called malignant [2]. Both rich and developing countries experience huge increases in morbidity and death as a result of it. Significant developments in fundamental cancer biology have been accomplished in recent decades, enabling tremendous advancements in cancer diagnosis and treatment. But, surprisingly, clinical translation of these breakthroughs lags far behind, and successful delivery of innovative therapeutic medicines to the target site while avoiding unwanted effects from systemic treatment is a key challenge [3 - 4].

There are instances of normal cells transforming to a neoplastic state from their normal state through six steps [5]:

- Proliferative signalling sustaining
- Bypassing growth suppressors
- Invasion and metastasis enabling
- Replicative immortality activation
- Angiogenesis induction
- Cell death resistance

Lung/bronchus cancer, colorectal cancer, breast cancer, and prostate cancer accounted for 56 percent of all cancer cases and 53 percent of all cancer deaths [1]. Approximately half of the cancer patients will progress to metastatic illness. Over 70% of cancer patients experience symptoms as a result of their primary or metastatic disease [6]. Prognosis is influenced by the total metastatic burden as well as the number and location of disease-affected locations [1].

Conventional cancer chemotherapy involves the blind delivery of the toxic anticancer agent to tumors and healthy tissues, resulting in unfavorable systemic side effects. Delivering anticancer medications selectively to places where cancer is likely to occur is one of the strategies to address these issues [7]. Several strategies can be utilized for the targeted delivery of anticancer agents. Exploiting the structural and pathophysiological defects of cancer tissue, particularly the cancer vasculature, and employing the enhanced permeability and retention (EPR) effect is one of the most successful approaches in the passive delivery of the drug [8 - 11].

The preferential delivery of nanocarrier-based anticancer medications to the cancer site with pinpointed accuracy has become a reality by utilizing this specific trait (EPR effect) of solid tumors. Most nanosized drug delivery technologies, such as nanoparticles and liposomal or micellar medicines, will benefit from the EPR effect, which will give selective cancer-targeting properties. These nanocarrier-based medications will stay in the tumor tissues for a long time after being given to the tumor [11 - 14].

In continuation of the above, different strategies exist for targeting the medicament viz active targeting, passive targeting, dual targeting, combination targeting, *etc*. Generally, the phenomenon of active and passive targeting occurs simultaneously [15]. It has also been noted that the surface functionalization of nano-carriers using proteins, aptamers, antibodies, *etc*., shows better interaction with the surface receptor, present on cell or tissue surface, which leads to better and more effective targeting [16]. The current chapter aims to summarize the different nanocarriers and the method of their surface modification which has shown their significance in the management of different ailments, specifically cancer.

Nanocarriers

Different forms of nanomaterial nanocarriers (NCs) are employed in pharmaceutical technology to carry medications throughout the bodily tissue. Although NCs have been certified in sizes scale from 1 to 1000 nm, nanoparticles have been approved in sizes varying from 1 to 100 nm [17]. A higher surface volume ratio, increased ability to penetrate the tissue, biological mobility, increased stability, and better control of the release of drug release make the NMs more useful for the delivery of drugs and in the development of suitable imaging in the pharmaceutical and medical field [18]. The concept behind the use of nanocarriers for its utilization for targeting purposes is highly influenced by the concept of the magic bullet proposed by Paul Ehrlich [19].

Since the emergence of nanocarriers, the use of these carriers has fascinated the research community for the management of various ailments, especially cancer, where targeting medicament to a specific site is believed to be most important, which increases the safety and efficacy by reducing the instances of toxicity associated with drugs and it is also a well-noted fact that recent advances in nanotechnology have a significant impact on treatment [20, 21]. For advanced drug delivery systems, a variety of nanocarriers have been developed as mentioned in Fig. (**1**) over the years, including lipid-based nanocarriers (liposome, noisome, lipoplexes, nanoemulsion, transferosomes, *etc*.), polymer-based nanocarriers (polymeric nanoparticles, polymeric micelles, polyplexes, *etc*.) and inorganic material based systems such as metallic nanoparticles (gold, silver, iron, silica, *etc.*) carbon-based materials such as nanotubes, graphene, *etc*. Some others, like dendrimers, virus-like materials, and hydrogels, have also been developed over time [22 - 25].

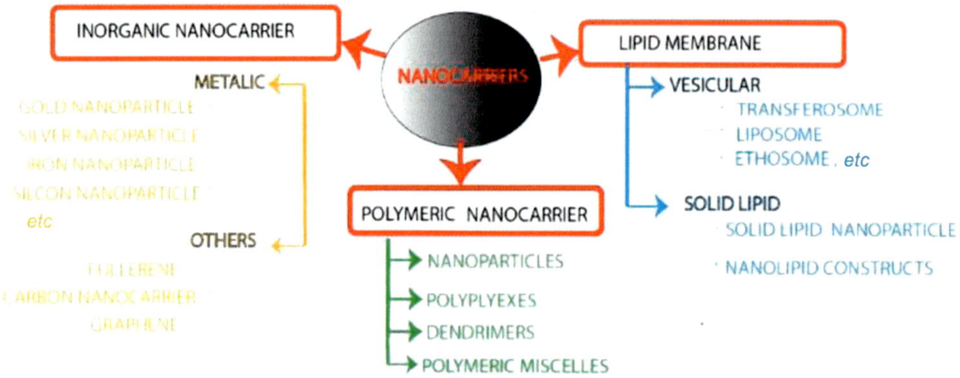

Fig. (1). Different Nanocarriers used for drug delivery and diagnostic materials.

Nanocarriers have proven their significance in the effective delivery of drug and diagnostic agent, but still, it suffers from certain problems, too, like poor drug loading, burst release in some cases, difficulty in designing an efficient system, *etc*. Targeting these carriers to a specific site is also very challenging and crucial for the development of an effective delivery system [26]. So, currently, the research related to nanocarrier (NCs) based delivery systems are aimed at preserving the chemical reactivity and targeting of NCs. It is necessary to create smart NCs that can deliver an active chemical to a specific location, evade biological protection systems, such as opsonization and RES clearance, and communicate and sense changes in their environment. Surface modification and functionalization may be suitably used for the site-specific delivery of medicament and attenuates the chance of uptake and related toxicity issues [16]. It might also affect their properties, including biocompatibility, stimuli-responsiveness, circulation time, targeting, intracellular penetration, therapeutic potential, *etc*. [27].

Several kinds of literature have reported several methods for surface modification and functionalization, which can successfully be used in the delivery of medicament and diagnostics during the management of cancer [27]. Several different molecules, like oligosaccharides, proteins, peptides, antibodies, aptamers, and many more, can be used for the surface modification of nanocarriers [16].

IMPORTANCE OF NANO-CARRIERS IN THE MANAGEMENT OF CANCER

To stop cancer cells from growing and multiplying, different diagnostic and therapeutic systems have been created. The most crucial aspect of cancer treatment is early and accurate diagnosis, which is generally accomplished by computed tomography (CT), magnetic resonance imaging (MRI), positron emission tomography (PET), ultrasound, and other methods [28]. Diagnostic nanoparticles are designed to aid in the visualization of pathologies and to better understand the important (patho-) physiological principles underlying various diseases and treatments [29]. It is well noted that nanosized drug delivery systems may get accumulated in the cancerous tissue in two major ways, *i.e.*, passive targeting and active targeting. As mentioned earlier, the permeability of vasculatures of cancerous tissue gets altered, leading to EPR, which is thought to be a major mechanism in case of targeted accumulation (passive targeting) of nano-particles or nano-carriers in vicinity of tumour tissue as shown in Fig. (**2**) [30, 31].

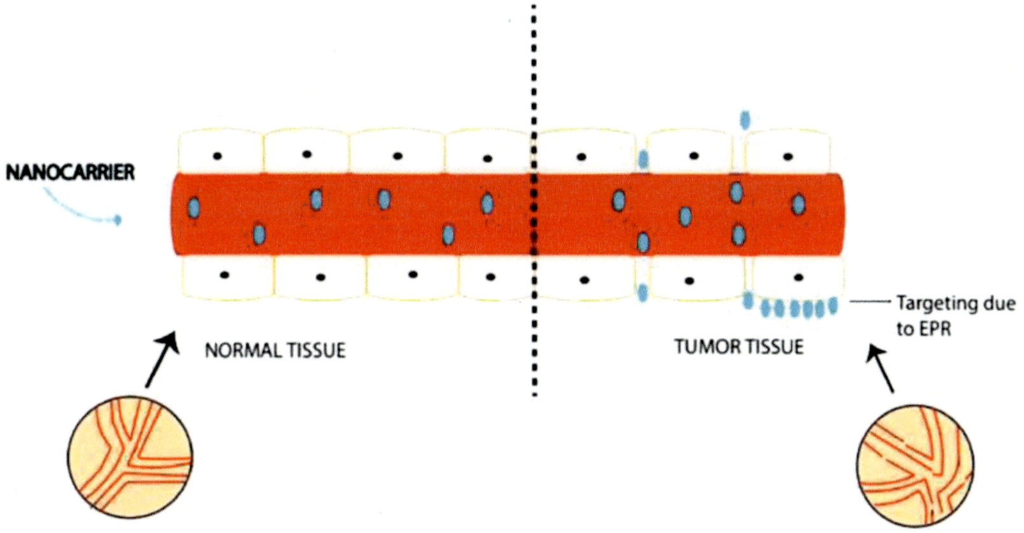

Fig. (2). Effect of EPR in targeting.

Modification and functionalization of the surface of nano-materials with different ligands which possess high affinity for the receptors, like transferrin, folate, nicotine, *etc.*, or molecules overexpressed on the tumor tissue, is the key component in the case of active targeting [32].

As mentioned earlier, targeting anticancer medicines to the specific side by using different surface modified/functionalized nano-carriers increases not only the circulation time but also decreases the chance of toxicity.

DIFFERENT APPROACHES TO SURFACE MODIFICATION OF NANOPARTICLES WITH THEIR SIGNIFICANCE IN THE MANAGEMENT OF CANCER

Several approaches are being used for the surface modification/functionalization of different nano-materials imparting better stability, safety, and efficacy. Some common approaches utilized for the purpose are as follows:

Surface Modification With Polyethylene Glycol(PEG)

Rapid clearance of medicaments from the systemic circulation and toxicity associated with cytotoxic drugs has always been a major issue in the case of cancer management. Loading such drugs in surface-modified nanocarriers with PEG may be a better choice to make them available in circulation for a longer time and so helpful in getting accumulated in the tumor tissue [33]. Pegylation is believed to be one of the most prominent approaches to avoid the chance of RES uptake along with improved antigenicity and anti-immunogenicity property.

In 1977, Davis and Abuchowski revealed that the covalent attachment of PEG to bovine liver catalase had increased the circulation time without any instance of immunogenicity [34]. Some different impacts of PEG attachments have been depicted in Fig. (**3**).

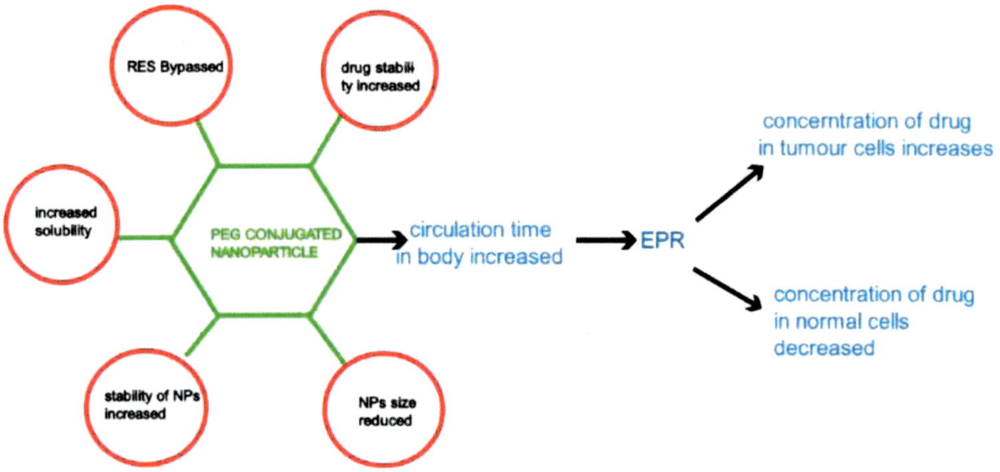

Fig. (3). Different effects of PEGylation on nanocarriers.

As NCs are recognized as foreign items, they are quickly removed from the systemic circulation by cells of the mononuclear phagocyte system (MPS), preventing accumulation in target cells and tissues. PEG coatings on NCs, like those on PEGylated proteins, protect the surface from aggregation, opsonization, and phagocytosis, allowing for longer circulation times. It has also been noted that stealth liposomes (Pegylated) show better accumulation in the tumor tissues [35]. Doxil®, the first FDA-approved PEGylated nanoparticle (NP) product, was approved in 1995. With a drug half-life of 72 hours and a circulation half-life of 36 hours, Doxil "Stealth®" liposomes enhanced doxorubicin bioavailability about 90-fold, 1 week after injection compared to free drug [36].

PEG chains substituted on NPs produce a hydrated structure with a huge omitted volume that spatially prevents NPs from interacting with adjacent nanoparticles(NPs)and/or blood components due to their water-loving nature [37]. Furthermore, the enormous conformational freedom given by PEG's flexibility makes nano-particles diffusion into the PEG corona thermodynamically unfavourable [38]. Surface modification with PEG extended the blood circulation half-life of systemically injected liposomes from 30 minutes up to 5 hours, according to Klibanov and colleagues [39]. Long-circulating PEGylated NPs have a unique chance to target tumors after systemic injection because of the increased permeability and retention (EPR) impact. PEG molecules can form a covalent linkage with different targeting moieties and work as a linker system. After the functionalization of the free end of the PEG chain with amine, carboxylic acid, or other groups, it can easily be linked with targeting moieties like thiamine, folate, transferring, RGD peptides, *etc*. leading to better targeting.

Modification of nano-carriers surface using PEG for the delivery of an anticancer drug is a well-established system and several polymer-like chitosan, poly (D, L-lactic acid) (PLA), poly(lactic-co-glycolic acid) (PLGA). Polyethyleneimine (PEI) *etc*, is being used for preparing such a system. Apart from it, several reports have been published regarding the use of different block polymers in this regard too.

Use of Pegylated Di-bock Polymers for the Formation of Nanocarrier

Diblock copolymers possess hydrophilic as well as hydrophobic parts with lower CMC [40] easily form micelle structure and hence better thermodynamic durability [40, 41] than triblock copolymers of the same molecular mass or HLB, as well as a greater drug-loading potential [40]. With their compact size and polydispersity in comparison to vesicular delivery systems, neutrally charged spherical micelles are considered powerful drug delivery methods that will not be quickly detected by the RES [42] and will remain in the circulation for a longer duration facilitating the accumulation of the drug in the tumor tissues. Several diblock polymers like PEG- PLL, PEG-PLA, PEG-PDLA, PEG-PAMA, PEG–PBLA, *etc* have been reported which possess PEG as one component for the development of nanoparticulate/ nanocarrier systems but PLA and PLGA are the most common polymers which are being used as the diblock polymer in their PEGylated form for the formulation of targeted nano-carrier/nanoparticulate system [27, 43]. Several formulations have been reported which utilize the different block polymers. Some of them are listed below in the Table **1**.

Table 1. Common example of PEG containing di-block polymer for the development of anticancer formulation.

S. No.	Polymers	Formulation	Drug	Purpose	References
1	Poly(ethylene glycol)-poly(γ-benzyl l-glutamate) PEG-PBLA	Micelles	Ellipticine	Better loading efficiency and controlled release profile	[44 - 54]
2	Poly(ethylene glycol)-poly(d,l-lactic acid) PEG-PDLLA	Nanovesicle	Doxorubicin	Better efficacy against human hepatocellular carcinoma	[55]
3	Poly(ethylene glycol)-poly(l-lactic acid) PEG-PLLA	Micelles	Docetaxel	Incorporating various agents and their ability to achieve multiple modifications to enhance cancer therapy.	[56]
4	Poly(ethylene glycol)-poly(- -caprolactone) PEG-PCL	Nanosphere	Camptothecin	Squamous cell carcinoma	[56]
5	Poly(ethylene glycol)-poly(d,l-lacti-e-co-glycolide) PEG-PLGA	Magnetic nanoparticle	Paclitaxel	Brain tumour	[57]
6	Poly(ethylene glycol)-poly(γ-benzyl l-glutamate) PEG-PBLG	Micelle	Doxorubicin and Paclitaxel	Increase in efficacy of anti-tumor drugs while reducing their systemic toxicity	[58]
7	poly(ethylene glycol)-poly(β-benzyl l-aspartate) PEG-PBLA	Micelle	Doxorubicin	Drug-loaded micelles with sufficient stability in dilute condition	[59]

(Table 1) cont.....

S. No.	Polymers	Formulation	Drug	Purpose	References
8	poly(ethylene glycol)-poly(α-benzyl carboxylate-ε-caprolactone) PEG-PBCL	Micelle	Silibinin	Narrowly distributed block copolymer micelle entrapping substantial amount of sustained drug for	[60]
9	poly(ethylene glycol)-poly(- -valerolactone) PEG-PVL	nanoparticle	oxaliplatin	Collateral cancer	[61]

Although the circulation time of prepared nanoparticles using PEGylated polymer gets increases significantly, at the same time, it may limit the interaction of these nanomaterials with targeted tissue, which leads to poor uptake. This limitation can be managed by coating the surface of these carriers with certain other materials like cationic electrolytes and protamine [62].

Use of Pegylated Tri-block Polymers for the Formation of Nanocarriers

Triblock polymers are another type of amphiphilic block copolymers (ABC) similar to di-block polymers having special capabilities which can be explored for drug delivery purposes. Based on the arrangement of hydrophobic and hydrophilic groups, these amphiphilic triblock polymers (ATBP) can be divided into symmetric and unsymmetric systems. Generally, ATBPS used for the delivery system contains PEG as a hydrophilic part, and depending on its position; three different arrangements can be made as mentioned in Fig. (**4**). Here arrangement B is utilized more efficiently for the development of the delivery system due to the high surface presence of PEG with increased stability [63]. Specific arrangements of the different blocks also lead to different structural variations including star and flower-like micelles or the formation of vesicles [64].

In their work, Ruan and Feng have prepared paclitaxel-loaded microspheres using PLA-PEG-PLA (Arrangement A) tri-block polymer and mentioned that the presence of PEG in the PLA chain may facilitate the drug release of such hydrophobic anti-cancer drug. They also assumed that the presence of PEG on the surface of microspheres may also add biocompatibility to the prepared formulation [65].

In case of arrangement B, the functional groups at the end can be decorated with either targeting moieties or imaging agents. One such doxorubicin micelle system was developed by Song *et al.* for metastatic breast cancer with improved drug loading capacity, drug release at a faster rate, and comparative improved cell toxicity as compared to the di-block polymers [66].

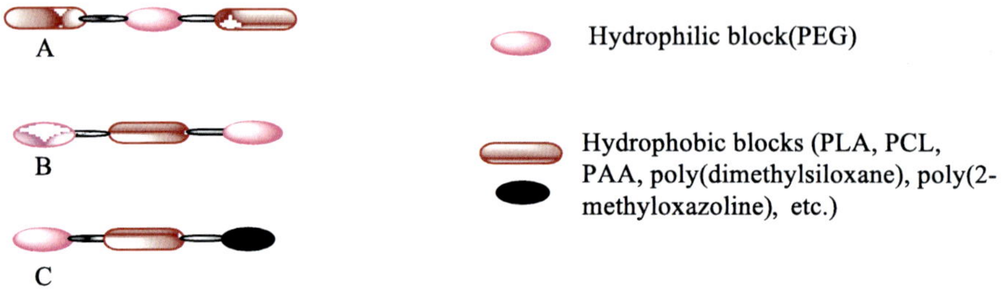

Fig. (4). Different arrangements of hydrophobic polymers with PEG (Hydrophilic block) forming triblock polymeric system.

Several other formulations have also been developed using such triblock polymers for the delivery of genes, drugs, and imaging agents. Some of them are listed below in the Table **2**.

Table 2. Different formulations prepared using tri-block polymers containing PEG.

S. No.	Polymers	Formulation	Purpose	Drug	Refs.
1.	Poly(lactic acid) Poly(ethylene glycol) (PEG-PLA-PEG)	Micelle	The blending method described here might be utilized as a nanoplatform for poorly water-soluble cancer medicines.	Doxorubicin and placitaxel	[67]
2.	Poly(lactic acid) Poly(ethylene glycol) (PLA-PEG-PLA)	Micelle	The micelles produced from these copolymers obviously include more hydrophobic medicines and considerably more efficiently regulate their release.	5-flurouracil	[68]
3.	Poly(glutamic acid) (PGA) and Poly(ethylene glycol) (PEG), (PGA-PEG-PGA)	Polymeor-somes	When Ptx and Pt were used together, they had a synergistic effect.	Paclitaxel andPlatinum(Pt)	[69]
4.	Poly(ε-caprolactone) Poly(ethylene glycol) (PCL-PEG-PCL)	Micelle	Promising dosage frequency decrease and compliance with patient	Dexamethasone	[70]

Pegylation of Already Formed Vesicles

Generally, pre-PEGylation is used to prepare different nanocarriers where PEG is either incorporated in form of a hydrophilic block, as in the case of di-block or triblock polymers already mentioned in the above sections, or in form of PEGylated lipid to prepare liposomes leading to enhanced stability and improved systemic circulation. But at the same time, the surface of already prepared nanocarriers can be modified by interaction (hydrophobic, electrostatic, or ligand binding) with PEG already dissolved in the aqueous system. The binding of cationic block polymers (PEG-PLL, PEG-PEI) on PLGA nanoparticles (negatively charged) may be a suitable example of electrostatic interaction. Chemical conjugation is another way by which PEG can be attached to the nanoparticle's surface [71].

For various kinds of NPs, different PEGylation methods were used. The nanoparticle composition determines the PEG conjugation technique used for each kind of NP. For example, PEG conjugation methods that work for organic liposomal NPs may not work for inorganic metal NPs [72].

Formulation of Stimuli-sensitive Nanocarrier

The stimulant conscious carriers react to a sensory signal or excitement that occurs in diseased tissue [73]. Tumour tissues demonstrate a lowered pH in solid tumors or inflammation [74] and at elevated temperatures [75] in comparison to the non-diseased cell [76, 77]. In addition, these tissues have a higher redox potential [78] as well as the presence of unusual enzyme systems that may be present in modest amounts or absent in normal tissue [79 - 81]. All of these are intrinsic stimulants as they are restricted to cancerous cells. Drug carriers may also be developed which show their movement and may carry the drug to a specific site under the influence of externally applied temperature, magnetic field, electrical field, ultrasonic or near-infrared light, *etc*. These externally applied stimuli are regarded as Extrinsic stimulants [82, 83]. When these stimuli (intrinsic and extrinsic) are applied, the sensitive carrier towards these stimuli goes under the change and releases the drug in the vicinity of the targeted tissue [84].

There are several such external and internal stimuli as mentioned in Fig. (**5**). which can be used for the development of a targeted nano-delivery system that has a comparatively better release system with the least chance of toxicity.

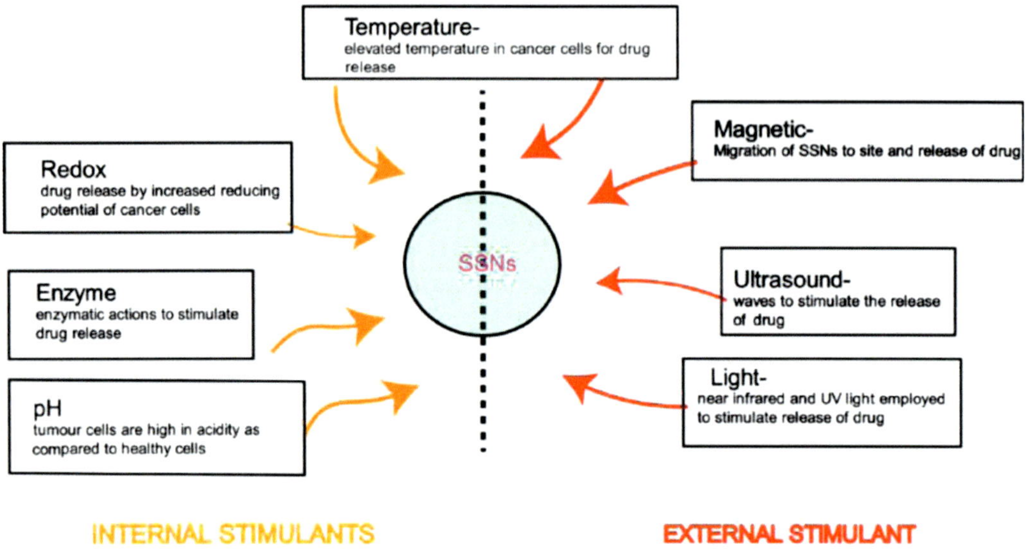

Fig. (5). Different stimuli used for the development of targeted nano-carriers.

pH-sensitive Nanocarriers

It is well evident that tumor tissue possesses an acidic environment as compared to a normal biological system probably due to the formation of lactic acid in a comparative hypoxic environment generated due to aggressive proliferation of tumor cells [83, 85, 86]. It has also been observed in certain cases of cancer cells that the extracellular pH can readily drop to 6-7, while in some cases it may be lower too [85] and this variability may be utilized for the development of site-specific drug delivery systems [86] as it has been noted that the following endocytosis, the nanocarrier system encounters extremely well-defined compartments with significantly varying pH levels. The pH of the early endosome is about 5-6, whereas the pH of the late lysosome, which is the most acidic compartment, is around 4-5 [87].

Several polymers show their response against the pH that can be utilized for the development of nanocarriers. Polymers having ionizable groups (amine or carboxylic group) and acid-labile linkage can be suitably used for the same. Polymers having ionizable groups may be of two types, the first which accepts the proton in an acidic medium and the other which donates the proton in a basic medium [88] and because of these characters, changes in the structure and hydrophobic character after protonation of these polymers which remains unprotonated at physiological pH, may be considered as a reason behind the loaded entity. Some commonly acidic group bearing (carboxylic acid, sulphuric acid, phosphonic acid, *etc.*) polymers for preparing such pH-responsive system are Poly glutamic acid(PGA), Polyacrylic acid(PAA), Poly(methacrylic acid)(PMAA), poly(2-acrylamido-2-methylpropane sulfonic acid) (PAMPS), poly(4-styrenesulfonic acid) (PSSA), polyvinylphenyl boronic acid(PVPBA), *etc.* [89] In a work, depending on the pH-responsive behavior of PAA, Liu *et al.* has developed Gambogenic acid (GNA) loaded micelles using PAA-b-PCL (polycaprolactone) showing very good transition in morphology with variation in pH and release of the drug [90].

Polymers containing tertiary amine group, morpholino, pyrrolidine, piperazine, pyridine, imidazole, *etc.* are regarded as basic polymers. Some common example of this category are poly[(2-diethylamino)ethyl methacrylate] (PDEA), poly[(2-diethylamino)ethyl methacrylate] (PDEA), poly[(2-diisopropylamino)ethyl methacrylate] (PDPA), poly(4-vinylpyridine) (P4VP), Poly[(2-N-morpholino) ethyl methacrylate] (PMEMA), Polyamido amine(PAMAM) *etc.* One such pH-responsive formulation based on basic polymer (PAMAM dendrimer) was developed by Zhang *et al.* for pH-dependent release of doxorubicin. [91] Some other examples of formulations developed using pH-responsive acidic and basic polymers are listed in Table **3**.

Table 3. Some examples of pH-responsive drug delivery systems.

S. No.	Polymers Used	Formulation	Drug Loaded	Refs.
1.	poly(methacrylic acid) (PMAA) and poly(N-vinylpyrrolidone) (PVPON)	Hydrogel cubes	Doxorubicin	[92]
2.	poly(*N,N*-diethyl acrylamide)	Thermo/pH-responsive (Pectin---PDEAAm/Chitosan) microcarriers	5-Fluorouracil	[93]
3.	PDEA-*block*-poly(ethylene glycol) copolymer	pH-responsive nano-particles	Cisplatin	[94]
4.	PDEA-mPEG	pH-responsive dendrimer nano-carrier	5-Fluorouracil	[95]
5.	PDMA-b-PDPA di-block copolymer/siRNA	Dual pH responsiveMicelleplexes	Amphotericin B	[96]
6.	PDPA as the inner core, lipid PEG as an outer shell,andiRGD peptide on surface	pH-responsive nano-particle with multi-functionality	Mitoxantrone	[97]

Another approach is to utilize detachable functionalities or to cover nanocarriers with a detachable protective polyethylene glycol (PEG) layer that dissolves when exposed to a low pH environment. The notion of shedding the connected PEG coat when exposed to particular pH levels is essential in some cases because the PEG coat can prevent encapsulated drug/DNA from the carrier from reaching the cytoplasm [98]. Inclusion of different bonds like orthoesters, hydrazones, oxime, hydroxide, vinyl esters [99], acetal [100], vinyl ethers, *etc*. during the formation of the drug-polymer conjugate or within di-block copolymers which are acid-labile linkages and breakdown at the lower pH values can be used for drug delivery to the specific site under the influence pH [88, 101].

Another option is to connect the medication to the hydrophobic part of the amphiphilic polymer *via* acid-degradable linker units. In context to it, Kataoka *et al.* has developed a micellar system having self-assembling block polymer (PEG-b-PAsp) possessing conjugation with Adriamycin through acid-labile hydrazone linkage. Drug release in this system occurs due to cleavage of hydrazones bond at lower pH [102].

The aforementioned pH–labile components have been used to create a variety of nanocarriers, including liposomes, micelles, dendrimers, and nanogels, to enable site-specific active delivery of anticancer drugs and genes in the targeted cancerous site [73].

Temperature Sensitive Nanocarrier

Nanocarrier system which shows their responsiveness towards the change in temperature of the vicinity where they are placed can be effectively used for targeting purposes. Any formulation should be designed in such a way that it does not release the activity component and remain stable at body temperature. Tumor cells have a higher temperature than normal cells because they are constantly reproducing and proliferating, a process that requires and releases energy [82]. The change in the micro-environment of tumor tissue like more blood flow, higher temperatures (40–45 °C), and enhanced vasculature permeability as compared to normal tissues (37 °C) can be utilized for the delivery of thermo-responsive nano-carrier systems [103].

Different thermo-responsive nano-carriers can be prepared using smart thermo-responsive polymers. The critical solution temperature, or the temperature above or below which the polymer behaviour is changed, is used to classify thermo-responsive polymers. Lower Critical Solution Temperature (LCST) and Upper Critical Solution Temperature (UCST) polymers are included here. Polymers containing LCST stay soluble below a certain temperature but become insoluble when heated. As a result, for polymers with LCST, solubility is inversely proportional to increase temperature. Polymers having UCST or HCST (Higher Critical Solution Temperature) have a phase transition above a certain temperature, meaning that as the temperature rises, so does the solubility [104].

Some common examples of polymers with lower LCST include poly(N-isopropylacrylamide) (PNIPAM), poly(N,N-diethyl acrylamide) (PDEAM), poly (methyl vinyl ether) [105], Poly(N-isopropylacrylamide) [106], Poly(N,N-diethy lacrylamide) [107], Poly(N-vinylcaprolactam) [108], Poly(2-(dimethylamino) ethyl methacrylate) [104, 109].

Dipalmitoyl phosphatidy lcholine (DPPC), which has an excellent gel-to-liquid crystalline transition temperature (Tg) of 41 °C, is one of the most widely utilized and researched lipids, which can be used for the thermo responsive liposome [103]. Many investigations have found that DPPC goes through a phase transition and conformational changes in response to hyperthermia, affecting the integrity of the liposomes and causing the payload to be released [110].

Surface Modification Using Different Ligands

Modification of Nano-carrier/Nanoparticles Surface With Transferrin

Transferrin, a 78-kDa monomeric glycoprotein with a primary role in serum iron transportation, is an important chelator [111]. It has a strong affinity for reversibly binding two atoms of ferric iron ($Fe3^{+}$). Following iron binding, the free transferrin peptide (apotransferrin) undergoes a conformational shift (di-ferric transferrin or holo-transferrin), which is important in transferrin receptor identification [112, 113]. Iron is necessary for a variety of biological activities, including DNA synthesis, cellular metabolism, and proliferation, and transferrin is the primary protein that regulates and distributes circulating iron [114, 115].

Transferrin receptors (TfRs), which are found on the outer cell membrane and are present at low levels in healthy cells, serve as a primary port of entry for iron into cells by cycling into acidic endosomes in a clathrin/dynamin-dependent manner. Meanwhile, in the rapidly expanding tumor microenvironment, TfRs expression was shown to be at least 100-fold greater, making this receptor an accessible gateway for drug targeting into tumor cells [116, 117]. Iron is an essential component of the ribonucleotide reductase enzyme required for the synthesis of DNA in rapidly proliferating cells, thus upregulation of transferrin in cancer may be due to higher iron demand [118]. This over-expression of transferrin receptor and higher demand of iron in a cancer cell is utilized for the targeted delivery of anticancer drugs to the specific required site by Modification of the nanoparticle/nanocarrier surface with transferrin. During the preparation of modified NPs, the Tf ligand can be conjugated to create TfR specific NPs using the post-insertion technique, which involves a reaction between the specific ligand and the group present on linker molecule attached on NPs surface in a specific reacting fluid under specified reaction conditions [119]. Jain *et al.* has prepared transferrin decorated long circulatory PEGylated nanoparticles loaded with paclitaxel. Initially, they PEGylated the drug-loaded nanoparticles, and then further transferrin was conjugated with surface PEG. In another work,

Doxorubicin-loaded poly D, L-lactic-co-glycolic acid (PLGA) nanoparticle was reported for lung cancer therapy which was initially coated with lipid, and then the surface was modified with transferrin. Better endocytosis of transferrin-modified nanocarrier was observed by the A549 cells [119].

Even the highly specialized blood-brain barrier can be overcome by utilizing these transferrin-modified carriers which is the major hurdle in case of brain-related diseases, especially brain tumors [115, 120]. One such attempt has been made by Zhang *et al* by preparing the transferrin-modified polyphosphoester hybrid micelles for effective delivery of paclitaxel across the BBB [121]. In another work, Vyas *et al.* reported the increased localization of Azidothymidine(an antiviral drug) when it was loaded in the PEGylated albumin nano-particle whose surface was modified with transferrin [122].

Apart from the effective use of transferrin in site-specific drug delivery, it can be used for the site-specific localization of imaging agents for diagnostic purposes too. In this context, Li *et al.* have reported almost six-time higher uptake of gold nanoparticles conjugated with transferrin during the therapy and imaging of breast cancer cells. Similarly, other imaging materials can also be utilized for effective diagnosis and theranostics purposes.

These transferrin-modified nano-carriers can also be utilized for the targeted delivery of DNA/RNA, enzymes, peptides, *etc* [123].

Modification of Nano-carrier/Nanoparticles Surface with Folate

Folic acid is a tiny (441 Da) molecule that is nonimmunogenic, required for optimum health, and acts as a cofactor for various enzymes especially involved in DNA/RNA synthesis [124]. The folate receptor, a glycosylphosphatidylinositol-anchored cellular receptor, is abundantly expressed in the vast range of tumor tissues, but not in non-tumorous cells and can be used as a biomarker of tumors [125, 126]. In the case of normal tissues, expression of folate receptors is generally restricted to the Kidney, placenta, and choroid plexus [124] but epithelial, ovarian, cervical, breast, lung, kidney, colorectal, and brain cancers are some common examples where folate receptors are abundantly expressed [127]. The previous literature levels that are due to the above-mentioned fact, folic acid can be utilized as an effective ligand for the targeting of nano-carriers loaded with drug/imaging agent/genetic material including liposomes [128], nanoparticles [129], lipoplexes [130], *etc.* to the cancerous tissues. One thing which is important during the targeting of the specific site *via* folate receptors is that the receptors should be abundant at the surface.

Among the three major types of folate receptors *i.e,* FRα, α, FRβ, and FRγ, the first two are supposed to be responsible for the endocytosis of the folate [131]. Beginning with compound attachment to a cell surface FR and ending with the release of at least part of the therapeutic payload into the cytoplasm, receptor-mediated uptake of folate-drug conjugates goes through several different stages as shown in Fig. (**6**) [131]. Stepwise it could be summarized as:

• Acidification of the endosomal segment to pH 5 leads to the liberation of some folate conjugates from their receptors after membrane invagination and internalization to form an endocytic vesicle [132, 133].

• Separation of membrane-bound FR from released conjugates/free drugs is then possible when the acidic endosome is sent to a recycling site. Through an unknown mechanism, released folate conjugates are seen to escape the endosome, resulting in drug deposition in the cytoplasm. Membrane-bound FR, on the other hand, primarily recycles back to the cell surface, allowing for the transport of more folate-linked medicines into the cell. The recycling rate in cancer cells ranges *in vivo* from one cycle every 4 hours to one cycle every 12 hours [134].

Several formulations have been developed for targeting different materials to the specific site using the concept of folate conjugation. Some of the reported work is listed in the Table **4**.

Table 4. Different folate conjugated formulations for different purposes (*In-vitro/In-vivo).*

S. No.	Component to be targeted	Formulation	Purpose	Refs.
1.	Interleukin-15 gene	Lipoplex	Colon cancer	[130]
2.	Curcumin	Dendritic magnetite nanocarriers	KB nasopharyngeal cancer cells	[135]
3.	Paclitaxel	Graphene oxide-methyl acrylate (GO-g-MA) nanocarrier	Breast Cancer cells	[136]
4.	Letrozole	Lipid hybrid nanoparticles	Breast Cancer	[137]
5.	Super-magnetic iron oxide	PEGylated nanoparticles	Imaging of Lung cancer	[138]
6.	Co-delivery of Cisplatin, paclitaxel	Nanoparticle of PEG-PLA diblock polymer	Non-small lung cancer	[139]
7.	Doxorubicin	PEGylated gold nanoparticels	Targeted delivery	[140]
8.	Paclitaxel	PLGA nanoparticles	Ovarian cancer	[141]
9.	Iron oxide	Dextran coated nanoparticles	MR Imaging	[142]
10.	Docetaxel and Ketoconazole	Solid lipid nanoparticles	Increased brain uptake	[143]

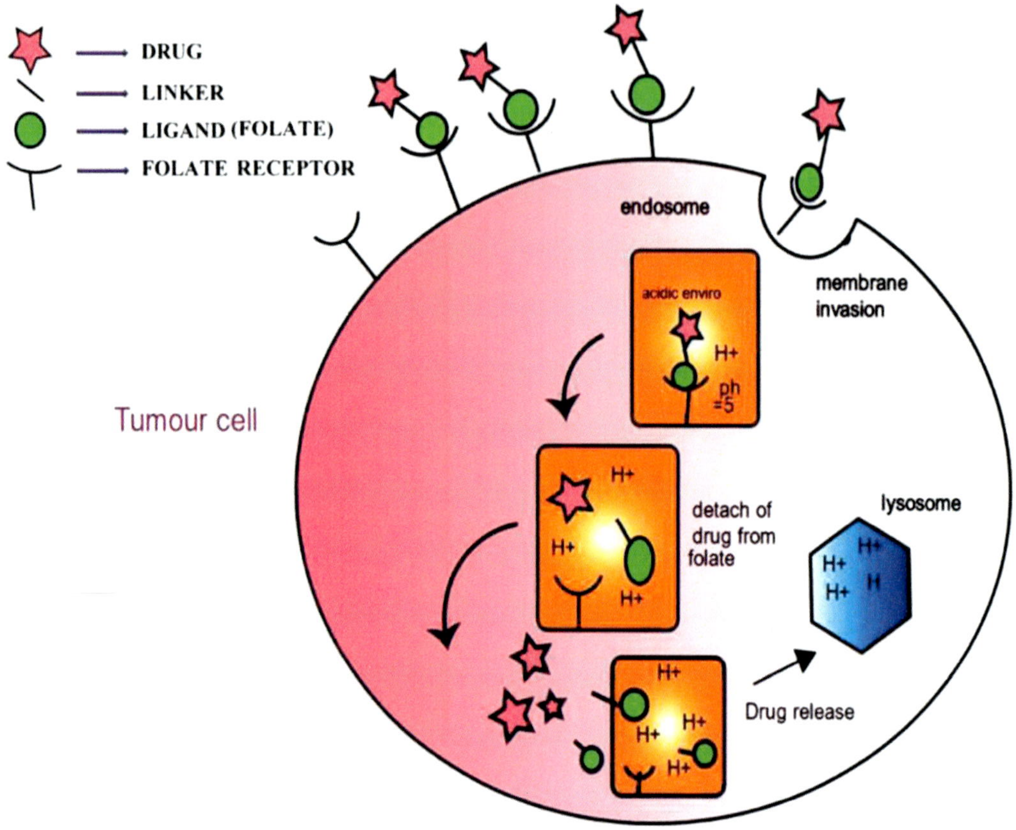

Fig. (6). Different steps during the invasion of folate-drug conjugate.

Modification of Nano-carrier/Nanoparticles Surface with Aptamers

Aptamers are unique three-dimensional structures having single-stranded oligonucleotides exhibiting specific binding to homologous targets (small or macromolecules or a complete cell) that can mimic antibodies in a different application [144]. In comparison to antibodies, these are small, less complex, and flexible structured systems with lower immunogenic properties and can bind to their targets with more specificity and high affinity even on hidden aptamers too [145]. Because of their extremely selective binding power for cancer-related chemicals and cells, aptamers have been widely investigated as cancer diagnostic tools. Aptamer's capacity to identify minute variations between proteins of similar structure allows them to distinguish malignant from non-cancerous cells based on their distinct cell-surface homology [146]. A variety of new aptamers that can affect tumor growth, signal transduction, and immunological function have been reported through aptamer selection technological advancements [147]. Specific characteristics and easier synthesis even in larger quantities with reproducibility and purity, the possibility of easier modification, and the ability of the conformation structure after denaturation due to higher temperature make it ideal in comparison to antibodies [146].

Aptamers are chosen from a nucleic acid library and then put through the SELEX *in vitro* screening procedure [148]. A beginning oligonucleotide pool is created with a huge number of random sequences (on the order of 1014-15) with a range of 22-100 nucleotides. Consider two primer-binding sequences identified on both sides of the sequences, enabling them to be amplified by PCR. To obtain particular aptamer sequences, 8-18 rounds of SELEX are usually required [148, 149].

Several applications of Aptamers are reported including the development of different types of sensors for cancer diagnosis such as optical and electrochemical aptasensors and targeting ligands for site-specific delivery of drugs and drug-loaded nanocarriers. Aptamers can also be utilized for different imaging techniques like fluorescence imaging, MR imaging, computed tomography, positron emission tomography, *etc.* during a cancer diagnosis [146].

Aptamers utilized in cancer therapy are now divided into three categories: free aptamers against particular cancer proteins, free aptamers against immunomodulatory components, and aptamers as anti-tumor drug carriers [147]. Aptamers like AS 1411 (unmodified guanosine-rich 26-mer DNA strand) as such can be utilized as a drug for the management of cancer [150]. While, apart from the therapeutic utility, as mentioned earlier, aptamers can be utilized as a ligand for targeting drug delivery. There are two major ways to utilize the aptamer for drug delivery, first by preparing drug-aptamer conjugate and second by modifying the surface of nanomaterials with the help of aptamers [151, 152]. In their work, Zhao *et al.* has developed Aptamer-methotrexate (APT-MTX) conjugate for the management of acute myeloid leukemia and observed the targeted and selective inhibition of acute myeloid leukemia cells [153]. In another work, Tan *et al.* initially prepared an aptamer-doxorubicin complex and further modified it by attaching the PEG to make the entire system long circulatory. He observed that in comparison to free doxorubicin, the complex was having almost six times more affectivity against the MUC1-expressing breast cancer cell line [154]. Similar to these, several drug-aptamer conjugates have been reported with improved efficacy and lower toxicity, which establishes the significance of aptamer-drug conjugates in drug delivery [155 - 157].

Modification of drug-loaded nanomaterial with aptamer is another way to achieve selective targeting. Li *et al.* has reported a liposomal complex, prepared by anchoring the surface of liposome with anti-EGFR aptamer-chitosan conjugate for co-delivery of oxygen and erlotinib for managing the hypoxia-associated drug resistance [158]. In another work reported by Yang *et al.*, aptamer-modified mesoporous silica nanoparticles for targeted delivery of doxorubicin to leukemia cells have been reported which utilizes the tumor-targeting ability of the aptamer Sgc8. [159] Several other works showing the ability of aptamer for the surface medication of various nanomaterials used for drug delivery and diagnosis have also been reported [160 - 162].

Modification of Nano-carrier/Nanoparticle Surface with Peptides and Monoclonal Antibodies

Receptor-mediated transport is one of the finest approaches, utilized for the targeting of drug-loaded carriers across a specific barrier by decorating it with a specific ligand such as aptamers, monoclonal antibodies, peptides, *etc*. The high diversity of peptide sequence, ability to identify biomolecules, biocompatibility, *etc*. make the peptide a very good ligand for the development of targeted delivery [163]. Peptides are smaller bio-molecules in comparison to proteins and due to their specific properties, they can penetrate across the cell and specific biological barriers and can effectively be used for drug delivery [164]. Drug delivery system using peptides mainly depends on the microenvironment of the tumor, the rapid growth of tumor endothelial cells, the presence of integrins, the presence of aminopeptidase (a multifunctional metallo-proteinase), tumor-associated macrophages related to lymph-angiogenesis, high expression of epidermal growth factor receptors and transferrin receptors, *etc*. and these are some key features which should be taken into account during the development of drug delivery system anchored with different peptides [165]. Drugs Some commonly used peptides include RGD, NGR, Lyp-1, CLT-1, OCT, cNGR, CD47 peptide, Phytochelatin, iRGD, PAVLG, CKS9, CTGKSC, *etc*. which can be used for modifying the nano-carrier surface in the therapy of cancer [164]. Li *et al.* has isolated one such peptide named as pep TGN and utilized it for modifying the surface of PEG-PLGA based nano-particle for the development of a carrier system that can cross BBB [166].

RGD peptide (Arg-Gly-Asp) is one of the very good ligands used for the modification of nano-carriers in course of targeting. These peptides show their selectivity for integrin which is present on almost all cell types and possesses an important role in cell adhesion. In context to it, Cai *et al.* has suggested the RGD-modified stearic acid-grafted chitosan loaded with anticancer drugs can be effectively targeted to the tumor cells where integrins are over-expressed [167].

The monoclonal antibody (mAb) production technique has been developed in 1975 and is currently a well-established system (11 for cancer treatment among

27mAb medications) for therapy based on antibodies [168]. The use of antibodies for the development of targeted nano-carriers is another very important dimension and requires in-depth knowledge about the carrier, antibodies (linker molecule used to attach the antibody at the nanomaterial (NM) surface, and method of conjugation [169]. Hydrazone linkers, disulfide linkers, and peptide linkers are some very commonly explored systems to attach mAbs at NM surface [168]. Among all the nano-based systems, liposomes may be regarded as the highly explored nano-carrier for antibody-based targeted systems. Several studies have been done to develop immune-liposomes, attachment of nucleosome (NS)-specific 2C5 antibody (mAb 2C5) on Doxorubicin loaded PEGlated liposomes is one of them. Adsorption, covalent binding or binding of antibody fragment by using adapter are some methods for the functionalization of nanocarriers using antibody fragment [170].

Cetuximab-immunoliposomes is another example that utilizes mAb [171]. Anti-VEGF antibody(bevacizumab), anti-EGFR antibody(cetuximab), anti-HER2 antibody(trastuzumab) are some very important and approved mAbs for therapeutic use [172].

Modification of Nano-carrier Surface with Anisamide

Surface Modification of nanocarriers with tumor-targeting ligands may improve specificity for cancer cells overexpressing the relevant ligand-binding homolog. Based on its claimed interaction with sigma receptors, anisamide, a low-molecular-weight structurally modified benzamide, is utilized as a tumor-directing moiety in functionalized Nano systems. The sigma-1 receptor, a potential but questionable cellular target of anisamide, is addressed in terms of its subcellular location and cancer implications. The effect of anisamide on the anticancer effects of adorned nano-systems differs significantly among published publications, according to data from in-vivo investigations [173].

Several ligands like peptides, antibodies, aptamer, *etc.* are already reported and show a significant impact on the targeting but an increase in the size of the formulation after the modification may be a major issue, especially concerning extravasations and penetrating capability which is expected to be addressed properly [174]. Anisamide may be a better alternative due to its specific properties. Several reports have been published regarding the use of this smaller molecule for the surface modification of different nanocarriers. Concerning it, a PEGylated liposomal system decorated with anisamide loaded with doxorubicin by Banerjee *et al.* for targeting prostate cancer. They mentioned that the presence of PEG may improve the targeting ability of ligand and increases the stability and circulation time of the system [175] In another work, Docetaxel (DTX) loaded solid lipid nanoparticle functionalized with anisamide has been reported with an aim that this system will have the better interaction over-expressed sigma receptors in prostate cancer [176]. Several other works have also been published showing the importance of anisamide in targeting the tissue with over-expressed sigma receptors. Some of them are listed in Table **5** .

Table 5. Some examples of formulations functionalized with anisamide.

S. No.	Formulation	Drug/Active material	Utility	Refs.
1.	Cyclodextrin Nanoparticles	siRNA	Targeted delivery to prostate cancer cells	[177]
2.	Gold nanoparticles	siRNA	Management of prostate cancer	[178]
3.	Nanoparticles of Chitosan/poly(ethylene glycol)	Gemcitabine	Increased anti-tumor activity non-small cell lung cancer with less toxicity in other organs	[179]
4.	pH-Sensitive Degradable ChimaericPolymersomes	Apoptotic protein, (Granzyme B)	Targeted therapy of lung cancer	[180]
5.	Polymeric nanocapsules (Eudragit S100)	Thymoquinone	Higher cytotoxicity against HT-29 cells (Colon cancer)	[181]
6.	PH-responsive micelles of *N*-octyl-*N,O*-maleoyl-*O*-phosphoryl chitosan	Paclitaxel	Higher accumulation in tumors (Prostate cancer)	[182]
7.	PEGylated Gold nanorods	Epirubicin	pH-dependent drug release and Decreased proliferation in human prostate cancer PC-3 cells	[183]

Modification of Nano-carrier Surface with Cell-penetrating Peptides

Targeted delivery to the specific site sometimes suffers from problems related to their penetration in the cell system as plasma membrane work as a very effective barrier, especially for the larger molecules. This problem can be overcome with the use of cell-penetrating peptides (CPPs) which may help in the targeting of nanocarriers [184]. CPPs are short peptides (less than 30 residues) with a net positive charge that operate independently of receptors and energy [185]. CPPs are generally of modest size, with an almost non-toxic and non-immunogenic activity, between 5-30 amino acids. Several of the peptide sequences so far found have been employed as flexible means to transport different cargoes intracellularly, such as tiny molecular medications, peptides, proteins, nucleic acids, or particles [186 - 188].

Based on their origin, CPPs may be classified as protein-derived CPPs (Tat protein and Penetratin), chimeric CPPs (Transportan) and synthetic CPPs (oligoarginines and numerous peptide nucleic acids). While based on their chemical and physical properties they may be classified as cationic (containing positive charges), amphipathic (MPG and Pep-1), and hydrophobic CPPs [186, 188, 189]. Apart from these classes of CPPs, several other CPPs including synthetic CPPS generated with chemical modifications are also mentioned in the literature which can be utilized for drug delivery purposes [186, 188]. Cai *et al.* have investigated the internalization efficiency of four different CPPs, namely low molecular weight protamine (LMWP), penetration, Tat, and R8, by noncovalently attaching them to the negatively charged surface of PLGA NPs *via* electrostatic forces and investigating their use for cochlear drug delivery applications [190]

CPPs can overcome the probability of drug resistance when used as a conjugate system with a particular drug [191]. Intracellular delivery of different nanocarriers/ like liposomes, micelles, nanoparticles, *etc*, and peptides can also be effectively achieved when coupled with TATp CCP [192]. Organelle (Mitochondria, nuclei, lysosomes, *etc*) targeting is another dimension for the effective management of certain diseases and can be achieved with CPP conjugate system [193]. CPPs can also be utilized for the delivery of genes by using specific carriers. Rudolph *et al.* has utilized TAT_2-modified solid lipid nanoparticles for optimizing the gene transfer *in vitro* [194]. Non-viral gene therapy for lung cancer has also been reported based on the TAT conjugated Polyethylenimine *via* PEG as a linker molecule [195].

Other Approaches to Surface Modification

Light-sensitive Nano Preparation

Because of its non-invasiveness and great remote Spatio-temporal control over the release of cargo from nanocarriers, light is an appealing choice for use as an external stimulus [84].

The photo-reactive groups, or chromophores, are usually enclosed within the nanocarriers or coupled to their surfaces. To allow the cargo to be released, all photoreactions cause structural changes in the polymeric matrix or side chains of the nanocarrier [199, 200]. One of the most researched photo-responsive groups is azobenzene and its derivatives. Their nitrogen double bond undergoes reversible UV–visible photo isomerization. Light converts the planer trans isomer to the non-planner cis isomer(easily forms the micelle), which may then be transformed back to the trans isomer using UV radiation [196, 197]. This photo-isomerization changes the polarity, which can change the microenvironment in polymers [198]. Incorporation of pyrene group in hydrophobic polymethacrylate part of a di-block co-polymer with poly(ethylene oxide) as hydrophilic part may also be utilized for such light-sensitive carrier system. When the polymer is exposed to UV radiation, pyrene moiety gets detached due to photo-solvolysis leading to the conversion of polymethacrylate into hydrophilic poly(methacrylic acid) which results in disruption of a micelle [199]. Similarly, several other light-responsive delivery systems have also been generated.

Ultrasound-Responsive Drug Delivery Systems

Ultrasound-responsive drug delivery system is another good example of a non-invasive system. Ultrasound may go deeper in the tissue and may activate the accumulated micelle to release the drug in the tumor vicinity. It is supposed that encapsulation of the drug in the micelle is not uptaken by the normal cells but gets accumulated in the tumor tissue through passive targeting [200].

Various physical variables might cause drug release when ultrasound is applied to the target area. Simple pressure variations, acoustic fluid streaming, cavitations, and local hyperthermia are among them [201]. Several nanocarrier systems like liposomes, nanoparticles, micelles, *etc*, are there that respond against the ultrasound and release the drug. Different types of organic and inorganic materials including proteins, lipids, and different types of polymers such as alginates, chitosan, PLA, PLGA, *etc* may be utilized for the generation of such systems [202 - 206]. Different di-block polymers having the capability of micelle formation can also be utilized for the generation of an ultrasound-triggered system for drug release [207].

Magnetic field-sensitive Nano Preparation-

The development of magnetic field-sensitive nano-formulation using different carriers such as microcapsules, liposomes, *etc.* can be prepared by adding the therapeutic payload(s) as well as a magnetically active component [76, 208]. These nano-preparations may then be controlled to regulate drug release under the influence of an applied magnetic field. Thermal ablation of cells where this preparation is accumulated may be achieved by application of a high-frequency alternating field resulting in the increased temperature of Magnetic nanoparticles resulting in a temperature rise, or both when used alternatively [82, 208].

Several other formulations may also be prepared which possess magnetic field responsive behavior. Such formulations can be utilized for therapy as well as MR imaging too due to the presence of magnetic nanoparticles [209, 210]. The development of an effective theranostics formulation using such a system is another dimension.

Role of Surface-modified Nano-carriers in the Diagnosis of Different Types of Cancer

Diagnosis of any disease in its early stages, especially cancer, is of utmost importance for the better management of a disease. There are several techniques like Computed tomography scan (CT scan), magnetic resonance imaging (MRI), positron emission tomography (PET), photo acoustic imaging (PAI), *etc*., being used for assessing the different pathophysiological conditions, including tumors [29]. The use of Nano-carrier based contrast (with special surface characteristics and integrated design) may add a better alternative to traditional molecular-based contrast agents. Targeting such newer nano-carriers (contrast) to specified locations may also be very important in various imaging [211]. Quantum dots, magnetic nano-particles, gold nano-particles, carbon nano-tubes, *etc*., are some common examples of nanomaterials that have been identified for in-vivo imaging of tumors [29, 212 - 214]. Several nanomaterials are also there, which may identify the cancer biomarkers in their early stage [215, 216]. It is well evident that surface functionalization of different nano-carriers, increases the chance of localization in specific targeted areas/tissue. Several works regarding the use of surface-functionalized nano-carriers, which can be used for diagnosis, have been reported. Some of such formulations are listed in the Table **6**.

Table 6. Different formulations with surface functionalization used for Diagnosis.

S. No.	Formulation	Surface Modifying Approach/ Ligand	Purpose	Refs.
1.	Micelles	Hydrophobic imaging markers (pH-Sensitive)	Cancer Diagnosis	[217]
2.	Polymeric Nanoparticle	Simultaneous tumor magnetic resonance imaging (MRI) (pH-sensitive)	Cancer Diagnosis	[218]
3.	Hemoglobin	Smart pH -Sensitive Nanocarrier	Enhanced tumor Retention	[219]
4.	Hydrogel Nanoparticles	Anchored with Poly(*N*-Isopropylacrylamide) (PNIPAM) (Temprature And pH Sensitive Nanocarriers)	Cancer Diagnosis	[220]
5.	Surface-Modified Gold Nanocarriers	Modified with folic acid (fa)-conjugated biocompatible block copolymers through a bidentate dihydrolipoic acid (dhla) linker	Cancer Diagnosis	[221]
6.	Poly(Lactic-*Co*-Glycolic Acid) (PLGA) Nanoparticles	Transferrin surface-modified PLGA nanoparticles	Pancreatic Cancer Cells	[222]

(Table 6) cont.....

S. No.	Formulation	Surface Modifying Approach/ Ligand	Purpose	Refs.
7.	Human Serum Albumin (HSA) Nanoparticles (Nps)	Modified with tumor necrosis Factor (TNF)-Inducing ligand (TRAIL) and transferrin	Various Tumors	[223]
8.	Aptamer-Modified Nanoparticles	Modified with stranded Deoxyribonucleic Acid (DNA) Or Ribonucleic Acid (RNA) oligonucleotides (Aptamers)	Cancer Diagnosis	[152]
9.	Folate-Modified Gold Nanoclusters	Folic Acid (FA) was immobilized on the surface of Au Ncs	Various Tumors	[224]
10.	Conjugated Quantum Dots	Anchored with SP90 peptide	Breast Cancer	[225]

CONCLUSION

Development of nanocarriers and their surface functionalization for improved bioavailability, ability to remain in the systemic circulation for a longer duration, ability to target the specific cell/tissue/organ, and reduction in toxicity of cytotoxic drug are some major objectives of a safe and efficacious delivery system. Several nanocarriers like lipid-based nanocarriers (liposome, lipoplexes, SLNs, *etc*), polymeric nanocarriers (Polymeric nanocarriers, polyplexes, dendrimers, polymeric micelle), and different Inorganic nano-particle (Gold, Silver, Silica, Carbon nanotubes, *etc*) as such and in their functionalized form have been explored a lot for the drug delivery as well as for diagnostic purposes. Several targeting sites (Biomolecules, receptors, *etc.*) and targeting ligands (Folate, aptamers, anisamide, lectins, and many more) have also been explored for the successful development of different target-oriented drug delivery systems. But still, a long way to go; understating the structure and physiology of different targeting sites and receptors in a more detailed way is the need of the hour. The impact of a biological system on such functionalized formulation is also needed to exploit. At the same time, the fate and clearance of such formulation in the biological system are also needed to understand in a more detailed manner. As mentioned earlier, exhaustive research is going on regarding the development of novel carrier systems for the delivery of therapeutics as well as diagnostics, but the conversion of such formulation at the clinical level is highly desirable. Although, some nano-formulation can deliver drug-like Doxil®, AmBisome®, DepoCyt®, and many more are already available on the floor and have marketing approvals. Some novel preparation to be used as diagnostics, such as Feridex®, SonoVue®, Optison®, *etc.*, are also available. But other dimensions concerning surface functionalization of nanocarriers/nanomaterials are still to be discovered for safe and efficacious formulations with improved target ability. Therefore, current exhaustive research builds a strong hope in this regard to have some newer formulations in the near future.

CONSENT FOR PUBLICATION

Not applicable.

CONFLICT OF INTEREST

The authors declare no conflict of interest, financial or otherwise.

ACKNOWLEDGMENT

We are thankful to the team at Bentham Science Publishers for giving us this opportunity and to everyone who supported us directly or indirectly during the writing of this book chapter.

REFERENCES

[1] Arain MR, Buggy DJ. Anaesthesia for cancer patients. Curr Opin Anaesthesiol 2007; 20(3): 247-53. [http://dx.doi.org/10.1097/ACO.0b013e32814f1c34] [PMID: 17479030]

[2] Chaturvedi VK, Singh A, Singh VK, Singh MP. Cancer nanotechnology: a new revolution for cancer diagnosis and therapy. Curr Drug Metab 2019; 20(6): 416-29. [http://dx.doi.org/10.2174/1389200219666180918111528] [PMID: 30227814]

[3] van Vlerken LE, Vyas TK, Amiji MM. Poly(ethylene glycol)-modified Nanocarriers for Tumor-targeted and Intracellular Delivery. Pharm Res 2007; 24(8): 1405-14. [http://dx.doi.org/10.1007/s11095-007-9284-6] [PMID: 17393074]

[4] Triozzi PL, Eng C, Singh AD. Targeted therapy for uveal melanoma. Cancer Treat Rev 2008; 34(3): 247-58. [http://dx.doi.org/10.1016/j.ctrv.2007.12.002] [PMID: 18226859]

[5] Hanahan D, Weinberg RA. Hallmarks of cancer: the next generation. Cell 2011; 144(5): 646-74. [http://dx.doi.org/10.1016/j.cell.2011.02.013] [PMID: 21376230]

[6] ARAZ C. Kanser hastalarında anestezi. Anestezi Dergisi 2014; 22(1): 3-12.

[7] Jain V, Jain S, Mahajan SC. Nanomedicines based drug delivery systems for anti-cancer targeting and treatment. Curr Drug Deliv 2015; 12(2): 177-91. [http://dx.doi.org/10.2174/1567201811666140822112516] [PMID: 25146439]

[8] Maeda H. SMANCS and polymer-conjugated macromolecular drugs: advantages in cancer chemotherapy. Adv Drug Deliv Rev 2001; 46(1-3): 169-85. [http://dx.doi.org/10.1016/S0169-409X(00)00134-4] [PMID: 11259839]

[9] Maeda H, Wu J, Sawa T, Matsumura Y, Hori K. Tumor vascular permeability and the EPR effect in macromolecular therapeutics: a review. J Control Release 2000; 65(1-2): 271-84. [http://dx.doi.org/10.1016/S0168-3659(99)00248-5] [PMID: 10699287]

[10] Yokoyama M. Drug targeting with nano-sized carrier systems. J Artif Organs 2005; 8(2): 77-84. [http://dx.doi.org/10.1007/s10047-005-0285-0] [PMID: 16094510]

[11] Iyer AK, Khaled G, Fang J, Maeda H. Exploiting the enhanced permeability and retention effect for tumor targeting. Drug Discov Today 2006; 11(17-18): 812-8. [http://dx.doi.org/10.1016/j.drudis.2006.07.005] [PMID: 16935749]

[12] Greish K. Enhanced permeability and retention of macromolecular drugs in solid tumors: A royal gate for targeted anticancer nanomedicines. J Drug Target 2007; 15(7-8): 457-64. [http://dx.doi.org/10.1080/10611860701539584] [PMID: 17671892]

[13] Torchilin VP. Targeted pharmaceutical nanocarriers for cancer therapy and imaging. AAPS J 2007; 9(2): E128-47.
[http://dx.doi.org/10.1208/aapsj0902015] [PMID: 17614355]

[14] Fang J, Sawa T, Maeda H. Factors and mechanism of "EPR" effect and the enhanced antitumor effects of macromolecular drugs including SMANCS. Polymer Drugs in the Clinical Stage 2004; pp. 29-49.
[http://dx.doi.org/10.1007/0-306-47932-X_2]

[15] Riaz M, Riaz M, Zhang X, *et al.* Surface functionalization and targeting strategies of liposomes in solid tumor therapy: A review. Int J Mol Sci 2018; 19(1): 195.
[http://dx.doi.org/10.3390/ijms19010195] [PMID: 29315231]

[16] Sanità G, Carrese B, Lamberti A. Nanoparticle surface functionalization: How to improve biocompatibility and cellular internalization. Front Mol Biosci 2020; 7: 587012.
[http://dx.doi.org/10.3389/fmolb.2020.587012] [PMID: 33324678]

[17] de Jong WH, Borm PJ. Drug delivery and nanoparticles: Applications and hazards. Int J Nanomedicine 2008; 3(2): 133-49.
[http://dx.doi.org/10.2147/IJN.S596] [PMID: 18686775]

[18] Siafaka P, Üstündağ Okur N, Karavas E, Bikiaris D. Surface modified multifunctional and stimuli-responsive nanoparticles for drug targeting: current status and uses. Int J Mol Sci 2016; 17(9): 1440.
[http://dx.doi.org/10.3390/ijms17091440] [PMID: 27589733]

[19] Kreuter J. Nanoparticles—a historical perspective. Int J Pharm 2007; 331(1): 1-10.
[http://dx.doi.org/10.1016/j.ijpharm.2006.10.021] [PMID: 17110063]

[20] Poon W, Zhang X, Nadeau J. Nanoparticle drug formulations for cancer diagnosis and treatment. Critical Reviews™in Oncogenesis. 2014; 19: 3-4.
[http://dx.doi.org/10.1615/CritRevOncog.2014011563]

[21] Estanqueiro M, Amaral MH, Conceição J, Sousa Lobo JM. Nanotechnological carriers for cancer chemotherapy: The state of the art. Colloids Surf B Biointerfaces 2015; 126: 631-48.
[http://dx.doi.org/10.1016/j.colsurfb.2014.12.041] [PMID: 25591851]

[22] Kumari P, Ghosh B, Biswas S. Nanocarriers for cancer-targeted drug delivery. J Drug Target 2016; 24(3): 179-91.
[http://dx.doi.org/10.3109/1061186X.2015.1051049] [PMID: 26061298]

[23] Peer D, Karp JM, Hong S, Farokhzad OC, Margalit R, Langer R. Nanocarriers as an emerging platform for cancer therapy. Nat Nanotechnol 2007; 2(12): 751-60.
[http://dx.doi.org/10.1038/nnano.2007.387] [PMID: 18654426]

[24] Hossen S, Hossain MK, Basher MK, Mia MNH, Rahman MT, Uddin MJ. Smart nanocarrier-based drug delivery systems for cancer therapy and toxicity studies: A review. J Adv Res 2019; 15: 1-18.
[http://dx.doi.org/10.1016/j.jare.2018.06.005] [PMID: 30581608]

[25] Shukla T, Upmanyu N, Pandey SP, Gosh D. Lipid nanocarriers Lipid Nanocarriers for Drug Targeting. Elsevier 2018; pp. 1-47.

[26] Attia MF, Anton N, Wallyn J, Omran Z, Vandamme TF. An overview of active and passive targeting strategies to improve the nanocarriers efficiency to tumour sites. J Pharm Pharmacol 2019; 71(8): 1185-98.
[http://dx.doi.org/10.1111/jphp.13098] [PMID: 31049986]

[27] Yu W, Zhang N. Surface modification of nanocarriers for cancer therapy. Curr Nanosci 2009; 5(2): 123-34.
[http://dx.doi.org/10.2174/157341309788185370]

[28] Kim D, Jeong YY, Jon S. A drug-loaded aptamer-gold nanoparticle bioconjugate for combined CT imaging and therapy of prostate cancer. ACS Nano 2010; 4(7): 3689-96.
[http://dx.doi.org/10.1021/nn901877h] [PMID: 20550178]

[29] Baetke SC, Lammers T, Kiessling F. Applications of nanoparticles for diagnosis and therapy of cancer. Br J Radiol 2015; 88(1054): 20150207.
[http://dx.doi.org/10.1259/bjr.20150207] [PMID: 25969868]

[30] Hirsjärvi S, Passirani C, Benoit JP. Passive and active tumour targeting with nanocarriers. Curr Drug Discov Technol 2011; 8(3): 188-96.
[http://dx.doi.org/10.2174/157016311796798991] [PMID: 21513482]

[31] Shukla T, Upmanyu N, Pandey SP, Sudheesh M. Site-specific drug delivery, targeting, and gene therapy Nanoarchitectonics in Biomedicine. Elsevier 2019; pp. 473-505.

[32] Torchilin VP. Passive and active drug targeting: drug delivery to tumors as an example. Handb Exp Pharmacol 2010; 197(197): 3-53.
[http://dx.doi.org/10.1007/978-3-642-00477-3_1] [PMID: 20217525]

[33] Kim CH, Lee SG, Kang MJ, Lee S, Choi YW. Surface modification of lipid-based nanocarriers for cancer cell-specific drug targeting. J Pharm Investig 2017; 47(3): 203-27.
[http://dx.doi.org/10.1007/s40005-017-0329-5]

[34] Abuchowski A, McCoy JR, Palczuk NC, van Es T, Davis FF. Effect of covalent attachment of polyethylene glycol on immunogenicity and circulating life of bovine liver catalase. J Biol Chem 1977; 252(11): 3582-6.
[http://dx.doi.org/10.1016/S0021-9258(17)40292-4] [PMID: 16907]

[35] Torchilin V. Tumor delivery of macromolecular drugs based on the EPR effect. Adv Drug Deliv Rev 2011; 63(3): 131-5.
[http://dx.doi.org/10.1016/j.addr.2010.03.011] [PMID: 20304019]

[36] Gabizon A, Shmeeda H, Barenholz Y. Pharmacokinetics of pegylated liposomal Doxorubicin: review of animal and human studies. Clin Pharmacokinet 2003; 42(5): 419-36.
[http://dx.doi.org/10.2165/00003088-200342050-00002] [PMID: 12739982]

[37] Yang Q, Lai SK. Anti-PEG immunity: emergence, characteristics, and unaddressed questions. Wiley Interdiscip Rev Nanomed Nanobiotechnol 2015; 7(5): 655-77.
[http://dx.doi.org/10.1002/wnan.1339] [PMID: 25707913]

[38] Vonarbourg A, Passirani C, Saulnier P, Benoit JP. Parameters influencing the stealthiness of colloidal drug delivery systems. Biomaterials 2006; 27(24): 4356-73.
[http://dx.doi.org/10.1016/j.biomaterials.2006.03.039] [PMID: 16650890]

[39] Klibanov AL, Maruyama K, Torchilin VP, Huang L. Amphipathic polyethyleneglycols effectively prolong the circulation time of liposomes. FEBS Lett 1990; 268(1): 235-7.
[http://dx.doi.org/10.1016/0014-5793(90)81016-H] [PMID: 2384160]

[40] Nagarajan R. Solubilization of Hydrophobic Substances by Block Copolymer Micelles in Aqeous Solutions Solvents and Self-organization of Polymers. Springer 1996; pp. 121-65.

[41] Allen C, Maysinger D, Eisenberg A. Nano-engineering block copolymer aggregates for drug delivery. Colloids Surf B Biointerfaces 1999; 16(1-4): 3-27.
[http://dx.doi.org/10.1016/S0927-7765(99)00058-2]

[42] Hussein Y, Youssry M. Polymeric micelles of biodegradable diblock copolymers: Enhanced encapsulation of hydrophobic drugs. Materials (Basel) 2018; 11(5): 688.
[http://dx.doi.org/10.3390/ma11050688] [PMID: 29702593]

[43] Yu JJ, Lee HA, Kim JH, *et al.* Bio-distribution and anti-tumor efficacy of PEG/PLA nano particles loaded doxorubicin. J Drug Target 2007; 15(4): 279-84.
[http://dx.doi.org/10.1080/10611860701357235] [PMID: 17487696]

[44] La SB, Okano T, Kataoka K. Preparation and characterization of the micelle-forming polymeric drug indomethacin-incorporated poly(ethylene oxide)-poly(β-benzyl L-aspartate) block copolymer micelles. J Pharm Sci 1996; 85(1): 85-90.

[http://dx.doi.org/10.1021/js950204r] [PMID: 8926590]

[45] Kwon GS, Naito M, Kataoka K, Yokoyama M, Sakurai Y, Okano T. Block copolymer micelles as vehicles for hydrophobic drugs. Colloids Surf B Biointerfaces 1994; 2(4): 429-34. [http://dx.doi.org/10.1016/0927-7765(94)80007-3]

[46] Kwon G, Naito M, Yokoyama M, Okano T, Sakurai Y, Kataoka K. Block copolymer micelles for drug delivery: loading and release of doxorubicin. J Control Release 1997; 48(2-3): 195-201. [http://dx.doi.org/10.1016/S0168-3659(97)00039-4]

[47] Kwon GS, Naito M, Yokoyama M, Okano T, Sakurai Y, Kataoka K. Physical entrapment of adriamycin in AB block copolymer micelles. Pharm Res 1995; 12(2): 192-5. [http://dx.doi.org/10.1023/A:1016266523505] [PMID: 7784332]

[48] Lavasanifar A, Samuel J, Kwon GS. Micelles of poly(ethylene oxide)-block-poly(N-alkyl stearateL-aspartamide): synthetic analogues of lipoproteins for drug delivery. J Biomed Mater Res 2000; 52(4): 831-5. [http://dx.doi.org/10.1002/1097-4636(20001215)52:4<831::AID-JBM29>3.0.CO;2-K] [PMID: 11033567]

[49] Fernandez AM, Van derpoorten K, Dasnois L, *et al.* N-Succinyl-(β-alanyl-L-leucyl-L--lanyl-L-leucyl)doxorubicin: an extracellularly tumor-activated prodrug devoid of intravenous acute toxicity. J Med Chem 2001; 44(22): 3750-3. [http://dx.doi.org/10.1021/jm0108754] [PMID: 11606140]

[50] Vickers NJ. Animal communication: when i'm calling you, will you answer too? Curr Biol 2017; 27(14): R713-5. [http://dx.doi.org/10.1016/j.cub.2017.05.064] [PMID: 28743020]

[51] Yu BG, Okano T, Kataoka K, Kwon G. Polymeric micelles for drug delivery: solubilization and haemolytic activity of amphotericin B. J Control Release 1998; 53(1-3): 131-6. [http://dx.doi.org/10.1016/S0168-3659(97)00245-9] [PMID: 9741920]

[52] Liaw J, Aoyagi T, Kataoka K, Sakurai Y, Okano T. Visualization of PEO-PBLA-pyrene polymeric micelles by atomic force microscopy. Pharm Res 1998; 15(11): 1721-6. [http://dx.doi.org/10.1023/A:1011908728838] [PMID: 9833994]

[53] Görner T, Gref R, Michenot D, Sommer F, Tran MN, Dellacherie E. Lidocaine-loaded biodegradable nanospheres. I. Optimization Of the drug incorporation into the polymer matrix. J Control Release 1999; 57(3): 259-68. [http://dx.doi.org/10.1016/S0168-3659(98)00121-7] [PMID: 9895413]

[54] Liu J, Xiao Y, Allen C. Polymer–drug compatibility: A guide to the development of delivery systems for the anticancer agent, ellipticine. J Pharm Sci 2004; 93(1): 132-43. [http://dx.doi.org/10.1002/jps.10533] [PMID: 14648643]

[55] Xiang G-H, Hong G-B, Wang Y, Cheng D, Zhou J-X, Shuai X-T. Effect of PEG-PDLLA polymeric nanovesicles loaded with doxorubicin and hematoporphyrin monomethyl ether on human hepatocellular carcinoma HepG2 cells *in vitro*. Int J Nanomedicine 2013; 8: 4613-22. [PMID: 24324333]

[56] Shi L, Song XB, Wang Y, *et al.* Docetaxel-conjugated monomethoxy-poly(ethylene glycol)---poly(lactide) (mPEG-PLA) polymeric micelles to enhance the therapeutic efficacy in oral squamous cell carcinoma. RSC Advances 2016; 6(49): 42819-26. [http://dx.doi.org/10.1039/C6RA03332F]

[57] Cui Y, Zhang M, Zeng F, Jin H, Xu Q, Huang Y. Dual-targeting magnetic PLGA nanoparticles for codelivery of paclitaxel and curcumin for brain tumor therapy. ACS Appl Mater Interfaces 2016; 8(47): 32159-69. [http://dx.doi.org/10.1021/acsami.6b10175] [PMID: 27808492]

[58] Li Y, Zhang T, Liu Q, He J. PEG-Derivatized Dual-Functional Nanomicelles for Improved Cancer

Therapy. Front Pharmacol 2019; 10: 808.
[http://dx.doi.org/10.3389/fphar.2019.00808] [PMID: 31379579]

[59] Kataoka K, Matsumoto T, Yokoyama M, *et al.* Doxorubicin-loaded poly(ethylene glycol)–poly(β-benzyl-l-aspartate) copolymer micelles: their pharmaceutical characteristics and biological significance. J Control Release 2000; 64(1-3): 143-53.
[http://dx.doi.org/10.1016/S0168-3659(99)00133-9] [PMID: 10640653]

[60] Hassankhani Rad A, Asiaee F, Jafari S, Shayanfar A, Lavasanifar A, Molavi O. Poly(ethylene glycol)-poly(ε-caprolactone)-based micelles for solubilization and tumor-targeted delivery of silibinin. Bioimpacts 2019; 10(2): 87-95.
[http://dx.doi.org/10.34172/bi.2020.11] [PMID: 32363152]

[61] Kadina YA, Razuvaeva EV, Streltsov DR, *et al.* Poly (Ethylene Glycol)-b-Poly (D, L-Lactide) nanoparticles as potential carriers for anticancer drug oxaliplatin. Molecules 2021; 26(3): 602.
[http://dx.doi.org/10.3390/molecules26030602] [PMID: 33498932]

[62] Gao N, Chen Z, Xiao X, *et al.* Surface modification of paclitaxel-loaded tri-block copolymer PLGA---PEG-b-PLGA nanoparticles with protamine for liver cancer therapy. J Nanopart Res 2015; 17(8): 347.
[http://dx.doi.org/10.1007/s11051-015-3121-3]

[63] Hoang NH, Lim C, Sim T, *et al.* Characterization of a triblock copolymer, poly(ethylene glycol)-polylactide-poly(ethylene glycol), with different structures for anticancer drug delivery applications. Polym Bull 2017; 74(5): 1595-609.
[http://dx.doi.org/10.1007/s00289-016-1791-3]

[64] Hoang NH, Lim C, Sim T, Oh KT. Triblock copolymers for nano-sized drug delivery systems. J Pharm Investig 2017; 47(1): 27-35.
[http://dx.doi.org/10.1007/s40005-016-0291-7]

[65] Ruan G, Feng SS. Preparation and characterization of poly(lactic acid)–poly(ethylene glycol)–poly(lactic acid) (PLA–PEG–PLA) microspheres for controlled release of paclitaxel. Biomaterials 2003; 24(27): 5037-44.
[http://dx.doi.org/10.1016/S0142-9612(03)00419-8] [PMID: 14559017]

[66] Song HT, Hoang NH, Yun JM, *et al.* Development of a new tri-block copolymer with a functional end and its feasibility for treatment of metastatic breast cancer. Colloids Surf B Biointerfaces 2016; 144: 73-80.
[http://dx.doi.org/10.1016/j.colsurfb.2016.04.002] [PMID: 27070054]

[67] Hoang NH, Sim T, Lim C, *et al.* A nano-sized blending system comprising identical triblock copolymers with different hydrophobicity for fabrication of an anticancer drug nanovehicle with high stability and solubilizing capacity. Int J Nanomedicine 2019; 14: 3629-44.
[http://dx.doi.org/10.2147/IJN.S191126] [PMID: 31190816]

[68] Venkatraman SS, Jie P, Min F, Freddy BYC, Leong-Huat G. Micelle-like nanoparticles of PLA–PEG–PLA triblock copolymer as chemotherapeutic carrier. Int J Pharm 2005; 298(1): 219-32.
[http://dx.doi.org/10.1016/j.ijpharm.2005.03.023] [PMID: 15946811]

[69] Callari M, Wong S, Lu H, Aldrich-Wright J, de Souza P, Stenzel MH. Drug induced self-assembly of triblock copolymers into polymersomes for the synergistic dual-drug delivery of platinum drugs and paclitaxel. Polym Chem 2017; 8(40): 6289-99.
[http://dx.doi.org/10.1039/C7PY01162H]

[70] Alami-Milani M, Zakeri-Milani P, Valizadeh H, Salehi R, Jelvehgari M. Preparation and evaluation of PCL-PEG-PCL micelles as potential nanocarriers for ocular delivery of dexamethasone. Iran J Basic Med Sci 2018; 21(2): 153-64.
[PMID: 29456812]

[71] Suk JS, Xu Q, Kim N, Hanes J, Ensign LM. PEGylation as a strategy for improving nanoparticle-based drug and gene delivery. Adv Drug Deliv Rev 2016; 99(Pt A): 28-51.

[http://dx.doi.org/10.1016/j.addr.2015.09.012] [PMID: 26456916]

[72] Mozar FS, Chowdhury EH. Impact of PEGylated nanoparticles on tumor targeted drug delivery. Curr Pharm Des 2018; 24(28): 3283-96.
[http://dx.doi.org/10.2174/1381612824666180730161721] [PMID: 30062957]

[73] Bhardwaj A, Kumar L, Mehta S, Mehta A. Stimuli-sensitive Systems-an emerging delivery system for drugs. Artif Cells Nanomed Biotechnol 2015; 43(5): 299-310.
[http://dx.doi.org/10.3109/21691401.2013.856016] [PMID: 26561681]

[74] Wu H, Zhu L, Torchilin VP. pH-sensitive poly(histidine)-PEG/DSPE-PEG co-polymer micelles for cytosolic drug delivery. Biomaterials 2013; 34(4): 1213-22.
[http://dx.doi.org/10.1016/j.biomaterials.2012.08.072] [PMID: 23102622]

[75] Li G, Meng Y, Guo L, Zhang T, Liu J. Formation of thermo-sensitive polyelectrolyte complex micelles from two biocompatible graft copolymers for drug delivery. J Biomed Mater Res A 2014; 102(7): 2163-72.
[http://dx.doi.org/10.1002/jbm.a.34894] [PMID: 23894021]

[76] Torchilin V. Multifunctional and stimuli-sensitive pharmaceutical nanocarriers. Eur J Pharm Biopharm 2009; 71(3): 431-44.
[http://dx.doi.org/10.1016/j.ejpb.2008.09.026] [PMID: 18977297]

[77] Kamaly N, Xiao Z, Valencia PM, Radovic-Moreno AF, Farokhzad OC. Targeted polymeric therapeutic nanoparticles: design, development and clinical translation. Chem Soc Rev 2012; 41(7): 2971-3010.
[http://dx.doi.org/10.1039/c2cs15344k] [PMID: 22388185]

[78] Russo A, DeGraff W, Friedman N, Mitchell JB. Selective modulation of glutathione levels in human normal versus tumor cells and subsequent differential response to chemotherapy drugs. Cancer Res 1986; 46(6): 2845-8.
[PMID: 2421885]

[79] Ghadiali JE, Stevens MM. Enzyme□responsive nanoparticle systems. Adv Mater 2008; 20(22): 4359-63.
[http://dx.doi.org/10.1002/adma.200703158]

[80] Zhu L, Kate P, Torchilin VP. Matrix metalloprotease 2-responsive multifunctional liposomal nanocarrier for enhanced tumor targeting. ACS Nano 2012; 6(4): 3491-8.
[http://dx.doi.org/10.1021/nn300524f] [PMID: 22409425]

[81] Zhao Y, Butler EB, Tan M. Stimuli-responsive nanocarriers for drug delivery. Nature materials 2013; 12(11): 991-1003.
[http://dx.doi.org/10.1038/cddis.2013.60]

[82] Mura S, Nicolas J, Couvreur P. Stimuli-responsive nanocarriers for drug delivery. Nat Mater 2013; 12(11): 991-1003.
[http://dx.doi.org/10.1038/nmat3776] [PMID: 24150417]

[83] Perche F, Torchilin VP. Recent trends in multifunctional liposomal nanocarriers for enhanced tumor targeting. J Drug Deliv 2013; 2013: 705265.
[http://dx.doi.org/10.1155/2013/705265]

[84] Fleige E, Quadir MA, Haag R. Stimuli-responsive polymeric nanocarriers for the controlled transport of active compounds: Concepts and applications. Adv Drug Deliv Rev 2012; 64(9): 866-84.
[http://dx.doi.org/10.1016/j.addr.2012.01.020] [PMID: 22349241]

[85] Vaupel P, Kallinowski F, Okunieff P. Blood flow, oxygen and nutrient supply, and metabolic microenvironment of human tumors: a review. Cancer Res 1989; 49(23): 6449-65.
[PMID: 2684393]

[86] Gao W, Chan JM, Farokhzad OC. pH-Responsive nanoparticles for drug delivery. Mol Pharm 2010; 7(6): 1913-20.

[http://dx.doi.org/10.1021/mp100253e] [PMID: 20836539]

[87] Mukherjee S, Ghosh RN, Maxfield FR. Endocytosis. Physiological Reviews 1997; 77(3): 759-803.

[88] Tang H, Zhao W, Yu J, Li Y, Zhao C. Recent development of pH-responsive polymers for cancer nanomedicine. Molecules 2018; 24(1): 4.
[http://dx.doi.org/10.3390/molecules24010004] [PMID: 30577475]

[89] Kocak G, Tuncer C, Bütün V. pH-Responsive polymers. Polym Chem 2017; 8(1): 144-76.
[http://dx.doi.org/10.1039/C6PY01872F]

[90] Liu H, Chen H, Cao F, Peng D, Chen W, Zhang C. Amphiphilic block copolymer poly (acrylic acid)-b-polycaprolactone as a novel pH-sensitive nanocarrier for anti-cancer drugs delivery: In-vitro and in-vivo evaluation. Polymers (Basel) 2019; 11(5): 820.
[http://dx.doi.org/10.3390/polym11050820] [PMID: 31067730]

[91] Zhang M, Zhu J, Zheng Y, *et al.* Doxorubicin-conjugated PAMAM dendrimers for pH-responsive drug release and folic acid-targeted cancer therapy. Pharmaceutics 2018; 10(3): 162.
[http://dx.doi.org/10.3390/pharmaceutics10030162] [PMID: 30235881]

[92] Kozlovskaya V, Chen J, Tedjo C, *et al.* pH-responsive hydrogel cubes for release of doxorubicin in cancer cells. J Mater Chem B Mater Biol Med 2014; 2(17): 2494-507.
[http://dx.doi.org/10.1039/C4TB00165F] [PMID: 32261419]

[93] Işıklan N, Tokmak Ş. Development of thermo/pH-responsive chitosan coated pectin-graft-poly(N-N-diethyl acrylamide) microcarriers. Carbohydr Polym 2019; 218: 112-25.
[http://dx.doi.org/10.1016/j.carbpol.2019.04.068] [PMID: 31221312]

[94] Xu P, Van Kirk EA, Murdoch WJ, *et al.* Anticancer efficacies of cisplatin-releasing pH-responsive nanoparticles. Biomacromolecules 2006; 7(3): 829-35.
[http://dx.doi.org/10.1021/bm050902y] [PMID: 16529420]

[95] Jin Y, Ren X, Wang W, *et al.* A 5-fluorouracil-loaded pH-responsive dendrimer nanocarrier for tumor targeting. Int J Pharm 2011; 420(2): 378-84.
[http://dx.doi.org/10.1016/j.ijpharm.2011.08.053] [PMID: 21925254]

[96] Yu H, Zou Y, Wang Y, *et al.* Overcoming endosomal barrier by amphotericin B-loaded dual pH-responsive PDMA-b-PDPA micelleplexes for siRNA delivery. ACS Nano 2011; 5(11): 9246-55.
[http://dx.doi.org/10.1021/nn203503h] [PMID: 22011045]

[97] Yao Y, Saw PE, Nie Y, *et al.* Multifunctional sharp pH-responsive nanoparticles for targeted drug delivery and effective breast cancer therapy. J Mater Chem B Mater Biol Med 2019; 7(4): 576-85.
[http://dx.doi.org/10.1039/C8TB02600A] [PMID: 32254791]

[98] Lo YL, Chang CH, Wang CS, *et al.* PEG-coated nanoparticles detachable in acidic microenvironments for the tumor-directed delivery of chemo- and gene therapies for head and neck cancer. Theranostics 2020; 10(15): 6695-714.
[http://dx.doi.org/10.7150/thno.45164] [PMID: 32550898]

[99] Boomer JA, Thompson DH. Synthesis of acid-labile diplasmenyl lipids for drug and gene delivery applications. Chem Phys Lipids 1999; 99(2): 145-53.
[http://dx.doi.org/10.1016/S0009-3084(99)00033-X] [PMID: 10390837]

[100] Gu Y, Zhong Y, Meng F, Cheng R, Deng C, Zhong Z. Acetal-linked paclitaxel prodrug micellar nanoparticles as a versatile and potent platform for cancer therapy. Biomacromolecules 2013; 14(8): 2772-80.
[http://dx.doi.org/10.1021/bm400615n] [PMID: 23777504]

[101] Alsehli M. Polymeric nanocarriers as stimuli-responsive systems for targeted tumor (cancer) therapy: Recent advances in drug delivery. Saudi Pharm J 2020; 28(3): 255-65.
[http://dx.doi.org/10.1016/j.jsps.2020.01.004] [PMID: 32194326]

[102] Bae Y, Jang WD, Nishiyama N, Fukushima S, Kataoka K. Multifunctional polymeric micelles with

folate-mediated cancer cell targeting and pH-triggered drug releasing properties for active intracellular drug delivery. Mol Biosyst 2005; 1(3): 242-50.
[http://dx.doi.org/10.1039/b500266d] [PMID: 16880988]

[103] Zhu L, Torchilin VP. Stimulus-responsive nanopreparations for tumor targeting. Integr Biol 2013; 5(1): 96-107.
[http://dx.doi.org/10.1039/c2ib20135f] [PMID: 22869005]

[104] Ward MA, Georgiou TK. Thermoresponsive polymers for biomedical applications. Polymers (Basel) 2011; 3(3): 1215-42.
[http://dx.doi.org/10.3390/polym3031215]

[105] Schmaljohann D. Thermo- and pH-responsive polymers in drug delivery. Adv Drug Deliv Rev 2006; 58(15): 1655-70.
[http://dx.doi.org/10.1016/j.addr.2006.09.020] [PMID: 17125884]

[106] Shibayama M, Mizutani S, Nomura S. Thermal properties of copolymer gels containing N-isopropylacrylamide. Macromolecules 1996; 29(6): 2019-24.
[http://dx.doi.org/10.1021/ma951390q]

[107] Idziak I, Avoce D, Lessard D, Gravel D, Zhu XX. Thermosensitivity of aqueous solutions of poly (N, N-diethylacrylamide). Macromolecules 1999; 32(4): 1260-3.
[http://dx.doi.org/10.1021/ma981171f]

[108] Van Durme K, Verbrugghe S, Du Prez FE, Van Mele B. Influence of poly (ethylene oxide) grafts on kinetics of LCST behavior in aqueous poly (N-vinylcaprolactam) solutions and networks studied by modulated temperature DSC. Macromolecules 2004; 37(3): 1054-61.
[http://dx.doi.org/10.1021/ma035319t]

[109] San Miguel V, Limer AJ, Haddleton DM, Catalina F, Peinado C. Biodegradable and thermoresponsive micelles of triblock copolymers based on 2-(N,N-dimethylamino)ethyl methacrylate and ε-caprolactone for controlled drug delivery. Eur Polym J 2008; 44(11): 3853-63.
[http://dx.doi.org/10.1016/j.eurpolymj.2008.07.056]

[110] Ta T, Porter TM. Thermosensitive liposomes for localized delivery and triggered release of chemotherapy. J Control Release 2013; 169(1-2): 112-25.
[http://dx.doi.org/10.1016/j.jconrel.2013.03.036] [PMID: 23583706]

[111] Huebers HA, Finch CA. The physiology of transferrin and transferrin receptors. Physiol Rev 1987; 67(2): 520-82.
[http://dx.doi.org/10.1152/physrev.1987.67.2.520] [PMID: 3550839]

[112] Richardson DR, Ponka P. The molecular mechanisms of the metabolism and transport of iron in normal and neoplastic cells. Biochim Biophys Acta Rev Biomembr 1997; 1331(1): 1-40.
[http://dx.doi.org/10.1016/S0304-4157(96)00014-7] [PMID: 9325434]

[113] Ogun AS, Adeyinka A. Biochemistry, Transferrin. StatPearls 2020. [Internet]

[114] Brandsma ME, Jevnikar AM, Ma S. Recombinant human transferrin: Beyond iron binding and transport. Biotechnol Adv 2011; 29(2): 230-8.
[http://dx.doi.org/10.1016/j.biotechadv.2010.11.007] [PMID: 21147210]

[115] Johnsen KB, Burkhart A, Thomsen LB, Andresen TL, Moos T. Targeting the transferrin receptor for brain drug delivery. Prog Neurobiol 2019; 181: 101665.
[http://dx.doi.org/10.1016/j.pneurobio.2019.101665] [PMID: 31376426]

[116] Daniels TR, Bernabeu E, Rodríguez JA, *et al.* The transferrin receptor and the targeted delivery of therapeutic agents against cancer. Biochim Biophys Acta, Gen Subj 2012; 1820(3): 291-317.
[http://dx.doi.org/10.1016/j.bbagen.2011.07.016] [PMID: 21851850]

[117] Lu Y, Zhu D, Gui L, *et al.* A dual-targeting ruthenium nanodrug that inhibits primary tumor growth and lung metastasis *via* the PARP/ATM pathway. J Nanobiotechnology 2021; 19(1): 115.
[http://dx.doi.org/10.1186/s12951-021-00799-3] [PMID: 33892746]

[118] Daniels TR, Delgado T, Rodriguez JA, Helguera G, Penichet ML. The transferrin receptor part I: Biology and targeting with cytotoxic antibodies for the treatment of cancer. Clin Immunol 2006; 121(2): 144-58.
[http://dx.doi.org/10.1016/j.clim.2006.06.010] [PMID: 16904380]

[119] Guo Y, Wang L, Lv P, Zhang P. Transferrin-conjugated doxorubicin-loaded lipid-coated nanoparticles for the targeting and therapy of lung cancer. Oncol Lett 2015; 9(3): 1065-72.
[http://dx.doi.org/10.3892/ol.2014.2840] [PMID: 25663858]

[120] Choudhury H, Pandey M, Chin PX, *et al.* Transferrin receptors-targeting nanocarriers for efficient targeted delivery and transcytosis of drugs into the brain tumors: a review of recent advancements and emerging trends. Drug Deliv Transl Res 2018; 8(5): 1545-63.
[http://dx.doi.org/10.1007/s13346-018-0552-2] [PMID: 29916012]

[121] Zhang P, Hu L, Yin Q, Zhang Z, Feng L, Li Y. Transferrin-conjugated polyphosphoester hybrid micelle loading paclitaxel for brain-targeting delivery: Synthesis, preparation and *in vivo* evaluation. J Control Release 2012; 159(3): 429-34.
[http://dx.doi.org/10.1016/j.jconrel.2012.01.031] [PMID: 22306333]

[122] Mishra V, Mahor S, Rawat A, *et al.* Targeted brain delivery of AZT *via* transferrin anchored pegylated albumin nanoparticles. J Drug Target 2006; 14(1): 45-53.
[http://dx.doi.org/10.1080/10611860600612953] [PMID: 16603451]

[123] Kakudo T, Chaki S, Futaki S, *et al.* Transferrin-modified liposomes equipped with a pH-sensitive fusogenic peptide: an artificial viral-like delivery system. Biochemistry 2004; 43(19): 5618-28.
[http://dx.doi.org/10.1021/bi035802w] [PMID: 15134436]

[124] Müller C, Schibli R. Folic acid conjugates for nuclear imaging of folate receptor-positive cancer. J Nucl Med 2011; 52(1): 1-4.
[http://dx.doi.org/10.2967/jnumed.110.076018] [PMID: 21149477]

[125] Yoo HS, Park TG. Folate-receptor-targeted delivery of doxorubicin nano-aggregates stabilized by doxorubicin–PEG–folate conjugate. J Control Release 2004; 100(2): 247-56.
[http://dx.doi.org/10.1016/j.jconrel.2004.08.017] [PMID: 15544872]

[126] Yoo J, Park C, Yi G, Lee D, Koo H. Active targeting strategies using biological ligands for nanoparticle drug delivery systems. Cancers (Basel) 2019; 11(5): 640.
[http://dx.doi.org/10.3390/cancers11050640] [PMID: 31072061]

[127] Velikyan I. Radionuclides for imaging and therapy in oncology. In: Chen X, Wong S, Eds. Cancer Theranostics. Amsterdam, The Netherlands: Elsevier 2014; pp. 285-325.

[128] Lee RJ, Low PS. Folate-mediated tumor cell targeting of liposome-entrapped doxorubicin *in vitro*. Biochim Biophys Acta Biomembr 1995; 1233(2): 134-44.
[http://dx.doi.org/10.1016/0005-2736(94)00235-H] [PMID: 7865538]

[129] Mansouri S, Cuie Y, Winnik F, *et al.* Characterization of folate-chitosan-DNA nanoparticles for gene therapy. Biomaterials 2006; 27(9): 2060-5.
[http://dx.doi.org/10.1016/j.biomaterials.2005.09.020] [PMID: 16202449]

[130] Liang X, Luo M, Wei XW, *et al.* A folate receptor-targeted lipoplex delivering interleukin-15 gene for colon cancer immunotherapy. Oncotarget 2016; 7(32): 52207-17.
[http://dx.doi.org/10.18632/oncotarget.10537] [PMID: 27438147]

[131] Fernández M, Javaid F, Chudasama V. Advances in targeting the folate receptor in the treatment/imaging of cancers. Chem Sci (Camb) 2018; 9(4): 790-810.
[http://dx.doi.org/10.1039/C7SC04004K] [PMID: 29675145]

[132] Lee RJ, Wang S, Low PS. Measurement of endosome pH following folate receptor-mediated endocytosis. Biochim Biophys Acta Mol Cell Res 1996; 1312(3): 237-42.
[http://dx.doi.org/10.1016/0167-4889(96)00041-9] [PMID: 8703993]

[133] Wileman T, Harding C, Stahl P. Receptor-mediated endocytosis. Biochem J 1985; 232(1): 1-14. [http://dx.doi.org/10.1042/bj2320001] [PMID: 2867759]

[134] Paulos CM, Reddy JA, Leamon CP, Turk MJ, Low PS. Ligand binding and kinetics of folate receptor recycling *in vivo*: impact on receptor-mediated drug delivery. Mol Pharmacol 2004; 66(6): 1406-14. [http://dx.doi.org/10.1124/mol.104.003723] [PMID: 15371560]

[135] Montazerabadi A, Beik J, Irajirad R, *et al.* Folate-modified and curcumin-loaded dendritic magnetite nanocarriers for the targeted thermo-chemotherapy of cancer cells. Artif Cells Nanomed Biotechnol 2019; 47(1): 330-40. [http://dx.doi.org/10.1080/21691401.2018.1557670] [PMID: 30688084]

[136] Vinothini K, Rajendran NK, Ramu A, Elumalai N, Rajan M. Folate receptor targeted delivery of paclitaxel to breast cancer cells *via* folic acid conjugated graphene oxide grafted methyl acrylate nanocarrier. Biomed Pharmacother 2019; 110: 906-17. [http://dx.doi.org/10.1016/j.biopha.2018.12.008] [PMID: 30572195]

[137] Hemati Azandaryani A, Kashanian S, Derakhshandeh K. Folate conjugated hybrid nanocarrier for targeted letrozole delivery in breast cancer treatment. Pharm Res 2017; 34(12): 2798-808. [http://dx.doi.org/10.1007/s11095-017-2260-x] [PMID: 29110284]

[138] Yoo MK, Park IK, Lim HT, *et al.* Folate–PEG–superparamagnetic iron oxide nanoparticles for lung cancer imaging. Acta Biomater 2012; 8(8): 3005-13. [http://dx.doi.org/10.1016/j.actbio.2012.04.029] [PMID: 22543005]

[139] He Z, Huang J, Xu Y, *et al.* Co-delivery of cisplatin and paclitaxel by folic acid conjugated amphiphilic PEG-PLGA copolymer nanoparticles for the treatment of non-small lung cancer. Oncotarget 2015; 6(39): 42150-68. [http://dx.doi.org/10.18632/oncotarget.6243] [PMID: 26517524]

[140] Asadishad B, Vossoughi M, Alemzadeh I. Folate-receptor-targeted delivery of doxorubicin using polyethylene glycol-functionalized gold nanoparticles. Ind Eng Chem Res 2010; 49(4): 1958-63. [http://dx.doi.org/10.1021/ie9011479]

[141] Luiz MT, Abriata JP, Raspantini GL, *et al.* In vitro evaluation of folate-modified PLGA nanoparticles containing paclitaxel for ovarian cancer therapy. Mater Sci Eng C 2019; 105: 110038. [http://dx.doi.org/10.1016/j.msec.2019.110038] [PMID: 31546359]

[142] Choi H, Choi SR, Zhou R, Kung HF, Chen IW. Iron oxide nanoparticles as magnetic resonance contrast agent for tumor imaging *via* folate receptor-targeted delivery1. Acad Radiol 2004; 11(9): 996-1004. [http://dx.doi.org/10.1016/j.acra.2004.04.018] [PMID: 15350580]

[143] Venishetty VK, Komuravelli R, Kuncha M, Sistla R, Diwan PV. Increased brain uptake of docetaxel and ketoconazole loaded folate-grafted solid lipid nanoparticles. Nanomedicine 2013; 9(1): 111-21. [http://dx.doi.org/10.1016/j.nano.2012.03.003] [PMID: 22426195]

[144] Urmann K, Modrejewski J, Scheper T, Walter J-G. Aptamer-modified nanomaterials: principles and applications 2017; 18: 1-2. [http://dx.doi.org/10.1515/bnm-2016-0012]

[145] Odeh F, Nsairat H, Alshaer W, *et al.* Aptamers chemistry: Chemical modifications and conjugation strategies. Molecules 2019; 25(1): 3. [http://dx.doi.org/10.3390/molecules25010003] [PMID: 31861277]

[146] Wu X, Chen J, Wu M, Zhao JX. Aptamers: active targeting ligands for cancer diagnosis and therapy. Theranostics 2015; 5(4): 322-44. [http://dx.doi.org/10.7150/thno.10257] [PMID: 25699094]

[147] Zhou G, Wilson G, Hebbard L, *et al.* Aptamers: A promising chemical antibody for cancer therapy. Oncotarget 2016; 7(12): 13446-63. [http://dx.doi.org/10.18632/oncotarget.7178] [PMID: 26863567]

[148] Phillips JA, Lopez-Colon D, Zhu Z, Xu Y, Tan W. Applications of aptamers in cancer cell biology. Anal Chim Acta 2008; 621(2): 101-8.
[http://dx.doi.org/10.1016/j.aca.2008.05.031] [PMID: 18573375]

[149] Dua P, Kim S, Lee D. Nucleic acid aptamers targeting cell-surface proteins. Methods 2011; 54(2): 215-25.
[http://dx.doi.org/10.1016/j.ymeth.2011.02.002] [PMID: 21300154]

[150] Ireson CR, Kelland LR. Discovery and development of anticancer aptamers. Mol Cancer Ther 2006; 5(12): 2957-62.
[http://dx.doi.org/10.1158/1535-7163.MCT-06-0172] [PMID: 17172400]

[151] Zhu G, Niu G, Chen X. Aptamer–Drug Conjugates. Bioconjug Chem 2015; 26(11): 2186-97.
[http://dx.doi.org/10.1021/acs.bioconjchem.5b00291] [PMID: 26083153]

[152] Reinemann C, Strehlitz B. Aptamer-modified nanoparticles and their use in cancer diagnostics and treatment. Swiss Med Wkly 2014; 144(0102): w13908.
[http://dx.doi.org/10.4414/smw.2014.13908] [PMID: 24395443]

[153] Zhao N, Pei SN, Qi J, *et al.* Oligonucleotide aptamer-drug conjugates for targeted therapy of acute myeloid leukemia. Biomaterials 2015; 67: 42-51.
[http://dx.doi.org/10.1016/j.biomaterials.2015.07.025] [PMID: 26204224]

[154] Tan L, Neoh KG, Kang ET, Choe WS, Su X. PEGylated anti-MUC1 aptamer-doxorubicin complex for targeted drug delivery to MCF7 breast cancer cells. Macromol Biosci 2011; 11(10): 1331-5.
[http://dx.doi.org/10.1002/mabi.201100173] [PMID: 21818856]

[155] Powell Gray B, Kelly L, Ahrens DP, *et al.* Tunable cytotoxic aptamer–drug conjugates for the treatment of prostate cancer. Proc Natl Acad Sci USA 2018; 115(18): 4761-6.
[http://dx.doi.org/10.1073/pnas.1717705115] [PMID: 29666232]

[156] Zhou F, Wang P, Peng Y, *et al.* Molecular Engineering□Based Aptamer–Drug Conjugates with Accurate Tunability of Drug Ratios for Drug Combination Targeted Cancer Therapy. Angew Chem Int Ed 2019; 58(34): 11661-5.
[http://dx.doi.org/10.1002/anie.201903807] [PMID: 31125154]

[157] Deng Z, Yang Q, Peng Y, *et al.* Polymeric Engineering of Aptamer–Drug Conjugates for Targeted Cancer Therapy. Bioconjug Chem 2020; 31(1): 37-42.
[http://dx.doi.org/10.1021/acs.bioconjchem.9b00715] [PMID: 31815437]

[158] Li F, Mei H, Gao Y, *et al.* Co-delivery of oxygen and erlotinib by aptamer-modified liposomal complexes to reverse hypoxia-induced drug resistance in lung cancer. Biomaterials 2017; 145: 56-71.
[http://dx.doi.org/10.1016/j.biomaterials.2017.08.030] [PMID: 28843733]

[159] Yang Y, Zhao W, Tan W, *et al.* An efficient cell-targeting drug delivery system based on aptamer-modified mesoporous silica nanoparticles. Nanoscale Res Lett 2019; 14(1): 390.
[http://dx.doi.org/10.1186/s11671-019-3208-3] [PMID: 31872318]

[160] Yazdian-Robati R, Arab A, Ramezani M, *et al.* Smart aptamer-modified calcium carbonate nanoparticles for controlled release and targeted delivery of epirubicin and melittin into cancer cells *in vitro* and *in vivo*. Drug Dev Ind Pharm 2019; 45(4): 603-10.
[http://dx.doi.org/10.1080/03639045.2019.1569029] [PMID: 30633594]

[161] Motaghi H, Ziyaee S, Mehrgardi MA, Kajani AA, Bordbar AK. Electrochemiluminescence detection of human breast cancer cells using aptamer modified bipolar electrode mounted into 3D printed microchannel. Biosens Bioelectron 2018; 118: 217-23.
[http://dx.doi.org/10.1016/j.bios.2018.07.066] [PMID: 30092457]

[162] Xu L, He XY, Liu BY, *et al.* Aptamer-functionalized albumin-based nanoparticles for targeted drug delivery. Colloids Surf B Biointerfaces 2018; 171: 24-30.
[http://dx.doi.org/10.1016/j.colsurfb.2018.07.008] [PMID: 30005287]

[163] Spicer CD, Jumeaux C, Gupta B, Stevens MM. Peptide and protein nanoparticle conjugates: versatile platforms for biomedical applications. Chem Soc Rev 2018; 47(10): 3574-620. [http://dx.doi.org/10.1039/C7CS00877E] [PMID: 29479622]

[164] Ghosh D, Peng X, Leal J, Mohanty RP. Peptides as drug delivery vehicles across biological barriers. J Pharm Investig 2018; 48(1): 89-111. [http://dx.doi.org/10.1007/s40005-017-0374-0] [PMID: 29963321]

[165] Tang SY, Wei H, Yu CY. Peptide-functionalized delivery vehicles for enhanced cancer therapy. Int J Pharm 2021; 593: 120141. [http://dx.doi.org/10.1016/j.ijpharm.2020.120141] [PMID: 33279713]

[166] Li J, Feng L, Fan L, *et al.* Targeting the brain with PEG–PLGA nanoparticles modified with phage-displayed peptides. Biomaterials 2011; 32(21): 4943-50. [http://dx.doi.org/10.1016/j.biomaterials.2011.03.031] [PMID: 21470674]

[167] Cai L-L, Liu P, Li X, *et al.* RGD peptide-mediated chitosan-based polymeric micelles targeting delivery for integrin-overexpressing tumor cells. Int J Nanomedicine 2011; 6: 3499-508. [PMID: 22282676]

[168] Julien DC, Behnke S, Wang G, Murdoch GK, Hill RA, Eds. Utilization of monoclonal antibody-targeted nanomaterials in the treatment of cancer MAbs. Taylor & Francis 2011.

[169] Polakis P. Arming antibodies for cancer therapy. Curr Opin Pharmacol 2005; 5(4): 382-7. [http://dx.doi.org/10.1016/j.coph.2005.04.008] [PMID: 15951239]

[170] Juan A, Cimas FJ, Bravo I, Pandiella A, Ocaña A, Alonso-Moreno C. An Overview of Antibody Conjugated Polymeric Nanoparticles for Breast Cancer Therapy. Pharmaceutics 2020; 12(9): 802. [http://dx.doi.org/10.3390/pharmaceutics12090802] [PMID: 32854255]

[171] Pan X, Wu G, Yang W, Barth RF, Tjarks W, Lee RJ. Synthesis of cetuximab-immunoliposomes *via* a cholesterol-based membrane anchor for targeting of EGFR. Bioconjug Chem 2007; 18(1): 101-8. [http://dx.doi.org/10.1021/bc060174r] [PMID: 17226962]

[172] Zhao M, Sun Y, Zhu X, Chen D, Feng S, Guo S, *et al.* Antibody-Targeted Immunocarriers for Cancer Treatment. Smart Drug Delivery System 2016; p. 139.

[173] Dasargyri A, Kümin CD, Leroux JC. Targeting Nanocarriers with Anisamide: Fact or Artifact? Adv Mater 2017; 29(7): 1603451. [http://dx.doi.org/10.1002/adma.201603451] [PMID: 27885719]

[174] Jain RK, Stylianopoulos T. Delivering nanomedicine to solid tumors. Nat Rev Clin Oncol 2010; 7(11): 653-64. [http://dx.doi.org/10.1038/nrclinonc.2010.139] [PMID: 20838415]

[175] Banerjee R, Tyagi P, Li S, Huang L. Anisamide-targeted stealth liposomes: A potent carrier for targeting doxorubicin to human prostate cancer cells. Int J Cancer 2004; 112(4): 693-700. [http://dx.doi.org/10.1002/ijc.20452] [PMID: 15382053]

[176] Jalilian M, Derakhshandeh K, Kurd M, Lashani H. Targeting Solid Lipid Nanoparticles with Anisamide for Docetaxel Delivery to Prostate Cancer: Preparation, Optimization, and *In-vitro* Evaluation. Iran J Pharm Res 2021; 20(1): 327-38. [PMID: 34400962]

[177] Fitzgerald KA, Malhotra M, Gooding M, *et al.* A novel, anisamide-targeted cyclodextrin nanoformulation for siRNA delivery to prostate cancer cells expressing the sigma-1 receptor. Int J Pharm 2016; 499(1-2): 131-45. [http://dx.doi.org/10.1016/j.ijpharm.2015.12.055] [PMID: 26721726]

[178] Fitzgerald KA, Rahme K, Guo J, Holmes JD, O'Driscoll CM. Anisamide-targeted gold nanoparticles for siRNA delivery in prostate cancer – synthesis, physicochemical characterisation and *in vitro* evaluation. J Mater Chem B Mater Biol Med 2016; 4(13): 2242-52.

[http://dx.doi.org/10.1039/C6TB00082G] [PMID: 32263220]

[179] Garg NK, Dwivedi P, Campbell C, Tyagi RK. Site specific/targeted delivery of gemcitabine through anisamide anchored chitosan/poly ethylene glycol nanoparticles: An improved understanding of lung cancer therapeutic intervention. Eur J Pharm Sci 2012; 47(5): 1006-14. [http://dx.doi.org/10.1016/j.ejps.2012.09.012] [PMID: 23041219]

[180] Lu L, Zou Y, Yang W, *et al.* Anisamide-decorated pH-sensitive degradable chimaeric polymersomes mediate potent and targeted protein delivery to lung cancer cells. Biomacromolecules 2015; 16(6): 1726-35. [http://dx.doi.org/10.1021/acs.biomac.5b00193] [PMID: 25938556]

[181] Ramzy L, Metwally AA, Nasr M, Awad GAS. Novel thymoquinone lipidic core nanocapsules with anisamide-polymethacrylate shell for colon cancer cells overexpressing sigma receptors. Sci Rep 2020; 10(1): 10987. [http://dx.doi.org/10.1038/s41598-020-67748-2] [PMID: 32620860]

[182] Qu D, Jiao M, Lin H, *et al.* Anisamide-functionalized pH-responsive amphiphilic chitosan-based paclitaxel micelles for sigma-1 receptor targeted prostate cancer treatment. Carbohydr Polym 2020; 229: 115498. [http://dx.doi.org/10.1016/j.carbpol.2019.115498] [PMID: 31826492]

[183] Wang L, Pei J, Cong Z, *et al.* Development of anisamide-targeted PEGylated gold nanorods to deliver epirubicin for chemo-photothermal therapy in tumor-bearing mice. Int J Nanomedicine 2019; 14: 1817-33. [http://dx.doi.org/10.2147/IJN.S192520] [PMID: 30880982]

[184] Gessner I, Neundorf I. Nanoparticles modified with cell-penetrating peptides: Conjugation mechanisms, physicochemical properties, and application in cancer diagnosis and therapy. Int J Mol Sci 2020; 21(7): 2536. [http://dx.doi.org/10.3390/ijms21072536] [PMID: 32268473]

[185] Deshayes S, Morris MC, Divita G, Heitz F. Cell-penetrating peptides: tools for intracellular delivery of therapeutics. Cell Mol Life Sci 2005; 62(16): 1839-49. [http://dx.doi.org/10.1007/s00018-005-5109-0] [PMID: 15968462]

[186] Borrelli A, Tornesello A, Tornesello M, Buonaguro F. Cell penetrating peptides as molecular carriers for anti-cancer agents. Molecules 2018; 23(2): 295. [http://dx.doi.org/10.3390/molecules23020295] [PMID: 29385037]

[187] Derakhshankhah H, Jafari S. Cell penetrating peptides: A concise review with emphasis on biomedical applications. Biomed Pharmacother 2018; 108: 1090-6. [http://dx.doi.org/10.1016/j.biopha.2018.09.097] [PMID: 30372809]

[188] Milletti F. Cell-penetrating peptides: classes, origin, and current landscape. Drug Discov Today 2012; 17(15-16): 850-60. [http://dx.doi.org/10.1016/j.drudis.2012.03.002] [PMID: 22465171]

[189] Pooga M, Langel Ü. Classes of cell-penetrating peptides Cell-Penetrating Peptides. Springer 2015; pp. 3-28. [http://dx.doi.org/10.1007/978-1-4939-2806-4_1]

[190] Cai H, Liang Z, Huang W, Wen L, Chen G. Engineering PLGA nano-based systems through understanding the influence of nanoparticle properties and cell-penetrating peptides for cochlear drug delivery. Int J Pharm 2017; 532(1): 55-65. [http://dx.doi.org/10.1016/j.ijpharm.2017.08.084] [PMID: 28870763]

[191] Lindgren M, Rosenthal-Aizman K, Saar K, *et al.* Overcoming methotrexate resistance in breast cancer tumour cells by the use of a new cell-penetrating peptide. Biochem Pharmacol 2006; 71(4): 416-25. [http://dx.doi.org/10.1016/j.bcp.2005.10.048] [PMID: 16376307]

[192] Torchilin VP. Tat peptide-mediated intracellular delivery of pharmaceutical nanocarriers. Adv Drug

Deliv Rev 2008; 60(4-5): 548-58.
[http://dx.doi.org/10.1016/j.addr.2007.10.008] [PMID: 18053612]

[193] Xiao Q, Dong X, Yang F, *et al.* Engineered Cell□Penetrating Peptides for Mitochondrion□Targeted Drug Delivery in Cancer Therapy. Chemistry 2021; 27(59): 14721-9.
[http://dx.doi.org/10.1002/chem.202102523] [PMID: 34436802]

[194] Rudolph C, Schillinger U, Ortiz A, *et al.* Application of novel solid lipid nanoparticle (SLN)-gene vector formulations based on a dimeric HIV-1 TAT-peptide *in vitro* and *in vivo*. Pharm Res 2004; 21(9): 1662-9.
[http://dx.doi.org/10.1023/B:PHAM.0000041463.56768.ec] [PMID: 15497694]

[195] Kleemann E, Neu M, Jekel N, *et al.* Nano-carriers for DNA delivery to the lung based upon a TAT-derived peptide covalently coupled to PEG–PEI. J Control Release 2005; 109(1-3): 299-316.
[http://dx.doi.org/10.1016/j.jconrel.2005.09.036] [PMID: 16298009]

[196] Zhao Y. Rational design of light-controllable polymer micelles. Chem Rec 2007; 7(5): 286-94.
[http://dx.doi.org/10.1002/tcr.20127] [PMID: 17924441]

[197] Fomina N, Sankaranarayanan J, Almutairi A. Photochemical mechanisms of light-triggered release from nanocarriers. Adv Drug Deliv Rev 2012; 64(11): 1005-20.
[http://dx.doi.org/10.1016/j.addr.2012.02.006] [PMID: 22386560]

[198] Tong R, Hemmati HD, Langer R, Kohane DS. Photoswitchable nanoparticles for triggered tissue penetration and drug delivery. J Am Chem Soc 2012; 134(21): 8848-55.
[http://dx.doi.org/10.1021/ja211888a] [PMID: 22385538]

[199] Jiang J, Tong X, Zhao Y. A new design for light-breakable polymer micelles. J Am Chem Soc 2005; 127(23): 8290-1.
[http://dx.doi.org/10.1021/ja0521019] [PMID: 15941255]

[200] Rapoport N, Christensen D, Fain H, Barrows L, Gao Z. Ultrasound-triggered drug targeting of tumors in vitro and in vivo 2004; 42(1-9): 943-50.
[http://dx.doi.org/10.1016/j.ultras.2004.01.087]

[201] Sirsi SR, Borden MA. State-of-the-art materials for ultrasound-triggered drug delivery. Adv Drug Deliv Rev 2014; 72: 3-14.
[http://dx.doi.org/10.1016/j.addr.2013.12.010] [PMID: 24389162]

[202] Baghbani F, Chegeni M, Moztarzadeh F, Mohandesi JA, Mokhtari-Dizaji M. Ultrasonic nanotherapy of breast cancer using novel ultrasound-responsive alginate-shelled perfluorohexane nanodroplets: In vitro and *in vivo* evaluation. Mater Sci Eng C 2017; 77: 698-707.
[http://dx.doi.org/10.1016/j.msec.2017.02.017] [PMID: 28532082]

[203] Sabourian P, Tavakolian M, Yazdani H, *et al.* Stimuli-responsive chitosan as an advantageous platform for efficient delivery of bioactive agents. J Control Release 2020; 317: 216-31.
[http://dx.doi.org/10.1016/j.jconrel.2019.11.029] [PMID: 31778742]

[204] Du J, Zhang Y, Ge H, *et al.* Ultrasound-degradable serum albumin nanoplatform for *in situ* controlled drug release. Chem Commun (Camb) 2020; 56(54): 7503-6.
[http://dx.doi.org/10.1039/D0CC01937B] [PMID: 32501465]

[205] Sciurti E, Primavera R, Di Mascolo D, *et al.* Ultrasound-induced deformation of PLGA-microPlates for on-command drug release. Microelectron Eng 2020; 229: 111360.
[http://dx.doi.org/10.1016/j.mee.2020.111360]

[206] Entzian K, Aigner A. Drug delivery by ultrasound-responsive nanocarriers for cancer treatment. Pharmaceutics 2021; 13(8): 1135.
[http://dx.doi.org/10.3390/pharmaceutics13081135] [PMID: 34452096]

[207] Xia H, Zhao Y, Tong R. Ultrasound-mediated polymeric micelle drug delivery. Therapeutic Ultrasound 2016; pp. 365-84.

[208] Nappini S, Fogli S, Castroflorio B, Bonini M, Baldelli Bombelli F, Baglioni P. Magnetic field responsive drug release from magnetoliposomes in biological fluids. J Mater Chem B Mater Biol Med 2016; 4(4): 716-25.
[http://dx.doi.org/10.1039/C5TB02191J] [PMID: 32262953]

[209] Singh RK, Patel KD, Kim JJ, *et al.* Multifunctional hybrid nanocarrier: magnetic CNTs ensheathed with mesoporous silica for drug delivery and imaging system. ACS Appl Mater Interfaces 2014; 6(4): 2201-8.
[http://dx.doi.org/10.1021/am4056936] [PMID: 24476195]

[210] Shi J, Yu X, Wang L, *et al.* PEGylated fullerene/iron oxide nanocomposites for photodynamic therapy, targeted drug delivery and MR imaging. Biomaterials 2013; 34(37): 9666-77.
[http://dx.doi.org/10.1016/j.biomaterials.2013.08.049] [PMID: 24034498]

[211] Sumer B, Gao J. Theranostic nanomedicine for cancer. Nanomedicine (Lond) 2008; 3(2): 137-40.
[http://dx.doi.org/10.2217/17435889.3.2.137]

[212] Lee SB. Focus on nanoparticles for cancer diagnosis and therapeutics. Nanomed 2007; 2(5).
[http://dx.doi.org/10.2217/17435889.2.5.647]

[213] Ghasemi Y, Peymani P, Afifi S. Quantum dot: magic nanoparticle for imaging, detection and targeting. Acta Biomed 2009; 80(2): 156-65.
[PMID: 19848055]

[214] Hainfeld JF, Smilowitz HM, O'Connor MJ, Dilmanian FA, Slatkin DN. Gold nanoparticle imaging and radiotherapy of brain tumors in mice. Nanomedicine (Lond) 2013; 8(10): 1601-9.
[http://dx.doi.org/10.2217/nnm.12.165] [PMID: 23265347]

[215] Luo Y, Wang Y, Yan H, *et al.* SWCNTs@GQDs composites as nanocarriers for enzyme-free dual-signal amplification electrochemical immunoassay of cancer biomarker. Anal Chim Acta 2018; 1042: 44-51.
[http://dx.doi.org/10.1016/j.aca.2018.08.023] [PMID: 30428987]

[216] Zhang H, Ba S, Yang Z, *et al.* Graphene quantum dot-based nanocomposites for diagnosing cancer biomarker APE1 in living cells. ACS Appl Mater Interfaces 2020; 12(12): 13634-43.
[http://dx.doi.org/10.1021/acsami.9b21385] [PMID: 32129072]

[217] Liu Y, Feng L, Liu T, *et al.* Multifunctional pH-sensitive polymeric nanoparticles for theranostics evaluated experimentally in cancer. Nanoscale 2014; 6(6): 3231-42.
[http://dx.doi.org/10.1039/c3nr05647c] [PMID: 24500240]

[218] Gao GH, Li Y, Lee DS. Environmental pH-sensitive polymeric micelles for cancer diagnosis and targeted therapy. J Control Release 2013; 169(3): 180-4.
[http://dx.doi.org/10.1016/j.jconrel.2012.11.012] [PMID: 23195533]

[219] Li H, Chen Y, Li Z, Li X, Jin Q, Ji J. Hemoglobin as a smart pH-sensitive nanocarrier to achieve aggregation enhanced tumor retention. Biomacromolecules 2018; 19(6): 2007-13.
[http://dx.doi.org/10.1021/acs.biomac.8b00241] [PMID: 29498829]

[220] Zhao Y, Shi C, Yang X, *et al.* pH-and temperature-sensitive hydrogel nanoparticles with dual photoluminescence for bioprobes. ACS Nano 2016; 10(6): 5856-63.
[http://dx.doi.org/10.1021/acsnano.6b00770] [PMID: 27232534]

[221] Zhao L, Kim TH, Ahn JC, Kim HW, Kim SY. Highly efficient "theranostics" system based on surface-modified gold nanocarriers for imaging and photodynamic therapy of cancer. J Mater Chem B Mater Biol Med 2013; 1(42): 5806-17.
[http://dx.doi.org/10.1039/c3tb20933d] [PMID: 32261238]

[222] Frasco MF, Almeida GM, Santos-Silva F, Pereira MC, Coelho MAN. Transferrin surface-modified PLGA nanoparticles-mediated delivery of a proteasome inhibitor to human pancreatic cancer cells. J Biomed Mater Res A 2015; 103(4): 1476-84.
[http://dx.doi.org/10.1002/jbm.a.35286] [PMID: 25046528]

[223] Bae S, Ma K, Kim TH, *et al.* Doxorubicin-loaded human serum albumin nanoparticles surface-modified with TNF-related apoptosis-inducing ligand and transferrin for targeting multiple tumor types. Biomaterials 2012; 33(5): 1536-46.
[http://dx.doi.org/10.1016/j.biomaterials.2011.10.050] [PMID: 22118776]

[224] Chen H, Li S, Li B, *et al.* Folate-modified gold nanoclusters as near-infrared fluorescent probes for tumor imaging and therapy. Nanoscale 2012; 4(19): 6050-64.
[http://dx.doi.org/10.1039/c2nr31616a] [PMID: 22930451]

[225] Lu RM, Chen MS, Chang DK, *et al.* Targeted drug delivery systems mediated by a novel Peptide in breast cancer therapy and imaging. PLoS One 2013; 8(6): e66128.
[http://dx.doi.org/10.1371/journal.pone.0066128] [PMID: 23776619]

CHAPTER 4

Importance of Surface-modified Nanocarriers (SMN) in the Management of Cancer

Meghna A. Singh[1], **Azmi Khan**[1], **Tarani P. Shrivastava**[2], **Firdos Khan**[3], **Ajay Sharma**[4] and **Madhu Gupta**[1,*]

[1] *Department of Pharmaceutics, Delhi Pharmaceutical Sciences and Research University, Pushp Vihar Sector 3, MB Road, New Delhi-110017, India*

[2] *Department of Pharmacology, Delhi Pharmaceutical Sciences and Research University, Pushp Vihar Sector 3, MB Road, New Delhi-110017, India*

[3] *Department of Pharmacology, BM College of Pharmaceutical Education and Research, Indore, MP – 452020, India*

[4] *Department of Pharmacognosy, Delhi Pharmaceutical Sciences and Research University, Pushp Vihar Sector 3, MB Road, New Delhi-110017, India*

Abstract: Cancer is among the leading causes of death worldwide, causing a significant rise in mortality and morbidity. In this regard, nanotechnology gained a plethora of attention from researchers, owing to its nano-size and larger surface area, leading to one of the most effective drug delivery systems for chemotherapeutic agents. Indeed, they enhance the bioavailability and targeting of antitumor drugs. The formulations developed utilizing nanotechnology have been used for a long to deliver anticancer drugs. Still, they greatly suffered from several restrictions to effectively deliver the incorporated drug at the specific site. Recently, an advanced technique of developing Surface Modified Nanocarriers (SMN) addressed the shortcomings of older nanotechnology-based formulations. Specifically, ligands or other conjugates attached to the nanocarriers for targeting site-specific tumor/s have been more successful in offering site-specific drug targeting and reducing cell toxicity coupled with prolonged and sustained drug delivery.

Keywords: Antitumor drugs, Cancer, Drug delivery, Nanocarrier, Nanotechnology.

INTRODUCTION

Cancer is a heterogeneous disease that develops through several pathophysiological processes and is characterized by uncontrolled growth of

* **Corresponding author Madhu Gupta:** Department of Pharmaceutics, Delhi Pharmaceutical Sciences and Research University,Pushp Vihar Sector 3, MB Road, New Delhi-110017, India; Tel: +91-9205916054;
E-mail: madhugupta98@gmail.com

Neeraj Mishra, Ashish Garg and Neeraj Upmanyu (Eds.)

cell/s [1]. Manifolds in the genetic alteration might be the reason for the inactivation of tumor suppressor genes or the triggering of oncogenes, which further leads to carcinoma [2]. According to WHO, 2018 recorded over 18 million fresh cancer cases and about 10 million deaths due to cancer. The reason behind rising cancer cases includes a dense population, aging, and the lifestyle of industrialized countries [3].

Conventional cancer chemotherapy has many limitations like patient compliance, severe side effects, cytotoxicity, drug resistance, *etc* [4]. Therefore, the modern drug delivery system has been introduced to overcome these problems. The advancement in nanotechnology shows tremendous management of cancer. The specific range of molecules in the field of nanotechnology fascinated the researchers, as the physical size of nanoparticles ranges between 1-100 nm, and the nanocarriers have a wider range, *i.e.*, 1-1000 nm. The construct of nanocarriers can involve different types of nanomaterials, which offer several functionalities as drug carriers with specific properties of better tissue penetration, large surface ratio, drug protection against degradation, *etc.* Indeed, various biodegradable and non-biodegradable polymers were used to develop liposomes, nanoparticles, solid lipid nanoparticles, dendrimers, and micelles. These formulations reduce the side effects and raise the therapeutic efficacy of the active pharmaceutical moiety [5].

In the present scenario of the nano-particulate system, various new chemical entities are introduced which have poor hydrophilicity and higher active macromolecule utilization in improving therapeutic efficacy. Therefore, the nanoparticulate system needs modification to facilitate drug delivery to the targeted site [6].

Although there are many advantages of nanocarriers, there is limitation also, such as after reaching through systemic circulation, there is cellular uptake that occurs by the reticular endothelial system (RES), which leads to poor transfection efficacy to the target site. Hence, surface-modified nanocarriers have been introduced to overcome these problems. This technique attaches different conjugate ligands to the nanocarriers for effective therapeutic outcomes. Firstly, the surface-modified conjugate-specific-ligands nanocarriers evade their identity by RES. Secondly, surface-modified ligand conjugates nanocarriers limit the intercellular disposition. Surface-modified pharmaceutical nanocarriers, such as liposomes, nanocapsules, niosomes, solid-lipid nanoparticles and many others, are there to manage the tasks, such as penetration through biological barriers, improving the capability of the target, longer duration of action, and contrast loading that permits them to complete therapeutic or diagnostic activities (Fig. **1**) [7, 8].

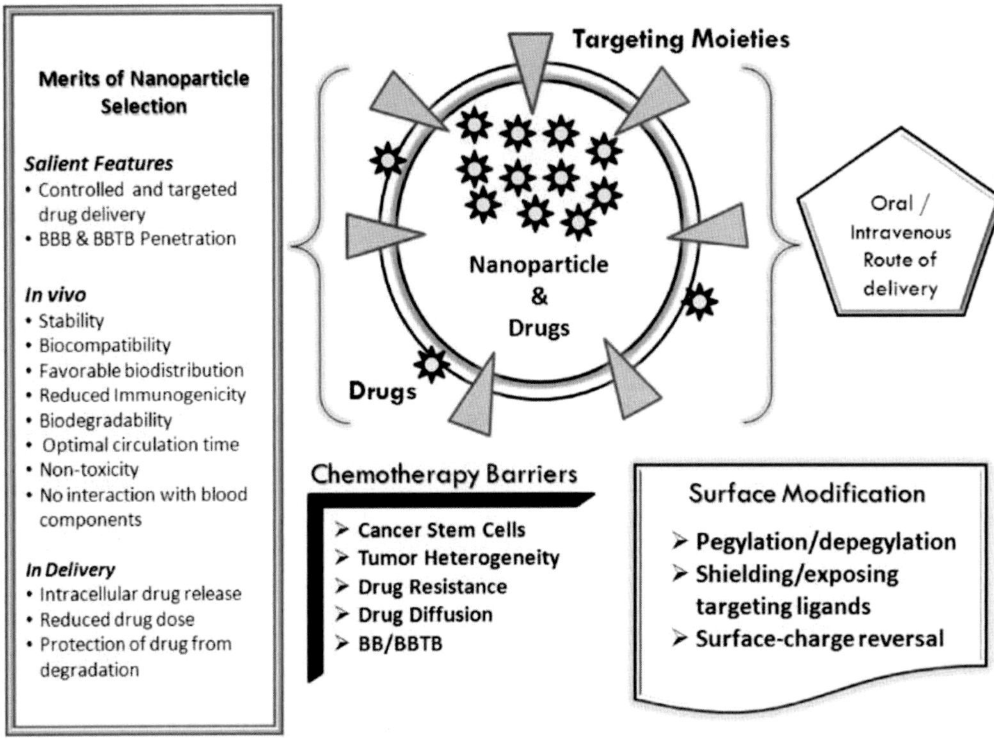

Fig. (1). Selection criteria, barriers to chemotherapy, and surface modification associated with NPs for drug delivery in selected solid tumors [8].

Scientists in the pharmaceutical domain have performed numerous research studies for devising nanocarriers that can effectively target tumor cells. Some of these successful candidates that have been clinically approved and available in the market, are listed in Table **1** [9 - 16].

Table 1. List of Available Marketed Formulations of Nanocarriers for Cancer Treatment.

S. No.	Drug/Product	Company	Year of Approval	Indication	Dose Required	Refs.
1.	Doxil®/Caelyx™	Schering Plough; Ortho-Biotech	1995	Kaposi's sarcoma; ovariancancer; multiple myeloma	20 mg/m^2; 50 mg/m^2; 30 mg/m^2	[9]
2.	Myocet®	Sopherion; Cephalon	2000	Metastatic breast cancer	Based on weight and height	[9]
3.	Lipodox®	Sunpharma		Ovarian cancer	2mg/ml	[10]
4.	DaunoXome®	Galen	2002	Kaposi's sarcoma	2mg/ml	[11]

(Table 1) cont.....

S. No.	Drug/Product	Company	Year of Approval	Indication	Dose Required	Refs.
5.	Marqibo®	Talon; Merrimack	2012	Acute lymphoblastic leukemia	1mg/ml	[9]
6.	Onivyde®	Ipsen	2019	Pancreatic cancer	43mg/10ml	[12]
7.	Oncaspar®	Enzon	2006	Acute lymphoblastic leukemia	5mg/ml	[10]
8.	Eligard®	Tolmar	2016	Prostate cancer	ELIGARD 7.5 mg: 1 month of therapy ELIGARD 22.5 mg: 3 months of therapy ELIGARD 30 mg: 4 months of therapy ELIGARD 45 mg: 6 months of therapy	[13]
9.	NanoTherm®	MagForce	2018	Brain tumors	112mg/ml	[14]
10.	Ontak®	Eisai	1999		9 or 18 mcg/kg/day over 30 to 60 minutes for 5 consecutive days	[15]
11.	Vyxeos	Jazz	2017	Acute myeloid leukemia	VYXEOS (daunorubicin 44 mg/m2 and cytarabine 100 mg/m2) over 90 minutes on days 1, 3, and 5	[16]

PHYSICOCHEMICAL AND BIOLOGICAL BARRIERS IN TUMOR TARGETING

For remedial and indicative reasons, nanocarrier or nanomedicine relies upon numerous natural frameworks or biological barriers of the human body. Firstly enrooting through gastrointestinal, skin or mucosal membrane where nanoparticle absorbs through the epithelium, the nanocarriers are transferred to the endothelium, the second cellular barrier involved in providing supplements to the cells. Later on, the cytomembrane fills in as a movable material or obstructive boundary to the therapeutic agents, limiting therapeutic agents' cellular absorption limits cellular absorption. Low molecular weight drugs and lipophilic drug particles absorb through the passive diffusion method to cross the lipid bilayer of the cytomembrane. However, for the absorption of macromolecular size, drug particles can not be absorbed by passive diffusion and require more complex and dynamic processes through which the drug can get entry inside the cells [17].

Hence, the nanocarriers which are loaded with genetic materials require extra support from more than 400 carriers present intracellularly coupled with help from surface carriers that facilitate the internalization of the nanomaterials [18]. Besides this, tumor cells also restrict the entry of nanomaterials by involving physiochemical barriers, such as molecular size and shape, surface charge, hydrophobicity, *etc.* One of the critical changes in cancer cells includes a negative charge on the cell surface which restricts the entry of nanocarriers; this also leads to increased secretion of lactate from the cell, which results from increased glucose metabolism in tumors. [19] It is also evident that there is an excess transfer of growth factors to cancer cells through blood vessels in the host tissues, which ultimately results in an angiogenic state due to increased demand for growth factors. [20] The growth factors which are present in high levels within the tumor microenvironment include Platelet-derived Growth Factors (PDGF), Fibroblast Growth Factor (FGF) and Vascular Endothelial Growth Factor (VEGF) and the overexpression of VEGF receptors (VEGFR), PDGF receptors (PDGFR) and FGF receptors (FGFR) in endothelial cells and vascular smooth muscle cells finally result into angiogenesis of tumor microvessels [21]. Another limiting factor is the presence of blood proteins, such as albumin, globulin and fibrinogen, which directly govern the fate of nanocarriers through the phagocytic system [22].

NEED OF NANO-FORMULATIONS IN CANCER TREATMENT

Until now, there are a few choices for strong tumor therapy, for example, chemotherapy, radiation and medical procedure. Chemotherapy is considered the best treatment for malignancies and metastatic tumors, particularly requiring chemotherapy as radiotherapy or medical procedure could not offer broad cytotoxic actions [23]. Despite numerous advances in traditional chemotherapy, successive difficulties are experienced at formulation design and tumor targeting levels. There are some major issues related to the use of chemotherapy, for example, the definition and biodistribution of the medication, their harmfulness towards ordinary cells with multidrug opposition of the malignant growth cells. Subsequently, the examination endeavors the improvement of an ideal malignancy chemotherapeutic based plan to conquer these issues. By and large, chemotherapy has a huge part in the field of clinical utilization of disease treatment, however, the sub-atomic intricacy connected with cytotoxic operators and the detachment of most physiological targets brought about a critical need to improve drug viability with a simple way to deal with targeting tumors [24]. Notwithstanding, a larger part of anticancer medications introduced the definition related issues attributable to their poor fluid dissolvability, subsequently, they ought to be disintegrated in a natural dissolvable to oversee as an injectable arrangement structure [17].

In any case, natural solvents have a few restrictionsand they are commonly harmful. The majority of the low atomic weight anticancer medications have an innate character to navigate all through veins unreservedly and bring about fast discharge with a low restorative record, requiring the incessant organization of dosages to the malignancy tolerant and eventually expanding the cytotoxicity with other serious results [25]. For example, a drug in an arrangement structure might have the option to unreservedly diffuse with vague development in the body and all the while unfit to amass at the tumor site. All the functions make the extremely lamentable circumstance for patients [26]. An anticancer medication in arrangement structure is administrated alone; at that point, the absence of particularity and wellspring of deadly harm to typical cells presents extreme poisonous impacts, including bone marrow concealment and alopecia [27].

The union of all issues related to traditional treatment has made examination interest in the medication conveyance field to upgrade their therapeutic potential and limit unfavorable impacts [28]. As of now, utilization of such novel conveyance frameworks can convey strong medications to the favored site in an exact way. The various pathophysiological states of illnesses dramatically affect the exploration of creative and novel remedial methodologies. Subsequently, utilizing such novel transporters may additionally upgrade the pharmacological properties of medications and be considered the next best elective decision [29]. The plan of nanomedicine made out of nanosystems is generally capable to control the arrival of destructive moiety straightforwardly inside malignancy cells [30]. The plan of nanomedicine made out of nanosystems is generally capable of controlling the arrival of destructive moiety straightforwardly inside malignancy cells [31].

At first, for malignant growth nanotechnology, drug transporters have been utilized for parenteral organization and are relied upon to be biodegradable, simple and sensibly modest alongside their particular amassing at the necessary destinations [32]. For example, Doxil and Abraxane are two nanocarriers, utilized for ovarian and metastatic bosom disease separately. Doxil has long flowing liposomal plan of doxorubicin with essentially improved remedial result when contrasted with the free medication, while Abraxane is an egg white bound nanoparticles of paclitaxel and reduce the touchiness response related to the standard paclitaxel dissolvable Cremophor EL [33, 34].

BIODEGRADABLE AND NON-BIODEGRADABLE POLYMERS

Biodegradable Polymers

Nanoformulations are generally composed of two types of polymers namely,

Biodegradable and Non-biodegradable polymers. Biodegradable polymers have recently gained hype in their scale of utilization which is due to their natural occurrence from biological sources like cOrn, wood cellulose, *etc.*, and they can also be synthesized in the laboratory with the help of microorganisms by utilizing butyric or valeric acids, *etc* [35]. These polymers are biologically degraded by microbial chain scission which results into mineralizing the polymer if the environmental condition like pH, humidity, 0xygenation and the presence of some metals are met sufficiently. Biodegradable polymers of both native and synthetic origin can be distinguished by their distinct molecular weights [36]. For an ideal biodegradable polymer, it must remain stable and composite until its application period, while it should also be disposed entirely of through easy breakdown. Contrary to this, biodegradable polymers are made of sturdy carbon backbones that are hard to break; hence, the side chains of these polymers are first exposed to degradation by chemical, light or organism offering them a higher surface area for easy breakdown. Biodegradable polymers are widely used for drug delivery in the treatment of diseases that require the presence of drugs at a specific site in a sustained and controlled manner for a longer duration of time [37]. Besides this, biodegradable polymers also offer specific advantages like;

- non-toxic nature

- capacity to maintain the mechanical strength of the formulation until degradation

- capacity to degrade in a sustained and controlled manner

Mechanism of the Breakdown of Biodegradable Polymers

The fate of biodegradable polymers is determined by the complete breakdown of a polymer moiety into monomers and finally mineralization to form gases, salts, and biomass. The process of biodegradation is influenced by various factors, including the type of chemical bonding, solubility of polymer units and presence of copolymers. The environmental factors present at the site of degradation, such as water, temperature, microorganism and pH, are also equally important in determining the rate and extent of breakdown of these polymers [38]. There are two primary ways of biodegradation, namely, physical decomposition by hydrolysis & photodegradation or through aerobic & anaerobic biological processes. These processes lead to the partial or complete breakdown of biodegradable polymers [38].

Examples of Biodegradable Polymers

Dextran

Simple repeated units of α-d-glycose combined with glycosidic bonds form Dextran's branched polysaccharides. It is a naturally occurring water-soluble polymer but can be acetylated to create a hydrophobic polysaccharide (AcDex). The formulations such as hydrogels can be synthesized by combining Dextran with crosslinkers. Dextran can be easily converted into amphiphilic micelles by linkinxg with hydrophilic polymers like Polylactide (PLA), PolycaprolactOne (PCL) and Polyethylyline Glyc0l (PEG), which act as copolymers and can effectively incorporate hydrophobic chemotherapeutic drugs [39].

Poly(L-lysine) (PLL)

PLL consists of lysine in a polymerized form which is bonded with cationic amino acid (L stereochemistry) for enzymatic degradation. PLL is highly promising in forming nanoparticulate systems as its positive charge offers the greater ability of particle uptake, further, a high density of positive charge of PLL also allows condensing of negatively charged molecules into nanoparticles. PLL is also compatible with synthesizing dendritic and linear forms for improved neutralizing capacity and optimal delivery of nucleic acids.

Poly[Lactide-co-Glycolide] (PLGA)

Poly-glycolic acid (PGA) and Poly-lactic acid (PLA) are combined to form a copolymer which is known as Poly[Lactide-co-Glycolide] (PLGA). PLGA is a highly versatile copolymer with high stability, low toxicity and degradation rate. It can be transformed easily into various requisite forms by varying the ratios of PLA and PGA monomers. Emulsification is the method of choice for synthesizing the nanoparticles using PLGA. The PLGA nanoparticles can easily incorporate drugs with lower molecular weight. By the method of surface modification (cationic ligands), PLGA can be effectively used for gene delivery, *e.g.,* siRNA delivery using cationic lipids.

Poly(ε-caprolactone) (PCL)

PCL is a semi-crystalline biodegradable polymer lipid soluble and shows a great drug binding capacity. PCL shows better physiological characteristics such as colloidal stability in biological fluids, low molecular toxicities, easy cellular uptake by endocytosis, *etc.* Due to its better physiological promise, PCL is preferred for tissue engineering scaffolds, biomedical devices and implantable drug delivery devices (*e.g.*, Capronor®). The combination of PCL with other polymers also enhances the rate of its bio-degradation. PCL, in combination with PEG, has been employed to generate micelles that can incorporate chemotherapeutic drugs [40].

Biodegradable polymers are widely used as biomedical devices, and in tissue engineering applications, they are used in controlled drug delivery systems such as liposomes, niosomes and have vast usage within nanotechnology, like, nanomedicine and nanocarrier. Therefore, they are widely used in the treatment of various types of cancers.

Non-Biodegradable Polymers

The non-biodegradable polymers are made up of inter-atomic solid bonding and are hence tough to break by microbes. Long chains of carbon and hydrogen atoms constitute this tough structure of non-biodegradable polymers, which requires more extended periods to decompose them properly.

Examples of Non-Biodegradable Polymers

The non-biodegradable polymers are widely utilized in pharmaceutical processes ranging from the binder, thickening agent, and tablet granulation to delivering drugs at the specific target site.

Polyethylene

These are one of the most widely applicable thermoplastics, which are durable in nature and can exist in variable crystalline structures. Physically Polyethylenes can be grouped into:

- Linear High-Density Polyethene (HDPE)
- Branched Low-Density Polyethene (LDPE)
- Ultra-High Molecular Weight Polyethylene (UHMWPE)

Poly (tetrafluoroethylene) (PTFE)

PTFE is commonly known as Teflon, which has a wide application as pharmaceutical coatings. Such product areas range from sampling probes, soft gel equipment, powder mills and tablet & capsule packaging equipment. They are chemically and biologically inert and have high lubricant nature.

Polystyrene (PS)

Polystyrene offers several benefits like lower physical weight, stability, cheaper cost, versatility and a higher insulation capacity. In pharmaceutical packaging, polystyrene holds a higher degree of acceptability and is used as insulation boxes for aseptic transport of medications, blood and its components, organs, specimens, *etc.*

Polycarbonate (PC)

Polycarbonate is one of the most versatile and transparent thermoplastic materials, and because of its inherent strength, excellent optical clarity, high heat distortion temperature, and dimensional stability, it is an ideal material for critical healthcare applications. PCs are widely used as hospital equipments like syringes, catheters, I.V. sets and other healthcare delivery products [40].

TARGETED DELIVERY FOR SMN IN THE MANAGEMENT OF CANCER

Surface Modified Nanocarriers (SMNc) have expressed themselves as excellent targeting drug delivery system for chemotherapeutic drugs without damaging normal cells. However, targeted delivery is dramatically challenging for pharmaceutical researchers because there has been an increase in new molecular entities, which range from lower to higher molecular weight, such as protein and genes. It is very difficult to achieve site-specific delivery by particular drug carriers. However, by identifying a particular drug's pharmacological action, the targeting homing drug will be site-specific [41]. Two targeting strategies can be employed, firstly, passive targeting, which flows the convection and diffusion processes for targeting the tumor. They require no specific attachment of ligand for the delivery of the active components. Secondly, active targeting requires an attachment of ligands and conjugates to nanoparticles to achieve the target.

Passive Targeting

Passive targeting efficiently contributes to improving the pathophysiological and bio-distribution condition of poorly water-soluble chemotherapeutic drugs [42]. The compromised condition of tissue has an enhanced permeability and retention (EPR) effect, which maintains nanoparticles such as liposomes, polymeric nanoparticles, and micelles for a longer duration at the tumor site [43]. The blood vessels bearing the tumor have leaky and unusually dense conditions. The endothelium cell lining of the tumor varies from 100-700nm, which is just double of normal distinct endothelium cells, *i.e.*, up to 10 nanometres [44]. The malignant tumor has a deficient lymphatic drainage system. This nature of tumor leads to the collection of nanocarriers at their specific site, which is beneficial for the targeted delivery of low molecular compounds (drugs) through nanocarriers. The targeting is based on the pathophysiological and immunochemical nature of the cancerous cell. This is also known as passive targeting [45]. The first generation of nanomedicine follows the passive targeting system. The modulation in the physicochemical properties of the active component, majorly relies on controlling bio-distribution and pharmacokinetics properties of nanomedicine. The clinically approved first-generation drugs were nab-paclitaxel (Abraxane®), and pegylated liposomal doxorubicin(Doxil®/Caelyx®) [46, 47]. The Genexol-PM®, a nanocarrier system, showed excellent results in terms of in-vitro and in-vivo correlation state, improved water solubility, and improved colloidal stability. It offers an effective bio-distribution profile, *i.e.*, three times higher than a normal drug [48].

Active Targeting

Active targeting is based on surface modification phenomena, mainly known ligands attached to nanoparticles for targeting site-specific tumors. These ligands can combine with targeted site receptors which are uttered by tumor cells. Substances like antibodies, vitamins, peptides, glycoproteins, and nucleic acid are used to enlarge the site specificity of ligand-bonded nanoparticles [49]. Boleta, 2011, developed a surface-modified silica nanoparticle (SMN) for delivering camptothecin (CPT). The synthesis process involved a covalent link between drug and nanoparticle, to maintain their stability and evade the free drug release. The *in-vitro* results explained that the surface-modified silica nanoparticles camptothecin entered the biological system *via* the endocytosis process and induced targeted cell death at a half-maximal inhibitory concentration (IC_{50}). The *in-vivo* test was performed on human colorectal cancer; the outcome showed that its surface-modified nanoparticle camptothecin enhances the drug concentration in the tumor cell and extensively reduces systemic toxicity. Although this accumulated in the reticular endothelium system, their results illustrated that this could be the strongest drug delivery system against tumors [50].

The surface-modified Gold nanoparticles (AuNPs) also have wide applications in the field of biomedical research. Their unique properties, like photothermal nature, convenient shape and size, and biological behavior, play an essential role in the targeted drug delivery system. The gold nanoparticles were modified by two main linkages non-covalent and covalent interactions. Both have pros and cons, but their study showed that they exclusively participate in diagnoses and treatment of cancer [51].

Another surface-modified polylactic-co-glycolic acid (PLGA) immuno-nanoparticles was developed for targeting breast tumor cells. They developed two types of nanoparticles, with or with Monoclonal antibody (mAb), for targeting MCF-10A neoT cells. The Monoclonal antibody (mAb) attaches to the nanoparticle either with a covalent or non-covalent bond to maintain its stability and targeted site of action. The study's outcome showed the immune nanoparticle is directly attached to the target while non-coated is distributed to all cells. Therefore, this has been proven that immune nanoparticles have a higher rate of targeting cancerous cells than non-coated nanoparticles. They developed an effective carrier system for micro or macromolecular active substances in the biological system [52].

CHALLENGES FOR SMNS IN CANCER DRUG TARGETING

The utilization of different nanomaterials with different properties and new approaches in the drug delivery field has uncovered exceptional challenges in malignant growth treatment and management through the biological barrier, physicochemical properties, toxicity and regulations, large scale-up production and many more. Further poor pharmacokinetic properties of anticancer drugs arise from low solubility, stability and metabolism and face different challenges like toxicity, low efficacy and limited biodistribution [53]. Once nanocarrier drugs are targeted at tumor tissue, where it faces the challenge first with the high interstitial fluid pressure as compared to normal tissue where the level of oxygen is low, it is responsible for inducing peritumoral condition induced. It is important for the good response of nanocarriers to act intracellularly [54]. Besides, the mucus is also an obstacle because its complex pattern can slow down or completely inhibit particle transport and drug absorption, making it difficult to treat. The physicochemical properties of nanocarriers play an important role in biocompatibility and toxicity in the biological system, which is the major challenge for the targeted drug delivery system. So to avoid unwanted toxicity of nanocarriers to a healthy cell is important to be careful in the synthesis and characterization of nanocarriers [55]. As well nanocarriers also interact with biological molecules and form protein corona, which may alter the function and effect of nanocarriers, making it difficult to manage cancer cell growth [56]. Nanocarrier stability and storage properties also affect pharmacological performance [57]. Besides, the large-scale manufacturing of nanomaterials is quite challenging compared to physicochemical properties because only a small quantity is used for preclinical and clinical studies. Additionally, multi-stage cycles of manufacturing nanomaterials and a high cost of crude materials is an expensive options for the delivery of nanocarriers [55]. Another key challenge is regulatory approval because the FDA has not set the proper guideline for Nanomedicines. The drug-loaded nanocarrier changes its pharmacokinetic and pharmacodynamic properties, increasing the drug efficacy and safety [58]. Although, nanomedicine formulation, approval, and commercialization must outline significant regulatory requirement guidelines [59]. Regulatory agencies often suggest that nanomedicine should be regulated as combination products since it is not straightforward to establish a boundary that disguises them from common pharmaceutical products, medical devices, or even biological agents. The challenges of the nanoparticle drug delivery system are represented in Fig. (**2**) [55].

CLINICALLY APPROVED/ PATENTED NANO-FORMULATIONS

Many nanomedicine compounds like viral vectors, drug conjugates, lipid-based nanocarriers, polymer-based nanocarriers, and inorganic nanoparticles have been used in cancer treatment and management. For the investigation of claims, nanomedicine patents can be used in the United States or the European state. The United States Patent and Trademark Office is a source of patent data that provides patent data using a patent view. In International Patent Classification, many classes or categories are divided for a particular technology, which is also one of class B82Y 5/00, where nanomedicine patents are classified along with nanobiotechnology [60]. In the nanotechnology category (1974–2016), 3,497 out of the total 48,212 nanomedicine patents were granted. During the filling of a patent, all information related to the material to patentability has to be revealed, which is a duty of the applicant, their lawyer and operators (Title 37 of the Code of Federal Regulations, §1.56[a]), some patents are listed in Table **2** [61 - 75]. The nanoparticulate system has several effective applications in cancer, such as diagnosis, imaging, sensing and targeting the therapeutic agents [76]. Surface-modified nanocarriers play an important role in drug targeting and maintaining the therapeutic efficacy of the drug. It also shows great results in the nose-to-brain drug delivery system; it directly targets the central nervous system for better and safer results in Alzheimer's disease [77].

Table 2. List of Clinically Approved and Patented Based Nano-Formulations for Targeting Various Cancers.

S. No.	Patent Number	Patent Title	Inventor	Filing Date	Publication Date	Remarks	Refs.
1.	EP3087974A1	Targeted nanocarriers for targeted drug delivery of gene therapeutics	Marcus Furch, Robert Gieseler	29.07.2015	02.11.2016	• Targeted nanocariers for delivering genes • Methods of preferentially, or actively, targeting and delivering a tool for gene transfer or genome editing (*i.e.*, a plasmid or a restriction enzyme - such as a zinc finger nuclease,	[61]

(Table 2) cont.....

S. No.	Patent Number	Patent Title	Inventor	Filing Date	Publication Date	Remarks	Refs.
						a CRISPR/Cas system, or a TALEN) • A tool for gene silencing or post-transcriptional regulation of gene expression (*i.e.*, a microRNA, a siRNA, a mRNA, an antisense oligonucleotide, or a sense oligonucleotide) to a range of mammalian cell species.	
2.	US10668024B2	Mesoporous silica nanoparticles for biomedical applications	Monty Liong, Jie Lu FuyuhikTamanoi, Jeffrey I. Zink Andre E. Nel	01.06.2018	02.06.2020	• A submicron structure includes a silica body defining a plurality of pores that are suitable to receive molecules therein • The silica body further defining an outer surface between pore openings of said plurality of pores • Several anionic molecules attached to the outer surface of the silica body • The submicron structure has a maximum dimension less than one micron.	[62]

(Table 2) cont.....

S. No.	Patent Number	Patent Title	Inventor	Filing Date	Publication Date	Remarks	Refs.
3.	US9579400B2	Nanocarriers for drug delivery	Kit S. Lam, JuntaoLuo	22.09.2009	28.02.2017	• A nanocarrier having an interior and an exterior surface • The nanocarrier comprising at least one conjugate, wherein each conjugate includes a polyethylene glycol (PEG) polymer • Each conjugate also includes at least two amphiphilic compounds having both a hydrophilic face and a hydrophobic face • Each conjugate also includes an oligomer, wherein at least 2 of the amphiphilic compounds are covalently attached to the oligomer which is covalently attached to the PEG.	[63]
4.	US20100076092A1	Lipid-derived nanoparticles for brain-targeted drug delivery	JayanthPanyam, Mahesh D. Chavanpatil	21.08.2007	25.03.2010	• Compositions and methods useful for the delivery of compounds across the Blood Brain Barrier (BBB) • Nanoparticles comprising lipids, such as brain lipids, are used to encapsulate drugs and to facilitate drug delivery to the brain.	[64]

(Table 2) cont.....

S. No.	Patent Number	Patent Title	Inventor	Filing Date	Publication Date	Remarks	Refs.
5.	US20150024033A1	Method and system for synthesizing nanocarrier based long acting drug delivery system for buprenorphine	MehrdadHamidi	21.07.2014	03.05.2016	• A nanocarrier system for delivering a long-acting injectable drug of buprenorphine and a method of synthesising the same • The drug entrapped nanoparticle formation is achieved by diffusion of the organic solvent within the aqueous solvent to obtain the nanoparticles • The drug gets entrapped within the nanoparticles *via* the anti-solvency effect of the aqueous matrix • The resulting drug nanocarriers are capable of releasing the drug in a slow rate upon injection. The synthesized drug carrying nanoparticles are cryopreserved for future administration • For better storage, the nanodispersion is dried to form a powder.	[65]

(Table 2) cont.....

S. No.	Patent Number	Patent Title	Inventor	Filing Date	Publication Date	Remarks	Refs.
6.	US20100255103A1	Mesoporous Silica Nanoparticles for Biomedical Applications	Monty Liong, Jie Lu, FuyuhikTamanoi, Jeffrey I. Zink, Andre Nel	08.12.2008	12.06.2018	• A submicron structure includes a silica body defining a plurality of pores that are suitable to receive molecules therein • The silica body further defining an outer surface between pore openings of said plurality of pores; and a plurality of anionic molecules attached to the outer surface of the silica body • Submicron structure has a maximum dimension less than one micron.	[66]
7.	US9629922B2	Nanoparticle-based tumor-targeted drug delivery	Ralph A. Reisfeld, Rong Xiang, YunpingLuo, Debbie Liao, Ze Liu Tingmei, Chen Si, Chen Dan Lu	02.09.2011	25.04.2017	• An aqueous tumor-targeting liposome nanoparticle composition comprising an aqueous dispersion of liposome nanoparticles • The nanoparticles preferably encapsulate an anti-cancer chemotherapeutic agent, which can be added to a pre-formed liposome composition or can be incorporated in the liposomes during the formation of the liposomes.	[67]

(Table 2) cont.....

S. No.	Patent Number	Patent Title	Inventor	Filing Date	Publication Date	Remarks	Refs.
8.	WO2009137592A3	Surface-modified nanoparticles	Neeraj Sharma, Choua C. Vu	06.05.2009	25.03.2010	• Surface-modified nanoparticles of at least one metal phosphate • The nanoparticles bear at least a portion of their surfaces • Surface modification comprising at least one organosilane surface modifier comprising at least one organic moiety comprising at least about six carbon atoms.	[68]
9.	US7641972B2	Surface-modified nanoparticles comprising polysiloxane modifier, their preparation and use	Ulrich Nolte, Alfred Bubat, KarlheinzHaubennestel, Thomas Sawitowski,	14.02.2006	14.02.2006	• Surface-modified nanoparticles composed of metal or semimetal oxides or hydroxides and having been reacted on their surface with a modifier, with formation of covalent bonds • The invention also relates to a process for preparing the nanoparticles, to their use as fillers in coating materials, plastics, foams and nail varnishes, and to dispersions which comprise the nanoparticles.	[69]
10.	US8642787B2	Surface modified nanoparticles, methods of their preparation, and uses thereof for gene and drug delivery	Kazuki Fukushima, James Lupton Hedrick, Alshakim Nelson Daniel, Paul Sanders	05.06.2012	04.02.2014	• Surface modified nanoparticle comprising a core material selected from the group consisting of organic materials, organometallic materials, inorganic materials, metals, metal oxides, and combinations	[70]

(Table 2) cont.....

S. No.	Patent Number	Patent Title	Inventor	Filing Date	Publication Date	Remarks	Refs.
11.	US5256395A	Affinity enhancement immunological reagents for *in vivo* detection and killing of specific target cells	Jacques Barbet; Michel Delaage; Jean-Marc Le Doussal, a	10.09.1987	26.10.2010	• Immunological reagents, consisting of an antibody or fragment conjugates having both an anti-cell specificity and an anti-hapten specificity • Synthetic tracers containing at least two hapten sites and at least one site suitable to attach radioactive isotopes, paramagnetic ions, drugs or toxins • Capable of binding to target cells in a specific way, and the tracer localizes preferentially on the membrane of antigen-bearing cells, even in the presence of excess antibody conjugate (affinity enhancement) • Usefully employed either *in-vitro* or *in-vivo*, to detect tumors, metastases, or other tissue injuries.	[71]
12.	US5543158A	Biodegradable injectable nanoparticles	RuxandraGref,Yoshiharu Minamitake, Robert S. Langer	23.07.1993	06.08.1996	• Biodegradable and injectable nanoparticles and microparticles for the controlled delivery of biologically active materials and diagnostic purposes.	[72]

(Table 2) cont.....

S. No.	Patent Number	Patent Title	Inventor	Filing Date	Publication Date	Remarks	Refs.
13.	US5024998A	Pharmaceutical formulations for parenteral use	Nicholas S. Bodor	11.12.1989	18.06.1991	• Aqueous parenteral solutions of drugs which are insoluble or only sparingly soluble in water and/or which are unstable in water • Combined with cyclodextrin selected from the group consisting of hydroxypropyl, hydroxyethyl, glucosyl, maltosyl and maltotriosyl derivatives of β- and γ-cyclodextrin • Provide a means for alleviating problems associated with drug precipitation at the injection site and/or in the lungs or other organs following parenteral administration.	[73]
14.	US9549901B2	Lipid-polymer hybrid particles	Jinjun Shi Zeyu Xiao Cristian Vilos Alexander Votruba Robert S. Langer Omid C. Farokhzad	02.09.2011	24.01.2017	• Include an aqueous core; a first amphiphilic layer surrounding the aqueous core; and a polymeric matrix surrounding the first amphiphilic layer.	[74]

(Table 2) cont.....

S. No.	Patent Number	Patent Title	Inventor	Filing Date	Publication Date	Remarks	Refs.
15.	JP2016053048A	Targeted synthetic nanocarrier with ph sensitive release of immunomodulatory agent	Zepp Charles, Yun Gao, J Keegan Mark, Sam Baldwin, Fen-Ni Fu, Lloyd Johnston, B Lipford Grayson	16.10.2015	22.11.2017	• Synthetic nanocarrier composition comprising an immunomodulator that separates from a synthetic nanocarrier in a pH sensitive manner • Targets a site of action in a cell, such as an antigen presenting cell (APC) • Protection of unstable immunomodulators by means of encapsulation within synthetic nanocarriers.	[75]

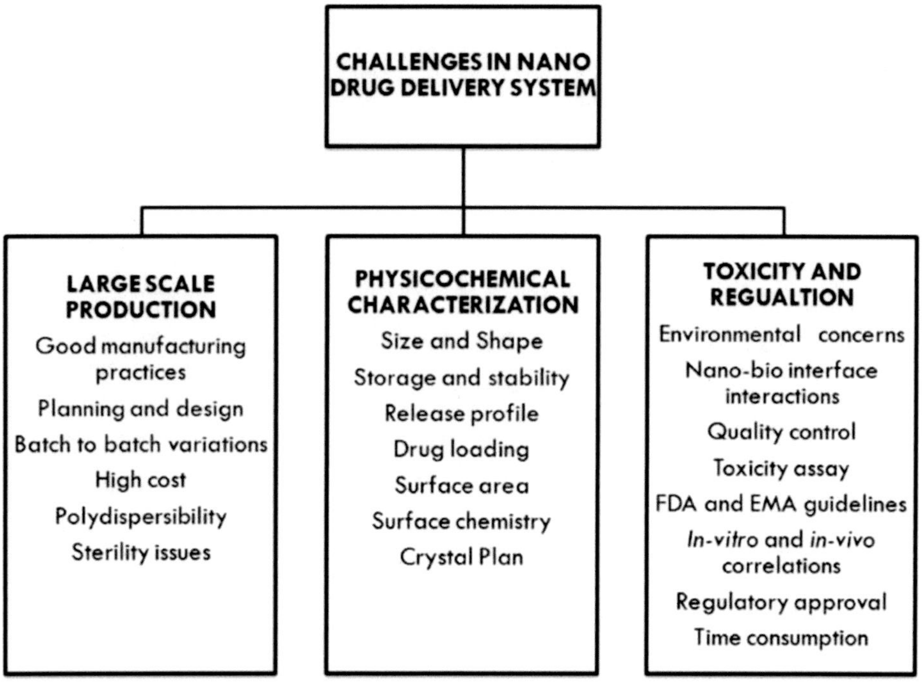

Fig. (2). Challenges in Nano Drug Delivery System [55].

CONCLUSION AND FUTURE PROSPECTIVE

Overall, nanotechnology opens a wide area of research for cancer treatment. The nanoparticulate system revolutionized drug delivery in cancer treatment by optimizing site-specific tumor cell targeting for effective therapeutic outcomes. SMN particularly interested in cancer drug delivery as they can easily incorporate low molecular weight chemotherapeutic compounds. Further, SMNs are also capable of reducing drug toxicity & improving the stability of a particular formulation. This unique nature of SMN expands the research area for the management of various types of cancers.

CONSENT FOR PUBLICATION

Not applicable.

CONFLICT OF INTEREST

The authors declare no conflict of interest, financial or otherwise.

ACKNOWLEDGEMENT

Declared none.

REFERENCE

[1] Luo J, Solimini NL, Elledge SJ. Principles of cancer therapy: oncogene and non-oncogene addiction. Cell 2009; 136(5): 823-37. [http://dx.doi.org/10.1016/j.cell.2009.02.024] [PMID: 19269363]

[2] Qiao W, Wang B, Wang Y, Yang L, Zhang Y, Shao P. 'Cancer therapy based on nanomaterials and nanocarrier systems'Journal of Nanomaterials, Volume 2010. Article ID 2010; 796303: 9. [In Press].

[3] International Agency for Research on Cancer. WHO,Geneva, Switzerland 2018; 263.

[4] Khan DR. The use of nanocarriers for drug delivery in cancer therapy. Journal of Cancer Science & Clinical Thereapeutics 2010; 2: 58-62. [http://dx.doi.org/10.4172/1948-5956.1000024]

[5] Wang YC, Liu XQ, Sun TM, Xiong MH, Wang J. Functionalized micelles from block copolymer of polyphosphoester and poly(ε-caprolactone) for receptor-mediated drug delivery. J Control Release 2008; 128(1): 32-40. [http://dx.doi.org/10.1016/j.jconrel.2008.01.021] [PMID: 18395283]

[6] Kwon IK, Lee SC, Han B, Park K. Analysis on the current status of targeted drug delivery to tumors. J Control Release 2012; 164(2): 108-14. [http://dx.doi.org/10.1016/j.jconrel.2012.07.010] [PMID: 22800574]

[7] Nkansah P, Antipas A, Lu Y, *et al.* Development and evaluation of novel solid nanodispersion system for oral delivery of poorly water-soluble drugs. J Control Release 2013; 169(1-2): 150-61. [http://dx.doi.org/10.1016/j.jconrel.2013.03.032] [PMID: 23570985]

[8] Wei QY, Xu YM, Lau ATY. Recent progress of nanocarrier-based therapy for solid malignancies. Cancers (Basel) 2020; 12(10): 2783. [http://dx.doi.org/10.3390/cancers12102783] [PMID: 32998391]

[9] Smith A. Big Moment for Nanotech: Oncology Therapeutics Poised for a Leap. OncLive 2013; 14(6).

[10] Bawa R, Audette GF, Rubinstein I. Copaxone® in the era of biosimilars and nanosimilars," Handbook of Clinical Nanomedicine.. Jenny Stanford Publishcation 2016; pp. 829-72. [http://dx.doi.org/10.1201/b19915-38]

[11] Chen L, Shiah H, Chao T, *et al.* Phase I study of liposome irinotecan (PEP02) in combination with weekly infusion of 5-FU/LV in advanced solid tumors. J Clin Oncol 2010; 28(15_suppl): e13024-4. [http://dx.doi.org/10.1200/jco.2010.28.15_suppl.e13024]

[12] Tran S, DeGiovanni PJ, Piel B, Rai P. Cancer nanomedicine: a review of recent success in drug delivery. Clin Transl Med 2017; 6(1): 44. [http://dx.doi.org/10.1186/s40169-017-0175-0] [PMID: 29230567]

[13] Rezvantalab S, Drude NI, Moraveji MK, *et al.* PLGA-based nanoparticles in cancer treatment. Front Pharmacol 2018; 9: 1260. [http://dx.doi.org/10.3389/fphar.2018.01260] [PMID: 30450050]

[14] Ledet G, Mandal TK. Nanomedicine: emerging therapeutics for the 21st century. US Pharm 2012; 37(3): 7-11.

[15] Bobo D, Robinson KJ, Islam J, Thurecht KJ, Corrie SR. Nanoparticle-based medicines: a review of FDA approved materials and clinical trials to date. Pharm Res 2016; 33(10): 2373-87. [http://dx.doi.org/10.1007/s11095-016-1958-5] [PMID: 27299311]

[16] Anselmo AC, Mitragotri S. Nanoparticles in the clinic: An update. Bioeng Transl Med 2019; 4(3): e10143. [http://dx.doi.org/10.1002/btm2.10143] [PMID: 31572799]

[17] Blanco E, Shen H, Ferrari M. Principles of nanoparticle design for overcoming biological barriers to drug delivery. Nat Biotechnol 2015; 33(9): 941-51. [http://dx.doi.org/10.1038/nbt.3330] [PMID: 26348965]

[18] Kou L, Bhutia YD, Yao Q, He Z, Sun J, Ganapathy V. Transporter-guided delivery of nanoparticles to improve drug permeation across cellular barriers and drug exposure to selective cell types. Front Pharmacol 2018; 9: 27. [http://dx.doi.org/10.3389/fphar.2018.00027] [PMID: 29434548]

[19] Chen B, Le W, Wang Y, *et al.* Targeting negative surface charges of cancer cells by multifunctional nanoprobes. Theranostics 2016; 6(11): 1887-98. [http://dx.doi.org/10.7150/thno.16358] [PMID: 27570558]

[20] Folkman J, Watson K, Ingber D, Hanahan D. Induction of angiogenesis during the transition from hyperplasia to neoplasia'Nature 1989; 339(6219): 58-61.

[21] Ballas MS, Chachoua A. Rationale for targeting VEGF, FGF, and PDGF for the treatment of NSCLC. OncoTargets Ther 2011; 4: 43-58. [http://dx.doi.org/10.2147/OTT.S18155] [PMID: 21691577]

[22] Lundqvist M, Stigler J, Elia G, Lynch I, Cedervall T, Dawson KA. Nanoparticle size and surface properties determine the protein corona with possible implications for biological impacts. Proc Natl Acad Sci USA 2008; 105(38): 14265-70. [http://dx.doi.org/10.1073/pnas.0805135105] [PMID: 18809927]

[23] Singhal S, Nie S, Wang MD. Nanotechnology applications in surgical oncology. Annu Rev Med 2010; 61(1): 359-73. [http://dx.doi.org/10.1146/annurev.med.60.052907.094936] [PMID: 20059343]

[24] Wang X, Wang Y, Chen ZG, Shin DM. Advances of cancer therapy by nanotechnology. Cancer Res Treat 2009; 41(1): 1-11. [http://dx.doi.org/10.4143/crt.2009.41.1.1] [PMID: 19688065]

[25] Kwon GS. Polymeric micelles for delivery of poorly water-soluble compounds. Crit Rev Ther Drug

Carrier Syst 2003; 20(5): 357-403.
[http://dx.doi.org/10.1615/CritRevTherDrugCarrierSyst.v20.i5.20] [PMID: 14959789]

[26] Walko CM, McLeod H. Pharmacogenomic progress in individualized dosing of key drugs for cancer patients. Nat Clin Pract Oncol 2009; 6(3): 153-62.
[PMID: 19174777]

[27] Maeda H, Bharate GY, Daruwalla J. Polymeric drugs for efficient tumor-targeted drug delivery based on EPR-effect. Eur J Pharm Biopharm 2009; 71(3): 409-19.
[http://dx.doi.org/10.1016/j.ejpb.2008.11.010] [PMID: 19070661]

[28] Luo Y, Prestwich G. Cancer-targeted polymeric drugs. Curr Cancer Drug Targets 2002; 2(3): 209-26.
[http://dx.doi.org/10.2174/1568009023333836] [PMID: 12188908]

[29] Vyas SP, Gupta M, Mishra N, Dube D. 2011.Block copolymer based nanoconstructs: importance in drug delivery. In: Felton GP, (Ed.) Biodegradable polymers: processing, degradation and applications Nova Science Publishers, USA, 2011; 273-324.

[30] Calderón M, Quadir MA, Strumia M, Haag R. Functional dendritic polymer architectures as stimuli-responsive nanocarriers. Biochimie 2010; 92(9): 1242-51.
[http://dx.doi.org/10.1016/j.biochi.2010.02.017] [PMID: 20211678]

[31] Bae Y, Kataoka K. Intelligent polymeric micelles from functional poly(ethylene glycol)-poly(amino acid) block copolymers. Adv Drug Deliv Rev 2009; 61(10): 768-84.
[http://dx.doi.org/10.1016/j.addr.2009.04.016] [PMID: 19422866]

[32] Torchilin VP. Targeted pharmaceutical nanocarriers for cancer therapy and imaging. AAPS J 2007; 9(2): E128-47.
[http://dx.doi.org/10.1208/aapsj0902015] [PMID: 17614355]

[33] Nishiyama N, Kataoka K. Current state, achievements, and future prospects of polymeric micelles as nanocarriers for drug and gene delivery. Pharmacol Ther 2006; 112(3): 630-48.
[http://dx.doi.org/10.1016/j.pharmthera.2006.05.006] [PMID: 16815554]

[34] Sparreboom A, Scripture CD, Trieu V, *et al.* Comparative preclinical and clinical pharmacokinetics of a cremophor-free, nanoparticle albumin-bound paclitaxel (ABI-007) and paclitaxel formulated in Cremophor (Taxol). Clin Cancer Res 2005; 11(11): 4136-43.
[http://dx.doi.org/10.1158/1078-0432.CCR-04-2291] [PMID: 15930349]

[35] Ray SS, Bousmina M. ' Biodegradable polymers and their layered silicate nanocomposites: In greening the 21st century materials world'. Prog Mater Sci 2006; 50(8): 962-1079.

[36] Albertsson A C, Karlsson S. Comprehensive Polymer Science and Supplements', Biodegradable Polymers 1989; 285-97.
[http://dx.doi.org/10.1016/B978-0-08-096701-1.00231-7]

[37] Ratner DB, Hoffman AS, Schoen FJ, Lemons JE. Biomaterials science: an introduction to materials in medicine. 2nd ed., San Diego, Calif.: Elsevier Academic Press 2004.

[38] Bastioli C. Handbook of biodegradable polymers ,1st ed, Shawbury, Shrewsbury, Shropshire. U.K., Rapra Technology Ltd. 2005.

[39] Karlsson J, Vaughan HJ, Green JJ, Green JJ. Biodegradable polymeric nanoparticles for therapeutic cancer treatments. Annu Rev Chem Biomol Eng 2018; 9(1): 105-27.
[http://dx.doi.org/10.1146/annurev-chembioeng-060817-084055] [PMID: 29579402]

[40] Archana George. ' A review on natural formulation basednanoformulations for drug delivery. Int J Pharm 2019; 20(561): 244-64.
[http://dx.doi.org/10.10.16/j.ijpharm.2019.03.011h]

[41] Petrak K. Essential properties of drug-targeting delivery systems. Drug Discov Today 2005; 10(23-24): 1667-73.
[http://dx.doi.org/10.1016/S1359-6446(05)03698-6] [PMID: 16376827]

[42] Owens D III, Peppas N. Opsonization, biodistribution, and pharmacokinetics of polymeric nanoparticles. Int J Pharm 2006; 307(1): 93-102.
[http://dx.doi.org/10.1016/j.ijpharm.2005.10.010] [PMID: 16303268]

[43] Acharya S, Sahoo SK. PLGA nanoparticles containing various anticancer agents and tumour delivery by EPR effect. Adv Drug Deliv Rev 2011; 63(3): 170-83.
[http://dx.doi.org/10.1016/j.addr.2010.10.008] [PMID: 20965219]

[44] Haley B, Frenkel E. Nanoparticles for drug delivery in cancer treatment. Urol Oncol 2008; 26(1): 57-64.
[http://dx.doi.org/10.1016/j.urolonc.2007.03.015] [PMID: 18190833]

[45] Torchilin V. Tumor delivery of macromolecular drugs based on the EPR effect. Adv Drug Deliv Rev 2011; 63(3): 131-5.
[http://dx.doi.org/10.1016/j.addr.2010.03.011] [PMID: 20304019]

[46] Golden PL, Huwyler JÖR, Pardridge WM. Treatment of large solid tumors in mice with daunomycin-loaded sterically stabilized liposomes. Drug Deliv 1998; 5(3): 207-12.
[http://dx.doi.org/10.3109/10717549809052036] [PMID: 19569986]

[47] Hobbs SK, Monsky WL, Yuan F, *et al.* Regulation of transport pathways in tumor vessels: Role of tumor type and microenvironment. Proc Natl Acad Sci USA 1998; 95(8): 4607-12.
[http://dx.doi.org/10.1073/pnas.95.8.4607] [PMID: 9539785]

[48] Kim TY, Kim DW, Chung JY, *et al.* Phase I and pharmacokinetic study of Genexol-PM, a cremophor-free, polymeric micelle-formulated paclitaxel, in patients with advanced malignancies. Clin Cancer Res 2004; 10(11): 3708-16.
[http://dx.doi.org/10.1158/1078-0432.CCR-03-0655] [PMID: 15173077]

[49] Pérez-Herrero E, Fernández-Medarde A. Advanced targeted therapies in cancer: Drug nanocarriers, the future of chemotherapy. Eur J Pharm Biopharm 2015; 93: 52-79.
[http://dx.doi.org/10.1016/j.ejpb.2015.03.018] [PMID: 25813885]

[50] Botella P, Abasolo I, Fernández Y, *et al.* Surface-modified silica nanoparticles for tumor-targeted delivery of camptothecin and its biological evaluation. J Control Release 2011; 156(2): 246-57.
[http://dx.doi.org/10.1016/j.jconrel.2011.06.039] [PMID: 21756949]

[51] Mugaka BP. Surface modification of goldnanoparticles for targeted drug delivery, YV Pathak(ed). book: surface modification of nanoparticles for targeted drug delivery. Springer Nature Switzerland AG 2019; pp. 391-403.

[52] Kocbek P, Obermajer N, Cegnar M, Kos J, Kristl J. Targeting cancer cells using PLGA nanoparticles surface modified with monoclonal antibody. J Control Release 2007; 120(1-2): 18-26.
[http://dx.doi.org/10.1016/j.jconrel.2007.03.012] [PMID: 17509712]

[53] Ruozi B, Belletti D, Sharma HS, *et al.* 2015; PLGA Nanoparticles Loaded Cerebrolysin: Studies on Their Preparation and Investigation of the Effect of Storage and Serum Stability with Reference to Traumatic Brain Injury 52(2): 899-912.
[http://dx.doi.org/10.1007/s12035-015-9235-x]

[54] Torosean S, Flynn B, Axelsson J, *et al.* Nanoparticle uptake in tumors is mediated by the interplay of vascular and collagen density with interstitial pressure. Nanomedicine 2013; 9(2): 151-8.
[http://dx.doi.org/10.1016/j.nano.2012.07.002] [PMID: 22841910]

[55] Navya PN, Kaphle A, Srinivas SP, Bhargava SK, Rotello VM, Daima HK. Current trends and challenges in cancer management and therapy using designer nanomaterials. Nano Converg 2019; 6(1): 23.
[http://dx.doi.org/10.1186/s40580-019-0193-2] [PMID: 31304563]

[56] Shi J, Kantoff PW, Wooster R, Farokhzad OC. Cancer nanomedicine: progress, challenges and opportunities', Nature Reviews Cancer 2016; 17(1): 20-7.

[57] Ma S, Zhou J, Zhang Y, *et al.* Highly Stable Fluorinated Nanocarriers with iRGD for Overcoming the Stability Dilemma and Enhancing Tumor Penetration in an Orthotopic Breast Cancer. ACS Appl Mater Interfaces 2016; 8(42): 28468-79.
[http://dx.doi.org/10.1021/acsami.6b09633] [PMID: 27712073]

[58] Pepic I, Hafner A, Lovric J, Perina Lakos G. Nanotherapeutics in the EU: an overview on current state and future directions. Int J Nanomedicine 2014; 19(9): 1005-23.
[http://dx.doi.org/10.2147/IJN.S55359]

[59] Rycroft T, Trump B, Poinsatte-Jones K, Linkov I. Nanotoxicology and nanomedicine: making development decisions in an evolving governance environment. J Nanopart Res 2018; 20(2): 52. [http://dx.doi.org/10.1007/s11051-018-4160-3]

[60] Jürgens B, Herrero-Solana V. Monitoring nanotechnology using patent classifications: an overview and comparison of nanotechnology classification schemes. J Nanopart Res 2017; 19(4): 151.
[http://dx.doi.org/10.1007/s11051-017-3838-2]

[61] Marcus Furch, Robert Gieseler. Targeted Nanocarriers for Targeted Drug Delivery Of Gene Therapeutics. 2016, EP3087974A1.

[62] Liong Monty, Lu Jie, Tamanoi F. Mesoporous silica nanoparticles for biomedical applications. applications. 2020, US10668024B2.

[63] Kit S. Juntao Luo. Nanocarriers for drug delivery. 2017, US9579400B2.

[64] Jayanthpanyam Mahesh D. Chavanpatil (2010), 'Lipid-Derived Nanoparticles for Brain-Targeted Drug Delivery' US20100076092A1.

[65] Hamidi Mehrdad. (2016), 'Method And System For Synthesizing Nanocarrier Based Long Acting Drug Delivery System for Buprenorphine, US20150024033A1.

[66] Liong Monty, Lu Jie, Fuyuhiktamanoi Jeffrey I. Zink, Andre Nel (2018) 'Mesoporous Silica Nanoparticles for Biomedical Applications', US20100255103A1. 2018.

[67] Ralph A. Reisfeld, Rong Xiang,Yunpingluo, Debbie Liao, Ze Liu, Tingmei Chen, Si Chen, Dan Lu(2017), 'Nanoparticle-Based Tumor-Targeted Drug Delivery', US9629922B2.

[68] Sharma Neeraj. Choua C. Vu(2010) 'Surface-Modified Nanoparticles', WO2009137592A3.

[69] Nolte Ulrich, Bubat Alfred, Haubennestel Karlheinz, Sawitowski Thomas. (2006), 'Surface-Modified Nanoparticles Comprising Polysiloxane Modifier, Their Preparation And Use', US7641972B2.

[70] Fukushima Kazuki, Hedrick James Lupton, Nelson Alshakim, Sanders Daniel Paul. (2014) 'Surface Modified Nanoparticles, Methods of their Preparation, and uses thereof for Gene And Drug Delivery', US8642787B2.

[71] Barbet Jacques, Delaage Michel, Le Doussal Jean-Marc. 2010.(2010), 'Affinity Enhancement Immunological Reagents for in Vivo Detection And Killing of Specific Target Cells', US5256395A.

[72] Ruxandragref Yoshiharu Minamitake, Langer Robert S. (1996), 'Biodegradable Injectable Nanoparticles' US5543158A

[73] Nicholas S Bodor. (1991), 'Pharmaceutical Formulations for Parenteral use' US5024998A

[74] Shi Jinjun, Xiao Zeyu. Cristian Vilos, Alexander Votruba, Robert S. Langer, Omid C. Farokhzad (2017), 'Lipid-Polymer Hybrid Particles' US9549901B2.

[75] Charles Zepp. Yun Gao, J Keegan Mark, Sam Baldwin, Fen-Ni Fu, Lloyd Johnston, B Lipford Grayson(2017), 'Targeted Synthetic Nanocarrier with pH Sensitive Release of Immunomodulatory Agent' JP2016053048A.

[76] Yu W, Zhang N. (2009), 'Surface Modification of Nanocarriers for Cancer Therapy', Current Nanoscience', 5, 123-134.

[77] Sonvico F, Clementino A, Buttini F, *et al.* Surface-modified nanocarriers for nose-to-brain delivery: from bioadhesion to targeting. Pharmaceutices, 2018; 10,34.

CHAPTER 5

Targeted Nanocarriers-based Approach For Prostate Cancer Therapy

Ashish Garg[1], Vijay Sagar Madamsetty[2], Sumel Ashique[3], Vinod Gauttam[4] and Neeraj Mishra[5,*]

[1] *Department of P.G. Studies and Research in Chemistry and Pharmacy, Rani Durgavati University, Jabalpur, M.P.482001 India.*

[2] *Department of Biochemistry and Molecular Biology, Mayo Clinic, Jacksonville, Florida 32224, USA*

[3] *Department of Pharmaceutics, Bharat Institute of Technology (BIT), School of Pharmacy, Meerut- 250103, UP, India*

[4] *IES Institute of Pharmacy, IES University, Bhopal 462044, India*

[5] *Amity Institute of Pharmacy, Amity University, , Gwalior 474005, MP, India*

Abstract: Prostate cancer is the most common malignancy in men, with elevated morbidity and mortality. The current management, along with dope, leads to chemo defiance. On molecular imaging, many researchers have assisted with staging, restaging, early diagnosis, and, particularly, prostate cancer healing. At the site of cancer, treatment of prostate cancer, including chemo, has encountered many difficulties, such as quick clearance of dope or defiance of drug and short accumulation. Nanotechnology applications and their use in biomedicine to deliver various therapeutic carriers fitted to relieve deputy chemotherapy for cancer treatment. The tumor-targeted dope delivery-related carriers are outlined for prostate cancer healing. Among them, the developing nanotechnology has introduced several innovative new testing technologies, and medications for prostate cancer nanotechnology can significantly increase the management operation of prostate cancer by using specific physical and chemical properties, targeting techniques, or anchoring with imaging / pharmacological substances to provide an innovative theranostics device. This chapter focused on the ultra-modern outgrowth in the observation of nanomaterial and the identity of prostate cancer, including the representation of modes used to point biomolecules operationalization and the various prostate cancers along with nanoparticles, multifunctional nanoplatforms, and nano-related methods of dope delivery in the administration.

Keywords: Cancer pointing, Chemo, Dope delivery, Nanoparticles, Prostate cancer.

* **Corresponding author Neeraj Mishra:** Amity Institute of Pharmacy, Amity University, Gwalior, 474005, MP, India; Tel: +91-8454746714; E-mail: neerajdops@gmail.com

Neeraj Mishra, Ashish Garg and Neeraj Upmanyu (Eds.)

INTRODUCTION

Worldwide, cancer is the main reason of death, and this disease leads up to the second position in all countries and has been considered a pandemic over time [1]. This is a kind of disease that was observed by cell multiplications. The lack of dead cells leads to unrestrained cell division, which produces tumors. To violate the various cells and body organs, the tumor forms, possessing the biological process, and gets metastatic. Malevolent growth has been fetched by multiple aspects, such as the changes to the genetic resource, obtained genetic merits, environmental variables such as toxic waste, life system, tobacco, anxiety, power, contaminants, energy, and absence of bodily actions. The approaches of growth therapy are based upon the process of medicinal, irradiation, or chemo. These can show more reasonableness for therapy, especially at subsequent stages. The prostate gland placed before the rectum excretes a solid white fluid mixed through the sperm of the gonads towards generating the semen. Together with the spermatozoa, white prostatic fluid is open and hooked onto the urethra on the central release division. Almost 30-50 little sacs can hold the white liquid inside the prostate. It also produces a protein known as Prostate-Specific Antigen or shortly known as PSA [2], and can convert semen into liquid. Fig. (**1**) shows that the prostate gland structure includes the cancerous prostate. This particular organ is placed in between the urethra or bladder and rectum. Through the circulatory system, the cancerous gland and the prostate organ spread to the human body [3].

All over the world, in many countries, Prostate malignant growth is the second on the whole cause on behalf of deadliness, and its frequency is also extended together. The potentiality of this disease is 1 in 6 in the United States of America. This disease is the most common among men. This particular disease is the reason for most of the deaths. While screening Prostate-Specific Antigen PSA, this disease production differs from country to country. In the west, this disease can be widespread in both ecology and lifestyle; the information has to be possessed by migrants. In its therapy, various advances are embarked upon. They added multiple dopes that give a boost to patients living capability, including the advanced stages of cancer. Many diseases called cancers are hormone-driven despite the type of castration resistance [4, 5].

Nonetheless, several areas of urgent unmet need remain a) a validated biomarker to complement PSA for screening; b) molecular differentiation of indolent and aggressive disease and prognostic biomarkers with clinical utility; c) molecular stratification methods and predictive biomarkers; d) adjuvant therapies to increase cure rates in higher-risk locally advanced disease; e) treatment of metastatic disease; f) imaging of bone metastasis for staging and response measures; and g) surrogate biomarkers for overall survival benefit.

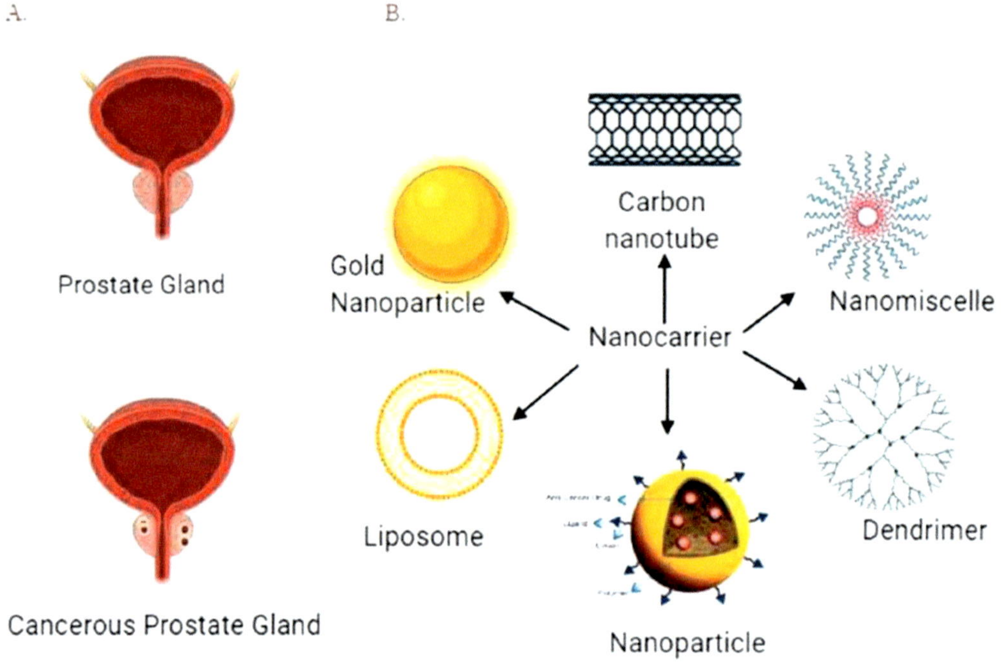

Fig. (1). (A) Structure of prostate gland and tumour in prostate gland; (B) Schematic representation of various nanocarriers applied for prostate tumour targeting and treatment [6]. (Reproduced with permission of Elsevier; Licence No. 5064700159505).

Cancer treatment can be reached by managing the anti-cancer dopes by the technique of systemic infusion. Systemic and Regional are the two techniques of chemotherapeutic delivery related to the coverage of the body area. Systemic delivery has major flaws because of its contradictory dispensation in the body. This dispensation has emerged in the dead cells. Such dead cells are bone marrow, hair follicles, gonads, and gastrointestinal mucosa. These dead cells are major to the acute complexities and systemic toxicity. The incompatible dopes are taken by the normal cells, and the content of the dopes has to be brought down and transferred to the malignant cells. So, to attain the powerful treatment, a large number of drugs must be shipped. Irradiation and chemo treatments are battled with the disease called cancer. The targeted approaches needed are that it helps to increase the treatment along with the side effects. In the stages of microscopic and macroscopic organelles, nanomedicine is utilized to spot cancer [7] *via* the functionalization of substances. Such substances are hormones, carbohydrates, vitamins, aptamers, antibodies, and oligopeptides. These have improved the effectiveness of nanomedicine biodistribution, pharmacokinetics, and therapy protocol [8]. While delivering the dopes to the tumor cells through the locoregional (local regions borders) techniques, nanomedicine is a choice that decreases the effects to a gripping level. In clinical trials, the locoregional dope delivery chemo treatment was examined to break the poisoning of anti-cancer medicines. In the cancer of pancreatic research, enduring the chemo treatment, the subject has to be found to be more potent than the systemic approach with the side effects. This shows average ratings of living conditions along with the highest partial response, including the fewest hematological complications [9].

PROSTATE CANCER NANOCARRIERS & NANOTECHNOLOGY

Nanocarriers, a particle's submicron size <500 nm, are considered the colloidal drug carrier for the management of prostate cancer [10]. In the past few decades, Nanocarriers have been examined significantly in the dope delivery areas. Nanocarriers can make the properties and dopes of bioactivities. Some features are incorporated into dope delivery methods. Such features include pharmacokinetics and biodistribution improvements, poisonous decreases, stability & solubility improvements, and discharge and site-specific delivery of controlled healing agents [11, 12]. By changing the physicochemical properties of nanocarriers compositions like organic and inorganic, sizes like small and large, shapes like a ball, rod, and dice, and surface possessions like surface charge, functional groups, PEGylation or pegylation, targeting moieties attachments, the nanocarriers properties of physicochemical, are attuned [13].

In drug delivery, the entire aim of the nanocarriers is to handle the particular disease productively along with lower side effects. The structural representation of prostate cancer and the nanoparticle-based targeting approach is depicted in Fig. (**2**). When shipped through the dope delivery methods, Anti-cancer chemotherapeutics can confer various issues with poor specificity, high poisoning, and drug resistance foundation [14]. These barriers can decrease the anti-cancer Dope healing merits. By utilizing the pathophysiology of tumor microhabitat, Nanocarrier related areas allow anti-cancer dopes delivery into the tumours. For oncological set-ups, consequently enhancing the results of the healings [16]. In the cells of the tumour surface, the overexpressed receptors are pointed with platforms of the nanocarriers. This can be modelled by targeting ligands. Various nanocarrier-related products are accepted for treating tumours, and others are in various stages of medical testing. In cancer treatments, the characteristics of the multiple nanocarriers are organic, inorganic, and hybrid. The targeting mechanisms can be extended, and the operationalized surface on nanocarriers enhances the identifiability. Nanotechnology is considered an emerging area that is used for nanoparticles. It is also used in the study and treatment of disease encouragements [17 - 19].

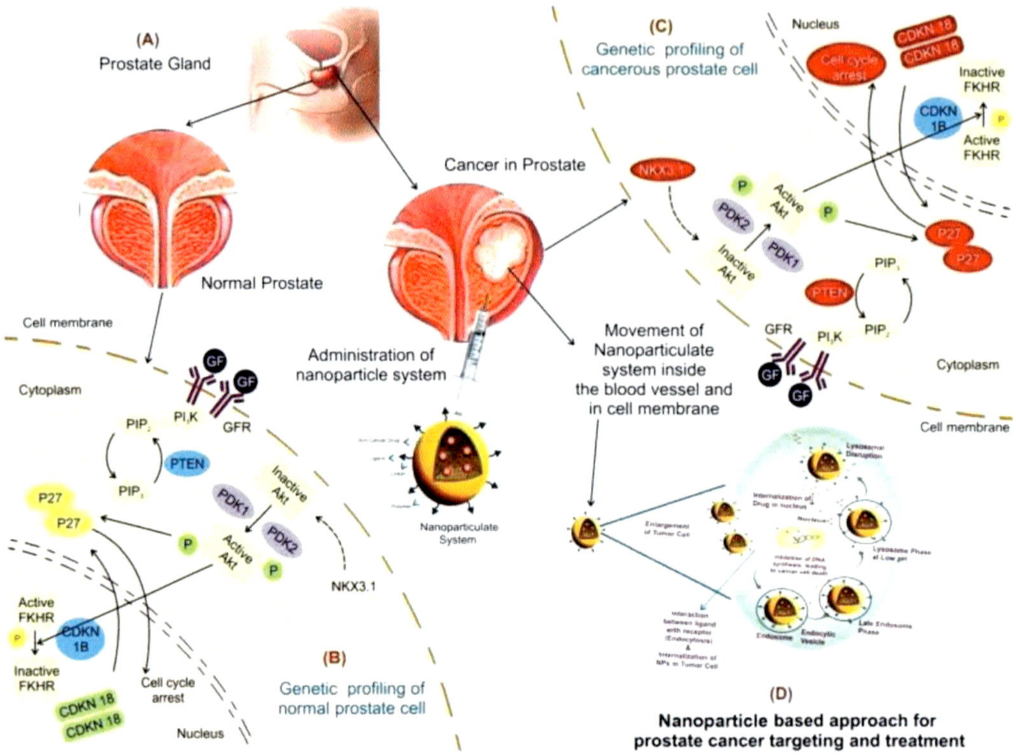

Fig. (2). Structure represents the (**A**) Prostate gland (normal and cancerous prostate); (**B** & **C**) Genetic profiling of normal and cancerous prostate and (**D**) Nanoparticle-based approach for prostate cancer targeting and therapy (Reproduce with permission of Elsevier; Licence No. 5064700159505 [15].

Due to their size and surface-to-volume proportions, nanoparticles give solutions to the remedies for malignant growth. In *vivo,* the nanoparticles' size, surface, and shape moderate their part in biodistribution [20]. It is possible to fulfill the issues by using the methods of nanotechnology, which include (a) water-solvent medications transportation improvements, (b) regarding the sub-atomic points and clear-cut organic, site-coordinated medications are transported, (c) emerging some surgical utensils and (d) mixture of confirmative experiments along with medicinal experts. A few remedial agents are entered into the medicinal developments for a few treatments; at the nanoscale stage, the nano's creation, including the substance's properties, progressed. Nanotechnology was the center stage in medicine on a molecular scale, along with nano-structure combinations. In cancer treatment, a new therapy has been created by utilizing nanomedicine to enhance medication delivery and 100 percent effectiveness with insignificant symptoms. The part of NT is Nanomedicine which applies to medication, assessing, preventing diseases, relieving pressure, protection, and improving human life, using utensils at a molecular stage, including the molecular information of the human body. Miniaturization impacts the essential characteristics of the substances compared to the growth stage. Due to the extension of the region of the surface to the size of the molecules, such impacts are formed. The arrangement of the atom is different along with the surface area. This can give the magnetic, electronic, and optical, thermal properties that affect the biological conveying. For example, the surface arrangements and the cell size use up [21]. Nanoparticles are custom-built to particular supplications. Nanoparticles are heaped along with atoms in detective agents [22].

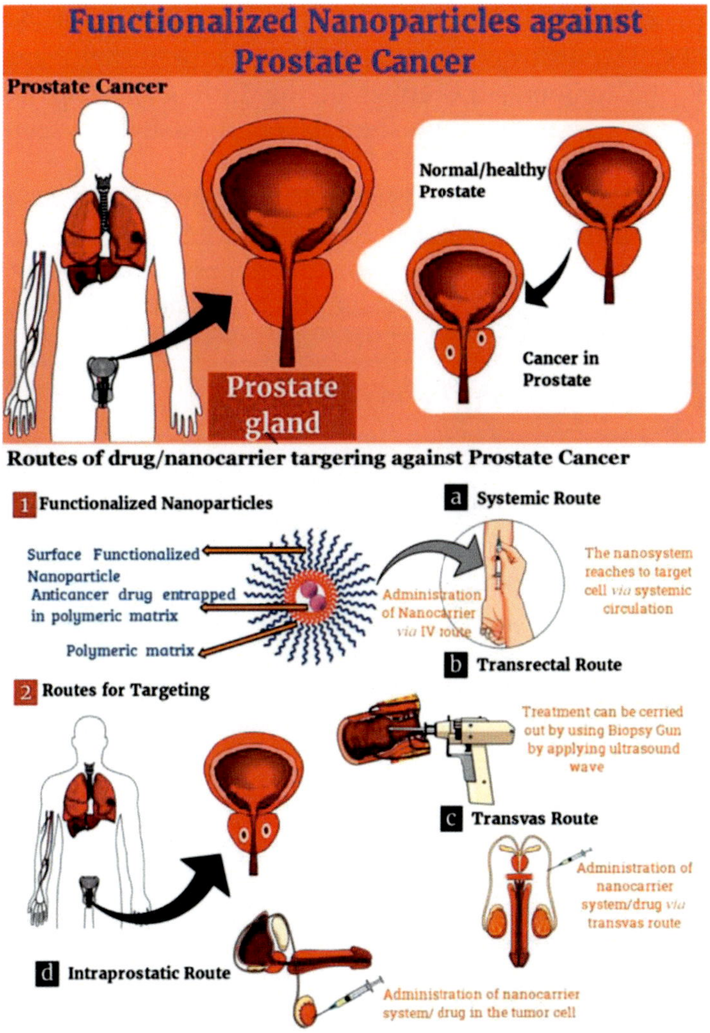

Fig. (3). Prostate cancer; Structure of functionalized nanoparticles and their targeting strategy against prostate cancer with different methods of targeting.

Forming an antineoplastic therapy is the most significant objection in medical science fields. Chemo treatment delivers the cytotoxic agent to the neoplastic cells. By changing the dispersion, NT chemo treatment is custom-built to provide a large amount of medication to the tissues of the tumour [23]. Furthermore, by using the mixed-type treatment, this process could enhance the effects of the medical [24]. For constructing the nanoparticles, elements are shown in Fig. (**3**).

In both active and passive ways, nanoparticle assemblages can be executed inside the tumours. The passive type of pointing is based on the phenomena like convection and diffusion. Throughout the pressure-driven blood movement, the convection procedure occurred. Convection is chargeable for the release of big-sized molecules. The diffusion is chargeable for expelling the lower molecular weight. Inside the tumours, the effect of the EPR stands up the nanocarrier aggregation [25]. By using the fluorescent nanoprobe and microscopy, this can be visualized in prostate malignancy [26]. In linking the carrier and target and through the receptors in the tumor sites, the surfaces of the nanoparticles are changed to obtain the specific interactions. Without the effects, the active pointing should not improve the gatherings of the dopes within the tumour cells. Centralizing the cells of the tumour, examples of ligands are galactosamine [27] and transferrin [28], including folate [29].

ROUTES OF DRUG DELIVERY TO THE PROSTATE

Routes of drug delivery towards prostate cancer related to 2 altered routes: locoregional route and systemic route, displayed in Fig. (**3**).

Systemic Route

The primary issue in the prostate tumor is using the animal as models; it was not occurring as in humans because of the differences in inherited parameters and dealings employing the gene-ecology. Most of the study was done only by prostate tumor cells of animal models rather than humans with or without any genetic changes by inducing the cells externally orthotopically or subcutaneously. Thus, it might stimulate the disease by hereditary, physiological prostate tumor cells in both animal and human systems. Generally, DD and NPs are utilized to revise the prostate disease in the study form. The significant drugs which were for systemic delivery were intraperitoneal [30], retro-orbital [31], intravenous [32], tail vein [33], and intravenous and subcutaneous [34]. These medications and nanoparticles will go into the blood, run through the body, and store in the tumor site. The ligand's effect intercedes the active and passive targeting that encouraged the dopes to attain the nanoparticles and locales of the tumor.

Locoregional Routes

Intraprostatic Route

Intraprostatic sedate was divided into two significant thoughts, such as the preclinical and clinical arrangement. The medication conveyance approaches utilized this chiefly. The medicated implant is considered in preclinical models, and brachytherapy was mainly used in the therapeutic area [35]. The intraprostatic organization delivered a large amount of medication to the tissue with little experience. It can lower the complete administration-based reactions and the toxicities of noncancerous tissues and organs. For the intraprostatic DD study, choosing the living models is more important than selecting the creative models because of the variations physically and anatomically. In locoregional therapy, the primary target is to fulfill the medication into different organs. Plasma plays a vital role altogether less than intravenously conveyed doxorubicin, which recommends the disclosure of the systemic for decreasing the conveyance of the medications to the tissue. Intraprostatic implantations of therapeutic goods are now available in the medicinal therapy suggested as brachytherapy.

Vas Deferens

It is used only for the sperms to modify the urethra and is from the testis [36]. RISUG AdvR, consisting of SMAh & SMAl, SMAl reacts as a model dope. While interpolated into the vas deferens, the wrapped chains of SMAl are changed into the prostate *via* vas in male rats for cancer precaution [37]; Guha SK: WO2009113108 A2). In another assignment, a Finasteride-SMAh+SMAl complex trial was performed in male rats to heal prostate hyperplasia (Guha SK: WO2013124865 A1). These technologies display that vas deferens are used as dope depots for NPs and DD and also NPs transference to the prostate gland.

Transrectal

The rectum is the proximal anatomical region of the prostate [38]. In such a manner, computerized rectal assessment and transrectal prostate biopsies are the broadly utilized urological strategies for prostate-related illness analysis [39]. Utilizing ultrasound, not just for analysis, however, its misuse as an outer methodology for either immediate or roundabout NPs DD to prostate builds ultrasound implication. For prostate-based infection therapy, the transrectal is a locoregional contender for growth healing [40]. The high-frequency and the low-frequency ultrasound emerged to be prospective. The low frequency exhibits a large tissue penetrant [41]. The rectal is placed following the path to obtain into the prostate noninvasively in humans.

NANOPARTICLES SYSTEM FOR PROSTATE TARGETING CLASSIFICATIONS

Prostate Cancer and Liposomal Nanoparticles

Liposomes are considered circular in shape and have different two-layered structures of the lipid, which gathered themselves in the methods of water [42]. From the circulatory system to the interstitial space, Liposomes appear at the site of activity *via* the eruption [43]. Liposomes are pointed at the tissues by the active and the passive diffusion procedure, through the surface of the lipid layer, the energetic kind of objective encouraged by counting the ligands. These are very useful for syndrome imaging and DD [44]. The nanotechnology method applies to the growth of the tumour, which analyses the liposomal bearers. Due to their humid nature, these can be considered biodegradable and bear up the hydrophilic and hydrophobic matter. Through the procedure of synthesis and composition, they can vary the size and structure. The size extends from 90 to 150 nm and should be natural. The phospholipids, including cholesterol, are the basic divisions [45]. Liposomes are connected with cells only to deliver their substances in four similar manners: adsorption, endocytosis, interchange and amalgamation. Endocytosis is significant for DD. The formation and size would affect the methods, like the cell and the microhabitat. Doxil® took up Ovarian cancer treatment instead of treating a prostate tumour in 1995 [46]. Myocet® was non-pegylated liposomal doxorubicin utilized in the therapy of the 2nd stage of breast cancer and prostate tumour. Montanari (2012) dealt with the studies contrasting the effects of Myocet® and Caelyx® on cells of prostate disease. A higher executable of Myocet® was envisioned than the structure of the pegylated.

Systems of Polymeric Nanoparticles for Cancer Treatment

Polymeric nanoparticles are vesicles that allude to the nanospheres and nanocapsules [47]. It can be shaped spherically, and also it can suck up molecules through the surface. The nanocapsules are also vesicles with cavity restrictions [48]. Several polymers have been generated for ligand-targeted and reflexive deliverance of healing formulations. Starting with the broad spread of polymers, Nanoparticles are gathered. It improves the pharmacokinetic properties of the bioavailability chemo treatment dopes for prostate tumours and can prompt progress in this ground [49]. Natural polysaccharides, such as chitosan and egg whites as polyesters, poly(d,l-lactic-co-glycolic acid)(PLGA) [50], poly(d,l-lactic corrosive) (PLA) [51] and poly (caprolactone) (PCL) [52] should be presently capable of being altered with PEG units determining pegylated co-polymers and are useful polymers for DD. They are considered biodegradable and biocompatible, and they personify the medications of varieties [53]. The

Nanoparticle carrier has various structures, such as dendrimers, nanospheres, nano-capsules, and micelles [54]. Nano-capsules are considered the vesicular structure that made the focal liquid or oily center which was closed by the polymeric shell. The basic modes used to shape these nanoparticles are emulsion polymerization or interfacial polycondensation and nanoprecipitation with emulsification [55]. Nanocapsules and nanospheres are in proper shape from the direct co-polymers or polymers. Remarkably, the pronged polymers form dendrimers. Dendrimer comes from the Greek word, dendron, which defines a tree.

System of Carbon-based

Carbon nanoparticles are used in luminous experiments of bioimaging [56]. The cause is that the inherent is luminous, including the large biodegradability [57]. Their lack of effectiveness and the way exogenous copied elements might exchange them, make them adequately used for luminous DD. Carbon nanotubes have commenced hyperthermia. This can be investigated in prostate growth xenografts in bare mice with the tumour response [58].

Dendrimeric Device

Dendrimers are considered a collection of polymeric materials [59, 60]. The formation of advanced generation is established as round and denser than the dendrimers of lesser production [61]. And its entire plan makes them used as DNA and drug delivery carriers with sensors [62, 63]. Lasker and his colleague formulated a camptothecin functionalized dendrimersomes system for redox-responsive and gene delivery and drug delivery toward prostate cancer cells; completing this method led to enhanced cellular uptake of DNA by near 1.6-fold with enlarged gene transfixion by near 2.4-fold in prostate cancer cells in contrast with the unchanged dendrimer so promising for single carrier related grouping cancer treatment. In this way, Somani (2019) prepared camptothecin functionalized dendrimersomes for redox responsiveness and gene deliverance. Another research study was done with prepared triazine dendrimers highlighted with 4, 16, and 64 PSMA-targeted ligands to improve tumour uptake [64]. Other clusters of researchers planned dendrimer-based platforms for efficient tumor cells subsequent to TGFβ1-induced epithelial-mesenchymal conversion, demonstrating the method's significantly improved feeling [65].

Quantum Dot Platform

Semiconductor nanocrystals are considered the position of atoms described from 2-6 or 3-5 clusters in the periodic table [66]. Quantum dots are covered, which could be utilized for fasteners to many diagnostic and healing agents for cancer findings [67]. Cai and his studies have labeled the human prostate tumour cells using quantum dots with PSMA antibody [68]. Twin colour magnetic-quantum dot nanobeads (MQBs) method urbanized, including the projected twin-color MQBs-based luminous side immunoassay, is a point-of-care diagnostics method for analyzing PCa even in the resource-limited locale [69]. The technique was urbanized by Wang, which acts as a biomarker and can detect the prognostic worth of prostate cancer. Wang and his research group, formed a quantum-do--related method for immune-fluorescent base imaging and finding of DNER, Delta/Notch-like Epidermal Growth Factor (EGF) based on the receptor [70].

System of Gold Nanoparticulate

Gold nanoparticles have properties such as a vast surface-to-volume proportion, unique biocompatibility, and low lethality [71]. A mixture of shape and size blends show altering properties that should be abused for theranostic reasons, such as optical properties that permit use as an agent for contrast, next to photothermal capabilities in the infrared range [72]. The unambiguously enhanced radiative properties like scattering, assimilation and a plasmonic field to the surface-upgraded Raman of close-by atoms create gold nanoparticles supportive for subatomic malignant growth diagnostics [73]. Gold nanoparticle tests discriminate against tuberculosis [74], just growth biomarkers in the ex vivo locale. In 2010, the writers functionalized the exterior of gold nanoparticles and RNA aptamer, which ties to prostate-explicit layer antigen with a developed subatomic CT imaging structure [75]. Gold nanoparticles are considered nontoxic and non-immunogenic and developed as DD vehicles in focusing on tumours, briefly recovering the collision of exact medication familiar to be forced by restrictions [76]. Brown (2010) pointed out that platinum-related anti-cancer medicine oxaliplatin, while conjugated to AuNPs, enhanced DD.

Platform for Metallic Nanoparticle

Metallic nanoparticles are considered flexible devices in biomedical research because of their potency with their small size and precious optical properties. For instance, radio healing enhancement [77], thermal ablation [78], analytical measurements [79], and DD is the central point of late investigations. In addition, the metal property is suitable for the healing and diagnostics in a related molecule, known as theranostics. The established biocidal impact of silver NPs (AgNPs) [80] appeared to be the exacting highlight used for malignant growth. For instance, silver NPs contain antiangiogenic properties that restrain cell extension in tumour enlargement. Gopinath *et al.,* examined the AgNPs cytotoxicity in tumour cells and pragmatic dead cells and a synergic impact with the chemotherapeutic operator 5-fluorouracil [81].

Amongst nanoparticles, superparamagnetic iron oxide nanoparticles are not declared by the FDA. But it was used as the pigmenting agent for liver, spleen and gut imaging due to the inalienable nanocomposite. These are mixed *via* the co-precipitation approach along with the dextran polymer. Non-hydrolytic strategies are used to give high crystalline iron oxide NPs. Pluronic polymers are envisioned as stability for nanoparticles, owing to the enhancing circulation, RES retention limitations, and tumour targeting enhancement by the effect of the EPR [82, 83]. Polymers, for instance, PVP [84], PVA [85], chitosan [86], and starch, used this sort of causing's. PLGA, PCL and its iron oxide nanoparticle-related combinations are examined as malignant growth DD systems [87]. Dextran is the stable and declared FDA plan of magnetic NP for imaging applications. Most of the dextran-based mixtures are used in the solutions. Egg whites are the most pliable covering for generating the NP [88]. Polymersomes [89, 90], dendrimer [91], and Pluronic® polymers [92] are suitable for stabilities. Chemo treatment experts use paclitaxel for the widespread use of malignancies. Docetaxel (Dtxl, Taxotere®) is another FDA-endorsed chemotherapeutic operator for prostate malignancy, and its dangerous symptoms have decreased its medical uses. The nanoparticle can enhance the conveyance and viability of docetaxel in the tumour of the prostate (LNCaP, DU 145, and PC3) [93]. This can also enhance the anti-cancer process of docetaxel, which was fulfilled with nanoparticle ideas decorated with layers of polymer vesicles. The NPs bearer are used to anti-cancer medication atoms, for instance, 5-fluorouracil (5-FU), zoledronate (anti osteoclastic properties) [94], flutamide [95], bicalutamide (antiandrogen) [96] and doxorubicin (DOX) [97]. In addition, lipid-based magnetic nanoparticles are proposed broadly due to medication capability in hydrophobic layers [98]. Iron oxide nanoparticles are composed of a centre and a hydrophilic level of dextran to extend their power [99]. The operators show that the size-subordinate super magnetism enhances them with the magnet field use. After the expulsion of the magnetic force, the particles don't have any combination. Superparamagnetic iron oxide NPs are used as T2-weighted MR staining agents to follow [100]. They provide advantages through gadolinium and advanced imaging affectability [101]. Ferumoxtran-10 is a monocrystalline superparamagnetic iron oxide consisting of solid coverage of dextrans which has been boosted by lymph hubs [102]. Ferumoxtran-10 is exploded into the interstitial space, and it is from the vascular space starting the point to lymph hubs through lymphatic vessels producing lower intensity inside the tissue of the lymph on T2*-weighted iron-delicate MRI successions [103]. The various nanocarrier systems utilized in the treatment of prostate cancer are depicted in Table **1**.

Table 1. Various nanocarriers utilized in the treatment of prostate cancer.

S. No.	Nanocarrier based System	Therapeutic approach	References
1.	Liposome	Resveratrol and curcumin enclosed into liposomal carriers for the reduction of the prostate adenocarcinoma	[104]
-	-	Curcumin-PSMA	[105]
-	-	Liposome nano vector with docetaxel	[106]
-	-	Liposome (surface functionalized) with PSMA for precise delivery of theranostics to $PSMA^+$ prostate cancer	[107]
-	-	Folate-conjugated liposomes	[108]
2	Nanoparticles Polymeric Nanoparticles	Cisplatin-PLGA-PEG-Apt nanoparticles	[109]
-	-	Docetaxel entrapped PLGA-PEG and PLA-PEG system	[110]
-	-	PEG-covered and Gd-stacked fluorescent silica nanoparticles	[111]
-	-	Salinomycin-typified lipid-PLGA nanoparticles	[112]
-	-	Plumbagin-stacked aptamer focused on poly D,L-lactic--o-glycolic corrosive b-polyethylene glycol nanoparticles	[113]
-	Gold Nanoparticles	AuNPs-thiolate polyethylene glycol (PEG)	[114]
-	-	AuNPs-L-aspartate with anti-cancer drugs (Cisplatin, Doxorubicin, and Capecitabine)	[115]
-	-	Gold nanoparticles-EGFRs antibodies	[116]
-	-	Goserelin-gold nanorods (gAuNRs) and pegylated-gold nanorods (pAuNRs).	[117]
-	Metal-based Nanoparticle system	Silver nanoparticles system for PC3 prostate cells	[118]
-	-	Glucose-bound AuNPs	[119]
-	Dendrimer	Chlorambucil-Ugi dendrimers with PAMAM-NH_2 Core system	[120]
-	-	Dendriplexes system against prostate cancer.	[121]
-	Quantum Dot	CdTe Quantum dot	[122]
-	-	Fluorometric immune device with quantum-dot labeled antibodies	[123]
-	Carbon Nanotube	Functionalized multi-walled carbon nanotubes with H3R6 polypeptide (MHR-CpG)	[124]
-	-	Carbon nanomaterials with docetaxel (DTX) and mitomycin C (MMC)	[125]

PROSTATE CANCER DIAGNOSIS AND NANOTECHNOLOGY APPROACH

The proportion of the biological markers concerning the prostate-specific antigen, for prostate tumour screening test biomarkers, are used in serum which is interrelated to a consequence of the functioning with the pathophysiology of prostatic epithelial cells. Though, investigators and physicians are focused on Prostate-specific antigen levels. Prostate-specific antigen device quality is a screening device for Prostate hateful development. For specific pointer reactions, treatments for prostate-specific antigens will be used, and those who have experienced radical prostatectomy will use it again for those patients.

A research group [126] utilized a wonder touch based on the things of nanotechnology, it is known as the "bio-standardized tag" construction, and it is used to identify an invisible degree of a prostate-specific antigen in prostate cruel growth patients. So Kattesh's has connected GNPs to a Prostate disease cell line to activate visual difficulty in growth cells of non-pigmented malignant cells and to empower the location of cells in a photoacoustic run meter, planned toward discovering coursing tumour cells in blood tests [127]. Finally, acoustic photo reaction from Prostate disease cells treated the white platters cells are flows and cells are undercurrent. According to the research, thermotherapy is used to biocompatible SPION in patients with locally repetitive prostate malignancy tumours. Another research group created an open plan of attractive liquid about hyperthermia based on the methodology of non-invasive figurings of the three-dimensional temperature [128]. Interstitial hyperthermia utilizing attractive NPs in patients with malignant prostate growth was the first clinically used with followers of radiotherapy with a therapeutic purpose. Weissleder bunch found the usage in a single circumstance of the utilization of exceptionally location-specific practice number that holds notable guarantees are permitted in the magnetic resonance imaging scan, which clinically strange lymph-node to the patients with Prostate tumour growth, these things are not identified by more non-invasive methodology. For Prostate malignant growth image, Lee has announced plans for the magneto fluorescent polymeric materials in vivo. In particular, gastric-discharging peptide receptors focused on BC-NAHis-GC are bombesin-conjugated N-acetyl histidine-glycol chitosan, and prostate disease cells are expressed about it. Bombesin-conjugated N-acetyl histidine-glycol chitosan designed with nitrophenyl sulfenyl checked all high authorities about the prostate growth cell surface compared with nitrophenyl sulfenyl, including bombesin. In the future, superparamagnetic iron oxide nanoparticles staked in the Bombesin-conjugated N-acetyl histidine-glycol chitosan nitrophenyl sulfenyl will be used for magnetic resonance imaging. Prostate disease imaging may be helpful with the framework before it was recommended for malignant prostate expansion; rats are enhanced tumours, as shown in the result [129]. PSA or prostate-specific antigen is a glycoprotein sent by prostatic epithelial cells and obtained by a progressive Prostate tumour development end [130, 131]. Prostate-specific antigen was obtained by typical prostate cells and carcinogenic prostate cells. Despite the statement that prostate-specific antigen levels will be used, as usual, showing materials used for Prostate tumour development discovery, and it is used for a specific marker of result to the treatment and do again for the patients who are already experienced in the radical prostatectomy. Silver nanoparticles show the lights are close to the surface plasmon reverberation (SPR), and its wavelengths are settled [132]. Dynamic light dissipating is combined with silver nanoparticles, and an appreciation and exploration were created by the protein biomarkers and serum biomarkers, which are simple nitrophenyl sulfenyl with the immunochemical assay. The nanoparticle of the immuno-chemical assay was revealed to help in the normal needed things for breaking down the serum biomarkers and protein biomarkers such as prostate-specific antigen and also discover the new biomarkers coherent with tumour and various human [133]. An ultra-delicate creation is also known as a bio-level framework, and that is based on silver nanoparticles. The test has been finished with the use of deoxyribonucleic acid and antibodies, which we can preserve and attach with prostate-specific antigen when it seems normal and low standard during the serum tests. This study has come many times and is reachable and economically available in prostate-specific antigen tests. Viator's (2010) bunch has been connected with AuPs to create Prostate disease cell lines to ensure non-pigmented malignant development of some sets of size (2.5×109) to stimulate the separation of tumour cells. As a result, prostate-specific antigens preserve the human prostate tumour development cells upto 50-cells standard. Another study [134] described human immunoglobulin in a detailed manner G(IgG) with the use of gold nanoparticle protein, which deals with the development of cancer patients' tumours, which is different from non-disease control. Prostate tumour development of bio-repository collects polycrystalline cubic boron nitride blood test has a 90-95%, which is used to identify the initial stage of Prostate disease, which deals with the development of the prostate-specific antigen test. The test will be more suitable for calculating the level of malignancy range from the initial to the final stage.

Prostate Cancer Fluorescence Diagnosis Using Nanotechnologies

Fluorescence Diagnosis method helps to identify the levels of cancer, and it helps to provide treatment according to the level. Molecular imaging helps calculate the stages of cancer from initial to final and also helps to give therapy for cancer according to the level of the tumour. Nanotechnology and fluorescence diagnosis helps to reach solutions for many parts. Nowadays, we have a lot of advanced equipment in the medical field. One of the advanced treatments is nanotechnology, through which we can analyze the level of malignancy and give treatment results in vivo. Many biomarkers were invented to know about the initial stage of cancer [135] and matriptase [136].

Targeted PSA Nanoprobe for Imaging Prostate Cancer

Prostate-specific antigen stimulates prostate gland. Produces PSA, and about thirty-three kDa deals with androgen-regulated serine protease. The specific biomarker can analyze prostate tumours and express it initially. In 2001, Lövgren stated an analytic view of equipment based on the country of europium and nanoparticles that complained about the mental picture and view of the prostate-specific antigen molecules with microscopy [137]. In 2009, Gao developed a new net promoter score or NPs system that helps to create an established acute exposure to prostate-specific antigen [138]. They are moving towards further action for QD preparation which comes under the nanoparticle difficulties in homogeneous solutions. In 2016, a new document was started by Chen that is the form of $Lu_6O_5F_8:Eu^{3+}$ nanoprobe and its analysis of prostate-specific antigens in the medical field. They also created nanoparticles such as non-living lanthanide fluoride based on a luminescent bioassay method to help the sensitivity and amplified signal.

Prostate-Specific Membrane Antigen (PSMA) Nanoprobes for Imaging Prostate Cancer

Prostate-specific membrane antigen was discovered in prostatic epithelial cells and caring cells, and it is also called tissues like the brain, liver and kidney. This prostate-specific membrane antigen collected 750 amino acids in the form of transmembrane attached in the form of 2 glycoproteins, which shows human prostate epithelium, including majorly the prostate malignant cells. In metastasis, it reacts poorly with distinguishable and hormone-refractory carcinomas [139]. Biotinylated anti-prostate-specific membrane antigen antibodies, such as streptavidin-labeled iron oxide nanoparticles, can be used for probe analysis and help find malignant prostate cells [140]. The development of prostate-specific membrane antigen focuses on gold nanoparticles, and it was complete with the use of 5 prostate-specific membrane antigen focused on gold nanoparticles was successes with the use of 5 nuclear medicine gold nanoparticles enclosed with streptavidin and inducting prostate-specific membrane antigen forbid that biotinylated. The end results advocate that prostate-specific membrane antigen focused on the gold nanoparticles and that focused on being well than non-specificity non-focused gold nanoparticles, which was praised about the gold nanoparticles that can be used for prostate-specific membrane antigen by distributing forbids.

RECENT AND ONGOING CLINICAL TRIALS FOR PROSTATE CANCER TREATMENT

In America, prostate cancer is a normally found cancer; in the second stage, cancer leads to death during this period, and population growth is greatly affected. In the United States, 174,650 people were affected by this prostate cancer, and 31,620 people died in 2019 [141]. This cancer affects adults according to their age. Accurate information of affected people is 30% of men aged 60 to 69 years and 67% of men were involved in aged starting from 60 to 80 years, and it was analyzed of prostate cancer. Most cancer comes from their family genetic disorder and the sexual affair between Africans and Americans; they also consume more fatty foods. Symptoms of prostate cancer are focal nodules, backbone pain, strength less bones that break easily and urinary difficulties. Before prostate cancer, we can take a test that helps to know about prostate cancer levels in human blood. Physicians take many tests and exams to enhance the level of prostate-specific antigens using magnetic resonance imaging. Especially for males, the newly analyzed prostate cancer took on difficulties in the beginning level of treatment. It may increase the disease if the molecules are present in the tumour and serum prostate-specific antigen level. The outcome comes with various treatment facilities and difficulties with patients' health conditions and age in every treatment. There are many treatments available in cancer options, such as operation and radiation method, hormonal unbalancing treatment combined of thalamus cells and gland levels in kidneys, therapy based on chemicals and therapy based on immune potential. Immunotherapy treatment is not recommended for males with no practice in that illness [142]. The recent and ongoing clinical trials for the management of prostate cancer are represented in Table **2**.

Table 2. Current & ongoing clinical trials for the treatment of prostate cancer.

S. No.	Clinical Trials for the Treatment of Prostate Cancer	Status/Phase	References/ Identification No.
1.	A Multi-modal, Physician-centered Intervention to Improve Guideline-concordant Prostate Cancer Imaging.	Active/ NA	[143]
2.	Outcomes of Focal Therapies for Prostate Cancer.	Recruiting/ -	[144]
3.	Imaging Studies to Check the Local Response of Prostate Cancer to Radiation Therapy	Recruiting/ -	[145]

(Table 2) cont.....

S. No.	Clinical Trials for the Treatment of Prostate Cancer	Status/Phase	References/ Identification No.
4.	PSMA-based 18F-DCFPyL PET/CT and PET/MRI Pilot Studies in Prostate Cancer	Recruiting/ Early Phase 1	[146]
5.	Stereotactic Body Radiation Therapy (SBRT) for Prostate Cancer.	Recruiting/ NA	[147]
6.	Imaging Studies to Check the Local Response of Prostate Cancer to Radiation Therapy.	Recruiting/ -	[148]
7.	PD-L1 Inhibition as Checkpoint Immunotherapy for Neuroendocrine Phenotype Prostate Cancer (PICK-NEPC).	Completed/ Phase 2	[149]
8.	A Study of Olaparib and Durvalumab in Prostate Cancer.	Recruiting/ Phase 2	[150]
9.	Prostate SBRT for Locally Recurrent Prostate Cancer After Prior Radiotherapy.	Recruiting/ Phase 1	[151]
10.	Nivolumab in Patients With High-Risk Biochemically Recurrent Prostate Cancer.	Recruiting/ Phase 2	[152]
11.	Trial of Curcumin to Prevent Progression of Low-risk Prostate Cancer Under Active Surveillance.	Recruiting/ Phase 3	[153]
12.	BrUOG 337: Olaparib Prior to Radical Prostatectomy For Patients With Locally Advanced Prostate Cancer and Defects in DNA Repair Genes (337).	Recruiting/ Phase 2	[154]
13.	Focal Laser Ablation of Prostate Cancer Tumors.	Recruiting/ NA	[155]
14.	Abiraterone With Discontinuation of Gonadotropin-Releasing Hormone Analogues in Metastatic Prostate Cancer.	Active/ Phase 2	[156]
15.	Prostate Cancer Intensive, Non-Cross Reactive Therapy (PRINT) for Castration-Resistant Prostate Cancer (CRPC).	Recruiting/ Phase 2	[157]
16.	Study of VERU-944 to Ameliorate Hot Flashes in Men With Advanced Prostate Cancer.	Completed/ Phase 2	[158]
17.	PreOperative RadioTherapy for High-Risk Prostate Cancer (PORT-PC Trial) (PORT-PC).	Recruiting/ NA	[159]
18.	Abiraterone Acetate, Niclosamide, and Prednisone in Treating Patients With Hormone-Resistant Prostate Cancer.	Recruiting/ Phase 2	[160]
19.	CART-PSMA-TGFÎ²RDN Cells for Castrate-Resistant Prostate Cancer.	Recruiting/ Phase 1	[161]
20.	Focal Radiation for Oligometastatic Castration-resistant Prostate Cancer (FORCE).	Recruiting/ Phase 2	[162]
21.	ESK981 in Treating Patients With Metastatic Castrate-Resistant Prostate Cancer.	Active/ Phase 2	[163]
22.	LEE011 (Ribociclib) in Combination With Docetaxel Plus Prednisone in mCRPC.	Active/ Phase 2	[164]

(Table 2) cont.....

S. No.	Clinical Trials for the Treatment of Prostate Cancer	Status/Phase	References/ Identification No.
23.	Fluciclovine F18 or Ga68-PSMA PET/CT to Enhance Prostate Cancer Outcomes.	Recruiting/ Phase 2	[165]

CONCLUSION

In the outline, dope release systems came under the NPs. They recommended malignant medications utilized for interacting with specific molecule actions and their involvedness and growth in the cancer cells. This method comes under the NPs to develop the particular cancer cell and provide treatment to make it a suitable cancer cell. Many difficulties and obstacles are present in the current period to solve these problems and give more valuable treatment for this type of PSA cancer. Compared with other studies, they have enough compositions of NPs agreed for cancer treatment. In the future, many innovative technologies will be essential for rebalancing the particle and increasing the target potential.

CONSENT FOR PUBLICATION

Not applicable.

CONFLICT OF INTEREST

The authors declare no conflict of interest, financial or otherwise.

ACKNOWLEDGMENTS

We are thankful to the team at Bentham Science Publishers for giving us this opportunity, the editor of this book, and everyone who supported us directly or indirectly while writing this book chapter.

REFERENCES

[1] Bray F, Ferlay J, Soerjomataram I, Siegel RL, Torre LA, Jemal A. Global cancer statistics 2018: GLOBOCAN estimates of incidence and mortality worldwide for 36 cancers in 185 countries. CA Cancer J Clin 2018; 68(6): 394-424.
[http://dx.doi.org/10.3322/caac.21492] [PMID: 30207593]

[2] Lilja H, Ulmert D, Vickers AJ. Prostate-specific antigen and prostate cancer: prediction, detection and monitoring. Nat Rev Cancer 2008; 8(4): 268-78.
[http://dx.doi.org/10.1038/nrc2351] [PMID: 18337732]

[3] Hodson R. Small organ, big reach. Nature 2015; 528(7582): S118-9.
[http://dx.doi.org/10.1038/528S118a] [PMID: 26672780]

[4] Chen CD, Wels birDS, Tran C, *et al.* Sawyers CL (2004) Molecular de te mi nants of resistance to anti androgen therapy. Nat Med 2004; 10: 33-9.

[5] Taplin ME, Bubley GJ, Shuster TD, *et al.* Mutation of the androgen-receptor gene in metastatic androgen-independent prostate cancer. N Engl J Med 1995; 332(21): 1393-8.

[http://dx.doi.org/10.1056/NEJM199505253322101] [PMID: 7723794]

[6] Garg A, Garg S, Swarnakar NK. Nanoparticles and prostate cancer. Nano Drug Delivery Strategies for the Treatment of Cancers 2021; 275-318.
[http://dx.doi.org/10.1016/B978-0-12-819793-6.00012-6]

[7] Hofheinz RD, Gnad-Vogt SU, Beyer U, Hochhaus A. Liposomal encapsulated anti-cancer drugs. Anticancer Drugs 2005; 16(7): 691-707.
[http://dx.doi.org/10.1097/01.cad.0000167902.53039.5a] [PMID: 16027517]

[8] Jha RK, Jha PK, Chaudhury K, Rana SVS, Guha SK. An emerging interface between life science and nanotechnology: present status and prospects of reproductive healthcare aided by nano-biotechnology. Nano Rev 2014; 5(1): 22762.
[http://dx.doi.org/10.3402/nano.v5.22762] [PMID: 24600516]

[9] Liu F, Tang Y, Sun J, *et al.* Regional intra-arterial vs. systemic chemotherapy for advanced pancreatic cancer: a systematic review and meta-analysis of randomized controlled trials. PLoS One 2012; 7(7): e40847.
[http://dx.doi.org/10.1371/journal.pone.0040847] [PMID: 22815840]

[10] Rawat M, Singh D, Saraf S, Saraf S. Nanocarriers: promising vehicle for bioactive drugs. Biol Pharm Bull 2006; 29(9): 1790-8.
[http://dx.doi.org/10.1248/bpb.29.1790] [PMID: 16946487]

[11] Mishra B, Patel BB, Tiwari S. Colloidal nanocarriers: a review on formulation technology, types and applications toward targeted drug delivery. Nanomedicine 2010; 6(1): 9-24.
[http://dx.doi.org/10.1016/j.nano.2009.04.008] [PMID: 19447208]

[12] Liu Y, Solomon M, Achilefu S. Perspectives and potential applications of nanomedicine in breast and prostate cancer. Med Res Rev 2013; 33(1): 3-32.
[http://dx.doi.org/10.1002/med.20233] [PMID: 23239045]

[13] Din F, Aman W, Ullah I, *et al.* Effective use of nanocarriers as drug delivery systems for the treatment of selected tumors. Int J Nanomedicine 2017; 12: 7291-309.
[http://dx.doi.org/10.2147/IJN.S146315]

[14] Wong H, Bendayan R, Rauth A, Li Y, Wu X. Chemotherapy with anticancer drugs encapsulated in solid lipid nanoparticles. Adv Drug Deliv Rev 2007; 59(6): 491-504.
[http://dx.doi.org/10.1016/j.addr.2007.04.008] [PMID: 17532091]

[15] Garg A, Garg S, Swarnakar NK. Nanoparticles and prostate cancer. Nano Drug Delivery Strategies for the Treatment of Cancers 2021; 275-318.
[http://dx.doi.org/10.1016/B978-0-12-819793-6.00012-6]

[16] Wang AZ, Langer R, Farokhzad OC. Nanoparticle delivery of cancer drugs. Annu Rev Med 2012; 63(1): 185-98.
[http://dx.doi.org/10.1146/annurev-med-040210-162544] [PMID: 21888516]

[17] Ferrari M. Cancer nanotechnology: opportunities and challenges. Nat Rev Cancer 2005; 5(3): 161-71.
[http://dx.doi.org/10.1038/nrc1566] [PMID: 15738981]

[18] Farokhzad OC, Langer R. Impact of nanotechnology on drug delivery. ACS Nano 2009; 3(1): 16-20.
[http://dx.doi.org/10.1021/nn900002m] [PMID: 19206243]

[19] Petros RA, DeSimone JM. Strategies in the design of nanoparticles for therapeutic applications. Nat Rev Drug Discov 2010; 9(8): 615-27.
[http://dx.doi.org/10.1038/nrd2591] [PMID: 20616808]

[20] Alexis F, Pridgen E, Molnar LK, Farokhzad OC. Factors affecting the clearance and biodistribution of polymeric nanoparticles. Mol Pharm 2008; 5(4): 505-15.
[http://dx.doi.org/10.1021/mp800051m] [PMID: 18672949]

[21] He C, Hu Y, Yin L, Tang C, Yin C. Effects of particle size and surface charge on cellular uptake and

biodistribution of polymeric nanoparticles. Biomaterials 2010; 31(13): 3657-66. [http://dx.doi.org/10.1016/j.biomaterials.2010.01.065] [PMID: 20138662]

[22] de Barros A, Tsourkas A, Saboury B, Cardoso V, Alavi A. Emerging role of radiolabeled nanoparticles as an effective diagnostic technique. EJNMMI Res 2012; 2(1): 39. [http://dx.doi.org/10.1186/2191-219X-2-39] [PMID: 22809406]

[23] Hu CMJ, Aryal S, Zhang L. Nanoparticle-assisted combination therapies for effective cancer treatment. Ther Deliv 2010; 1(2): 323-34. [http://dx.doi.org/10.4155/tde.10.13] [PMID: 22816135]

[24] Chow EKH, Ho D. Cancer nanomedicine: from drug delivery to imaging. Sci Transl Med 2013; 5: 216. [http://dx.doi.org/10.1126/scitranslmed.3005872] [PMID: 24353161]

[25] Danhier F, Feron O, Préat V. To exploit the tumor microenvironment: Passive and active tumor targeting of nanocarriers for anti-cancer drug delivery. J Control Release 2010; 148(2): 135-46. [http://dx.doi.org/10.1016/j.jconrel.2010.08.027] [PMID: 20797419]

[26] Sandanaraj BS, Gremlich HU, Kneuer R, Dawson J, Wacha S. Fluorescent nanoprobes as a biomarker for increased vascular permeability: implications in diagnosis and treatment of cancer and inflammation. Bioconjug Chem 2010; 21(1): 93-101. [http://dx.doi.org/10.1021/bc900311h] [PMID: 19958018]

[27] Xu X, Xie K, Zhang XQ, *et al.* Enhancing tumor cell response to chemotherapy through nanoparticle-mediated codelivery of siRNA and cisplatin prodrug. Proc Natl Acad Sci USA 2013; 110(46): 18638-43. [http://dx.doi.org/10.1073/pnas.1303958110] [PMID: 24167294]

[28] Tortorella S, Karagiannis T. The significance of transferrin receptors in oncology: the development of functional nano-based drug delivery systems. Curr Drug Deliv 2014; 11(4): 427-43. [http://dx.doi.org/10.2174/1567201810666140106115436] [PMID: 24387131]

[29] Wang L, Zhang M, Tan K, *et al.* Preparation of nanobubbles carrying androgen receptor siRNA and their inhibitory effects on androgen-independent prostate cancer when combined with ultrasonic irradiation. PLoS One 2014; 9(5): e96586. [http://dx.doi.org/10.1371/journal.pone.0096586] [PMID: 24798477]

[30] Hine CM, Seluanov A, Gorbunova V. Rad51 promoter-targeted gene therapy is effective for *in vivo* visualization and treatment of cancer. Mol Ther 2012; 20(2): 347-55. [http://dx.doi.org/10.1038/mt.2011.215] [PMID: 22008909]

[31] Zhu Y, Sun Y, Chen Y, *et al.* In vivo molecular MRI imaging of prostate cancer by targeting PSMA with polypeptide-labeled superparamagnetic iron oxide nanoparticles. Int J Mol Sci 2015; 16(12): 9573-87. [http://dx.doi.org/10.3390/ijms16059573] [PMID: 25927579]

[32] Thomas S, Waterman P, Chen S, *et al.* Development of secreted protein and acidic and rich in cysteine (SPARC) targeted nanoparticles for the prognostic molecular imaging of metastatic prostate cancer. J Nanomed Nanotechnol 2011; 2(4): 2157-7439-2-112. [http://dx.doi.org/10.4172/2157-7439.1000112] [PMID: 22319675]

[33] Wadajkar AS, Menon JU, Tsai YS, *et al.* Prostate cancer-specific thermo-responsive polymer-coated iron oxide nanoparticles. Biomaterials 2013; 34(14): 3618-25. [http://dx.doi.org/10.1016/j.biomaterials.2013.01.062] [PMID: 23419645]

[34] Ghosh D, Lee Y, Thomas S, *et al.* M13-templated magnetic nanoparticles for targeted *in vivo* imaging of prostate cancer. Nat Nanotechnol 2012; 7(10): 677-82. [http://dx.doi.org/10.1038/nnano.2012.146] [PMID: 22983492]

[35] Wolinsky JB, Colson YL, Grinstaff MW. Local drug delivery strategies for cancer treatment: Gels, nanoparticles, polymeric films, rods, and wafers. J Control Release 2012; 159(1): 14-26.

[http://dx.doi.org/10.1016/j.jconrel.2011.11.031] [PMID: 22154931]

[36] Koslov DS, Andersson KE. Physiological and pharmacological aspects of the vas deferens—an update. Front Pharmacol 2013; 4: 101.
[http://dx.doi.org/10.3389/fphar.2013.00101] [PMID: 23986701]

[37] Guha SK, Chauhan V, Banerjee S. Designed self assembly of nano–liposomes in the male reproductive tract for model drug delivery to the prostate. The Open Nanoscience Journal 2011; 5(1).
[http://dx.doi.org/10.2174/1874140101105010011]

[38] Schutzer ME, Orio PF, Biagioli MC, Asher DA, Lomas H, Moghanaki D. A review of rectal toxicity following permanent low dose-rate prostate brachytherapy and the potential value of biodegradable rectal spacers. Prostate Cancer Prostatic Dis 2015; 18(2): 96-103.
[http://dx.doi.org/10.1038/pcan.2015.4] [PMID: 25687401]

[39] Penzkofer T, Tempany-Afdhal CM. Prostate cancer detection and diagnosis: the role of MR and its comparison with other diagnostic modalities - a radiologist's perspective. NMR Biomed 2014; 27(1): 3-15.
[http://dx.doi.org/10.1002/nbm.3002] [PMID: 24000133]

[40] Kosheleva OK, Lai TC, Chen NG, Hsiao M, Chen CH. Selective killing of cancer cells by nanoparticle-assisted ultrasound. J Nanobiotechnology 2016; 14(1): 46.
[http://dx.doi.org/10.1186/s12951-016-0194-9] [PMID: 27301243]

[41] George AK, Turkbey B, Valayil SG, *et al.* A urologist's perspective on prostate cancer imaging: past, present, and future. Abdom Radiol (NY) 2016; 41(5): 805-16.
[http://dx.doi.org/10.1007/s00261-016-0751-6] [PMID: 27138438]

[42] Torchilin VP. Recent advances with liposomes as pharmaceutical carriers. Nat Rev Drug Discov 2005; 4(2): 145-60.
[http://dx.doi.org/10.1038/nrd1632] [PMID: 15688077]

[43] Malam Y, Loizidou M, Seifalian AM. Liposomes and nanoparticles: nanosized vehicles for drug delivery in cancer. Trends Pharmacol Sci 2009; 30(11): 592-9.
[http://dx.doi.org/10.1016/j.tips.2009.08.004] [PMID: 19837467]

[44] Park JH, Cho HJ, Yoon HY, *et al.* Hyaluronic acid derivative-coated nanohybrid liposomes for cancer imaging and drug delivery. J Control Release 2014; 174: 98-108.
[http://dx.doi.org/10.1016/j.jconrel.2013.11.016] [PMID: 24280260]

[45] Medina O, Zhu Y, Kairemo K. Targeted liposomal drug delivery in cancer. Curr Pharm Des 2004; 10(24): 2981-9.
[http://dx.doi.org/10.2174/1381612043383467] [PMID: 15379663]

[46] Hubert A, Lyass O, Pode D, Gabizon A. Doxil (Caelyx): an exploratory study with pharmacokinetics in patients with hormone-refractory prostate cancer. Anticancer Drugs 2000; 11(2): 123-7.
[http://dx.doi.org/10.1097/00001813-200002000-00009] [PMID: 10789595]

[47] Thakor AS, Gambhir SS. Nanooncology: The future of cancer diagnosis and therapy. CA Cancer J Clin 2013; 63(6): 395-418.
[http://dx.doi.org/10.3322/caac.21199] [PMID: 24114523]

[48] Rao JP, Geckeler KE. Polymer nanoparticles: Preparation techniques and size-control parameters. Prog Polym Sci 2011; 36(7): 887-913.
[http://dx.doi.org/10.1016/j.progpolymsci.2011.01.001]

[49] Sanna V, Sechi M. Nanoparticle therapeutics for prostate cancer treatment. Maturitas 2012; 73(1): 27-32.
[http://dx.doi.org/10.1016/j.maturitas.2012.01.016] [PMID: 22341739]

[50] Makadia HK, Siegel SJ. Poly lactic-co-glycolic acid (PLGA) as biodegradable controlled drug delivery carrier. Polymers (Basel) 2011; 3(3): 1377-97.
[http://dx.doi.org/10.3390/polym3031377] [PMID: 22577513]

[51] Riley T, Stolnik S, Heald CR, *et al.* Physicochemical evaluation of nanoparticles assembled from Poly (lactic acid)– Poly (ethylene glycol)(PLA– PEG) block co-polymers as drug delivery vehicles. Langmuir 2001; 17(11): 3168-74. [http://dx.doi.org/10.1021/la001226i]

[52] Pohlmann AR, Fonseca FN, Paese K, *et al.* Poly(ϵ-caprolactone) microcapsules and nanocapsules in drug delivery. Expert Opin Drug Deliv 2013; 10(5): 623-38. [http://dx.doi.org/10.1517/17425247.2013.769956] [PMID: 23387432]

[53] Chen Z, Tai Z, Gu F, Hu C, Zhu Q, Gao S. Aptamer-mediated delivery of docetaxel to prostate cancer through polymeric nanoparticles for enhancement of antitumor efficacy. Eur J Pharm Biopharm 2016; 107: 130-41. [http://dx.doi.org/10.1016/j.ejpb.2016.07.007] [PMID: 27393562]

[54] Soppimath KS, Aminabhavi TM, Kulkarni AR, Rudzinski WE. Biodegradable polymeric nanoparticles as drug delivery devices. J Control Release 2001; 70(1-2): 1-20. [http://dx.doi.org/10.1016/S0168-3659(00)00339-4] [PMID: 11166403]

[55] Couvreur P, Barratt G, Fattal E, Vauthier C. Nanocapsule technology: a review. Critical Reviews™ in Therapeutic Drug Carrier Systems 2002; 19: 2. [http://dx.doi.org/10.1615/CritRevTherDrugCarrierSyst.v19.i2.10]

[56] Bhunia SK, Saha A, Maity AR, Ray SC, Jana NR. Carbon nanoparticle-based fluorescent bioimaging probes. Sci Rep 2013; 3(1): 1473. [http://dx.doi.org/10.1038/srep01473] [PMID: 23502324]

[57] Kumar V, Toffoli G, Rizzolio F. Fluorescent carbon nanoparticles in medicine for cancer therapy. ACS Med Chem Lett 2013; 4(11): 1012-3. [http://dx.doi.org/10.1021/ml400394a]

[58] Krishnan S, Diagaradjane P, Cho SH. Nanoparticle-mediated thermal therapy: Evolving strategies for prostate cancer therapy. Int J Hyperthermia 2010; 26(8): 775-89. [http://dx.doi.org/10.3109/02656736.2010.485593] [PMID: 20858069]

[59] Nanjwade BK, Bechra HM, Derkar GK, Manvi FV, Nanjwade VK. Dendrimers: Emerging polymers for drug-delivery systems. Eur J Pharm Sci 2009; 38(3): 185-96. [http://dx.doi.org/10.1016/j.ejps.2009.07.008] [PMID: 19646528]

[60] Wu L, Ficker M, Christensen JB, Trohopoulos PN, Moghimi SM. Dendrimers in Medicine: Therapeutic Concepts and Pharmaceutical Challenges. Bioconjug Chem 2015; 26(7): 1198-211. [http://dx.doi.org/10.1021/acs.bioconjchem.5b00031] [PMID: 25654320]

[61] Cheng Y, Wang J, Rao T, He X, Xu T. Pharmaceutical applications of dendrimers: promising nanocarriers for drug delivery. Front Biosci 2008; 13(13): 1447-71. [http://dx.doi.org/10.2741/2774] [PMID: 17981642]

[62] Wang Y, Li P, Chen L, Gao W, Zeng F, Kong LX. Targeted delivery of 5-fluorouracil to HT-29 cells using high efficient folic acid-conjugated nanoparticles. Drug Deliv 2015; 22(2): 191-8. [http://dx.doi.org/10.3109/10717544.2013.875603] [PMID: 24437926]

[63] Svenson S, Chauhan AS. Dendrimers for enhanced drug solubilization. Nanomedicine (Lond) 2008; 3(5): 679-702. [http://dx.doi.org/10.2217/17435889.3.5.679]

[64] Lim J, Guan B, Nham K, Hao G, Sun X, Simanek EE. Tumor uptake of triazine dendrimers decorated with four, sixteen, and sixty-four PSMA-targeted ligands: Passive versus active tumor targeting. Biomolecules 2019; 9(9): 421. [http://dx.doi.org/10.3390/biom9090421] [PMID: 31466360]

[65] Myung JH, Cha A, Tam KA, *et al.* Dendrimer-based platform for effective capture of tumor cells after TGFβ1-induced epithelial–mesenchymal transition. Anal Chem 2019; 91(13): 8374-82. [http://dx.doi.org/10.1021/acs.analchem.9b01181] [PMID: 31247718]

[66] Chan WCW, Maxwell DJ, Gao X, Bailey RE, Han M, Nie S. Luminescent quantum dots for multiplexed biological detection and imaging. Curr Opin Biotechnol 2002; 13(1): 40-6. [http://dx.doi.org/10.1016/S0958-1669(02)00282-3] [PMID: 11849956]

[67] Gao X, Yang L, Petros JA, Marshall FF, Simons JW, Nie S. In vivo molecular and cellular imaging with quantum dots. Curr Opin Biotechnol 2005; 16(1): 63-72. [http://dx.doi.org/10.1016/j.copbio.2004.11.003] [PMID: 15722017]

[68] Cai W, Chen X. Nanoplatforms for targeted molecular imaging in living subjects. Small 2007; 3(11): 1840-54. [http://dx.doi.org/10.1002/smll.200700351] [PMID: 17943716]

[69] Rong Z, Bai Z, Li J, *et al.* Dual-color magnetic-quantum dot nanobeads as versatile fluorescent probes in test strip for simultaneous point-of-care detection of free and complexed prostate-specific antigen. Biosens Bioelectron 2019; 145: 111719. [http://dx.doi.org/10.1016/j.bios.2019.111719] [PMID: 31563066]

[70] Wang L, Wu Q, Zhu S, *et al.* Quantum dot-based immunofluorescent imaging and quantitative detection of DNER and prognostic value in prostate cancer. Cancer Biomark 2018; 22(4): 683-91. [http://dx.doi.org/10.3233/CBM-171107] [PMID: 29843212]

[71] Yeh YC, Creran B, Rotello VM. Gold nanoparticles: preparation, properties, and applications in bionanotechnology. Nanoscale 2012; 4(6): 1871-80. [http://dx.doi.org/10.1039/C1NR11188D] [PMID: 22076024]

[72] Arvizo R, Bhattacharya R, Mukherjee P. Gold nanoparticles: opportunities and challenges in nanomedicine. Expert Opin Drug Deliv 2010; 7(6): 753-63. [http://dx.doi.org/10.1517/17425241003777010] [PMID: 20408736]

[73] Huang XH. El Sayed, IH; Qian; El Sayed, MA Am. InChem. Soc 2006; Vol. 128: p. 2115.

[74] Soo PC, Horng YT, Chang KC, *et al.* A simple gold nanoparticle probes assay for identification of Mycobacterium tuberculosis and Mycobacterium tuberculosis complex from clinical specimens. Mol Cell Probes 2009; 23(5): 240-6. [http://dx.doi.org/10.1016/j.mcp.2009.04.006] [PMID: 19463945]

[75] Kim D, Jeong YY, Jon S. A drug-loaded aptamer-gold nanoparticle bioconjugate for combined CT imaging and therapy of prostate cancer. ACS Nano 2010; 4(7): 3689-96. [http://dx.doi.org/10.1021/nn901877h] [PMID: 20550178]

[76] Connor EE, Mwamuka J, Gole A, Murphy CJ, Wyatt MD. Gold nanoparticles are taken up by human cells but do not cause acute cytotoxicity. Small 2005; 1(3): 325-7. [http://dx.doi.org/10.1002/smll.200400093] [PMID: 17193451]

[77] Berbeco RI, Ngwa W, Makrigiorgos GM. Localized dose enhancement to tumor blood vessel endothelial cells *via* megavoltage X-rays and targeted gold nanoparticles: new potential for external beam radiotherapy. International Journal of Radiation Oncology* Biology* Physics 2011; 81(1): 270-6.

[78] Cardinal J, Klune JR, Chory E, *et al.* Noninvasive radiofrequency ablation of cancer targeted by gold nanoparticles. Surgery 2008; 144(2): 125-32. [http://dx.doi.org/10.1016/j.surg.2008.03.036] [PMID: 18656617]

[79] Chandra P, Singh J, Singh A, Srivastava A, Goyal RN, Shim YB. Gold nanoparticles and nanocomposites in clinical diagnostics using electrochemical methods. J Nanopar 2013; 2013: 1-12. [http://dx.doi.org/10.1155/2013/535901]

[80] Rai M, Yadav A, Gade A. Silver nanoparticles as a new generation of antimicrobials. Biotechnol Adv 2009; 27(1): 76-83. [http://dx.doi.org/10.1016/j.biotechadv.2008.09.002] [PMID: 18854209]

[81] Gopinath P, Gogoi SK, Chattopadhyay A, Ghosh SS. Implications of silver nanoparticle induced cell

apoptosis for *in vitro* gene therapy. Nanotechnology 2008; 19(7): 075104. [http://dx.doi.org/10.1088/0957-4484/19/7/075104] [PMID: 21817629]

[82] Lu AH. Salabas EeL, Schüth F. Angew Chem Int Ed 2007; 46: 1222-44. [http://dx.doi.org/10.1002/anie.200602866]

[83] Martina MS, Fortin JP, Fournier L, *et al.* Magnetic targeting of rhodamine-labeled superparamagnetic liposomes to solid tumors: *in vivo* tracking by fibered confocal fluorescence microscopy. Mol Imaging 2007; 6(2): 7290.2007.00004. [http://dx.doi.org/10.2310/7290.2007.00004] [PMID: 17445508]

[84] Rose PA, Praseetha PK, Bhagat M, Alexander P, Abdeen S, Chavali M. Drug embedded PVP coated magnetic nanoparticles for targeted killing of breast cancer cells. Technol Cancer Res Treat 2013; 12(5): 463-72. [http://dx.doi.org/10.7785/tcrt.2012.500333] [PMID: 23547975]

[85] Petri-Fink A, Chastellain M, Juillerat-Jeanneret L, Ferrari A, Hofmann H. Development of functionalized superparamagnetic iron oxide nanoparticles for interaction with human cancer cells. Biomaterials 2005; 26(15): 2685-94. [http://dx.doi.org/10.1016/j.biomaterials.2004.07.023] [PMID: 15585272]

[86] Parsian M, Unsoy G, Mutlu P, Yalcin S, Tezcaner A, Gunduz U. Loading of Gemcitabine on chitosan magnetic nanoparticles increases the anti-cancer efficacy of the drug. Eur J Pharmacol 2016; 784: 121-8. [http://dx.doi.org/10.1016/j.ejphar.2016.05.016] [PMID: 27181067]

[87] Ling Y, Wei K, Luo Y, Gao X, Zhong S. Dual docetaxel/superparamagnetic iron oxide loaded nanoparticles for both targeting magnetic resonance imaging and cancer therapy. Biomaterials 2011; 32(29): 7139-50. [http://dx.doi.org/10.1016/j.biomaterials.2011.05.089] [PMID: 21726899]

[88] Zeybek A, Şanlı-Mohamed G, Ak G, Yılmaz H, Şanlıer ŞH. In vitro evaluation of doxorubicin-incorporated magnetic albumin nanospheres. Chem Biol Drug Des 2014; 84(1): 108-15. [http://dx.doi.org/10.1111/cbdd.12300] [PMID: 24524300]

[89] Bleul R, Thiermann R, Marten GU, *et al.* Continuously manufactured magnetic polymersomes – a versatile tool (not only) for targeted cancer therapy. Nanoscale 2013; 5(23): 11385-93. [http://dx.doi.org/10.1039/c3nr02190d] [PMID: 23820598]

[90] Hickey RJ, Koski J, Meng X, Riggleman RA, Zhang P, Park SJ. Size-controlled self-assembly of superparamagnetic polymersomes. ACS Nano 2014; 8(1): 495-502. [http://dx.doi.org/10.1021/nn405012h] [PMID: 24369711]

[91] Sun W, Mignani S, Shen M, Shi X. Dendrimer-based magnetic iron oxide nanoparticles: their synthesis and biomedical applications. Drug Discov Today 2016; 21(12): 1873-85. [http://dx.doi.org/10.1016/j.drudis.2016.06.028] [PMID: 27388223]

[92] Jain TK, Morales MA, Sahoo SK, Leslie-Pelecky DL, Labhasetwar V. Iron oxide nanoparticles for sustained delivery of anticancer agents. Mol Pharm 2005; 2(3): 194-205. [http://dx.doi.org/10.1021/mp0500014] [PMID: 15934780]

[93] Sato A, Itcho N, Ishiguro H, *et al.* Magnetic nanoparticles of Fe3O4 enhance docetaxel-induced prostate cancer cell death. Int J Nanomedicine 2013; 8: 3151-60. [PMID: 23990723]

[94] Benyettou F, Lalatonne Y, Sainte-Catherine O, Monteil M, Motte L. Superparamagnetic nanovector with anti-cancer properties: γFe2O3@Zoledronate. Int J Pharm 2009; 379(2): 324-7. [http://dx.doi.org/10.1016/j.ijpharm.2009.04.010] [PMID: 19457625]

[95] Licciardi M, Scialabba C, Fiorica C, Cavallaro G, Cassata G, Giammona G. Polymeric nanocarriers for magnetic targeted drug delivery: preparation, characterization, and in vitro and *in vivo* evaluation. Mol Pharm 2013; 10(12): 4397-407.

[http://dx.doi.org/10.1021/mp300718b] [PMID: 24168360]

[96] Lee KJ, An JH, Shin JS, Kim DH. Synthesis and characterization of bicalutamide-loaded magnetic nanoparticles as anti-tumor drug carriers. J Nanosci Nanotechnol 2012; 12(2): 1611-5. [http://dx.doi.org/10.1166/jnn.2012.4632] [PMID: 22630012]

[97] Ranney D, Antich P, Dadey E, *et al.* Dermatan carriers for neovascular transport targeting, deep tumor penetration and improved therapy. J Control Release 2005; 109(1-3): 222-35. [http://dx.doi.org/10.1016/j.jconrel.2005.09.022] [PMID: 16290245]

[98] Huang HC, Chang PY, Chang K, *et al.* Formulation of novel lipid-coated magnetic nanoparticles as the probe for *in vivo* imaging. J Biomed Sci 2009; 16(1): 86. [http://dx.doi.org/10.1186/1423-0127-16-86] [PMID: 19772552]

[99] Weissleder R, Elizondo G, Wittenberg J, Rabito CA, Bengele HH, Josephson L. Ultrasmall superparamagnetic iron oxide: characterization of a new class of contrast agents for MR imaging. Radiology 1990; 175(2): 489-93. [http://dx.doi.org/10.1148/radiology.175.2.2326474] [PMID: 2326474]

[100] Bulte JW, Kraitchman DL. Noninvasive detection of clinically occult lymph-node metastases in prostate cancer. NMR Biomed 2004; 17: 484-99. [http://dx.doi.org/10.1002/nbm.924] [PMID: 15526347]

[101] Talelli M, Rijcken CJF, Lammers T, *et al.* Superparamagnetic iron oxide nanoparticles encapsulated in biodegradable thermosensitive polymeric micelles: toward a targeted nanomedicine suitable for image-guided drug delivery. Langmuir 2009; 25(4): 2060-7. [http://dx.doi.org/10.1021/la8036499] [PMID: 19166276]

[102] Harisinghani MG, Saini S, Weissleder R, *et al.* MR lymphangiography using ultrasmall superparamagnetic iron oxide in patients with primary abdominal and pelvic malignancies: radiographic-pathologic correlation. AJR Am J Roentgenol 1999; 172(5): 1347-51. [http://dx.doi.org/10.2214/ajr.172.5.10227514] [PMID: 10227514]

[103] Fortuin AS, Smeenk RJ, Meijer HJM, Witjes AJ, Barentsz JO. Lymphotropic nanoparticle-enhanced MRI in prostate cancer: value and therapeutic potential. Curr Urol Rep 2014; 15(3): 389. [http://dx.doi.org/10.1007/s11934-013-0389-7] [PMID: 24430170]

[104] Narayanan NK, Nargi D, Randolph C, Narayanan BA. Liposome encapsulation of curcumin and resveratrol in combination reduces prostate cancer incidence in PTEN knockout mice. Int J Cancer 2009; 125(1): 1-8. [http://dx.doi.org/10.1002/ijc.24336] [PMID: 19326431]

[105] Thangapazham R, Puri A, Tele S, Blumenthal R, Maheshwari R. Evaluation of a nanotechnology-based carrier for delivery of curcumin in prostate cancer cells. Int J Oncol 2008; 32(5): 1119-23. [http://dx.doi.org/10.3892/ijo.32.5.1119] [PMID: 18425340]

[106] Shao L, Kahraman N, Yan G, Wang J, Ozpolat B, Ittmann M. Targeting the TMPRSS2/ERG fusion mRNA using liposomal nanovectors enhances docetaxel treatment in prostate cancer. Prostate 2020; 80(1): 65-73. [http://dx.doi.org/10.1002/pros.23918] [PMID: 31614005]

[107] Yari H, Nkepang G, Awasthi V. Surface modification of liposomes by a lipopolymer targeting prostate specific membrane antigen for theranostic delivery in prostate cancer. Materials (Basel) 2019; 12(5): 756. [http://dx.doi.org/10.3390/ma12050756] [PMID: 30841602]

[108] Patil Y, Shmeeda H, Amitay Y, Ohana P, Kumar S, Gabizon A. Targeting of folate-conjugated liposomes with co-entrapped drugs to prostate cancer cells *via* prostate-specific membrane antigen (PSMA). Nanomedicine 2018; 14(4): 1407-16. [http://dx.doi.org/10.1016/j.nano.2018.04.011] [PMID: 29680672]

[109] Dhar S, Kolishetti N, Lippard SJ, Farokhzad OC. Targeted delivery of a cisplatin prodrug for safer and

more effective prostate cancer therapy in vivo. Proc Natl Acad Sci USA 2011; 108(5): 1850-5. [http://dx.doi.org/10.1073/pnas.1011379108] [PMID: 21233423]

[110] Kolishetti N, Dhar S, Valencia PM, *et al.* Engineering of self-assembled nanoparticle platform for precisely controlled combination drug therapy. Proc Natl Acad Sci USA 2010; 107(42): 17939-44. [http://dx.doi.org/10.1073/pnas.1011368107] [PMID: 20921363]

[111] Jiang W, Fang H, Liu F, *et al.* PEG-coated and Gd-loaded fluorescent silica nanoparticles for targeted prostate cancer magnetic resonance imaging and fluorescence imaging. Int J Nanomedicine 2019; 14: 5611-22. [http://dx.doi.org/10.2147/IJN.S207098] [PMID: 31413566]

[112] Azandeh SS, Abbaspour M, Khodadadi A, Khorsandi L, Orazizadeh M, Heidari-Moghadam A. Anticancer activity of curcumin-loaded PLGA nanoparticles on PC3 prostate cancer cells. Iranian journal of pharmaceutical research. Iran J Pharm Res 2017; 16(3): 868-79. [PMID: 29201078]

[113] Pan M, Li W, Yang J, *et al.* Plumbagin-loaded aptamer-targeted poly D,L-lactic-co-glycolic acid---polyethylene glycol nanoparticles for prostate cancer therapy. Medicine (Baltimore) 2017; 96(30): e7405. [http://dx.doi.org/10.1097/MD.0000000000007405] [PMID: 28746182]

[114] Patra CR, Bhattacharya R, Mukhopadhyay D, Mukherjee P. Fabrication of gold nanoparticles for targeted therapy in pancreatic cancer. Adv Drug Deliv Rev 2010; 62(3): 346-61. [http://dx.doi.org/10.1016/j.addr.2009.11.007] [PMID: 19914317]

[115] Tomuleasa C, Soritau O, Orza A, *et al.* Gold nanoparticles conjugated with cisplatin/doxorubicin/capecitabine lower the chemoresistance of hepatocellular carcinoma-derived cancer cells. J Gastrointestin Liver Dis 2012; 21(2): 187-96. [PMID: 22720309]

[116] Huang X, Jain PK, El-Sayed IH, El-Sayed MA. Determination of the minimum temperature required for selective photothermal destruction of cancer cells with the use of immunotargeted gold nanoparticles. Photochem Photobiol 2006; 82(2): 412-7. [http://dx.doi.org/10.1562/2005-12-14-RA-754] [PMID: 16613493]

[117] Wolfe T, Chatterjee D, Lee J, *et al.* Targeted gold nanoparticles enhance sensitization of prostate tumors to megavoltage radiation therapy in vivo. Nanomedicine 2015; 11(5): 1277-83. [http://dx.doi.org/10.1016/j.nano.2014.12.016] [PMID: 25652893]

[118] Firdhouse MJ, Lalitha P. Biosynthesis of silver nanoparticles using the extract of *Alternanthera sessilis*—antiproliferative effect against prostate cancer cells. Cancer Nanotechnol 2013; 4(6): 137-43. [http://dx.doi.org/10.1007/s12645-013-0045-4] [PMID: 26069509]

[119] Zhang X, Xing JZ, Chen J, *et al.* Enhanced radiation sensitivity in prostate cancer by gold-nanoparticles. Clinical and Investigative Medicine 2008 Jun 1:E160-7. 2008; E160-7. [http://dx.doi.org/10.25011/cim.v31i3.3473]

[120] Seixas N, Ravanello B, Morgan I, Kaluđerović G, Wessjohann L. Chlorambucil Conjugated Ugi Dendrimers with PAMAM-NH2 Core and Evaluation of Their Anticancer Activity. Pharmaceutics 2019; 11(2): 59. [http://dx.doi.org/10.3390/pharmaceutics11020059] [PMID: 30717083]

[121] Sánchez-Milla M, Muñoz-Moreno L, Sánchez-Nieves J, *et al.* Anti-cancer activity of dendriplexes against advanced prostate cancer from protumoral peptides and cationic carbosilane dendrimers. Biomacromolecules 2019; 20(3): 1224-34. [http://dx.doi.org/10.1021/acs.biomac.8b01632] [PMID: 30669830]

[122] Jigyasu AK, Siddiqui S, Jafri A, Arshad M, Lohani M, Khan IA. Biological Synthesis of CdTe Quantum Dots and Their Anti-Proliferative Assessment Against Prostate Cancer Cell Line. J Nanosci Nanotechnol 2020; 20(6): 3398-403. [http://dx.doi.org/10.1166/jnn.2020.17316] [PMID: 31748032]

[123] Chen Y, Guo X, Liu W, Zhang L. Paper-based fluorometric immunodevice with quantum-dot labeled antibodies for simultaneous detection of carcinoembryonic antigen and prostate specific antigen. Mikrochim Acta 2019; 186(2): 112.
[http://dx.doi.org/10.1007/s00604-019-3232-0] [PMID: 30643993]

[124] Xia Q, Gong C, Gu F, *et al.* Functionalized multi-walled carbon nanotubes for targeting delivery of immunostimulatory CpG oligonucleotides against prostate cancer. J Biomed Nanotechnol 2018; 14(9): 1613-26.
[http://dx.doi.org/10.1166/jbn.2018.2605] [PMID: 29958555]

[125] Erdmann K, Ringel J, Hampel S, Wirth MP, Fuessel S. Carbon nanomaterials sensitize prostate cancer cells to docetaxel and mitomycin C *via* induction of apoptosis and inhibition of proliferation. Beilstein J Nanotechnol 2017; 8(1): 1307-17.
[http://dx.doi.org/10.3762/bjnano.8.132] [PMID: 28690966]

[126] Thaxton CS, Elghanian R, Thomas AD, *et al.* Nanoparticle-based bio-barcode assay redefines "undetectable" PSA and biochemical recurrence after radical prostatectomy. Proc Natl Acad Sci USA 2009; 106(44): 18437-42.
[http://dx.doi.org/10.1073/pnas.0904719106] [PMID: 19841273]

[127] Viator JA, Gupta S, Goldschmidt BS, *et al.* Gold nanoparticle mediated detection of prostate cancer cells using photoacoustic flowmetry with optical reflectance. J Biomed Nanotechnol 2010; 6(2): 187-91.
[http://dx.doi.org/10.1166/jbn.2010.1105] [PMID: 20738074]

[128] Johannsen M, Gneveckow U, Thiesen B, *et al.* Thermotherapy of prostate cancer using magnetic nanoparticles: feasibility, imaging, and three-dimensional temperature distribution. Eur Urol 2007; 52(6): 1653-62.
[http://dx.doi.org/10.1016/j.eururo.2006.11.023] [PMID: 17125906]

[129] Lee CM, Jeong HJ, Cheong SJ, *et al.* Prostate cancer-targeted imaging using magnetofluorescent polymeric nanoparticles functionalized with bombesin. Pharm Res 2010; 27(4): 712-21.
[http://dx.doi.org/10.1007/s11095-010-0072-3] [PMID: 20182773]

[130] Azzawi M, Seifalian A, Ahmed W. Nanotechnology for the diagnosis and treatment of diseases. Nanomed 2016; 11(16).
[http://dx.doi.org/10.2217/nnm-2016-8000]

[131] Bharali DJ, Mousa SA. Emerging nanomedicines for early cancer detection and improved treatment: Current perspective and future promise. Pharmacol Ther 2010; 128(2): 324-35.
[http://dx.doi.org/10.1016/j.pharmthera.2010.07.007] [PMID: 20705093]

[132] Yguerabide J, Yguerabide EE. Light-scattering submicroscopic particles as highly fluorescent analogs and their use as tracer labels in clinical and biological applications. Anal Biochem 1998; 262(2): 157-76.
[http://dx.doi.org/10.1006/abio.1998.2760] [PMID: 9750129]

[133] Huo Q, Colon J, Cordero A, *et al.* A facile nanoparticle immunoassay for cancer biomarker discovery. J Nanobiotechnology 2011; 9(1): 20.
[http://dx.doi.org/10.1186/1477-3155-9-20] [PMID: 21605409]

[134] Zhang T, Xue X, He D, Hsieh JT. A prostate cancer-targeted polyarginine-disulfide linked PEI nanocarrier for delivery of microRNA. Cancer Lett 2015; 365(2): 156-65.
[http://dx.doi.org/10.1016/j.canlet.2015.05.003] [PMID: 26054847]

[135] Constantinou J, Feneley MR. PSA testing: an evolving relationship with prostate cancer screening. Prostate Cancer Prostatic Dis 2006; 9(1): 6-13.
[http://dx.doi.org/10.1038/sj.pcan.4500838] [PMID: 16314892]

[136] Saleem M, Adhami VM, Zhong W, *et al.* A novel biomarker for staging human prostate adenocarcinoma: overexpression of matriptase with concomitant loss of its inhibitor, hepatocyte

growth factor activator inhibitor-1. Cancer Epidemiol Biomarkers Prev 2006; 15(2): 217-27. [http://dx.doi.org/10.1158/1055-9965.EPI-05-0737] [PMID: 16492908]

[137] Ferguson RA, Yu H, Kalyvas M, Zammit S, Diamandis EP. Ultrasensitive detection of prostate-specific antigen by a time-resolved immunofluorometric assay and the Immulite immunochemiluminescent third-generation assay: potential applications in prostate and breast cancers. Clin Chem 1996; 42(5): 675-84. [http://dx.doi.org/10.1093/clinchem/42.5.675] [PMID: 8653891]

[138] Gao X, Luo Y, Wang Y, *et al.* Prostate stem cell antigen-targeted nanoparticles with dual functional properties: *in vivo* imaging and cancer chemotherapy. Int J Nanomedicine 2012; 7: 4037-51. [http://dx.doi.org/10.2147/IJN.S32804] [PMID: 22888241]

[139] O'Keefe DS, Bacich DJ, Heston WDW. Comparative analysis of prostate-specific membrane antigen (PSMA) versus a prostate-specific membrane antigen-like gene. Prostate 2004; 58(2): 200-10. [http://dx.doi.org/10.1002/pros.10319] [PMID: 14716746]

[140] Kasten BB, Liu T, Nedrow-Byers JR, Benny PD, Berkman CE. Targeting prostate cancer cells with PSMA inhibitor-guided gold nanoparticles. Bioorg Med Chem Lett 2013; 23(2): 565-8. [http://dx.doi.org/10.1016/j.bmcl.2012.11.015] [PMID: 23232055]

[141] Papadakis GZ, Marias K, Millo C, Karantanas AH. 18F-NaF PET/CT imaging versus 99mTc-MDP scintigraphy in assessing metastatic bone disease in patients with prostate cancer. Hellenic Journal of. Radiology 2019; 4(4).

[142] https://www.cancernetwork.com/view/current-clinical-trials-prostate-cancer2021.

[143] ClinicalTrials.gov Identifier: NCT03445559.

[144] ClinicalTrials.gov Identifier: NCT03492424.

[145] ClinicalTrials.gov Identifier: NCT01834001.

[146] ClinicalTrials.gov Identifier: NCT03232164. 2021.

[147] ClinicalTrials.gov Identifier: NCT03889119. 2021.

[148] ClinicalTrials.gov Identifier: NCT01834001. 2021.

[149] ClinicalTrials.gov Identifier: NCT03179410. 2021.

[150] ClinicalTrials.gov Identifier: NCT03810105. 2021.

[151] ClinicalTrials.gov Identifier: NCT03253744. 2021.

[152] ClinicalTrials.gov Identifier: NCT03637543. 2021.

[153] ClinicalTrials.gov Identifier: NCT03769766. 2021.

[154] ClinicalTrials.gov Identifier: NCT03432897. 2021.

[155] 2021.ClinicalTrials.gov Identifier: NCT02600156.

[156] 2021.ClinicalTrials.gov Identifier: NCT03565835.

[157] 2021.ClinicalTrials.gov Identifier: NCT02903160.

[158] 2021.ClinicalTrials.gov Identifier: NCT03646162.

[159] 2021.ClinicalTrials.gov Identifier: NCT03663218.

[160] 2021.ClinicalTrials.gov Identifier: NCT02807805.

[161] 2021.ClinicalTrials.gov Identifier: NCT03089203.

[162] 2021.ClinicalTrials.gov Identifier: NCT03556904.

[163] 2021.ClinicalTrials.gov Identifier: NCT03456804.

[164] 2021.ClinicalTrials.gov Identifier: NCT02494921.

[165] 2021.ClinicalTrials.gov Identifier: NCT03762759.

CHAPTER 6

Nanocarriers and their Role in the Treatment of Breast Cancer

Sidhartha S. Kar[1], **Arghya Kusum Dhar**[2,*] and **Shvetank Bhatt**[3]

[1] *Institute of Pharmacy & Technology, Salipur, Cuttack, Odisha, India*

[2] *School of Pharmacy, Neotia University, Sarisa, D.H. Road, 24 Pgs (South) West Bengal 743368, India*

[3] *Amity Institute of Pharmacy, Amity University, Gwalior 474005, India*

Abstract: Breast cancer is the most common disease in women worldwide, yet current pharmacological therapy is far from ideal due to the high mortality rate among breast cancer patients. Emerging nanomedicine is a viable therapy option for breast cancer. Various potential organic and inorganic nanoparticles are promising drug nanocarriers developed for targeted delivery in breast cancer therapy over the years, with evidence established. Nanocarriers have passive and ligand-based targeting mechanisms that allow them to accumulate preferentially in breast tumours. Besides many conventional nanocarriers, polymer-based nanocarriers include the application of dendrimers, polymersomes, polymeric nanoparticles, polymer micelles, polyplexes, polymer–lipid hybrid systems, and polymer-drug/Polymer-protein conjugates to improve breast cancer therapeutic efficacy, has expanded in the recent past. However, the concept of nanocarriers with drug conjugates is constrained to the lab size. They must be scaled up to generate active-targeted nanomedicine for clinical use against breast cancer. As a result, the current chapter focuses on research that has recently been reported in the exploration of emerging nanocarriers for breast cancer therapy.

Keywords: Breast cancer, Drug conjugates, Inorganic nanoparticles, Lipid-based nanocarriers, Nanocarriers, Targeted delivery, Therapeutic efficacy, Polymeric nanoparticles.

INTRODUCTION

The second leading cause of death among women is breast cancer, estimated to cause more than 600,000 deaths per year worldwide [1]. As per the WHO cancer profile 2020, around 269,792 new breast cancer cases were detected in 2018, and

* **Corresponding author Arghya Kusum Dhar:** School of Pharmacy, Neotia University, Sarisa, D.H. Road, 24 Pgs (South) West Bengal 743368, India; Tel: +91-9785977595; E-mail: dhararghyakusum@gmail.com

Neeraj Mishra, Ashish Garg and Neeraj Upmanyu (Eds.)

an additional 2,778,850 cases are predicted to be diagnosed by 2040. Breast cancer is typically categorized into two major subtypes based on their histological constituents: ductal and lobular carcinomas. Additionally, as per the human epidermal growth factor receptor 2 (HER2), estrogen receptor (ER) and progesterone receptor (PR) expression levels, breast tumours are classified into luminal A (ER+ PR+, and HER2-), luminal B (ER+/PR+ and HER2+/-), HER2 positive (ER+/PR- and HER2+), triple-negative/basal-like (ER+, PR+, and HER2+), and claudin-low [2 - 4]. Moreover, the American Joint Committee on Cancer (AJCC) identified eight phases of breast cancer according to the presence of tumour-node metastasis (TNM) [5, 6]. Chemotherapy is the most widely used treatment, and it now includes the use of two or more anticancer drugs (Fig. **1**) in combination to combat drug resistance. However, chemotherapy has a number of drawbacks, such as multidrug resistance, drug toxicity, limited bioavailability, poor water solubility, and suboptimal pharmacokinetic characteristics. Nanocarriers are promising technologies for delivering drugs to specific locations. Their capacity to overcome the limitations of anticancer agents is encouraging. Nanocarriers are used in drug delivery systems that are formulated to provide both hydrophilic and hydrophobic drugs to the targeted biological environment. In addition, nanocarrier systems offer numerous advantages, such as improved drug solubility, enhanced biodegradability and bioavailability, improved patient compliance, controllable release kinetics, retention of drug efficacy throughout plasma circulation, decreased drug toxicity as well as overcoming drug resistance.

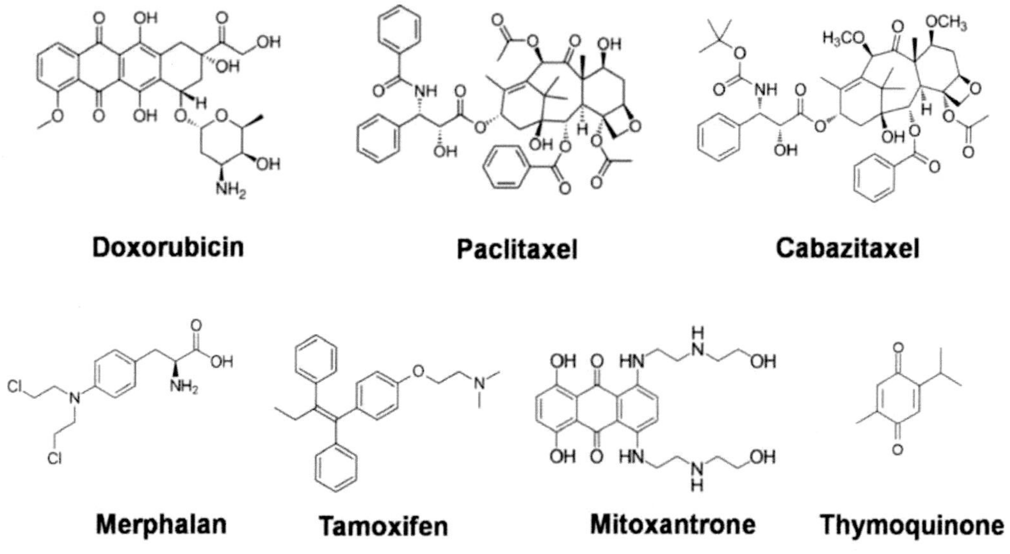

Fig. (1). Chemical structures of anti-breast cancer drugs.

CONVENTIONAL DIAGNOSIS AND TREATMENT OF BREAST CANCER

Breast cancer diagnosis depends on clinical investigation and imaging and is confirmed through pathology. Manual testing of the lymph nodes and breasts is included in the clinical assessment, as is the testing of distant metastasis (bones, liver, lungs, and neurological examination in the case of symptoms). A comprehensive family and personal history are also carried out, along with a menopausal assessment, a physical investigation, a blood count analysis, tests on the liver and renal function, and screening of alkaline phosphate and calcium [7].

The treatment strategy for breast cancer is based on molecular heterogeneity, receptor expression, amount of lesions and number and involvement of the lymph node, stage of cancer, and other parameters, for instance, age, lifestyle and overall health state of the patient. Early breast cancers are most of the time not fatal and treatable (72–80 percent), however advanced breast cancers are fatal and are the main reason for mortality due to the metastases of remote essential organisms such as liver, lung, brain, lymphatic nodes and bones [8].

Breast cancer treatment has been aimed at prolonging life span by minimizing unwanted side effects to improve quality of life. Two approaches are localized treatment and systemic therapy. Surgery is the first therapeutic choice for non-metastatic individuals with early-stage breast cancer. Other minimally invasive early-stage breast cancer treatments have also been developed, including cryotherapy, laser ablation, and radiofrequency ablation (RFA) [9]. Locally advanced breast cancer can be treated using mastectomy or lumpectomy, chemotherapy and high-energy radiation [8]. Depending on the breast cancer type and stage, systemic therapies like endocrine therapy, targeted therapy and immunotherapy have been introduced to improve the therapeutic effectiveness [8].

LIMITATIONS OF THE CURRENT BREAST CANCER TREATMENTS

Solid tumours have high interstitial fluid pressure (IFP), which limits transcapillary movement and increases the blood volume, resulting in suboptimal drug distribution and penetration [7]. The half-life of the drug in circulation is an important factor in deciding its tissue distribution. The distribution of a drug with a longer half-life is more uniform, even if its extravasation and permeation of tissues are slow compared to its short half-life counterparts [7]. Furthermore, tumour vasculature is heterogeneous, and is equipped with fenestrations that facilitate the extravasation of drugs [7].

It has been established that the accumulation of anticancer drugs is greater in normal viscera than tumour by a factor of 10 to 20, and 40–50 mm (the combined diameter of three to five cells) is the limit of penetration of most of the anticancer drugs from the vascular system [7, 10]. These factors cause inadequate tumour response, multi-drug resistance (MDR), and treatment failure [7, 10]. MDR is usually based on the over-expression of efflux proteins by tumour cells and is thus a serious problem for breast cancer treatment. When tumour cells are treated with a single anti-cancer agent, they develop resistance to a wide variety of drugs [7]. The absence of selective toxicity, resulting in a lower therapeutic index and compromising the clinical forecast, is a serious difficulty for cancer therapy. Therefore, suboptimal doses of anticancer chemical therapy are frequently used in order to lessen the destruction of normal tissues [7].

NANODELIVERY SYSTEMS IN THE TREATMENT OF BREAST CANCER

Anticancer drug delivery systems based on nanotechnology can provide a versatile platform for transporting therapeutic medicines and delivering them to the targeted tissue. Nanocarriers are versatile in that they can be made to have high compatibility, site-specific targeting ability, immunogenicity, or therapeutic loading. Liposomes, nanoparticles, micelles, dendrimers, and nanotubes (Fig. **2**) are examples of nanodelivery systems, and they can be constituted of a wide range of materials, including inorganic materials, polymers, proteins, lipids, phospholipids, and a combination of them.

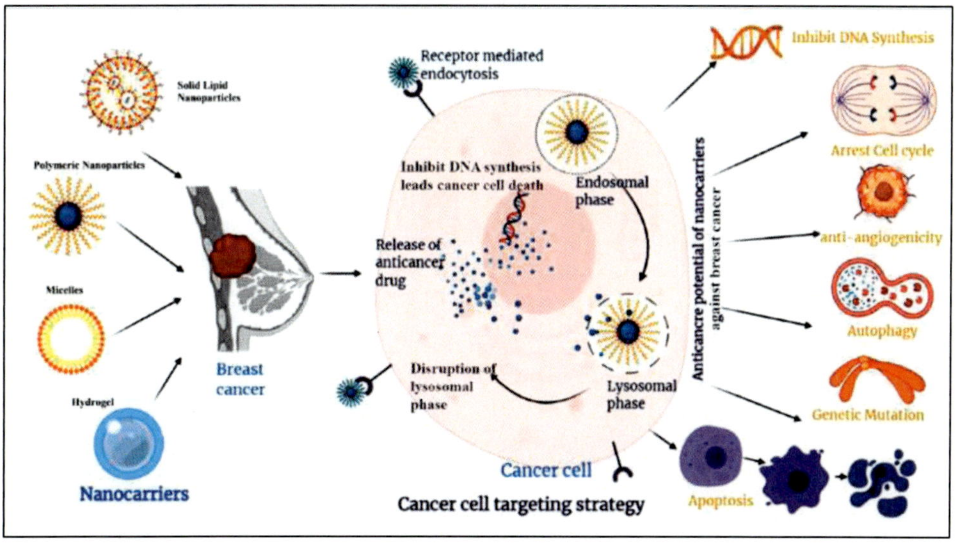

Fig. (2). Various applications of nanocarrier systems are used in breast cancer.

IDEAL CHARACTERISTICS OF NPS

Some important features must be considered in order to develop a suitable nanocarrier for fast and efficient clinical translation. The size and charge of nanoparticle systems are critical factors because they determine the nanoparticles' *in vivo* distribution, targeting ability, and biological destination. The nanocarriers should be constructed from a biocompatible material, easily functionalizable, well characterized, soluble, with extended circulatory capacities, no aggregation, and high target cell uptake efficiency.

Kidney clearance of NPs with hydrodynamic dimensions of 10 nm or less is dramatically accelerated. Research indicates that most injected nanoparticles travel to the liver and spleen. Existing macrophages phagocytose nanoparticles, which results in the phagocytosis of a small percentage of the nanoparticles, degradation of the nanoparticles, and the release of both the degraded and undamaged nanoparticles. To reduce the risk of mechanical filtration by the liver and spleen, the size of nanoparticles must not be smaller than 200 nm [7].

A relationship between the surface charge of nanoparticles and nanoparticle movement within tumours has been observed. Cationic nanoparticles may improve the absorption and binding of positively charged nanoparticles due to interactions with negatively charged cell membranes. Due to the smaller number of electrostatic contacts between charged cell membranes and nanoparticles, neutral particles have shown lesser interactions with the cell membrane than their counterparts with the same size and charge [7]. Additionally, the use of nanoparticles with a diameter of 30-40 nm and 70 nm and a slightly negative surface charge showed the transportation of nanoparticles into tumours and away from blood vessels in mice [7].

Neutral polymers reduce nanoparticle surface charge. The polymers are utilized to decrease particle-particle aggregation as well as electrostatic interactions with other components of circulation, such as plasma membranes of cells (negative charge). If the nanoparticle surface charge is raised positively and negatively, the chance of macrophage removal increases [7]. When nanomaterials are injected into the blood, they are quickly phagocytized by mononuclear phagocytes (MPS). Adding PEG to the surface of nanomaterials prevents opsonization. This enhances the blood half-life of all nanomaterials regardless of surface charge, boosting circulation and tissue accumulation. Long-circulating nanoparticles have a diameter of 30–200 nm [7]. Targeting ligands are added to the nanoparticle surface. The targeting ligand is included because the homologous receptor is increased on the cell surface of target cancer cells as compared to normal cells [7]. Surface coating provides biocompatibility, the biodistribution of nanoparticles, and the modulation of nanoparticle interactions with cells, tissues, and biomolecules [7].

TYPES OF NANOCARRIERS

Nanocarriers can be categorized depending on their composition: lipid-based, polymeric, and inorganic. Various uses have been identified for these nanocarriers, including delivery of drugs, imaging and detection of apoptosis, radiation sensitizers, and photothermal tumour destruction [11 - 13]. Below, several of these nanocarriers for breast cancer therapy are discussed.

Lipid-based Nanocarriers

All nanocarriers do have the capacity to solubilize, encapsulate, and distribute drugs in a specified order to achieve bioavailability and prevent side effects. Still, lipid-based nanocarriers have by far the most. Biocompatible lipids such as cholesterol, phospholipids, and triglycerides constitute these drug carriers. Lipid-based nanocarriers are an excellent drug delivery approach because of several advantages of the lipid matrix. These systems' biocompatibility and biodegradability elements make them safer than other drug delivery strategies like polymeric nanoparticles [14].

Features of Lipid-based Nanocarriers

- Allows exploitation of the rich chemical biodiversity in a simple and economical way.
- Increased safety by reducing cytotoxicity, hepatotoxicity and nephrotoxicity.
- High encapsulation capacity.
- Improves the aqueous solubility and bioavailability of existing drugs.
- Improves stability of drugs
- Biocompatibility and biodegradable materials.

The following is a list of nanocarriers that have already been employed as diagnostic and therapeutic tools in breast cancer research.

- Liposomes
- Solid lipid nanoparticles

• Nanostructured lipid carriers

• Lipid polymer hybrid nanoparticles.

Liposomes

Liposomes are quite old and renounced amongst the lipid nanocarriers designed to date. These colloidal carriers are biodegradable, biocompatible, non-immunogenic natural phospholipids that can encapsulate water-soluble, fat-soluble, amphiphilic, biphasic insoluble anti-breast cancer drugs in their aqueous core, which is surrounded by unilamellar/multilamellar membranes [15]. Liposomes have caught the considerable interest of established breast cancer chemotherapeutics because, as a drug delivery method, they can enhance drug concentration at tumour locations while decreasing it in normal tissues [16]. A few examples of liposomes used to target breast cancer are demonstrated in Table **1**.

Table 1. Liposomes to target breast cancer [17].

Drug	Target Ligand	Cell Surface Target
Doxorubicin	Chlorotoxin	Matrix metalloproteinases
	Estrone	Estrogen receptor
	Cetuximab	Epidermal growth factor receptor
Paclitaxel	Herceptin	HER2
Mitoxantrone	Luteinizing hormone-releasing hormone analog	Luteinizing hormone-releasing hormone receptor
Merphalan	Siale	Lectins
Melittin	Herceptin	HER2
Curcumin, Resveratrol	Trastuzumab	HER2

Advantages

• Formulation of pegylated (Stealth) liposomes becomes simple.

• Multidrug-resistant breast cancers can be treated efficiently from this approach.

• The systemic circulation time is extended by using a stealth coating.

• Diminishes cardio-toxicities.

• Pharmacokinetics properties of the drug can be modulated.

• The lipids utilized are suitable for parenteral delivery.

Disadvantages

- Liposomes are less stable.

- The presence of ligands in actively targeted liposomes may impact the formulation's stability.

Solid lipid Nanoparticles (SLNs)

SLNs are biocompatible, sub-micron-sized colloidal drug delivery technologies that replace oil in emulsions with solid lipids. They have higher entrapment efficiency, a higher loading capacity, a larger surface area, are easier to scale-up and manufacture, and are less hazardous than polymers, which amplify the drug's activity in the lipid core. SLNs have a longer drug release time and are more stable than liposomes, and they can even circumvent the sterilizing process used in liposome manufacturing. SLNs can overcome the therapeutic utility of nanoemulsions, hampered by erratic drug release, and nanocrystals, by poor drug solubilization in biological fluids. High-purity triglycerides, waxes, calixarenes, and sterols are among the lipids found in SLNs. Lipophilic medications have challenges with solubility and bioavailability, which can be solved by using SLNs to distribute them. SLNs can load hydrophilic/hydrophobic chemicals, release drugs in a regulated and protracted manner, bypass the reticuloendothelial system, and deliver chemotherapeutics directly to the breast cancer site. Preclinical research for the SLNs in breast cancer therapy, such as *in vitro* cell line studies or *in vivo* experiments, was promising, but this technology should be significant clinically.

Advantages

- Decreases systemic toxicity

- Protects the drug from degradation

- Has long-term stability

- Both lipophilic and hydrophilic drugs can be loaded

- Scale-up is simple

Disadvantages

- Low drug loading capacity due to the crystalline form of solid lipids.

- Expulsion from drug use

• Unpredictable agglomeration

• Polymorphic transitions occur more frequently

Tamoxifen SLNs used to have a longer duration of intact drug release in plasma, which elevated drug bioavailability. However, *in vitro* anti-cancer tests on MCF-7 cell lines revealed that the drug-loaded SLNs had a substantially higher cytotoxic effect than the free drug without compromising bioavailability [18].

Nanostructured Lipid Carriers (NLCs)

The second generations of SLNs are nanostructured lipid carriers (NLCs), a blend of multiple lipids, *i.e.*, a solid lipid matrix with a specified content of a liquid lipid [19]. Controlled drug release, site-specific targeting, and drug accumulation at the site of action are among the properties. Due to the presence of physiological and biocompatible lipids, this carrier system has a high tolerance level [20]. Due to lipid polymorphism, NLCs have a greater drug loading capacity, a reduced likelihood of gelation, and a lesser chance of drug leakage during storage. It can boost the therapeutic benefit of anticancer drugs by lengthening breast tumour cell exposure to anti-tumour drugs through the EPR effect [21].

Advantages

Enhanced drug payload

• Drug expulsion during storage

• The high water content of SLN dispersions

• This drug delivery system has been developed to avoid the challenges associated with SLNs.

Disadvantages

• Use of a significant volume of the aqueous phase may result in increased dispersion dilution

• Not appropriate for heat-sensitive drugs

• Metal contamination during the process of probe sonication.

Tamoxifen is one of the chemotherapeutic drugs that pass through first-pass metabolism more rapidly (524 hours). The use of NLC encapsulation enabled a longer duration for drugs to circulate in the body, bypassing first-pass metabolism and allowing for better absorption *via* lymphatic uptake. Curcumin was delivered using a similar folate targeting strategy. The conjugate of folic acid, PEG, and DSPE was created to actively target breast cancer cells. Folic acid-conjugated curcumin-NLCs have 3.5-fold more significant cytotoxicity than curcumin-NLCs [22].

Lipid-polymer Hybrid Nanoparticles

Polymeric nanoparticles and liposomes for breast cancer therapy are among the clinically cleared and commercially marketed nanoparticles/nanocarriers. Researchers combined lipid and polymer to create novel drug delivery systems known as lipid polymer hybrid nanoparticles LPN to address the issues with both technologies. A hybrid drug delivery system was developed by combining polymer's architectural features and lipids' biomimetic properties. Robustness, serum stability, sustained drug release, more significant drug loading, and tissue targeting are all features of this drug delivery method [23].

Advantages

- Optimum particle size
- Surface modification provision
- Entrapment of hydrophilic and lipophilic medicines
- Drug release pattern that is flexible
- High serum stability

Disadvantages

- Preparation on a lab scale is tedious
- Inappropriate for large-scale production
- Expensive to process aseptically

Due to the low partition coefficient in the lipid phase, encapsulating the ionic and highly water-soluble drug Doxorubicin into a lipid carrier is challenging. Doxorubicin encapsulated in an LPN nanoparticulated system had a superior cytotoxic effect, drug absorption, and retention than Doxorubicin-loaded SLNs [24]. Doxorubicin-loaded LPN was tested against multidrug-resistant breast cancer cell lines, and it was observed that Doxorubicin encapsulated in nanoparticles bypasses membrane-associated Pgp and is retained better within Pgp-overexpressing cells than the drug alone.

Nanoemulsions

Oils and surfactants are used in nanoemulsions, and their safety limits are well established. As a result, nanoemulsions could be utilized with far less complications. Nanoemulsions are colloidal dispersions of two immiscible liquids that are stabilized by emulsifying agents and have a mean diameter of less than a nanometer. Regardless of the preparation method, Nanoemulsions are heterogeneous dispersions of two immiscible liquids (oil-in-water or water-in-oil) with mean droplet size on the nanometric scale [25]. Positively charged nanoemulsion systems are expected to interact more effectively with negatively charged cell surfaces, and this feature of positively charged nanoemulsions has been investigated for the transport of oligonucleotides to cancer cells [26].

Three types of nanoemulsions are most likely to be formed depending on the composition:

• Bi-continuous nanoemulsions, in which oil and water microdomains are interspersed within the system

• Water-in-oil nanoemulsions, in which water droplets are dispersed in a continuous oil phase

• Oil-in-water nanoemulsions, in which oil droplets are dispersed in a continuous aqueous phase

An adequate combination of surfactants and/or co-surfactants stabilizes the interface in all three forms of nanoemulsions.

Advantages

• Drugs are delivered to specific locations

• Droplet size is small, optical clarity is good, and physical stability is good

• Able to dissolve vast amounts of hydrophobic compounds.

• Long-term stability and the capacity to preserve pharmaceuticals from deterioration.

• Improved bioavailability, non-toxicity and non-irritability

• Protects from hydrolysis and oxidation

Disadvantages

• To be used in pharmaceutical applications, the surfactant must be nontoxic.

• Solubilizing capacity for high-melting compounds is limited.

• A high concentration of surfactant and co-surfactant is required for nanodroplet stabilization.

• Environmental factors such as temperature and pH have an impact on nanoemulsion stability. When patients are given nanoemulsion, these metrics change.

Example

In the HTB-20 breast cancer cell line, nanoemulsions of TAM with mean particle sizes of 47 nm suppressed cell growth 20-fold and increased cell death 4-fold. As a result, when a nanoemulsion of TAM is compared to a suspension preparation of TAM, its breast cancer activity is increased [27].

Polymeric Nanoparticles

Natural, synthetic, or semisynthetic polymers constitute polymeric nanoparticles (Fig. **3**). The use of polymeric nanoparticles is characterized by their constrained form and wide size distribution. Although the ultimate size of polymeric NP can be adjusted during the synthesis process, they are normally spherical. To optimize the final product, polymeric NP characteristics, as well as the amount, pace, and pathway employed for cellular uptake of the encapsulated drug molecule, can be changed. These NPs have the potential to penetrate biological barriers, protect therapeutic cargo, and effectively transport it to sick tissue as promising biomaterials. The albumin-based nanoparticle, protein-bound paclitaxel (Abraxane), is the only polymer-based delivery method registered by the FDA for clinical use in the treatment of breast, pancreatic and non-small cell lung cancer [28]. To prepare both targeted and nontargeted hypoxia-responsive polymersomes, doxorubicin (DOX) was encapsulated in the polymersomes (DOX-iPs and DOX-Ps, respectively). Under normoxic circumstances (21 percent oxygen), the polymeric nanoparticles released less than 30% of their encapsulated DOX within 12 hours, however, under hypoxia (% oxygen), doxorubicin release surged to almost 95%. The targeted polymersomes considerably reduced triple-negative breast cancer cells [29].

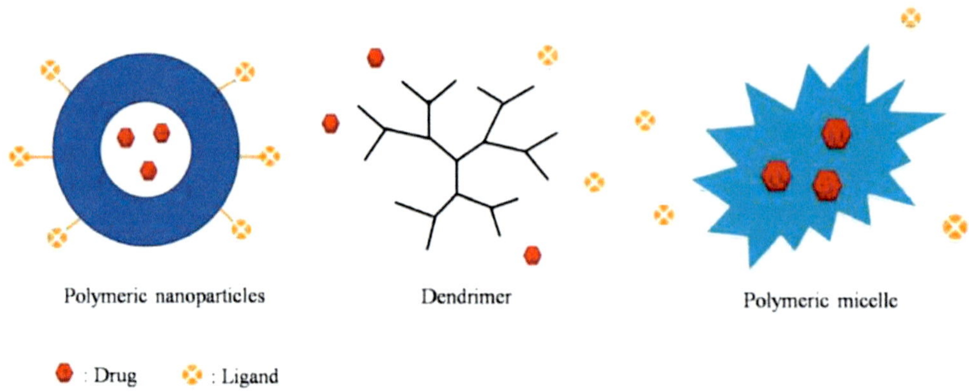

Fig. (3). Schematic representation of selected polymeric nanocarriers.

Dendrimers

Dendrimers are "onion skin-like" branched layers of globular macromolecules sized 1–100 nm with a selected number of functional groups to act as a monodispersed system for various biomedical applications [30]. A dendrimer is comprised of three domains: a central core, a hyperbranched mantle, and a corona with reactive functional groups on the periphery (Fig. **3**). Dendrimers are virtually perfect (spherical) nanocarriers with predictable features due to the high level of control over the synthesis of dendritic architecture. Dendrimers have been developed as nanodevices, either as nanocarriers for pharmaceuticals or as medications in their own right. Dendrimers' biological action is caused by terminal moieties, which are also responsible for their overall effectiveness.

Dendrimers are successful in overcoming the physicochemical limits of traditional pharmaceuticals (for example, solubility, specificity, stability, bio-distribution, and therapeutic efficiency) due to their correct, repeatable, and optimized design parameters [31]. Dendrimers have a specific homogeneity that allows them to cross the membrane of cancer cells. The anticancer medication can be non-covalently encapsulated in the dendrimer's core or covalently attached to its surface, with controlled depolarization processes allowing for customized drug release profiles [32]. Anticancer drugs are linked to the surface groups of the dendrimer *via* covalent chemical bonds, which have several advantages over non-covalent encapsulation. It is possible to attach a variety of hydrophobic anti-breast cancer drugs in addition to improving drug solubilization, and the regulated release is maintained [33].

For breast cancer therapy, several anticancer drugs have been incorporated into dendrimers. DEP® docetaxel is one of the anticancer dendrimer formulations that have progressed from preclinical testing to phase I clinical trials. In clinical trials, signifying the effectiveness of dendrimer systems, DEP® docetaxel manufactured from PEGylated poly(l-lysine) (PLL) dendrimer has shown encouraging results (Table **2**) [34]. DEP®cabazitaxel, ImDendrim, and MAG-Tn3 are three other dendrimers now in clinical trials (Table **2**) [35].

Table 2. Clinical status of dendrimers targeting breast cancer [37].

Product/Trade Name	Copolymer Composition	Entrapped Drug	Clinical Phase
DEP® docetaxel	PEGylated PLL	Docetaxel	Phase I
DEP®cabazitaxel	Polylysine	Cabazitaxel	Phase I
MAG-Tn3	Carbohydrate peptide lysine	Vaccine composed of tri Tnglycotope	Phase I

To study the radiopharmaceutical potential for targeted radiotherapy and the simultaneous detection of FA receptors and gastrin-releasing peptide receptors overexpressed in T47D breast cancer cells, investigators used 177Lu-DOT--dendrimer-FA-bombesin with Au NPs entrapped within the dendrimers [36].

Polymeric Micelles

Micelles are colloidal particles with a size usually within a range of 5–100 nm. Polymeric micelles (PMs) are nano-sized colloidal particles with a core-shell structure that develop spontaneously in a block selective solvent by self-assembly of amphiphilic macromolecules into nanoaggregates (Fig. **2**) above a critical micelle concentration (CMC). PMs are good systems for encapsulating hydrophobic compounds because their hydrophobic core can accommodate these drugs, while their hydrophilic corona, usually poly(ethylene glycol), allows PMs to circulate in the bloodstream for an extended period of time, allowing them to reach breast tumour tissues *via* the enhanced permeability and retention (EPR) effect [38]. The use of polymeric micelles for the delivery of polycyclic anticancer agents, which have poor aqueous solubility, is advantageous because it allows for the safe, contemporaneous, or sequential intravenous infusion of numerous drugs, which is becoming the norm in aggressive therapy models. There have been difficulties in the development of PMs because of issues with stability and low drug loading [39]. However, because of the chemical flexibility given by amphiphilic block co-polymers, polymeric micelles can be designed to circumvent these obstacles. To achieve the aforementioned goals, various strategies have been used, including non-covalent (hydrophobic and – interactions) and chemical (covalent binding of the drug to the polymer backbone and/or cross-linking of the core/shell) strategies to improve circulation stability and retain the loaded drug in the PM. This will cause the drug to accumulate at the target site to a larger extent than in healthy tissues, resulting in a better therapeutic outcome [40]. South Korea approved the first micellar formulation for the treatment of breast and non-small cell lung cancer in 2007. GenexolTM-PM is a formulation based on the mPEG-b-poly (D,L-lactic acid) block copolymer with paclitaxel encapsulated in the micelles' core [41].

Polymer-drug Conjugates

Polymer conjugates are water-soluble polymers conjugated to anticancer drugs or proteins. These have a distinct pharmacokinetic profile than the parent medication and are thus classified as new chemical entities [42]. Depending on the synthesis method, the drug is either covalently bonded or physically entrapped in a polymer matrix. Natural and synthetic polymers are the two types of polymers available. Polymers such as chitosan, albumin, and heparin are naturally occurring polymers used to carry DNA, protein, oligonucleotides, and drugs. Gradishar *et al.* developed a nanoparticle formulation using a paclitaxel-serum albumin combination. Metastatic breast cancer has successfully been treated with this drug-polymer conjugate [43].

N-(2-hydroxypropyl)-methacrylamide copolymer (HPMA), poly-1-glutamic acid (PGA), polystyrene maleic anhydride copolymer, and polyethylene glycol (PEG) are among the most prevalent synthetic polymers. In nanodelivery, polycaprolactone and polyalkyl cyanoacrylates are often utilized polymers. The biodegradable polymer PGA was the first to be employed in conjugate synthesis. The most widely used synthetic polymers are HPMC and PEG, non-biodegradable [44].

Inorganic Nanoparticles

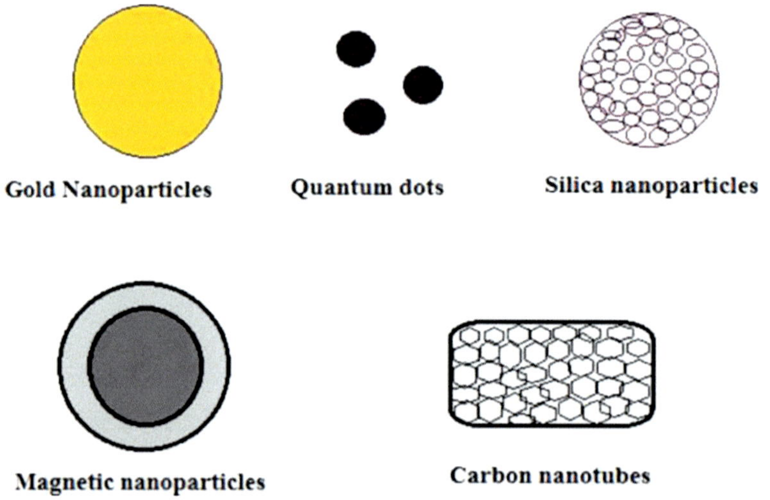

Fig. (4). Schematic representation of selected inorganic nanocarriers.

Gold nanoparticles, magnetic nanomaterials, carbon nanotubes, silica nanoparticles, and quantum dots (Fig. **4**) are all considered inorganic nanoparticles [7]. The following are some of the key reasons for the rise in the use of inorganic nanocarriers: chemical characteristics, size, form, excellent stability, the efficiency of functionalization, and greater surface-to-volume ratios.

Gold Nanoparticles (AuNPs)

Gold nanoparticles (AuNPs) are small gold particles, 1 to 100 nm in diameter, which, when disseminated in water, are also referred to as colloidal gold. Their various forms and sizes giveAuNPs distinct physical and chemical capabilities [45].AuNP's gold core is essentially non-reactive and non-toxic. Additionally, synthesizing AuNPs is simple, and it is possible to adjust the size to a controllable range from 1 to 150 nm. AuNPs can also function as drug transporters because the size and characteristics of the nanoparticles govern the release of drugs in various areas [45].

Various combinations of gold and phytochemicals have been used as "Swarna Bhasma" ("Swarna" means gold, "Bhasma" means ash) as ancient Indian anticancer medicine [46]. Gold NPs have some advantages such as simple, -efficient and reliable methodologies and different forms, like spheres, shells, rods and cages [47].AuNPs have strong surface plasmonresonanace and dialectal strength [47]. The presence of negative charge and strong binding capability of gold with functional groups such as thiols, disulfides, phosphines, and amines [47] makes gold NPs useful for modification and functionalization with various biomolecules. In addition, they are a valuable tool for cancer treatment due to their biocompatibility and non-toxicity [47].Chloroauric acid can be reduced to produce AuNPs with a diameter of 1 to 100 nm for imaging and radiation sensitization [45]. The gold nano shell (AuNS) is a spherical structure composed of a silica core and a thin gold shell of 50-150 nm diameters. By adjusting the core diameter and shell thickness, the optical characteristics of AUNSs can be changed. The reaction of chloroauric acid to the gold seed with ceyltromethylammonium bromide (CTAB) as a stabilizer [45], is commonly used to generate Gold nanorods (AusNRs).

Gold NPs were used as a probe for near-infrared induced hyperthermia [48] in photothermal therapy of cancer. *In vitro* and *in vivo* photothermal treatment of breast cancer by the use of silica-gold nanoshell has also been reported [49]. Induced hyperthermia or photothermal therapy technique involves the systemic administration of AuNP to a patient, leading to the accumulation of NPs in the tumour [50, 51], and to subsequent exposure of the tumour to a source of excitation, like near-infrared [NIR] laser light [49] or alternating magnetic field

[52]. The gold NPs transform the absorbed energy from the excitation source into heat, which increases tumour tissue temperature. The heat generated in this way kills cancer cells by damaging the cell membrane [50, 53]. This procedure prevents the negative effects of conventional cancer treatment because of minimal irradiation at the tumour site.

Using light-stimulated photothermal treatment, functionalized gold nanorods coated with the AS1411 DNA aptamer and doxorubicin [DOX] have been used to target breast cancer cells [47, 54]. When these conjugated NPs were grown with cells, over 20% cytotoxicity was observed, indicating some DOX leakage. While NIR irradiation resulted in the hybridization of DNA aptamers, which resulted in increased DOX release in up to 90% of MCF-7 cells [47, 55]. In addition, numerous other approaches, such as pH-dependent DOX release ligands, have been demonstrated that induce DOX release from golden nano-cages [47, 53]. or gold nanoshells [47, 56]. MDA-MB-231 breast cancer tumours in mice are studied with the help of gold–silica conjugate to check if it is capable of destroying the tumour cells with the help of NIR [47, 57]. As SK-BR-3 breast cancer cells were incubated with PEGylated AuNSs and then exposed to 820 nm NIR laser, the growth of the cells was significantly reduced when compared to that of the cells treated without PEGylated AuNSs [47, 49]. SK-BR-3 cells took up more PEGylated AuNSs conjugated with HER-2 antibodies [58]. When used against HER-2 overexpressing SKBR-3 breast cancer cells, using PEGylated AuNPs loaded with trastuzumab leads to DNA breakage that is 1.1 times greater than using PEGylated AuNPs alone [59].

Quantum Dots

Quantum dots (QDs) are luminous semiconductor crystals with a size of 1.5 nm to 10 nm, and their size and compact structure are unique in terms of chemicals and physical properties [60, 61]. Most QDs have a metal core that emits light ranging from visible to near-infrared (IR). The shell will often contain various metal doped materials or semiconductor layers depending on the purpose [62].QDs can be produced using a range of materials. Zinc sulphide, lead sulphide, cadmium selenide and indium phosphide are the most often utilized compounds [63]. Owing to robust quantum rates, easy surface modifications and customizable optical characteristics, these have been used as multi-function nanocarriers for PDT [63]. They also provide excellent donors for applications of fluorescent resonance transfer energy (FRET) [64]. Monroe *et al.* (2019) conducted spectrophotometric testing of Methylene Blue (MB) PS linked Grapheme QDs (GQD) using *in vitro* cultivated MCF-7 breast cancer cell to evaluate the cell absorption, anticancer activity, and ROS formation [65]. The investigation showed, relative to a 1:1 GQD: MB ratio, that the MB improved the cytotoxicity and ROS generation [65]. *In vitro* PDT activity in human breast cancer *in vitro* MCF-7 cell line was examined for the Zn(II) phthalocyanine (ZnPc)-GQDs conjugates, and it was found that compared to Pc administration alone, Pc-GQDs conjugates improved therapeutic outcomes [66].

Researchers have been aiming to develop a variety of targeted QDs against breast cancer. Under UV irradiation, it has been observed that QDs may exhibit cytotoxicity, allowing them to function as efficient PSs [63]. In comparison to small molecule-based PSs administered alone, NIR fluorescent QDs were found to increase PS water solubility, chemical resistance, and optical interaction with living tissues in PDT cancer therapies [67]. Additionally, due to the wide surface area of QDs, several PSs and ligands can be conjugated for targeted photodynamic imaging [63].

QDs that have multiple emissions were explored in a study of MCF-7 and BT-474 cell lines. The expression levels of five biomarkers such as ER, PR, EGFR, mTOR, and HER2 in these two cell lines was found to vary [68]. In order to carry out quantitative and multicolor protein marker analysis simultaneously, the primary antibodies for these biomarkers were combined with QDs [68]. A CuInS2/ZnS QDs-based water-soluble imaging agent capable of detecting breast cancer cells, coupled with an anti-Ki-67 monoclonal antibody, a nuclear protein related to the cell cycle, Ki-67, was reported by Sun *et al.* [69].

One major drawback of QDs is the presence of toxic heavy metals like cadmium ions in the inner core [63]. Therefore, the use of cadmium-free QDs, like indium and zinc-made QDs or their inclusion in polymeric NPs, has been suggested to improve their diagnostic uses and clinical studies involving PDT [70]. QDs tend to be highly hydrophobic. Therefore, polymers or multilayer ligand shells are required to provide particular water solubility to their surface [71].PEG coupling lowers the possible harmful accumulation of QDs in the reticular endothelial system and allows greater decoration of the surface [9, 72].

Carbon-based Nanoparticles

This category includes allotropes of carbon, such as carbon nanotube, carbon dots, fullerenes, and graphene oxide, commonly used in biomedical science [61, 73]. In hopes of eliminating poisonous heavy-metal comprising QDs and other metallic NPs, carbon-based NPs research was developed. NPs made of carbon atoms are characterized by numerous positive attributes, such as their optical and thermal properties, lesser size, greater surface area, multifunctional exterior, and gentle biocompatibility [61, 73]. This makes carbon-based NPs a promising drug delivery system to be used in the treatment of breast cancer.

Carbon nanomaterials have interesting optical, mechanical, electrical, and physicochemical properties. Due to their shape, they are good scaffolds for drugs, fluorophores, radionuclides, and good controllers of drug release [61]. They can cause toxicity because of their high *in vivo* stability and low aqueous solubility, but further functionalization can overcome these drawbacks [61].

Carbon nanotubes, carbon dots, fullerene, and graphene are all under consideration for managing breast cancer owing to their distinctive physical, optical, and biological properties.

Carbon-based nanomaterials are frequently used as photosensitizer (PS) nanocarriers in photodynamic therapy (PDT) [74 - 76]. Phenol, 1,1'-carbonyldiimidazole (CDI) and diisopropylcarbodiimide (DICDI) can be used to attach PSs to functionalized carbon-based nanomaterials, resulting in better solubility and biocompatibility when performing PDT treatments. Fullerenes are nanomaterials made of carbon that form into tubes, ellipsoids, or spheres and, upon exposure to light of a suitable wavelength, generate reactive oxygen species (ROS) [9, 77]. There are two additional forms of PS nanocarriers commonly used in PDT of cancer: single-walled carbon nanotubes (SWCNTs) and multi-walled carbon nanotubes (MWCNTs) [9, 77]. Since carbon nanotubes (CN) are useful due to their favorable properties, they are particularly beneficial as PS nanocarriers in PDT [9, 77]. In addition, the large surface areas of grapheme nanomaterials promote therapeutic loading, increasing the uptake of PS in tumour cells [78].

Carbon Nanotubes

Carbon nanotubes (CNTs) are spherical allotropes of buckminsterfullerene (C60) with a tubular shape full of elongated, hollow tubes constructed from a graphene layer that is rolled at a specific angle. Graphene sheets, on their own or in conjunction with multi-walled nanotubes, categorize CNTs as single-walled nanotubes (SWNTs) or multi-walled nanotubes (MWNTs). CNTs are still being developed, and a host of extraordinary properties remain to be explored, such as their thermal conductivity and optical and electrical properties [61]. Furthermore, due to the versatility of CNTs, they have seen tremendous application in nanomedicine, particularly in cancer-targeting nanomedicine applications [61].

Owing to the adjustable surface and exceptional thermal characteristics, CNTs can be used to create a particularly effective optical absorber in the NIR range (near-infrared light). This allows for increased penetration into biological systems, which are incredibly transparent in that region [61]. The treatment of cancer cells by using this approach that uses bio-functionalized CNTs is known as nano-photothermolysis [61].

He *et al.*, discovered that SWNTs displayed two exclusive optical characteristics [79]. A cancer cell exhibited a strong Raman signal and NIR absorbance, which were correlated with the selective photothermal ablation of tumours [79]. Following coupling with HER2 Ig Y, the combination displayed dual functionality, using an *in vitro* model with HER2-expressing SK-BR-3 cells and HER2-negative MCF-7 cells for recognition and selective cell damage. According to researchers, the protein annexin V (AV) is specific to anionic phospholipids expressed outside the tumour and endothelial cell surface, which are the liners of the tumour vasculature [61, 80, 81]. In a conjugate of SWNTs and AV, it was possible to treat breast cancer through photothermal therapy utilizing a 980 nm laser [61, 81].

As CNTs are pre-formed supramolecular nanotubes, drug loading is difficult. The filament method involves directly loading the drug onto the surface. Organic and inorganic chemotherapeutic drugs can be filled into CNTs *via* capillarity [82 - 84]. Nonetheless, loadable content is as low as 5% (w/w) [84]. While pre-functionalized CNTs allow direct attachment of certain small hydrophobic drugs to the coating-polymers, increasing loading capacity hinders hydrophobic drug attachment and thus reduces loading capacity. The coating polymer technique increased Dox loading capacity by 400% (w/w) [85]. The deficiency of space on the polymer surface limits the conjugation of other ligands, preventing multifunctional DDSs from doing their job [86]. The conjugate PTX-Long-Cha-n-Lipid-Docosanol was created by hydrophobic interactions between PTX and CNTs [87].

A novel drug delivery system comprised of antibody-coupled SWNTs, Dox, and SPIONs was proposed by Faraj *et al.* [88]. CNTs with -rich functional groups on the surface had a superior inhibitory effect on breast cancer cell proliferation when HIF-1α was down-regulated under hypoxia [89]. In contrast, this study failed to discuss any possible side effects of PTX. The effectiveness of breast cancer treatment can be limited by hypoxia as this enhances the tumour's resistance to chemo or radiotherapy.

MWNTs are CNTs used to treat breast cancer. SWCNTs are more cytotoxic to alveolar macrophages than MWCNTs. However, MWCNTs had the same effect at higher doses, indicating that SWCNTs are more toxic than MWCNTs [90]. As a result, MWCNTs for breast cancer treatments have been studied more recently [91]. Risi *et al.* studied MTX cytotoxicity, internalization, and loading in MDA-MB-231. The internalization of MWCNTs was confirmed by imaging [92]. A study on MWCNT-MTX cytotoxicity found linear kinetics with a 24-hour period and concentration-dependent MWCNT-MTX cytotoxicity. However, cancerous and non-cancerous cells were not clearly distinguished by MWCNT-MTX DDS

[92].

Functionalization of MWCNTs could better facilitate drug loading and targeted drug delivery. MWCNTs were functionalized with glucosamine in two patterns by Singh *et al.* [93]. They prepared the MWCNTs in two ways: covalent attachment of glucosamine and non-covalent covering MWCNTs with phospholipid-glucosamine [93]. The precise contact with the glucose transporters was required for the binding of MWCNTs. Glyco-MWCNTs prepared by the noncovalent coating of MWCNTs with phospholipid-glucosamine exhibited delayed urinary clearance, increased blood circulation time and increased breast cancer tumour accumulation than conventional MWCNTs. Hence, CNTs are a good drug delivery carrier.

Nonetheless, preparing CNTs is not as simple as it might seem. Solubility and biodegradability limitations have also been reported for CNTs [94]. Drug loading could also be complex in various ways. Carbon nanotubes have the ability to cause carcinogenic, asbestos-like inflammation [9, 95], thus, their distinct toxicity required to be comprehensively studied [9, 96].

Carbon Dots

In 2004, carbon dots (CDs) were discovered to be another type of carbon-based NPs [61]. The primary research into photoluminescence (PL) involved using various synthetic approaches, starting materials, and surface modifications in the early stages of the development of CDs [61]. In PL, surface doping improved fluorescence quantum yield (QY) up to 93.3% [61]. Further investigation and optimization of PL properties (especially for imaging *in vivo*) are obtained for CDs, through the addition of the PL-enhancing QY. CDs have specific properties such as water-dispersion, ease of production, high PL and bio-compatibility, large surface area and plenty of functional groups on the surface. Due to these properties CDs have been used as drug nanocarriers for *in vitro* and *in vivo* studies [61]. While these properties have made CDs particularly attractive for use in treating breast cancer, it was only in 2013 that CDs were first applied to breast cancer treatment.

According to Hsu *et al.* in 2013, green tea-derived CDs exhibited anti-cancer activity [97]. The cancer cell lines MDA-MB-231, HeLa, and MCF-7 have been used in the study. As the concentration of CDs increased, the cell viability decreased. To test the efficacy of CD cells on HeLa, MDA-MB-231, and MCF-7 cancer cells, the cell viability percentages were as follows: for HeLa, it was 20%; for MDA-MB-231, it was 18%; and for MCF-7, it was 68%. This clearly showed that CDs had a greater inhibitory effect on breast cancer cell lines. It was proposed that exposure to H_2O_2 and ROS results in the reduction of viability [97].

The researchers demonstrated green-emitting CDs synthesized from urea and citric acid, using a microwave-mediated method as the Dox-carrying nanocarrier [98]. Dox was released in cancer cells by means of a pH-dependent mechanism that began with the conjugation of Dox with CDs using basic electrostatic force or hydrogen bonds. These CDs were explored for anticancer activity using MCF-7 breast cancer cell lines. When exposed to the cancer cells, the CDs-Dox conjugate resulted in the decline of cell viability, which showed a significant clinical effect. In addition, Zhao and his colleagues explored MCF-7 in contrast to MDA-M--231 cells to identify the ability of CDs to detect and target acidic extracellular tumour conditions [99]. A follow-up study was reported in which CD-nanocarrier was utilized by Kong *et al.*, and Dox and CDs were conjugated using electrostatic interactions. The resulting conjugate obtained superior cellular uptake and anti-tumour efficacy on MCF-7 cells than free Dox [100].

CDs represent a promising nanocarrier in breast cancer drug delivery because their non-toxicity, excellent water dispersion, good biocompatibility and excellent PL make imaging and tracking possible. However, there have been only a few studies. Detailed studies about CDs that can be used as DDS for breast cancer are, therefore, necessary to clarify these new options [61].

Fullerene and Graphene

Fullerene-iron oxide NPs (IONP) for active tumour targeting were synthesized and functionalized with PEG, Ce6, and FA (c60-IONP-PEG-FA) by Shi *et al.* [101].

In vitro MCF-7 breast cancer cells and *in vivo* breast cancer mice models were used to investigate the PDT effect, radiofrequency thermal therapy(RTT), and magnetic targeting performance of these multifunctional NPs [9, 101].

Transferrin-targeted graphene oxide nanoparticles demonstrated a high loading capacity of docetaxel (37%), which was released pH-dependently and sustainably in physiological conditions, killing MCF-7 cells [9]. Additionally, grapheme nano dots destroyed MDA-MB-231 cells and xenografts *via* thermal ablation and enabled imaging of deep cancerous tissue when irradiated with a 670 nm laser [9].

The GO(HPPH)-PEG-HK was designed and functionalized with PEG-GO, so that an HK peptide could be attached to graphene oxide (GO) by benefiting from the highly significant loading volume of graphene oxide (GO) *via* pi-pi stacking and hydrophobic interactions [102].

A photochlorine (2-[1-hexyloxyethyl]-2-devinyl pyropheophorbidealpha, HPPH) PS was subsequently coated onto this nanoconjugate [103]. The huge GO region permits several HK peptides to combine and high HPPH levels, allowing for better *in vivo* breast cancer treatment outcomes [103].

In general, very few studies of the active PDT targeting of breast cancer were performed by using carbon-based nanomaterials. However, studies indicated the possibility of improving the effectiveness of breast cancer-PDT treatment with a blend of the synergistic effects of carbon-made NPs and PSs [74]. Furthermore, in PDT applications, fullerenes, like C60 [104] and CNTs [105], can operate on their own as PSs, thereby auto-generating ROS from photons by means of their electrons in the pi bond [106]. Fullerene derivatives alone are, therefore, modest PS for either *in vivo* or preclinical PDT treatment [107] as there are no requirements for additional PS to generate ROS and therefore, further breast cancer treatment research involving fullerenes should be undertaken [9].

Magnetic Nanoparticles

Magnetic nanoparticles are a form of magnetic field-compatible nanoparticles. These particles are made up of chemical compounds magnetic from nickel, cobalt and iron magnetic material [108].

Magnetic NPs (MNPs) are characterized as having two variants, one of which is magnetite (Fe_3O_4) and the other of which is maghemite (Fe_2O_3). These MNPs have found widespread use in cancer research, as they help limit systemic circulation, which results in their propensity to target specific sites and aid in drug encapsulation, slow drug suspension during delivery, and better dissolution, which allows for lower dosing of cytotoxic drugs and reduces side effects [108]. Drugs like mitoxantrone, tamoxifen, cefradine, doxorubicin, daunorubicin, cisplatin, gemcitabine, paclitaxel, Adriamycin, *etc*., are encapsulated into MNPs [108]. MNPs coated with oleic acid-pluronic led to sustained release of doxorubicin and exhibited anti-proliferative action on breast cancer cell lines [109]. As an advisable therapeutic strategy in breast cancer treatment, MNPs have been established. Iron NPs enhanced damage of tumour cells when exposed to an external magnetic field by producing efficient heat [110]. Magnetic hyperthermia offers a minimally intrusive means of transferring a therapeutic heat dose exactly to the cancer site compared to conventional hyperthermic procedures [111]. Trastuzumab-targeted HER2 functionalized MNPs have also been employed to detect breast xenografts overexpressing HER2 receptors [112]. Narsireddy *et al.* (2014) synthesized chitosan-coated Fe_3O_4 NPs that were then deposited with gold NPs and conjugated with lipoic acid [9, 116]. Additionally, a 5,10,15,20-tetrakis(4-hydroxyphenyl)-21H,23H-porphyrin PS was covalently linked to gold NPs to generate Fe_3O_4-Au-LA-PS (MGPS) [9, 113].To enhance the targeting of this nanoconjugate, a human epidermal growth factor receptor-specific peptide

(Affibody HER-2) was covalently attached to its chitosan coat, resulting in Aff-MGPS [9, 113]. The PDT outcomes of Aff-MGPS were next investigated *in vitro* using HER-2 positive SK-OV-3 breast cancer cells [9, 113]. The tailored Aff-MGPS had much higher uptake efficiency than free PS or NPs controls alone [9.113]. Additionally, MGPS or Aff-MGPS nanoplatforms exhibited no dark toxicity, but free PS exhibited a substantial level of dark toxicity [9, 113]. Moreover, compared to group controls, the Aff-MGPS nanoplatforms demonstrated increased targeted peptide uptake in breast cancer cells [9, 113]. The photodynamic anticancer properties of magnetic Fe_3O_4 nanoparticles on breast cancer were further studied by conjugating Ce6 and FA to create Fe_3O4-Ce6-FA [9, 114]. The produced nanoconjugate was capable of producing 1O2 and ROS with no evidence of dark toxicity [9, 114]. MCF-7 *in vitro* breast cancer cells demonstrated a concentration-dependent decrease in viability and an increase in apoptotic cell death in PDT Fe_3O_4-Ce6-FA 660 nm studies [9, 114].

Superparamagnetic Iron Oxide (SPIO)

The size of superparamagnetic iron oxide nanoparticles (SPIONs) is between 1 and 100 nm. The inner core of these NPs is made up of Magnetite, Fe_3O_4, or maghemite, γ-Fe_2O_3. Maghemite is generally regarded as one of the more appropriate internal core materials for SPIONs because of its low likelihood of toxicity from Fe (III) [61].

Biofouling and agglomeration of SPIONs in blood plasma constitute a significant drawback from their direct use in therapeutic and biomedical applications [61]. Thus, a hydrophilic stabilizing coating like polymers is covered for this magnetic core, which enables biomolecules to be targeted to a specific location. Polysaccharides, PEG, dextran, alginate and polyacrylic acid are the most commonly used biopolymers for stabilization [61].

SPIONs are simultaneously utilized in tissue reparation, immunoassay, magnet field cell imaging, and drug release systems [115]. Furthermore, in the processing of MRI and macrophages, SPIO is also one of the most efficient nanoparticles [115].

The chemical and physical properties of particles can be controlled, such as their surface chemistry, shape, and size, with SPIO nanoparticles. Additionally, these nanoparticles can be used to detect inflammatory diseases and are efficient at locating surface tumour markers. Iron oxide NPs with antibodies bound to polyethylene glycol polymers (SPION IL4Ra) were explored in a 4T1 breast cancer cell [115]. Blocking IL4Ra receptors triggered apoptosis in 4T1 cells, leading to a significant decrease in 4T1 cell viability. These results show that combining SPION-IL4Ra or doxorubicin alone, combining SPIONIL4Ra and doxorubicin, causes increased oxidative stress, cell death, and apoptosis [115].

A SPION of about 8–10 nm diameter was produced by Marcu *et al.* using laser pyrolysis with uniform particle size [116]. After additional coating of the NPs with the anthracycline antibiotic violamycine B1, the SPIONs showed anti-tumour activity on MCF-7 cells.

Poller *et al.* found that three different types of SPIONs, with different sizes, shapes, zeta potentials, and surface coatings, have different cell-killing effects. Magnetic properties, cellular uptake, and cytotoxicity of SPIONs were compared when analyzing their impact on cellular uptake, magnetic characteristics, and cytotoxicity [117]. The three SPIONs used for breast cancer treatment: dextran coated (SPIONDEX), lauric acid coated (SPIONLA), and SPIONLA with the addition of human serum albumin (SPIONLA-HSA).SPIONLA demonstrated the maximum cellular uptake and breast cancer cell damage [117].

Streptavidin-conjugated SPIONs were explored as a contrasting agent for targeted MRI in the quantification of tyrosine kinase HER2/neu receptor in breast cancer cells [118]. SPIONs were targeted to a panel of MCF-7 breast cancer cells with different concentrations of the receptors, which were pre-coated with biotinylated monoclonal antibodies [118]. The images observed showed that HER2/new receptor expression level is commensurate with the contrast. The study indicated that SPIONs were only attached to the breast cancer cell's surface without entering the cell, which was advantageous for *in vivo* imaging [118]. SPIONs have the potential to enhance contrast in imaging, especially when compared to conventional imaging techniques [119].

Silica Nanoparticles

Silica, a silicon oxide, is one of the best resources for controlled drug delivery. Due to the polymerization of silica, mesoporous silica nanoparticles (MSNs) have unique properties, such as the ability to tune pore size (providing extraordinary therapeutic drug loading abilities) [9] and enormous surface area to volume ratio, making drug release spontaneous [9]. As a result, silica NPs can be coated with covalently linked or encapsulated photosensitizers (PSs) for improved cancer treatment outcomes [9].MSNs with covalently attached anionic porphyrin PS and mannose targeting breast cancer were reported [9].

Based on two-photon absorption (TPE) with silica nanotechnology [9], PSs absorb a single photon equal to their band gap energy [9].TPE also has the effect of increasing light penetration and reducing photobleaching of the original PS. This allows for greater spatial control in three-dimensional (3D) tumour models and reduces off-target phototoxicity in healthy tissues [9].

Photodynamic therapy (PDT) and imaging potentials of porphyrin-functionalized silica NPs (pSiNP) were evaluated in cultured MCF-7 breast cancer cells [120]. pSiNPs appear to be biodegradable *in vivo* [121], as the silicon components of pSiNPs break down to silicic acid, which can be excreted by the kidneys [120, 121]. PDT phototoxicity showed a 2.3-fold better outcome when compared to one-photon excitation PDT at 650 nm in breast cancer cells modified with pSiNP mannose moieties [120].

Cao *et al.* (2014) used MSCs to deliver PS directly to *in vitro* cultured MCF-7 cells to increase PS accumulation [122]. The high affinity of MSCs for tumours *in vivo* has allowed them to be easily separated from the bone marrow and adapted to deliver the required drug. They can also be embedded to prevent immune clearance by the patient [123 - 126]. They were then subjected to *in vivo* PDT in modified MCF-7 mouse models with purpurin-18 PS conjugated (PS-SiO2NP--MSCs) [122]. After laser irradiation, intercellular ROS generation increased proportionally when a bond was formed between PS-SiO2NPs-MSCs, according to the study. *In vivo* breast cancer tumours retained the PS. PDT studies should also be considered in this review. This suggests that MSCs cells have a high affinity for PS-SiO2 NPs when compared to unmodified MSCs in these studies [122].

It was found that silica-Ce6-FA coated silica NPs increased significantly *in vitro* in MDA-MB-231 breast cancer cells compared to free Ce6 [127]. However, at 680 nm PDT, the data revealed that the presence of the folate receptor on the nanoconjugate improved PS uptake in breast cancer cells, resulting in a higher cell death rate [127].

The clinically accepted PSs have very little absorption in this range, which means their penetration depth is less than one centimeter [128]. As X-ray sources can penetrate deeper tissues, a study has already begun to explore X-ray-mediated PDT (X-PDT), also known as X-ray-puncture PDT (X-PDT). Because PSs cannot absorb X-ray photons directly [120], they require a system for converting X-rays into UV–visible photons. Rare-earth doped lanthanide nanoparticles have been created as energy transducers for this transformation and X-PDT treatment [129 - 131].

Sengar *et al.* (2018) explored the deep penetration of X-PDT into breast cancer tumours [132]. Y2.99Pr0.01Al5O12-based (YP) mesoporous silica (MS) coated NPs were produced and functionalized with protoporphyrin IX (PpIX) and folic acid (FA) (YPMS@PpIX@FA) for the X-PDT therapy of breast cancer cells with overexpressed folate receptors (Folr 1) [132]. PyMT-R221A mouse BC cells (with elevated amounts of folate receptors) and 4T1 BC cells (with low folate expression) were used as breast cancer *in vitro* cell lines [132]. PyMT-R221A mouse breast cancer cells had a greater uptake of YPMS@PpIX@FA than 4T1 breast cancer cells, indicating that FA targeting of this nanoconjugate was effective [132]. In addition, nonactivated YPMS@PpIX@FA exhibited modest cytotoxicity at concentrations below 25 g/ml, however, upon light activation at 365 nm, PyMT-R221A mouse breast cancer cells decreased significantly [132]. Lastly, administration of YPMS@PpIX@FA suspension at a single dose of up to 125 mg/kg to infected CD1 mice did not result in mortality or any observable behavior [132]. Overall, silica NPs appear favorable for PDT of breast cancer, and the use of these NPs in clinical practice is justified.

Titanium Oxide Nanoparticles

In addition to being resistant to corrosion and bacteriological contamination, titanium dioxide (TiO_2) is also photostable, has strong antimicrobial properties, and maintains stability within biomedical applications [9]. Additionally, the ability of TiO_2 to release highly reactive oxygen species (ROS) upon being excited with ultraviolet (UV) radiation between 390 and 400 nm can induce apoptosis in breast cancer cells [9].

TiO_2 NPs with 7, 8-dihydroxy coumarin PS chromophore and chlorambucil (Ti-DBMC-Cmbl NPs) were combined with FA (Ti-FA-DBMC-Cmbl NPs) and explored in PDT/chemotherapy treatments of MDA-MB breast cancer cells *in vitro* [9].

While the targeted PDT and well-established anti-cancer drug chlorambucil yielded positive results for the destruction of MDA-MB-231 breast cancer cells, overall, these results suggested that the synergic effect of both approaches was adequate for the treatment of MDA-MB-breast cancers [9]. Ceramic NPs are highly chemically inert and resistant to heat; therefore, these are excellent carriers for photodynamic therapy (PDT) treatment of targeted breast cancer tumours.

Other Inorganic Nanoparticles

Lanthanide metal oxide NPs are regarded as having a lanthanide metal oxide-based absorber that is useful for ultraviolet (UV) wavelengths [9]. Cerium oxide NPs (or nanoceria/ceria NPs) are viewed as having a lanthanide metal oxide-based absorber that may be utilized for UV wavelengths. These have strong antioxidant properties at physiological pH, but their oxides work ideally in an acidic microenvironment [9]. They are usually polymer-coated to increase the solubility, biocompatibility, and stability of nanoceria NPs [9].

A multifunctional drug delivery system of Ce6/FA-loaded branched polyethylenimine–PEGylation ceria NPs (PPCNPs) for the potential PDT targeting of drug-resistant *in vitro* breast cancer MCF-7/ADR cells was created by Li *et al.* [9]. In terms of the efficiency of internalization and the distribution of the synthesized NPs with positive surface charges to breast cancer cells, the results showed that the degree of internalization and distribution of the Ce6-based nanoplatform was much higher than free Ce6 [9].

Studies have indicated that treatment options, such as chemotherapy, radiation and operative procedures, are unproductive in treating metastatic triple-negative breast cancer (mTNBC). Thus, researchers have turned to immunotherapy as a possible treatment for mTNBC. The success of tumour immunotherapy depends on the suppression of breast cancer cells by $CD8^+$ cytotoxic T cells [9].

Immunotherapy based on blocking checkpoints may help manage primary *in vitro* 4T1 breast cancer tumours [9].ZnP@pyro NPs were made by placing Zn and pyrophosphate (ZnP) in a microscale reactor, and a pyrolipid PS was introduced as the core, whereas a PD-L1 antibody was introduced for checkpoint blockade immunotherapy [9]. It was found that the non-toxic ZnP@pyro NPs were able to elicit an immune response when exposed to light [9]. ZnP@pyro NPs could completely eradicate *in vitro* breast cancer cells upon 670 nm irradiation through apoptotic and necrotic cell death [9].

Antibody-conjugated Nanoparticles

Antibody conjugated nanoparticles (ACNPs) combine both nanoparticle and antibody conjugation (Fig. **5**) to achieve the highest potential of each technique [133]. It is possible to use membrane proteins expressed in tumour cells to develop antibodies linked to the nanoparticle (NP) as a vector. ACNPs can control the release of drugs and keep their structures intact, reducing side effects and toxicity.

Conjugation with membrane protein antibodies mainly expressed on tumour cells may produce vectorized NPs [133]. The interaction between ligand and receptor induces the internalization of the NPs through a receptor-facilitated endocytosis and the release of drugs inside the cell [133]. Because of their high specificity and affinity, antibodies are the most commonly used tumour cell ligands [133]. IgG is the most abundant human serum antibody and the most extensively-used NP vector antibody. Smaller fragments of antibodies are also used to improve the uptake of tumour [133]. The enzyme cleavage of a full-size antibody generates antigen-binding fragments (Fab) [133].

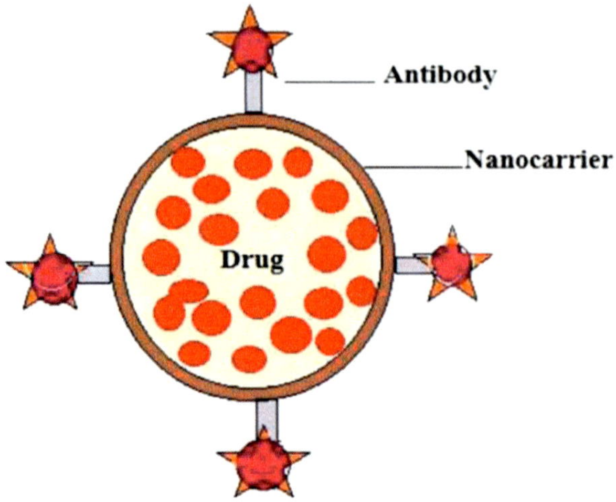

Fig. (5). Schematic representation of antibody-conjugated nanoparticle.

Antibodies or antibody fragments may be functionalized with NPs by adsorption or covalent attachment. This will guarantee the correct quantity of biomolecules per NP, and their positioning will be fixed, as the antibodies will remain immobile [133]. Higher ratio of antibody molecules to NP exterior results in lowering the spatial accessibility of the present antigen [133]. Another requirement for the coupling approach is retaining the antibody's biological action [133]. Physical adsorption and ionic binding are non-covalent immobilization strategies [133]. Physical adsorption involves the connection of antibodies to the surface of the NP employing weak interactions like electrostatic, hydrogen bonding, hydrophobic and van der Waals forces [133]. In contrast, the ionic interaction of differently charged antibody sites and NPs provides the basis for ionic binding [133]. Covalent binding means that nanoparticles must be activated in advance [133]. Carbodiimide, maleimide, or "click chemistry" are the most frequent covalent techniques. The use of carbodiimide is a straightforward procedure that does not require any chemical modification of antibodies. Interactions between cross-linkers and functional groups are not, however, selective. This is a significant drawback that results in a lack of control over antibody orientation onto the surface of NPs [133].

Various nanocarriers have been described as innovative therapies for the production of ACNPs. The most frequently assessed ACNPs include inorganic, polymeric ACNPs and immunoliposomes [133].

The Immunoliposomes have antibodies attached to the surface of liposomes. The use of several targeting ligands for targeted liposomes has been reported in the literature. Apart from doxorubicin (DOX), other anticancer drugs such as docetaxel (DTX) and paclitaxel (PTX) have been incorporated into immunoliposomes targeting the HER2 and EGFR antigens to treat breast cancer [133]. The majority of studies employed trastuzumab as the conjugating antibody intending to target HER2-overexpressing tumours. Other antibodies have also been conjugated to immunoliposomes to circumvent drug resistance mechanisms [133].

Taxanes have shown high toxicity for breast cancer treatment in ordinary tissue, as in the usage of DOX. The quality of life of the patient is affected by side effects greatly. Immunoliposomes provide significant advantages in comparison with conventional liposomes and antibody drug conjugates (ADCs) in this context. The antitumour efficacy and mechanisms of action in several breast cancer cells and nude mouse xenograft models have been evaluated for the PTX loaded trastuzumab immunoliposomes [134]. Immunoliposomes demonstrated improved efficacy greater tissue distribution of PTX in the BT-474 xenograft models as compared to taxol and non-target liposomes. Breast cancer cells use the mammalian target of rapamycin pathway to develop [135]. As a result, rapamycin has been intensively explored for treating breast cancer [136]. PTX and rapamycin co-delivery from trastuzumab-targeted immunoliposomes suppressed tumour growth *in vivo*. Curcumin and resveratrol co-delivery from trastuzumab-targeted immunoliposomes was also investigated for HER2 breast cancer [137].

Breast cancer treatment with inorganic ACNPs includes early detection, thermotherapy, and biomarker discovery. ACNPs based on SPIONs, gold, and QDs have also been proposed as drug and siRNA delivery systems [138 - 140]. SPIONs and DOX were encapsulated into a poly (lactic-co-glycolic acid) (PLGA) core using a nanoemulsion technique and then conjugated with trastuzumab using EDC/NHS chemistry [134]. PTX, DOX, and siRNA were effectively incorporated in SPION-based ACNPs, resulting in selective breast cancer cell destruction [141 - 143]. Anti-HER2 ACNPs for siRNA delivery were generated using a polyethyleneimine coating [142]. The ACNPs demonstrated the delivery of vascular endothelial growth factor (VEGF) siRNA into cancer cells and its therapeutic benefits. DOX was encapsulated in dextrane-modified SPIONs through ionic gelation and HER2 monoclonal antibody was attached to the surface of the NPs *via* EDC/NHS chemistry [143]. Zhang *et al.* reported the transport of HER2 siRNA through modified chitosan surface modifications to over-expressing SKBR3 breast cancer cells using ACNPs coupled with HER2 antibodies [144].

For gold ACNPs, HER2-conjugated gold ACNPs were described as a theranostic probe for imaging and the therapy of breast cancer [145]. Strong therapeutic benefits have been reported in combination with trastuzumab for administering cisplatin utilizing hybrid Au-Fe3O4 nanoparticles [146]. DOX was encapsulated in a PLGA core using nanoemulsion techniques and then conjugated with trastuzumab [147 - 149]. Additionally, PLGA ACNPs conjugated with trastuzumab were developed to entrap rapamycin 150 and DTX [150]. Utilizing polyvinylpyrrolidone coating and subsequent trastuzumab conjugation through EDC activation were achieved in the knowledge that trastuzumab tamoxifen combination increased treatment effectiveness for metastatic breast cancers that are HER2- and ER-positive [151]. A higher inhibition rate for ACNPs than the non-targeted NPs and free tamoxifen has been demonstrated *in vivo*. The limitations are the limitations of lack of understanding of nanocarrier-biological system interactions, poor accumulation at the tumour site, poor pharmacokinetics, and the safety concerns of raw materials for generating ACNPs and minimal *in vivo* studies to develop ACNP [133].

Exosomes as Nanocarrier

Exosomes are membranous vesicles with multiple biological functions. They were initially used for cancer detection or identification in the human body. Later, exosomes were further investigated as a drug delivery system, with some benefits such as non-immunogenicity and improved circulation time. Exosomes are composed of proteins and lipids in the human body [152]. Exosomes were developed for delivering Doxrubicin, which targeted and delivered to αv integrin-positive breast cancer cells. Doxrubicin-loaded exosomes administered through IV route reached tumour tissues, inhibiting tumour growth without toxicity. The external surface of exosomes can be modified to obtain significant target specificity, which is similar to other lipid-based nanometric devices [152]. Resistance can emerge over time with drugs such as Adriamycin and DTX, which are used as chemotherapeutic agents in breast cancer. Possibly exosome-mediated, miRNA- or protein-based propagation of resistant cancer cells to other sensitive cancer cells occurs [152]. Endogenous exosomes' primary utility is delivering therapies based on nucleic acids or peptides directly to cancer cells. Cationic bovine serum albumin (CBSA) was linked to siS100A4 following this concept. Exosome-mediated RNAi down-regulated the expression of S100A4, resulting in significant suppression of postoperative mTNBC. It was demonstrated by Singh *et al.* that micro-RNA (miR-10b) could also shuttle into metastatic breast cancer cells (MDA-MB-231) [152]. These studies show that exosome membrane-packaged core-shell NPs are a proficient clinical strategy for breast cancer prevention and treatment [152].

Virus-based NPs

Viral NPs are a subset of NPs that resemble viral capsids or protein envelopes. Because these viral NPs lack viral genomes, they cannot replicate and thus cannot infect. Plants quickly produce nucleic acid nanoparticles *via* viral envelope, capsid protein expression, and recombination. Transient plant tissue transformation produces recombinant proteins or products within days of activity, allowing rapid commercial production [61]. Viral NPs also have highly ordered repetitive surfaces that are ideal for drug conjugation [61]. Because viral NPs are becoming more versatile, they will be used for targeted drug delivery in the future.

Trastuzumab is presently used as a virus-delivered treatment for HER2+ breast cancer patients. Esfandiari *et al.* in 2015 discovered breast cancer cell death caused by PVX, a strain of potato virus X [61]. Based on these findings, they combined trastuzumab monoclonal antibody with PVX, which inhibits breast cancer cell multiplication and signal transduction [61]. The study also showed that Dox was conjugated to PVX and given to athymic mice with human MDA-M--231 breast cancer xenografts. Treatment with PVX-Dox slowed tumour growth [61]. This also applies to viral NPs derived from plants. Thus, PVX, a plant-originated viral NP, paves the way for viral NPs to treat cancer. In a mouse breast cancer model, influenza NPs with aglycosyl phosphatidylinositol (GPI) anchor and HER2 antigen accelerated the growth of HER2-positive tumours. Vaccination with GPI-HER2-modified influenza viral NPs increased HER2-specific IgG generation and Th1-type immunity [61].

This type of drug delivery system is ideal for a viral NP because it is biocompatible and biodegradable. Plant virus and bacteriophage-derived NPs are superior because they are less likely to cause unwanted side effects in humans [61]. The knowledge of this technique's capabilities is limited due to the lack of such studies. Nevertheless, viral NPs are predicted to be found in clinics very soon. Synthesizing viral NPs is sometimes more difficult and costly than creating other NPs so the method of synthesis should be made more accessible and straightforward [61].

NANOCARRIERS AND MULTIDRUG RESISTANCE

One of the most significant challenges in the treatment of breast cancer is drug resistance. Multiple factors contribute to this highly complex process, including P-glycoprotein overexpression, alterations in drug-binding sites such as microtubule, gene mutations, HER2 overexpression, and many more. Many nanocarriers (Table **3**) can alleviate some of these problems in part by overcoming the cell membrane barrier *via* endocytosis and achieving high intracellular drug concentrations even with passive targeting. Combination therapy is another popular technique for dealing with these problems. One or more cytotoxic chemotherapeutic drugs and a novel "helper" that either interferes with a drug resistance pathway or regulates a specific cell population that improves drug resistance are usually included [153].

Table 3. Nanocarriers to target multidrug resistance in human breast cancer [154].

Drug	Nanocarriers	Targeting Ligand
Thymoquinone	Gold niosome	siRNAAkt
Doxorubicin	Mesoporous silica	siRNA P-gp
	CdSe/ZnSe	siRNA P-gp
	Mesoporous silica	siRNA P-gp
	Graphene oxide	Molecular beacon MDR1 and ETS1
	Polymeric	shRNASurvivin
	Polymeric micelle	Folate
Adriamycin	Graphene oxide	siRNA miR-21
Vincristine sulfate	Polymeric	R7 peptide,folate

APPLICATIONS OF NANOCARRIERS IN BREAST CANCER STEM CELL THERAPY

Breast cancer stem cells or breast tumour initiating cells are a small fraction of cancer cells that can undergo self-renewal and differentiation to multiple cancer cell types. These cells are very often drug-resistant and act as seeds for the generation of full-grown tumours aggressively. Several nanocarriers have been used to develop formulations for highly expressed targets such as CD44 and CD133 of breast stem cells (Table **4**). Studies have shown that paclitaxel as a drug can effectively inhibit breast cancer cells' growth, but the cancer cells relapse quickly once the drug is withdrawn. However, PLGA nanoparticles with anti-CD133 antibody for paclitaxel delivery could successfully encounter this issue [155]. Hence, it can be a prospective strategy to be explored further.

Table 4. Nanocarriers used in breast cancer stem cell therapy [153].

Drug	Nanocarrier	Target
Paclitaxel	PLGA-co-PEG micelles decorated with anti-CD44 antibodies	CD44
	PLGA nanoparticles decorated with anti-CD133 antibody	CD133
Salinomycin and paclitaxel	PLGA nanoparticles coated with hyaluronic acid	CD44
Doxorubicin	Chitosan-decorated Pluronic F127 nanoparticles	CD44
Doxorubicin and irinotecan	Nanoparticles consist of four polymers PLGA Pluronic F127, chitosan and hyaluronic acid	CD44

CLINICAL TRIALS FOR NANOPARTICLES TARGETING BREAST CANCER

Oncology-based nanomedicinal therapeutic candidates are promising from the nanomedicine industry's perspective. An improved therapeutic index for anticancer drugs has been demonstrated by improving their pharmacokinetics and tissue distribution in order to improve targeted delivery.

Doxil™/Caelyx™ [156] was the first FDA-approved anticancer nanomedicine in 1995 and is currently permitted for numerous applications, including breast cancer, based on improved safety and efficacy *versus* standard conventional anticancer therapies. Polymeric NPs, liposomes, polymeric micelles, and polymeric conjugates are generally regarded as the main nanomedicines presently being explored in clinical trials for treating or diagnosing breast cancer.

Nanoparticles in various stages of clinical development for the treatment of breast cancer are summarized in Table **5**.

Table 5. Breast cancer nanotherapeutics in different stages of clinical trials [10, 157].

Type of nanoparticle	Drug /product	Sponsor company/Institute	Indication	Trial status
Non-PEGylated liposome	Doxorubicin	Elan Pharmaceuticals, Spherion Therapeutics	HER2-positive metastatic BC	Phase III (Approved in Canada and Europe)
Liposomal	Paclitaxel (EndoTAG-1)	Medigene/SynCore Biotechnology	Metastatic BC	Phase II
Liposomal	Paclitaxel	Fresenius Kabi Oncology Ltd.	Advanced BC	Phase 1
Albumin-Stabilized Nanoparticle	Adjuvant concurrent bevacizumab and dose-dense doxorubicin hydrochloride and cyclophosphamide followed by dose-dense paclitaxel NP	Memorial Sloan Kettering Cancer Center	Treatment of patients who have undergone surgery for early-stage BC	NA
Polymeric conjugates	Irinotecan (NKTR102 (PEG))	Nektar	Metastatic BC	Phase III
Polymeric micelles	Paclitaxel (NK105/NanoCarrier™)	-	BC	Phase III
Liposomes	Paclitaxel (EndoTAG-1)	MediGene	BC	Phase II

(Table 5) cont.....

Liposomes	Paclitaxel (LEP—ETU)	Insys	BC	Phase II
Albumin-stabilized nanoparticles	Paclitaxel	City of Hope Medical Center	Metastatic BC	Phase II
Carbon nanoparticles	Carbon nanoparticles labelled lymph nodes	The First Affiliated Hospital with Nanjing Medical University	cN+ BC	NA
Nanoparticles Albumin-Bound (Nab)	Paclitaxel/Cyclophosphamide	SCRI Development Innovations, LLC	Early-Stage BC	Phase II
Liposomal	Cisplatin	Regulon	BC	Phase III
Topical Fluorescent Nanoparticles	Somatostatin Analog	Al-Azhar University	Suppression and Bioimaging of BC	Phase 1
Albumin bound NP	Paclitaxel	EpiAxis Therapeutics	Metastatic or advanced BC (epi-primed)	Phase 1
Albumin-stabilized nanoparticle formulation	Carboplatin and paclitaxel	Sidney Kimmel Comprehensive Cancer Center at Johns Hopkins	Treatment of newly diagnosed operable BC	Phase II
Albumin-stabilized nanoparticles formulation	Paclitaxel (Doxorubicin hydrochloride, cyclophosphamide, and filgrastim followed by paclitaxel albumin-stabilized nanoparticles formulation with or without trastuzumab)	University of Washington	Patients with BC previously treated with surgery	Phase II
Albumin-stabilized nanoparticle formulation	Nab paclitaxel (paclitaxel and bevacizumab followed by bevacizumabanderlotinib)	University of Washington	Treatment of metastatic BC	Phase II
Pegylatedliposome and albumin-bound NP	Doxorubicin And paclitaxel	Arcus Biosciences,Inc.	Advanced metastatic TNBC	Phase I
Albumin-stabilized nanoparticle formulation	Paclitaxel (Paclitaxel AndCarboplatin with bevacizumab or trastuzumab)	University of California, Irvine	Stage I-III BC	Phase II
Albumin-bound NP	nab-Paclitaxel (Abraxane®)	International Breast cancer Study Group	Metastatic BC	Phase II
Albumin Bound NP	nab-paclitaxel plus lapatinib	Novartis Pharmaceuticals	Metastatic BC	Phase II

(Table 5) cont.....

Albumin Bound NP	paclitaxel (pembrolizumab in combination with nab-paclitaxel)	InstitutfuerFrauengesundheit	TNBC	Phase II
Albumin Bound NP	Paclitaxel (Nab-paclitaxel and Alpelisib)	M.D. Anderson Cancer Center	TNBC	Phase II
Albumin Bound NP	Paclitaxel (atezolizumab, and nab-paclitaxel)	Mayo Clinic	Advanced or metastatic TNBC	Early Phase 1
Albumin Bound NP	Nab-paclitaxel and durvalumab	National Cancer Institute (NCI)	Metastatic TNBC	Phase II
PEGylated liposome	Irinotecan	Nektar therapeutics	BC	Phase III
Polymeric micelle PEG-poly(D,L-lactide)	Paclitaxel	Samyang Biopharmaceuticals	Metastatic BC	Phase III (Approved inEuropeand Korea)
Liposomal	Paclitaxel	INSYS Therapeutics, Neopharma	Advanced BC	PhaseII
Polymeric micelle PEG-poly(D,L-lactide)	Docetaxel	Fresenius Kabi Oncology	Advanced BC	Phase I
Liposomal	Cisplatin	LiPlasomePharma	Metastatic BC	Phase I/II
Albumin Bound NP	Rapamycin	Mayo Clinic	Advanced BC	Early Phase 1
Targeted silica nanoparticles	cRGDY-PEG-Cy5.5-C dots	Memorial Sloan Kettering Cancer Center	Real-time image-guided intraoperative mapping of nodal metastases	Phase I/II

CONTINUING CHALLENGES IN NANOCARRIERS DEVELOPMENT

Nanoparticles provide advanced tumour targeting approaches with higher efficacy and lower toxicity. A plethora of inorganic nanomaterials (*e.g.*, iron oxide nanoparticles, gold nanoparticles, quantum dots, mesoporous silica nanoparticles, carbon nanotubes) and organic nanomaterials (*e.g.*, liposomes, polymeric nanoparticles, micelles, dendrimers) have all been studied. Despite the fact that some organic-based nanomaterials have made it into clinical trials, much more research is needed to comprehend the full potential and limitations of nanoformulations completely. It is vital to create nanoformulations that can sufficiently permeate these places without producing too many side effects.

Nanocarriers that follow passive drug delivery systems have limited usefulness for breast cancer therapy. To preferentially connect with breast cancer cells, nanoparticles must be functionalized with appropriate targeting ligands. The harmful impact of nanocarriers on healthy cells will be reduced. Moreover, large-scale manufacture of nanocarriers with precise drug ratios is always challenging, and further research is needed before they can be used in breast cancer therapy.

CONCLUSION AND FUTURE PERSPECTIVE

Human breast cancer is a complex and severe illness with many unanswered concerns. Breast cancer frequently spreads to the bone, lung, liver, and brain, yet the majority of anticancer therapies are inaccessible to these locations. Nanotechnology is a rapidly developing field of research that has the potential to revolutionize imaging, monitoring, diagnosis, and drug delivery of drugs to specifically targeted tumour cells. However, the existing multistep nanoformulations for co-loading multiple anticancer medications to treat breast cancer are too complex to be industrialized from a production standpoint. Beyond the proof-of-concept, more research should be conducted, emphasizing scale-up challenges and production. Though there are still a lot of unknowns about the toxicity, absorption and uptake of these nanomaterials, the recent data demonstrates clearly that in nanomedicine, nanomaterials have a bright future for the treatment of breast cancer.

CONSENT FOR PUBLICATION

Not applicable.

CONFLICT OF INTEREST

The authors declare no conflict of interest, financial or otherwise.

ACKNOWLEDGEMENT

Declared none.

REFERENCES

[1] Bray F, Ferlay J, Soerjomataram I, Siegel RL, Torre LA, Jemal A. Global cancer statistics 2018: GLOBOCAN estimates of incidence and mortality worldwide for 36 cancers in 185 countries. CA Cancer J Clin 2018; 68(6): 394-424. [http://dx.doi.org/10.3322/caac.21492] [PMID: 30207593]

[2] Amjad E, Asnaashari S, Sokouti B, Dastmalchi S. Systems biology comprehensive analysis on breast cancer for identification of key gene modules and genes associated with TNM-based clinical stages. Sci Rep 2020; 10(1): 10816. [http://dx.doi.org/10.1038/s41598-020-67643-w] [PMID: 32616754]

[3] Tran P, Lee SE, Kim DH, Pyo YC, Park JS. Recent advances of nanotechnology for the delivery of

anticancer drugs for breast cancer treatment. J Pharm Investig 2020; 50(3): 261-70. [http://dx.doi.org/10.1007/s40005-019-00459-7]

[4] Mittal P, Singh S, Singh A, Singh IK. Current advances in drug delivery systems for treatment of Triple negative breast cancer (TNBC). Chem Biol Lett 2020; 7: 1-12.

[5] Koh J, Kim MJ. Introduction of a new staging system of breast cancer for radiologists: An emphasis on the prognostic stage. Korean J Radiol 2019; 20(1): 69-82. [http://dx.doi.org/10.3348/kjr.2018.0231] [PMID: 30627023]

[6] Cserni G, Chmielik E, Cserni B, Tot T. The new TNM-based staging of breast cancer. Virchows Arch 2018; 472(5): 697-703. [http://dx.doi.org/10.1007/s00428-018-2301-9] [PMID: 29380126]

[7] Rocha M, Chaves N, Báo S. Breast cancer-From Biology to Medicine. London: IntechOpen 2017.

[8] Jahan S, Karim ME, Chowdhury EH. Nanoparticles Targeting Receptors on Breast Cancer for Efficient Delivery of Chemotherapeutics. Biomedicines 2021; 9(2): 114. [http://dx.doi.org/10.3390/biomedicines9020114] [PMID: 33530291]

[9] Montaseri H, Kruger CA, Abrahamse H. Inorganic Nanoparticles Applied for Active Targeted Photodynamic Therapy of Breast Cancer. Pharmaceutics 2021; 13(3): 296. [http://dx.doi.org/10.3390/pharmaceutics13030296] [PMID: 33668307]

[10] Grewal KI, Singh S, Arora S, Sharma N. Polymeric Nanoparticles for Breast cancer Therapy: A Comprehensive Review. Biointerface Res Appl Chem 2021; 11(4): 11151-71.

[11] Ferrari M. Cancer nanotechnology: opportunities and challenges. Nat Rev Cancer 2005; 5(3): 161-71. [http://dx.doi.org/10.1038/nrc1566] [PMID: 15738981]

[12] Duncan R. The dawning era of polymer therapeutics. Nat Rev Drug Discov 2003; 2(5): 347-60. [http://dx.doi.org/10.1038/nrd1088] [PMID: 12750738]

[13] LaVan DA, McGuire T, Langer R. Small-scale systems for *in vivo* drug delivery. Nat Biotechnol 2003; 21(10): 1184-91. [http://dx.doi.org/10.1038/nbt876] [PMID: 14520404]

[14] Fenske DB, Cullis PR. Liposomal nanomedicines. Expert Opin Drug Deliv 2008; 5(1): 25-44. [http://dx.doi.org/10.1517/17425247.5.1.25] [PMID: 18095927]

[15] Lammers T, Hennink WE, Storm G. Tumour-targeted nanomedicines: principles and practice. Br J Cancer 2008; 99(3): 392-7. [http://dx.doi.org/10.1038/sj.bjc.6604483] [PMID: 18648371]

[16] Gabizon AA, Shmeeda H, Zalipsky S. Pros and cons of the liposome platform in cancer drug targeting. J Liposome Res 2006; 16(3): 175-83. [http://dx.doi.org/10.1080/08982100600848769] [PMID: 16952872]

[17] Talluri SV, Kuppusamy G, Karri VVSR, Tummala S, Madhunapantula SV. Lipid-based nanocarriers for breast cancer treatment – comprehensive review. Drug Deliv 2016; 23(4): 1291-305. [http://dx.doi.org/10.3109/10717544.2015.1092183] [PMID: 26430913]

[18] Fontana G, Maniscalco L, Schillaci D, Cavallaro G, Giammona G. Solid lipid nanoparticles containing tamoxifen characterization and in vitro antitumoral activity. Drug Deliv 2005; 12(6): 385-92. [http://dx.doi.org/10.1080/10717540590968855] [PMID: 16253954]

[19] Esposito E, Mariani P, Ravani L, *et al.* Nanoparticulate lipid dispersions for bromocriptine delivery: Characterization and *in vivo* study. Eur J Pharm Biopharm 2012; 80(2): 306-14. [http://dx.doi.org/10.1016/j.ejpb.2011.10.015] [PMID: 22061262]

[20] Luo Q, Zhao J, Zhang X, Pan W. Nanostructured lipid carrier (NLC) coated with Chitosan Oligosaccharides and its potential use in ocular drug delivery system. Int J Pharm 2011; 403(1-2): 185-91. [http://dx.doi.org/10.1016/j.ijpharm.2010.10.013] [PMID: 20951778]

[21] Saupe A, Gordon KC, Rades T. Structural investigations on nanoemulsions, solid lipid nanoparticles and nanostructured lipid carriers by cryo-field emission scanning electron microscopy and Raman spectroscopy. Int J Pharm 2006; 314(1): 56-62. [http://dx.doi.org/10.1016/j.ijpharm.2006.01.022] [PMID: 16574354]

[22] Lin M, Teng L, Wang Y, Zhang J, Sun X. Curcumin-guided nanotherapy: a lipid-based nanomedicine for targeted drug delivery in breast cancer therapy. Drug Deliv 2016; 23(4): 1420-5. [http://dx.doi.org/10.3109/10717544.2015.1066902] [PMID: 26203688]

[23] Zhang L, Chan JM, Gu FX, *et al.* Self-assembled lipid--polymer hybrid nanoparticles: a robust drug delivery platform. ACS Nano 2008; 2(8): 1696-702. [http://dx.doi.org/10.1021/nn800275r] [PMID: 19206374]

[24] Wong HL, Rauth AM, Bendayan R, *et al.* A new polymer-lipid hybrid nanoparticle system increases cytotoxicity of doxorubicin against multidrug-resistant human breast cancer cells. Pharm Res 2006; 23(7): 1574-85. [http://dx.doi.org/10.1007/s11095-006-0282-x] [PMID: 16786442]

[25] Nirmala MJ, Nagarajan R. Nanoemulsions in Cancer Therapeutics. J Nanomed Nanotechnol 2016; 7: 2.

[26] Praveen Kumar G, Divya A. Nanoemulsion Based Targeting in Cancer Therapeutics. Med Chem 2015; 5: 272-84.

[27] Tagne JB, Kakumanu S, Ortiz D, Shea T, Nicolosi RJ. A nanoemulsion formulation of tamoxifen increases its efficacy in a breast cancer cell line. Mol Pharm 2008; 5(2): 280-6. [http://dx.doi.org/10.1021/mp700091j] [PMID: 18171014]

[28] Colone M, Calcabrini A, Stringaro A. Drug delivery systems of natural products in oncology. Molecules 2020; 25(19): 4560. [http://dx.doi.org/10.3390/molecules25194560] [PMID: 33036240]

[29] Mamnoon B, Loganathan J, Confeld MI, *et al.* Targeted polymeric nanoparticles for drug delivery to hypoxic, triple-negative breast tumors. ACS Appl Bio Mater 2021; 4(2): 1450-60. [http://dx.doi.org/10.1021/acsabm.0c01336] [PMID: 33954285]

[30] Xiong Z, Shen M, Shi X. Dendrimer-based strategies for cancer therapy: Recent advances and future perspectives. Sci China Mater 2018; 61(11): 1387-403. [http://dx.doi.org/10.1007/s40843-018-9271-4]

[31] Pietryga IF, Ziemba B, Messmer B, Krawczyk DS. Dendrimers - Fundamentals and Applications. IntechOpen 2018.

[32] Pérez-Herrero E, Fernández-Medarde A. Advanced targeted therapies in cancer: Drug nanocarriers, the future of chemotherapy. Eur J Pharm Biopharm 2015; 93: 52-79. [http://dx.doi.org/10.1016/j.ejpb.2015.03.018] [PMID: 25813885]

[33] Li MH, Choi SK, Thomas TP, *et al.* Dendrimer-based multivalent methotrexates as dual acting nanoconjugates for cancer cell targeting. Eur J Med Chem 2012; 47(1): 560-72. [http://dx.doi.org/10.1016/j.ejmech.2011.11.027] [PMID: 22142685]

[34] StarPharmaDEP.Docetaxel. https://starpharma.com/drug_delivery/dep_docetaxel

[35] Dias AP, da Silva Santos S, da Silva JV, *et al.* Dendrimers in the context of nanomedicine. Int J Pharm 2020; 573: 118814. [http://dx.doi.org/10.1016/j.ijpharm.2019.118814] [PMID: 31759101]

[36] Mendoza-Nava H, Ferro-Flores G, Ramírez FM, *et al.* Fluorescent, plasmonic, and radiotherapeutic properties of the ^{177}Lu–dendrimer-AuNP–folate–bombesin nanoprobe located inside cancer cells. Mol Imaging 2017; 16. [http://dx.doi.org/10.1177/1536012117704768] [PMID: 28654384]

[37] Alven S, Aderibigbe BA. The therapeutic efficacy of dendrimer and micelle formulations for breast

cancer treatment. Pharmaceutics 2020; 12(12): 1212.
[http://dx.doi.org/10.3390/pharmaceutics12121212] [PMID: 33333778]

[38] Maeda H, Wu J, Sawa T, Matsumura Y, Hori K. Tumor vascular permeability and the EPR effect in macromolecular therapeutics: a review. J Control Release 2000; 65(1-2): 271-84.
[http://dx.doi.org/10.1016/S0168-3659(99)00248-5] [PMID: 10699287]

[39] Kim S, Shi Y, Kim JY, Park K, Cheng JX. Overcoming the barriers in micellar drug delivery: loading efficiency, *in vivo* stability, and micelle–cell interaction. Expert Opin Drug Deliv 2010; 7(1): 49-62.
[http://dx.doi.org/10.1517/17425240903380446] [PMID: 20017660]

[40] Varela-Moreira A, Shi Y, Fens MHAM, Lammers T, Hennink WE, Schiffelers RM. Clinical application of polymeric micelles for the treatment of cancer. Mater Chem Front 2017; 1(8): 1485-501.
[http://dx.doi.org/10.1039/C6QM00289G]

[41] Cabral H, Kataoka K. Progress of drug-loaded polymeric micelles into clinical studies. J Control Release 2014; 190: 465-76.
[http://dx.doi.org/10.1016/j.jconrel.2014.06.042] [PMID: 24993430]

[42] Prabhu RH, Patravale VB, Joshi MD. Polymeric nanoparticles for targeted treatment in oncology: current insights. Int J Nanomedicine 2015; 10: 1001-18.
[PMID: 25678788]

[43] Gradishar WJ, Tjulandin S, Davidson N, *et al.* Phase III trial of nanoparticle albumin-bound paclitaxel compared with polyethylated castor oil-based paclitaxel in women with breast cancer. J Clin Oncol 2005; 23(31): 7794-803.
[http://dx.doi.org/10.1200/JCO.2005.04.937] [PMID: 16172456]

[44] Sharma A, Jain N, Sareen R. Nanocarriers for diagnosis and targeting of breast cancer. BioMed Res Int 2013; 2013: 1-10.
[http://dx.doi.org/10.1155/2013/960821] [PMID: 23865076]

[45] Peng J, Liang X. Progress in research on gold nanoparticles in cancer management. Medicine (Baltimore) 2019; 98(18): e15311.
[http://dx.doi.org/10.1097/MD.0000000000015311] [PMID: 31045767]

[46] Daniel MC, Astruc D. Gold nanoparticles: assembly, supramolecular chemistry, quantum-size-related properties, and applications toward biology, catalysis, and nanotechnology. Chem Rev 2004; 104(1): 293-346.
[http://dx.doi.org/10.1021/cr030698+] [PMID: 14719978]

[47] Naz S, Shahzad H, Ali A, Zia M. Nanomaterials as nanocarriers: a critical assessment why these are multi-chore vanquisher in breast cancer treatment. Artif Cells Nanomed Biotechnol 2018; 46(5): 899-916.
[http://dx.doi.org/10.1080/21691401.2017.1375937] [PMID: 28914553]

[48] Sam M, Hwang JH, Chanfreau G, Abu-Omar MM. Hydroxyl radical is the active species in photochemical DNA strand scission by bis(peroxo)vanadium(V) phenanthroline. Inorg Chem 2004; 43(26): 8447-55.
[http://dx.doi.org/10.1021/ic0486419] [PMID: 15606193]

[49] Hirsch LR, Stafford RJ, Bankson JA, *et al.* Nanoshell-mediated near-infrared thermal therapy of tumors under magnetic resonance guidance. Proc Natl Acad Sci USA 2003; 100(23): 13549-54.
[http://dx.doi.org/10.1073/pnas.2232479100] [PMID: 14597719]

[50] Kennedy LC, Bickford LR, Lewinski NA, *et al.* Photothermal Therapy: A New Era for Cancer Treatment: Gold-Nanoparticle-Mediated Thermal Therapies. Small 2010; 7: 1-15.

[51] Jain RK. Transport of molecules, particles, and cells in solid tumors. Annu Rev Biomed Eng 1999; 1(1): 241-63.
[http://dx.doi.org/10.1146/annurev.bioeng.1.1.241] [PMID: 11701489]

[52] Johannsen M, Gneveckow U, Eckelt L, *et al.* Clinical hyperthermia of prostate cancer using magnetic

nanoparticles: Presentation of a new interstitial technique. Int J Hyperthermia 2005; 21(7): 637-47. [http://dx.doi.org/10.1080/02656730500158360] [PMID: 16304715]

[53] Tong L, Zhao Y, Huff TB, Hansen MN, Wei A, Cheng JX. Gold nanorods mediate tumor cell death by compromising membrane integrity. Adv Mater 2007; 19(20): 3136-41. [http://dx.doi.org/10.1002/adma.200701974] [PMID: 19020672]

[54] Yang X, Liu X, Liu Z, Pu F, Ren J, Qu X. Near-infrared light-triggered, targeted drug delivery to cancer cells by aptamer gated nanovehicles. Adv Mater 2012; 24(21): 2890-5. [http://dx.doi.org/10.1002/adma.201104797] [PMID: 22539076]

[55] Shi P, Qu K, Wang J, Li M, Ren J, Qu X. pH-responsive NIR enhanced drug release from gold nanocages possesses high potency against cancer cells. Chem Commun (Camb) 2012; 48(61): 7640-2. [http://dx.doi.org/10.1039/c2cc33543c] [PMID: 22735385]

[56] Ma Y, Liang X, Tong S, Bao G, Ren Q, Dai Z. Gold nanoshell nanomicelles for potential magnetic resonance imaging, light-triggered drug release, and photothermal therapy. Adv Funct Mater 2013; 23(7): 815-22. [http://dx.doi.org/10.1002/adfm.201201663]

[57] Lin J, Wang S, Huang P, *et al.* Photosensitizer-loaded gold vesicles with strong plasmonic coupling effect for imaging-guided photothermal/photodynamic therapy. ACS Nano 2013; 7(6): 5320-9. [http://dx.doi.org/10.1021/nn4011686] [PMID: 23721576]

[58] Lowery AR, Gobin AM, Day ES, Halas NJ, West JL. Immunonanoshells for targeted photothermal ablation of tumor cells. Int J Nanomedicine 2006; 1(2): 149-54. [http://dx.doi.org/10.2147/nano.2006.1.2.149] [PMID: 17722530]

[59] Chattopadhyay N, Cai Z, Pignol JP, *et al.* Design and characterization of HER-2-targeted gold nanoparticles for enhanced X-radiation treatment of locally advanced breast cancer. Mol Pharm 2010; 7(6): 2194-206. [http://dx.doi.org/10.1021/mp100207t] [PMID: 20973534]

[60] Kamila S, McEwan C, Costley D, *et al.* Diagnostic and Therapeutic Applications of Quantum Dots in Nanomedicine. Top Curr Chem 2016; 370: 203-24. [http://dx.doi.org/10.1007/978-3-319-22942-3_7] [PMID: 26589510]

[61] Liyanage PY, Hettiarachchi SD, Zhou Y, *et al.* Nanoparticle-mediated targeted drug delivery for breast cancer treatment. Biochim Biophys Acta Rev Cancer 2019; 1871(2): 419-33. [http://dx.doi.org/10.1016/j.bbcan.2019.04.006] [PMID: 31034927]

[62] Kairdolf BA, Smith AM, Stokes TH, Wang MD, Young AN, Nie S. Semiconductor quantum dots for bioimaging and biodiagnostic applications. Annu Rev Anal Chem (Palo Alto, Calif) 2013; 6(1): 143-62. [http://dx.doi.org/10.1146/annurev-anchem-060908-155136] [PMID: 23527547]

[63] Tripathi SK, Kaur G, Khurana RK, Kapoor S, Singh B. Quantum dots and their potential role in cancer theranostics. Crit Rev Ther Drug Carrier Syst 2015; 32(6): 461-502. [http://dx.doi.org/10.1615/CritRevTherDrugCarrierSyst.2015012360] [PMID: 26559550]

[64] Samia ACS, Dayal S, Burda C. Quantum dot-based energy transfer: perspectives and potential for applications in photodynamic therapy. Photochem Photobiol 2006; 82(3): 617-25. [http://dx.doi.org/10.1562/2005-05-11-IR-525] [PMID: 16475871]

[65] Monroe JD, Belekov E, Er AO, Smith ME. Anticancer photodynamic therapy properties of sulfur-doped graphene quantum dot and methylene blue preparations in MCF -7 breast cancer cell culture. Photochem Photobiol 2019; 95(6): 1473-81. [http://dx.doi.org/10.1111/php.13136] [PMID: 31230353]

[66] Nene LC, Managa ME, Oluwole DO, Mafukidze DM, Sindelo A, Nyokong T. The photo-physicochemical properties and *in vitro* photodynamic therapy activity of differently substituted-zinc (II)-phthalocyanines and graphene quantum dots conjugates on MCF7 breast cancer cell line. Inorg

Chim Acta 2019; 488: 304-11.
[http://dx.doi.org/10.1016/j.ica.2019.01.012]

[67] Anas A, Akita H, Harashima H, Itoh T, Ishikawa M, Biju V. Photosensitized breakage and damage of DNA by CdSe-ZnS quantum dots. J Phys Chem B 2008; 112(32): 10005-11.
[http://dx.doi.org/10.1021/jp8018606] [PMID: 18582008]

[68] Yezhelyev MV, Al-Hajj A, Morris C, *et al. In situ* molecular profiling of breast cancer biomarkers with multicolor quantum dots. Adv Mater 2007; 19(20): 3146-51.
[http://dx.doi.org/10.1002/adma.200701983]

[69] Sun G, Xing W, Xing R, Cong L, Tong S, Yu S. Targeting breast cancer cells with a $CuInS_2$/ZnS quantum dot-labeled Ki-67 bioprobe. Oncol Lett 2018; 15(2): 2471-6.
[PMID: 29434960]

[70] Zrazhevskiy P, Sena M, Gao X. Designing multifunctional quantum dots for bioimaging, detection, and drug delivery. Chem Soc Rev 2010; 39(11): 4326-54.
[http://dx.doi.org/10.1039/b915139g] [PMID: 20697629]

[71] Shanmugam V, Selvakumar S, Yeh CS. Near-infrared light-responsive nanomaterials in cancer therapeutics. Chem Soc Rev 2014; 43(17): 6254-87.
[http://dx.doi.org/10.1039/C4CS00011K] [PMID: 24811160]

[72] Shen X, Li S, Li L, Yao SQ, Xu QH. Highly efficient, conjugated-polymer-based nano-photosensitizers for selectively targeted two-photon photodynamic therapy and imaging of cancer cells. Chemistry 2015; 21(5): 2214-21.
[http://dx.doi.org/10.1002/chem.201404378] [PMID: 25469739]

[73] Yan QL, Gozin M, Zhao FQ, Cohen A, Pang SP. Highly energetic compositions based on functionalized carbon nanomaterials. Nanoscale 2016; 8(9): 4799-851.
[http://dx.doi.org/10.1039/C5NR07855E] [PMID: 26880518]

[74] Hong G, Diao S, Antaris AL, Dai H. Carbon Nanomaterials for Biological Imaging and Nanomedicinal Therapy. Chem Rev 2015; 115(19): 10816-906.
[http://dx.doi.org/10.1021/acs.chemrev.5b00008] [PMID: 25997028]

[75] Huang P, Wang S, Wang X, *et al.* Surface Functionalization of Chemically Reduced Graphene Oxide for Targeted Photodynamic Therapy. J Biomed Nanotechnol 2015; 11(1): 117-25.
[http://dx.doi.org/10.1166/jbn.2015.2055] [PMID: 26301305]

[76] Liu Q, Xu L, Zhang X, *et al.* Enhanced photodynamic efficiency of an aptamer-guided fullerene photosensitizer toward tumor cells. Chem Asian J 2013; 8(10): 2370-6.
[http://dx.doi.org/10.1002/asia.201300039] [PMID: 23907978]

[77] Colombeau L, Acherar S, Baros F, *et al.* Inorganic Nanoparticles for Photodynamic Therapy. Top Curr Chem 2016; 370: 113-34.
[http://dx.doi.org/10.1007/978-3-319-22942-3_4] [PMID: 26589507]

[78] Mosinger J, Lang K, Kubát P. Photoactivatable Nanostructured Surfaces for Biomedical Applications. Top Curr Chem 2016; 370: 135-68.
[http://dx.doi.org/10.1007/978-3-319-22942-3_5] [PMID: 26589508]

[79] Xiao Y, Gao X, Taratula O, *et al.* Anti-HER2 IgY antibody-functionalized single-walled carbon nanotubes for detection and selective destruction of breast cancer cells. BMC Cancer 2009; 9(1): 351-61.
[http://dx.doi.org/10.1186/1471-2407-9-351] [PMID: 19799784]

[80] Neves LFF, Krais JJ, Van Rite BD, Ramesh R, Resasco DE, Harrison RG. Targeting single-walled carbon nanotubes for the treatment of breast cancer using photothermal therapy. Nanotechnology 2013; 24(37): 375104-15.
[http://dx.doi.org/10.1088/0957-4484/24/37/375104] [PMID: 23975064]

[81] Tait JF, Gibson D. Phospholipid binding of annexin V: Effects of calcium and membrane

phosphatidylserine content. Arch Biochem Biophys 1992; 298(1): 187-91. [http://dx.doi.org/10.1016/0003-9861(92)90111-9] [PMID: 1388011]

[82] Liu Z, Yanagi K, Suenaga K, Kataura H, Iijima S. Imaging the dynamic behaviour of individual retinal chromophores confined inside carbon nanotubes. Nat Nanotechnol 2007; 2(7): 422-5. [http://dx.doi.org/10.1038/nnano.2007.187] [PMID: 18654326]

[83] Meyer RR, Sloan J, Dunin-Borkowski RE, *et al.* Discrete atom imaging of one-dimensional crystals formed within single-walled carbon nanotubes. Science 2000; 289(5483): 1324-6. [http://dx.doi.org/10.1126/science.289.5483.1324] [PMID: 10958773]

[84] Hampel S, Kunze D, Haase D, *et al.* Carbon nanotubes filled with a chemotherapeutic agent: a nanocarrier mediates inhibition of tumor cell growth. Nanomedicine (Lond) 2008; 3(2): 175-82. [http://dx.doi.org/10.2217/17435889.3.2.175] [PMID: 18373424]

[85] Liu Z, Sun X, Nakayama-Ratchford N, Dai H. Supramolecular chemistry on water-soluble carbon nanotubes for drug loading and delivery. ACS Nano 2007; 1(1): 50-6. [http://dx.doi.org/10.1021/nn700040t] [PMID: 19203129]

[86] Liu Z, Chen K, Davis C, *et al.* Drug delivery with carbon nanotubes for *in vivo* cancer treatment. Cancer Res 2008; 68(16): 6652-60. [http://dx.doi.org/10.1158/0008-5472.CAN-08-1468] [PMID: 18701489]

[87] Shao W, Paul A, Zhao B, Lee C, Rodes L, Prakash S. Carbon nanotube lipid drug approach for targeted delivery of a chemotherapy drug in a human breast cancer xenograft animal model. Biomaterials 2013; 34(38): 10109-19. [http://dx.doi.org/10.1016/j.biomaterials.2013.09.007] [PMID: 24060420]

[88] Al Faraj A, Pasha Shaik A, Sultana Shaik A. Magnetic single-walled carbon nanotubes as efficient drug delivery nanocarriers in breast cancer murine model: noninvasive monitoring using diffusion-weighted magnetic resonance imaging as sensitive imaging biomarker. Int J Nanomedicine 2014; 10: 157-68. [http://dx.doi.org/10.2147/IJN.S75074] [PMID: 25565811]

[89] Wang Y, Wang C, Jia Y, *et al.* Oxygen-carbon nanotubes as a chemotherapy sensitizer for paclitaxel in breast cancer treatment. PLoS One 2014; 9(8): e104209-14. [http://dx.doi.org/10.1371/journal.pone.0104209] [PMID: 25089613]

[90] Jia G, Wang H, Yan L, *et al.* Cytotoxicity of carbon nanomaterials: single-wall nanotube, multi-wall nanotube, and fullerene. Environ Sci Technol 2005; 39(5): 1378-83. [http://dx.doi.org/10.1021/es048729l] [PMID: 15787380]

[91] Kavosi A, Hosseini Ghale Noei S, Madani S, *et al.* The toxicity and therapeutic effects of single-and multi-wall carbon nanotubes on mice breast cancer. Sci Rep 2018; 8(1): 8375-86. [http://dx.doi.org/10.1038/s41598-018-26790-x] [PMID: 29849103]

[92] Risi G, Bloise N, Merli D, *et al.* *In vitro* study of multiwall carbon nanotubes (MWCNTs) with adsorbed mitoxantrone (MTO) as a drug delivery system to treat breast cancer. RSC Advances 2014; 4(36): 18683-93. [http://dx.doi.org/10.1039/C4RA02366H]

[93] Fahrenholtz CD, Hadimani M, King SB, Torti SV, Singh R. Targeting breast cancer with sugar-coated carbon nanotubes. Nanomedicine (Lond) 2015; 10(16): 2481-97. [http://dx.doi.org/10.2217/nnm.15.90] [PMID: 26296098]

[94] Mehra NK, Jain AK, Lodhi N, *et al.* Challenges in the use of carbon nanotubes for biomedical applications. Crit Rev Ther Drug Carrier Syst 2008; 25(2): 169-206. [http://dx.doi.org/10.1615/CritRevTherDrugCarrierSyst.v25.i2.20] [PMID: 18540838]

[95] Zottel A, Videtič Paska A, Jovčevska I. Nanotechnology meets oncology: nanomaterials in brain cancer research, diagnosis and therapy. Materials (Basel) 2019; 12(10): 1588. [http://dx.doi.org/10.3390/ma12101588]

[96] Wolfram J, Zhu M, Yang Y, *et al.* Safety of Nanoparticles in Medicine. Curr Drug Targets 2015; 16(14): 1671-81.
[http://dx.doi.org/10.2174/1389450115666140804124808] [PMID: 26601723]

[97] Hsu PC, Chen PC, Ou CM, Chang HY, Chang HT. Extremely high inhibition activity of photoluminescent carbon nanodots toward cancer cells. J Mater Chem B Mater Biol Med 2013; 1(13): 1774-81.
[http://dx.doi.org/10.1039/c3tb00545c] [PMID: 32261141]

[98] Zeng Q, Shao D, He X, *et al.* Carbon dots as a trackable drug delivery carrier for localized cancer therapy *in vivo.* J Mater Chem B Mater Biol Med 2016; 4(30): 5119-26.
[http://dx.doi.org/10.1039/C6TB01259K] [PMID: 32263509]

[99] Feng T, Ai X, Ong H, Zhao Y. Dual-responsive carbon dots for tumour extracellular microenvironment triggered targeting and enhanced anticancer drug delivery. ACS Appl Mater Interfaces 2016; 8(29): 18732-40.
[http://dx.doi.org/10.1021/acsami.6b06695] [PMID: 27367152]

[100] Kong T, Hao L, Wei Y, Cai X, Zhu B. Doxorubicin conjugated carbon dots as a drug delivery system for human breast cancer therapy. Cell Prolif 2018; 51(5): e12488-96.
[http://dx.doi.org/10.1111/cpr.12488] [PMID: 30039515]

[101] Shi J, Wang L, Gao J, *et al.* A fullerene-based multi-functional nanoplatform for cancer theranostic applications. Biomaterials 2014; 35(22): 5771-84.
[http://dx.doi.org/10.1016/j.biomaterials.2014.03.071] [PMID: 24746227]

[102] Tian B, Wang C, Zhang S, Feng L, Liu Z. Photothermally enhanced photodynamic therapy delivered by nano-graphene oxide. ACS Nano 2011; 5(9): 7000-9.
[http://dx.doi.org/10.1021/nn201560b] [PMID: 21815655]

[103] Yu X, Gao D, Gao L, *et al.* Inhibiting metastasis and preventing tumor relapse by triggering host immunity with tumor-targeted photodynamic therapy using photosensitizer-loaded functional nanographenes. ACS Nano 2017; 11(10): 10147-58.
[http://dx.doi.org/10.1021/acsnano.7b04736] [PMID: 28901740]

[104] Yamakoshi Y, Umezawa N, Ryu A, *et al.* Active oxygen species generated from photoexcited fullerene (C60) as potential medicines: O2-* *versus* 1O2. J Am Chem Soc 2003; 125(42): 12803-9.
[http://dx.doi.org/10.1021/ja0355574] [PMID: 14558828]

[105] Murakami T, Nakatsuji H, Inada M, *et al.* Photodynamic and photothermal effects of semiconducting and metallic-enriched single-walled carbon nanotubes. J Am Chem Soc 2012; 134(43): 17862-5.
[http://dx.doi.org/10.1021/ja3079972] [PMID: 23083004]

[106] Zakharian TY, Seryshev A, Sitharaman B, Gilbert BE, Knight V, Wilson LJ. A fullerene-paclitaxel chemotherapeutic: synthesis, characterization, and study of biological activity in tissue culture. J Am Chem Soc 2005; 127(36): 12508-9.
[http://dx.doi.org/10.1021/ja0546525] [PMID: 16144396]

[107] Sharma SK, Chiang LY, Hamblin MR. Photodynamic therapy with fullerenes *in vivo* : reality or a dream? Nanomedicine (Lond) 2011; 6(10): 1813-25.
[http://dx.doi.org/10.2217/nnm.11.144] [PMID: 22122587]

[108] Naz S, Shahzad H, Ali A, Zia M. Nanomaterials as nanocarriers: a critical assessment why these are multi-chore vanquisher in breast cancer treatment. Artif Cells Nanomed Biotechnol 2018; 46(5): 899-916.
[http://dx.doi.org/10.1080/21691401.2017.1375937] [PMID: 28914553]

[109] Jain TK, Morales MA, Sahoo SK, Leslie-Pelecky DL, Labhasetwar V. Iron oxide nanoparticles for sustained delivery of anticancer agents. Mol Pharm 2005; 2(3): 194-205.
[http://dx.doi.org/10.1021/mp0500014] [PMID: 15934780]

[110] Gazeau F, Lévy M, Wilhelm C. Optimizing magnetic nanoparticle design for nanothermotherapy.

Nanomedicine (Lond) 2008; 3(6): 831-44.
[http://dx.doi.org/10.2217/17435889.3.6.831] [PMID: 19025457]

[111] Sanson C, Diou O, Thévenot J, *et al.* Doxorubicin loaded magnetic polymersomes: theranostic nanocarriers for MR imaging and magneto-chemotherapy. ACS Nano 2011; 5(2): 1122-40.
[http://dx.doi.org/10.1021/nn102762f] [PMID: 21218795]

[112] Lee JH, Huh YM, Jun Y, *et al.* Artificially engineered magnetic nanoparticles for ultra-sensitive molecular imaging. Nat Med 2007; 13(1): 95-9.
[http://dx.doi.org/10.1038/nm1467] [PMID: 17187073]

[113] Narsireddy A, Vijayashree K, Irudayaraj J, Manorama SV, Rao NM. Targeted *in vivo* photodynamic therapy with epidermal growth factor receptor-specific peptide linked nanoparticles. Int J Pharm 2014; 471(1-2): 421-9.
[http://dx.doi.org/10.1016/j.ijpharm.2014.05.063] [PMID: 24939618]

[114] Choi KH, Nam K, Cho G, Jung JS, Park B. Enhanced photodynamic anticancer activities of multifunctional magnetic nanoparticles (Fe_3O_4) conjugated with chlorin e6 and folic acid in prostate and breast cancer cells. Nanomaterials (Basel) 2018; 8(9): 722.
[http://dx.doi.org/10.3390/nano8090722]

[115] Allahverdiyev A M, Parlar E, Dinparvar S, Bagirova M, Abamor E S. Current aspects in treatment of breast cancer based of nanodrug delivery systems and future prospects 2018; 46.
[http://dx.doi.org/10.1080/21691401.2018.1511573]

[116] Marcu A, Pop S, Dumitrache F, *et al.* Magnetic iron oxide nanoparticles as drug delivery system in breast cancer. Appl Surf Sci 2013; 281: 60-5.
[http://dx.doi.org/10.1016/j.apsusc.2013.02.072]

[117] Poller J, Zaloga J, Schreiber E, *et al.* Selection of potential iron oxide nanoparticles for breast cancer treatment based on *in vitro* cytotoxicity and cellular uptake. Int J Nanomedicine 2017; 12: 3207-20.
[http://dx.doi.org/10.2147/IJN.S132369] [PMID: 28458541]

[118] Artemov D, Mori N, Okollie B, Bhujwalla ZM. MR molecular imaging of the Her-2/neu receptor in breast cancer cells using targeted iron oxide nanoparticles. Magn Reson Med 2003; 49(3): 403-8.
[http://dx.doi.org/10.1002/mrm.10406] [PMID: 12594741]

[119] Arbab AS, Bashaw LA, Miller BR, *et al.* Characterization of biophysical and metabolic properties of cells labeled with superparamagnetic iron oxide nanoparticles and transfection agent for cellular MR imaging. Radiology 2003; 229(3): 838-46.
[http://dx.doi.org/10.1148/radiol.2293021215] [PMID: 14657318]

[120] Secret E, Maynadier M, Gallud A, *et al.* Two-photon excitation of porphyrin-functionalized porous silicon nanoparticles for photodynamic therapy. Adv Mater 2014; 26(45): 7643-8.
[http://dx.doi.org/10.1002/adma.201403415] [PMID: 25323443]

[121] Park JH, Gu L, von Maltzahn G, Ruoslahti E, Bhatia SN, Sailor MJ. Biodegradable luminescent porous silicon nanoparticles for *in vivo* applications. Nat Mater 2009; 8(4): 331-6.
[http://dx.doi.org/10.1038/nmat2398] [PMID: 19234444]

[122] Cao B, Yang M, Zhu Y, Qu X, Mao C. Stem cells loaded with nanoparticles as a drug carrier for *in vivo* breast cancer therapy. Adv Mater 2014; 26(27): 4627-31.
[http://dx.doi.org/10.1002/adma.201401550] [PMID: 24890678]

[123] Kidd S, Spaeth E, Dembinski JL, *et al.* Direct evidence of mesenchymal stem cell tropism for tumor and wounding microenvironments using in vivo bioluminescent imaging. Stem Cells 2009; 27(10): 2614-23.
[http://dx.doi.org/10.1002/stem.187] [PMID: 19650040]

[124] Ren YJ, Zhang H, Huang H, *et al.* *In vitro* behavior of neural stem cells in response to different chemical functional groups. Biomaterials 2009; 30(6): 1036-44.
[http://dx.doi.org/10.1016/j.biomaterials.2008.10.028] [PMID: 19026444]

[125] Zhu H, Cao B, Zhen Z, *et al.* Controlled growth and differentiation of MSCs on grooved films assembled from monodisperse biological nanofibers with genetically tunable surface chemistries. Biomaterials 2011; 32(21): 4744-52.
[http://dx.doi.org/10.1016/j.biomaterials.2011.03.030] [PMID: 21507480]

[126] Sonabend AM, Ulasov IV, Tyler MA, Rivera AA, Mathis JM, Lesniak MS. Mesenchymal stem cells effectively deliver an oncolytic adenovirus to intracranial glioma. Stem Cells 2008; 26(3): 831-41.
[http://dx.doi.org/10.1634/stemcells.2007-0758] [PMID: 18192232]

[127] Bharathiraja S, Moorthy MS, Manivasagan P, Seo H, Lee KD, Oh J. Chlorin e6 conjugated silica nanoparticles for targeted and effective photodynamic therapy. Photodiagn Photodyn Ther 2017; 19: 212-20.
[http://dx.doi.org/10.1016/j.pdpdt.2017.06.001] [PMID: 28583295]

[128] Ntziachristos V, Bremer C, Weissleder R. Fluorescence imaging with near-infrared light: new technological advances that enable *in vivo* molecular imaging. Eur Radiol 2003; 13(1): 195-208.
[http://dx.doi.org/10.1007/s00330-002-1524-x] [PMID: 12541130]

[129] Bulin AL, Truillet C, Chouikrat R, *et al.* X-ray-Induced Singlet Oxygen Activation with Nanoscintillator-Coupled Porphyrins. J Phys Chem C 2013; 117(41): 21583-9.
[http://dx.doi.org/10.1021/jp4077189]

[130] Chen H, Wang GD, Chuang YJ, *et al.* Nanoscintillator-mediated X-ray inducible photodynamic therapy for *in vivo* cancer treatment. Nano Lett 2015; 15(4): 2249-56.
[http://dx.doi.org/10.1021/nl504044p] [PMID: 25756781]

[131] Kaščáková S, Giuliani A, Lacerda S, *et al.* X-ray-induced radiophotodynamic therapy (RPDT) using lanthanide micelles: Beyond depth limitations. Nano Res 2015; 8(7): 2373-9.
[http://dx.doi.org/10.1007/s12274-015-0747-5]

[132] Sengar P, Juárez P, Verdugo-Meza A, *et al.* Development of a functionalized UV-emitting nanocomposite for the treatment of cancer using indirect photodynamic therapy. J Nanobiotechnology 2018; 16(1): 19.
[http://dx.doi.org/10.1186/s12951-018-0344-3] [PMID: 29482561]

[133] Juan A, Cimas FJ, Bravo I, Pandiella A, Ocaña A, Alonso-Moreno C. Antibody Conjugation of Nanoparticles as Therapeutics for Breast Cancer Treatment. Int J Mol Sci 2020; 21(17): 6018.
[http://dx.doi.org/10.3390/ijms21176018] [PMID: 32825618]

[134] Yang T, Choi MK, Cui FD, *et al.* Antitumor effect of paclitaxel-loaded PEGylated immunoliposomes against human breast cancer cells. Pharm Res 2007; 24(12): 2402-11.
[http://dx.doi.org/10.1007/s11095-007-9425-y] [PMID: 17828616]

[135] Vicier C, Dieci MV, Arnedos M, Delaloge S, Viens P, Andre F. Clinical development of mTOR inhibitors in breast cancer. Breast Cancer Res 2014; 16(1): 203.
[http://dx.doi.org/10.1186/bcr3618] [PMID: 25189767]

[136] Seto B. Rapamycin and mTOR: a serendipitous discovery and implications for breast cancer. Clin Transl Med 2012; 1(1): 29.
[http://dx.doi.org/10.1186/2001-1326-1-29] [PMID: 23369283]

[137] Catania A, Barrajón-Catalán E, Nicolosi S, Cicirata F, Micol V. Immunoliposome encapsulation increases cytotoxic activity and selectivity of curcumin and resveratrol against HER2 overexpressing human breast cancer cells. Breast Cancer Res Treat 2013; 141(1): 55-65.
[http://dx.doi.org/10.1007/s10549-013-2667-y] [PMID: 23959397]

[138] Farahavar G, Abolmaali SS, Gholijani N, Nejatollahi F. Antibody-guided nanomedicines as novel breakthrough therapeutic, diagnostic and theranostic tools. Biomater Sci 2019; 7(10): 4000-16.
[http://dx.doi.org/10.1039/C9BM00931K] [PMID: 31355391]

[139] Arruebo M, Valladares M, González-Fernández Á. Antibody-Conjugated Nanoparticles for Biomedical Applications. J Nanomater 2009; 2009: 1-24.

[http://dx.doi.org/10.1155/2009/439389]

[140] Ko NR, Van SY, Hong SH, *et al.* Dual pH- and GSH-Responsive Degradable PEGylated Graphene Quantum Dot-Based Nanoparticles for Enhanced HER2-Positive Breast Cancer Therapy. Nanomaterials (Basel) 2020; 10(1): 91.
[http://dx.doi.org/10.3390/nano10010091] [PMID: 31906509]

[141] Kievit FM, Stephen ZR, Veiseh O, *et al.* Targeting of primary breast cancers and metastases in a transgenic mouse model using rationally designed multifunctional SPIONs. ACS Nano 2012; 6(3): 2591-601.
[http://dx.doi.org/10.1021/nn205070h] [PMID: 22324543]

[142] Bae KH, Lee K, Kim C, Park TG. Surface functionalized hollow manganese oxide nanoparticles for cancer targeted siRNA delivery and magnetic resonance imaging. Biomaterials 2011; 32(1): 176-84.
[http://dx.doi.org/10.1016/j.biomaterials.2010.09.039] [PMID: 20934746]

[143] Tarvirdipour S, Vasheghani-Farahani E, Soleimani M, Bardania H. Functionalized magnetic dextran-spermine nanocarriers for targeted delivery of doxorubicin to breast cancer cells. Int J Pharm 2016; 501(1-2): 331-41.
[http://dx.doi.org/10.1016/j.ijpharm.2016.02.012] [PMID: 26875475]

[144] Tan WB, Jiang S, Zhang Y. Quantum-dot based nanoparticles for targeted silencing of HER2/neu gene *via* RNA interference. Biomaterials 2007; 28(8): 1565-71.
[http://dx.doi.org/10.1016/j.biomaterials.2006.11.018] [PMID: 17161865]

[145] Day ES, Bickford LR, Slater JH, Riggall NS, Drezek RA, West JL. Antibody-conjugated gold-gold sulfide nanoparticles as multifunctional agents for imaging and therapy of breast cancer. Int J Nanomedicine 2010; 5: 445-54.
[http://dx.doi.org/10.2147/IJN.S10881] [PMID: 20957166]

[146] Falvo E, Tremante E, Fraioli R, *et al.* Antibody–drug conjugates: targeting melanoma with cisplatin encapsulated in protein-cage nanoparticles based on human ferritin. Nanoscale 2013; 5(24): 12278-85.
[http://dx.doi.org/10.1039/c3nr04268e] [PMID: 24150593]

[147] Kocbek P, Obermajer N, Cegnar M, Kos J, Kristl J. Targeting cancer cells using PLGA nanoparticles surface modified with monoclonal antibody. J Control Release 2007; 120(1-2): 18-26.
[http://dx.doi.org/10.1016/j.jconrel.2007.03.012] [PMID: 17509712]

[148] Yang J, Lee CH, Park J, *et al.* Antibody conjugated magnetic PLGA nanoparticles for diagnosis and treatment of breast cancer. J Mater Chem 2007; 17(26): 2695-9.
[http://dx.doi.org/10.1039/b702538f]

[149] Shi M, Ho K, Keating A, Shoichet MS. Doxorubicin-Conjugated Immuno-Nanoparticles for Intracellular Anticancer Drug Delivery. Adv Funct Mater 2009; 19(11): 1689-96.
[http://dx.doi.org/10.1002/adfm.200801271]

[150] Takeda M, Tada H, Higuchi H, *et al. In vivo* single molecular imaging and sentinel node navigation by nanotechnology for molecular targeting drug-delivery systems and tailor-made medicine. Breast Cancer 2008; 15(2): 145-52.
[http://dx.doi.org/10.1007/s12282-008-0037-0] [PMID: 18317884]

[151] Vivek R, Thangam R, NipunBabu V, *et al.* Multifunctional HER2-antibody conjugated polymeric nanocarrier-based drug delivery system for multi-drug-resistant breast cancer therapy. ACS Appl Mater Interfaces 2014; 6(9): 6469-80.
[http://dx.doi.org/10.1021/am406012g] [PMID: 24780315]

[152] Jain V, Kumar H, Anod HV, *et al.* A review of nanotechnology-based approaches for breast cancer and triple-negative breast cancer. J Control Release 2020; 326: 628-47.
[http://dx.doi.org/10.1016/j.jconrel.2020.07.003] [PMID: 32653502]

[153] Wu D, Si M, Xue HY, Wong HL. Nanomedicine applications in the treatment of breast cancer: current state of the art. Int J Nanomedicine 2017; 12: 5879-92.

[http://dx.doi.org/10.2147/IJN.S123437] [PMID: 28860754]

[154] Martinelli C, Biglietti M. Nanotechnological approaches for counteracting multidrug resistance in cancer. Cancer Drug Resist 2020; 3(4): 1003-20.
[http://dx.doi.org/10.20517/cdr.2020.47] [PMID: 35582219]

[155] Swaminathan SK, Roger E, Toti U, Niu L, Ohlfest JR, Panyam J. CD133-targeted paclitaxel delivery inhibits local tumor recurrence in a mouse model of breast cancer. J Control Release 2013; 171(3): 280-7.
[http://dx.doi.org/10.1016/j.jconrel.2013.07.014] [PMID: 23871962]

[156] Barenholz YC. Doxil® — The first FDA-approved nano-drug: Lessons learned. J Control Release 2012; 160(2): 117-34.
[http://dx.doi.org/10.1016/j.jconrel.2012.03.020] [PMID: 22484195]

[157] Mirza Z, Karim S. Nanoparticles-based drug delivery and gene therapy for breast cancer: Recent advancements and future challenges. Semin Cancer Biol 2021; 69: 226-37.
[http://dx.doi.org/10.1016/j.semcancer.2019.10.020] [PMID: 31704145]

CHAPTER 7

Importance of Surface-modified Nanocarriers in the Management of Cervical Cancer

Hari Krishnareddy Rachamalla[1] and **Vijay Sagar Madamsetty**[1,*]

[1] *Department of Biochemistry and Molecular Biology,Mayo Clinic,4500 San Pablo Road, Jacksonville, FL-32224, USA*

Abstract: Cervical cancer (CC) is women's fourth most occurring malignancy, with a high death rate. Every CC patient is related to infection with high-risk human papillomaviruses (HPV), predominantly transmitted through sexual contact. Early diagnosis of CC helps treat surgical removal of tumours, leading to an increased patient life span. However, existing detection methods of CC, like Pap smear test, have very low sensitivity. Even though preventive vaccines for CC are doing well, they cannot protect against all HPV cancers and potential side effects. Additionally, chemotherapy for CC has had a detrimental impact because of the lack of selective tumour cell toxicity, resulting in higher adverse effects. Despite significant progress in oncology research, efficient CCs treatment is still challenging, and target-selective drug delivery formulations with a systematic release mechanism potentially avoid and reduce bio-toxicity. Recent developments in nanomedicine and nanotechnology are creating more interest in developing new treatment strategies for CC treatment. Materials used in nanomedicine development are made up of synthetic or natural. These nanoparticles pointedly impacted therapeutic applications with enhanced specificity and unique personalized assets. Surface-engineered nanoparticles offer a massive possibility for compatibility with biological agents, including nucleic acids, proteins, *etc.* Surface fictionalization nanoparticles with targeting ligands further help in selective targeting. The present study summarizes recent advancements in surface-modified nanoparticle-based CC treatment methodologies.

Keywords: Active targeting, Cervical cancer, Nanotechnology, Passive targeting, Surface modifications.

INTRODUCTION

Cervical cancer (CC) has resulted from one of the deadliest malignancies in women because it is diagnosed at the advanced/later stage [1]. Over 70% of newly diagnosed CC cases are locally persistent or metastatic. Surgical removal of tumours was effective in early-stage patients with a high survival rate. On the

* **Corresponding author Vijay Sagar Madamsetty:** Department of Biochemistry and Molecular Biology, Mayo Clinic, 4500 San Pablo Road, Jacksonville, FL-32224, USA; Tel: +1 (904) 881-9890; E-mail: sagarchemistry@gmail.com

Neeraj Mishra, Ashish Garg and Neeraj Upmanyu (Eds.)

other hand, metastatic CCs have a 5-year endurance rate of only about 50%. Like this, additional upgrades in the analysis and treatment of CCs should be effectively sought to build the endurance rate [2]. All CCs are brought about by human papillomaviruses (HPVs). More than 100 different HPVs discovered after revealing the relationship between HPVs and CCs in the 1970s by Zur Hausen [3]. HPV16 and HPV18 are accountable for triggering more than 70% of CCs, but their mechanisms are partly illustrated [4]. For CCs, Gardasil®9 and Cervarix™ are available vaccines on the market; these vaccines have HPV late protein 1 (L1) of HPV16, HPV18, and these vaccines potentially prevent most of the CCs [5] [6]. However, other CCs triggering HPVs are still inducing cancer [7].

Consequently, the importance of this HPV against vaccines can decrease the pervasiveness of CC but can't eradicate it permanently. Moreover, these HPV vaccines are ineffective in persons already infected with HPVs [8]. Thus, the therapy of CC is still a most important medical challenge. After surgery, advanced-stage CCs are taken out and treated with different anti-tumour drugs, targeted therapy, immunotherapy, and radiotherapy [9, 10]. Nevertheless, all these therapeutic modalities could not attain acceptable results despite fast improvement in understanding the biology of HPVs and CC cells.

Chemotherapy for CC has had minimal success because of the non-specific interactions of the anticancer drugs. Consequently, higher medicines need to be injected to improve the therapeutic efficacy. However, higher doses result in adverse side effects, rapid clearance, and the development of drug resistance [11]. Local delivery of chemotherapeutic agents can escape some of these obstacles. However, delivery of drugs to the female reproductive tract can affect fast vaginal clearance, and hence very difficult to continue drug concentration in the cervix [12]. The pharmacokinetics of the drugs mainly depends on the tumour cell density and intercellular tight junction within solid tumours [13]. Effective nano delivery systems have been designed to selectively deliver drugs to the tumour site and improve drug concentration in the tumour microenvironment. Nanotechnology emerged as a promising alternative in cancer therapy that offers numerous benefits and helps avoid problems associated with conventional treatments, such as low target specificity, lack of stability, poor solubility, inadequate dose administration at the tumour site, and low survival rate [14, 15].

Nanotechnology employs a wide variety of soft and hard nanoparticles at a range of 1-100 nm, poses unique physiochemical properties, and has a larger surface area-to-volume ratio than macroparticles [16]. Nanotechnology aims at improving therapeutic efficacy while reducing toxicity to normal and healthy cells. Furthermore, nano-bio interface interactions help identify molecular changes in a tumour cell to alter the physicochemical properties of anticancer drugs [17]. The two main objectives involved in cancer nanotechnology are 1) increasing target selectivity through conjugation of nanoparticles with active recognizing moieties on their surface and 2) increasing tumour penetration capacity of nanomedicine by overcoming physiological barriers (such as non-specific macrophage uptake, presence of thick stroma, high interstitial pressure) helps to direct conjugated nanoparticles towards target site and increases the rate of drug delivery at malignant tissues rather than normal ones [18, 19]. In addition, the u nanoparticles increase solubility and stability of anticancer drugs, improve half-life and bio-distribution, and enable multi-drug delivery at the tumour site, which helps promote enhanced permeation and retention (EPR) of drugs, eventually reducing the multi-drug resistance [20]. All these progress in nanotechnology brought nano-based formulations forward in nanomedicine as a potential approach to cancer treatment.

Surface engineering of nanoparticles with functional moieties targeting ligands, therapeutic agents, and fluorescent dyes aided nano-based modalities as a valuable tool in bio-imaging and theragnostic applications [21]. In comparison, nanoparticles and other therapeutic agents like chemotherapeutics, immune therapeutics, cancer vaccines, and nucleic acids produce synergistic effects to achieve treatment efficacy [22]. Surface modification of nanoparticles with appropriate ligands improves therapeutic response with limited side effects by extending blood circulation. It also helps escape lysosomal degradation and enhances stimuli-responsive drug release [23]. Nanoparticles are functionalized with specific targeting ligands depending on their application [24]. Chemical interactions in conjugating ligands to PEGylated liposomes are 1) amide bond formation between the amino and carboxyl groups, 2) di-sulphide bond construction between pyridyl dithiols and thiol groups, and 3) thioester bond formation between MAL and thiol group. Different ligands involved in the functionalization of nanocarriers are antibodies and their fragments, aptamers, peptides, small molecules *etc*, [25].

TYPES OF NANOPARTICLES LOCALIZATION INTO THE TUMOR

Passive Targeting: Passive targeting depends on the pathophysiological conditions of the tumour microenvironment and the physicochemical properties of nanoparticles [26]. Tumour accumulation of drug-loaded nanoparticles increases due to leaky vasculature of the tumour, accumulation of extravasated molecules in the interstitial places, and poor lymphatic drainage, *i.e.*, Enhanced Permeation and Retention (EPR) effect [27]. It was identified as a unique feature offered by tumour tissue by Matsumura and Maeda in the 1980s, helping to develop a practical approach to passive targeting using nano-formulations (Fig. **1**).

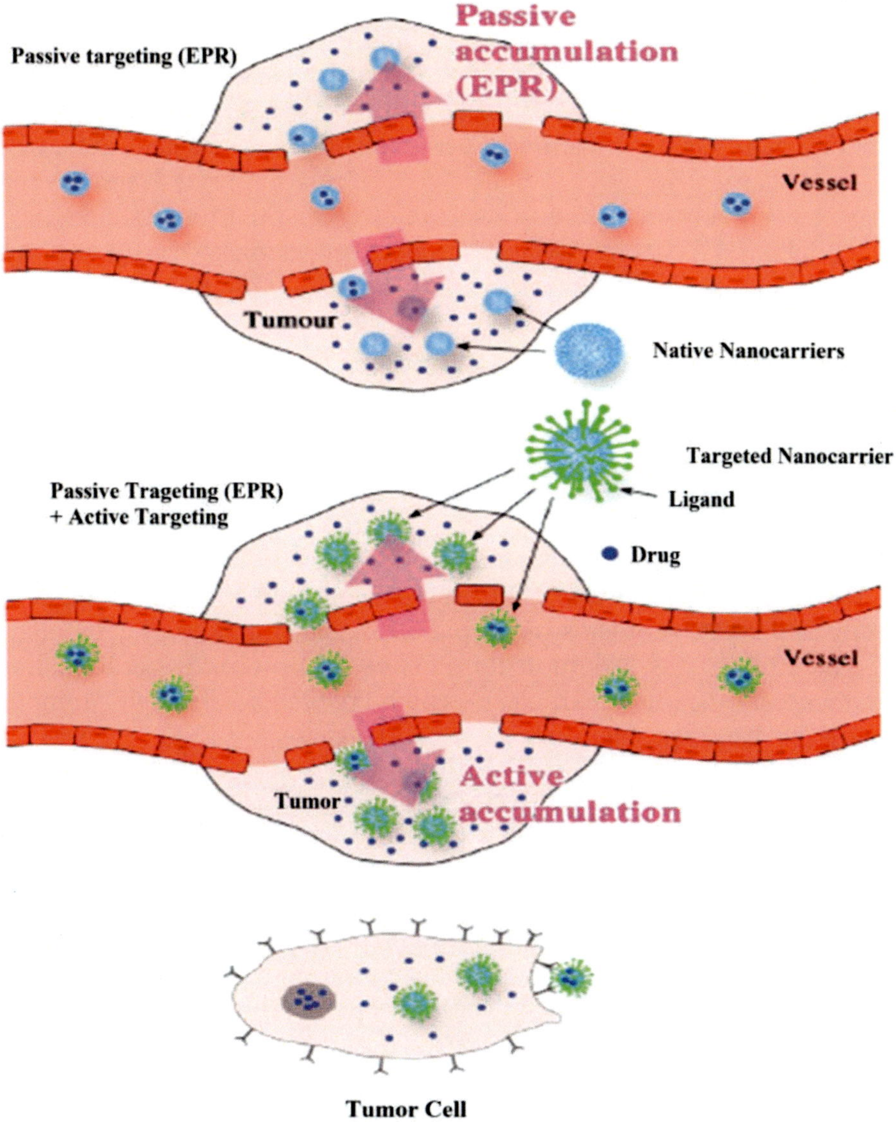

Fig. (1). Schematic diagram of the passive targeting (EPR) and the active targeting into a tumor. Reproduced from cited ref paper [27].

Due to their short circulation, low-molecular-weight drug molecules are easily eliminated from tumours *via* diffusion. Encapsulating drug molecules in nanocarriers increases circulation time, interact with tumour cells, and help achieve the EPR effect [28, 29].

The physicochemical properties of nanoparticles, such as size and surface charge, dramatically influence circulation time, tumour uptake, and targeting efficiency [30, 31]. Particle size is a key factor for effective drug delivery, which improves infusion and circulation and decreases renal clearance. The lower-sized nanoparticles provide high cellular localization, making them interact with cellular tissues more significantly to achieve specific biological outcomes [32]. The surface charge also plays a vital role in circulation time. Here, hydrophobic particles or positively charged particles are often marked for opsonization by the reticuloendothelial system and macrophages, namely positively charged liposomes, which persuade non-specific interactions with blood components, and aggregation of liposomes results in the decrease of EPR effect and augments renal clearance. In contrast, anionic charged and neutral particles escape the renal clearance [33, 34]. Polyethylene glycol (PEG) prolongs nanoparticles' circulation time and stability [35]. These PEG-coating develops steric stabilization by creating hydrophilicity on nanoparticles' surfaces, shielding surface charge, and protecting blood components.

Further PEG coating also prevents aggregation of nanoparticles and opsonization [36]. However, larger PEG-coated nanoparticles develop PEG-specific IgM antibodies and create problems like rapid clearance from systemic circulation on repeated administrations. Additionally, PEG coating produces steric hindrance on the surface of the nanoparticles, which prevents effective tumour cell internalization. These problems may reduce by using short PEG chains [37, 38].

Active Targeting: Although conventional nanoparticles improve the concentration of the drugs at the tumour site by the EPR effect, lack of targeting often decreases therapeutic efficacy. This could be overcome by employing a targeted drug delivery approach [39]. Nanoparticles surfaces are fabricated by targeting ligands like small peptide fragments, antibodies, small molecules, aptamers, proteins, *etc.* This helps internalize tumour cells by interacting with the cell surface receptors (Fig. **1**) [40]. These receptors are overexpressed in tumour cells more than in normal cells [41]. The affinity of the ligand to surface receptors primarily depends on the nature and concentration of the ligand. In addition, the optimum density of ligand and covalent bonding enhances tumour interaction and drug delivery [42]. Active drug delivery targeting depends on the nature of drug carriers and ligands linked to the nanoparticle surface [43].

Targeting cell surface receptors expressed by tumour cells is the most common strategy in the active targeting approach. Nanoparticles with specific cell receptor ligands enhance cellular uptake and therapeutic efficiency [44]. For example, the cancer cells overexpress folate receptors, transferrin receptors [45, 46], and folic acid transferring binding peptides are used for targeting [47]. Drug release from endocytosed folate-conjugated nanoparticles depends on the pH of tumour cells, where low pH conditions favour nanoparticle's internalization into tumour cells. Therefore, designing pH-sensitive folate-targeted particles like folate-LPDII enhances therapeutic efficiency [48]. Holo-Lf, the ligand of transferrin receptors conjugated with nanoparticles and chemotherapeutic agents like daunorubicin and docetaxel, increases therapeutic efficiency in liver cancer compared to free drug molecules in the blood [49]. Monoclonal antibodies are used as EGFR targeting ligand coated on the nanoparticle's surface [50]. Cetuximab, an antibody of EGFR linked to biotin liposomes encapsulating doxorubicin, showed a high binding capacity to SKOV-3, *i.e.*, 22-38 folds to that of non-targeted doxorubicin, thus inducing high cytotoxicity to ovarian cancer cells [51]. Shmeeda *et al.* reported that HER-2 targeted PEGylated doxorubicin liposomes in the J6456 ascitic lymphoma model showed high therapeutic efficacy by increasing binding capacity and accumulation of liposomes in cancer cells [52]. Overexpression of cluster of differentiation (CD44) is observed in several cancers, and hyaluronic acid acts as a ligand for CD44. In addition, monoclonal antibodies and aptamers are also being used to design CD44 targeting nanoparticles [53]. Liposomes, polymeric nanoparticles, carbon-based nanopariticles and dendrimers are promising nanomaterials to deliver various chemotherapeutic drugs to treat CC (Fig. **2**).

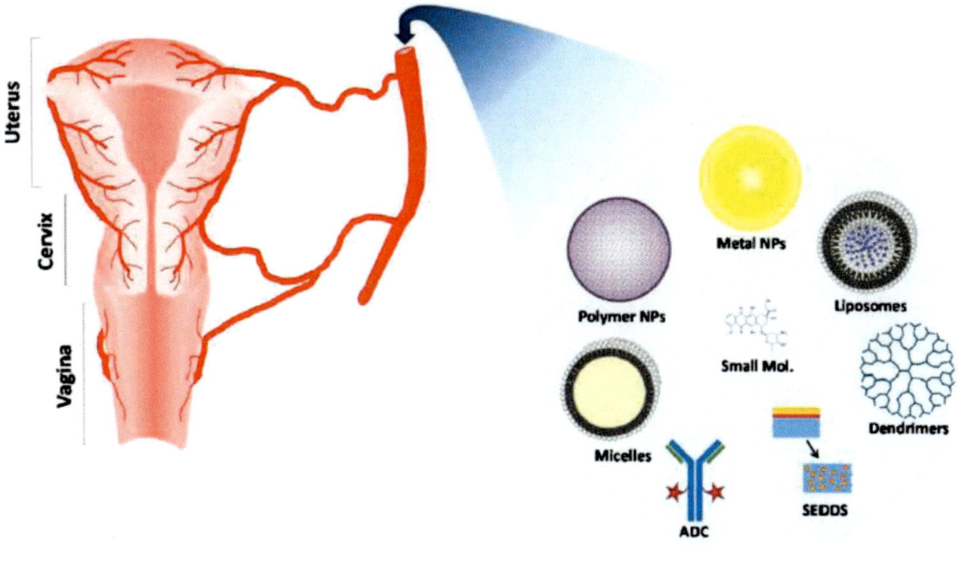

Fig. (2). Different drug delivery systems such as metal nanoparticles, polymer nanoparticles, liposomes, micelles, Antibody–Drug Conjugated, Self-Emulsifying Drug Delivery Systems, and dendrimers used in cervical cancer treatment. Reproduced from cited ref paper [54].

ROLE OF SURFACE-ENGINEERED LIPOSOMES IN CERVICAL CANCER

Liposomes are well-known circular-shaped lipid bilayer drug delivery particles that contain interior hydrophilic core and exterior hydrophobic phospholipid bilayers. The nanometer-sized liposomal particles offer substantial advantages, such as biodegradability, biocompatibility, robust manufacturing, less off-target effects, the systematic release of anticancer drugs, and the ability to integrate both hydrophilic and hydrophobic agents [55]. Many liposomal-based nanoformulations are approved for cancer, inflammation, infectious diseases, antibiotic drugs, and anesthetics, and many are undergoing clinical trials [56 - 59]. Sriraman *et al.* developed a doxorubicin-loaded liposomal system surface tethered with folic acid and transferrin ligands. The dual-targeted liposomal formulation showed 7-folds higher in cervical cancer cell association and showed 79% tumour growth inhibition in a HeLa xenograft model in nude mice compared to the untreated group [60]. Rosalva *et al.* designed an IL-2 protein-coated cationic liposomal system, and this formulation helps infiltrate many lymphocytes, significantly cytotoxic CD8(+) cells on cervical cancer tumours. Subsequently, these lymphocytes inhibited cervical cancer growth in mouse tumour models [61]. Chen MX *et al.* developed paclitaxel-loaded multilayered liposomes. Stearyl amine was used to provide a positive charge to the liposomal surface and subsequently coated with anionic polyacrylic acid (PAA), followed by cationic chitosan. This liposome formulation was stable in simulated gastrointestinal fluids, sustained the release of paclitaxel, and showed selective cytotoxicity in human cervical cancer cells [62]. Developed a liposomal delivery system, in which surfaces were decorated with CD59 antibody and miRNA1284; cisplatin drug was encapsulated inside the liposomes to increase the selectivity and therapeutic effect against the CCs. CD59 antibody tethered liposomes showed prolonged circulation in the blood and enhanced the drug bioavailability, subsequently improving the therapeutic effects against the CCs [63].

ROLE OF SURFACE ENGINEERED METAL NANOCARRIERS IN CERVICAL CANCER

Metal nanoparticles (MNPs) have proven useful in the biomedical field because of their unique attributes, such as sample preparation methods, easy surface functionalization, comprehensive optical properties, and high surface-to-volume ratios. MNPs are used in various biomedical applications, including drug delivery systems, bio-diagnostics, imaging agents, photothermal therapy, and enhancers of radiotherapy [64]. The anticancer properties of MNPs against various cancers have been reported. Their efficiency and biocompatibility come from their interactions with biological entities and their cytotoxic mechanisms toward cancer cells. However, most MNP's mechanisms are still unidentified [65]. Most conventional MNPs show promising results against cervical cancers. MNPs were not successfully translated from bench side to bedside [66].

To increase the specific delivery of therapeutic agents to specific tissues or organs, surfaces of MNPs are conjugated or absorbed with various targeting ligands like proteins, peptides, antibodies, and small molecular ligands, which permits superior accumulation of the MNPs in cervical cancers selectively [67]. Ye *et al.* developed a gold nanoparticle, and the surface was functionalized with PEGylated retinoic acid. They observed that nanoparticle conjugates exhibited 6-fold higher drug potency against cervical carcinoma than retinoic acid [68]. Polyphenol-coated platinum nanoparticles showed enhanced inhibition of human cervical cancer proliferation by introducing chromatin condensation and nuclear fragmentation [69]. Daduang *et al.* developed gold nanoparticles, conjugating their surface with gallic acid. They observed that gallic acid tethered gold nanoparticles enhanced the inhibition of CC cell proliferation and showed less toxicity towards healthy cells than pristine gallic acid and gold nanoparticles [70].

ROLE OF SURFACE ENGINEERED POLYMERIC NANOPARTICLES IN CERVICAL CANCER

Polymeric nanoparticles (PNPs) have attained massive importance in the regime of nanomedicine for cancer treatment. Because of their immense drug encapsulating efficiency, high stability, higher cellular localization, biocompatibility towards biological entities, and biodegradable and deliver hydrophilic and hydrophobic drugs [71]. Nevertheless, the stealth polymers around the nanoparticles extend the stability and circulation time in the biological fluids. Conventional PNPs mainly depend on physicochemical attributes like particle size, morphology, surface zeta potentials, and pathophysiological settings of the tumor microenvironment [72]. Many of the PNPs are showing valiant biomedical applications in various fields. However, intravenously injected PNP disperses throughout the body and accumulates in the healthy tissues, causing organ toxicity [73]. To overcome this non-specific toxicity, PNPs are functionalized on their outer surface by targeting moieties which helps more internalization into cancer cells by interacting with cell surface receptors [74]. Compared to normal healthy cells, cell surface receptors that are significantly overexpressed in cervical cancer cells provide a potential target for actively targeted drug delivery and help reduce off-target effects [75].

In human cervical cancer, folate receptors are over-expressed because folate receptors are a potential therapeutic target for treating cervical cancer. Andrew J. Ditto *et al.* developed L-tyrosine polyphosphate-based PNP; their surface was decorated with PEGylated folic acid and encapsulated silver-based drug, improving the cervical cancer cell accumulation improved the selective cytotoxicity of the medications up to 10-folds compared to control groups [76]. Liu *et al.* developed an anti-EGFR MAb conjugate of gold nanoparticles that can be localized explicitly into the human cervical cancer cells, modulating apoptosis-induced proteins and increasing the G2/M phase arrest when combined with radiotherapy [77].

ROLE OF SURFACE ENGINEERED CARBON-BASED NANOPARTICLES IN CERVICAL CANCER

Carbon-based nanoparticles (CNPs) are a novel class of materials extensively used in various biomedical applications such as drug delivery, imaging, biosensors, and cancer therapy [78]. CNPs are divided into single-walled carbon nanotubes and multiple-walled carbon nanotubes. They have been broadly studied in nanomedicine. For example, CNPs have been used for drug and gene delivery in cervical cancer and diagnosis [79].

ROLE OF SURFACE ENGINEERED POLYMERIC MICELLES (PMS) IN CERVICAL CANCER

PMs are nanometer-sized particles that are self-assembled by amphipathic polymers. The extensive accessibility of interior lipophilic lipid core and exterior lipophobic polymeric blocks permit scientists to explore different PMs formulations to enhance drug stability, drug circulation time in biological fluids, high biocompatibility, and drugs that can deliver to the specific target tissue. Moreover, PMs surface can be tethered with various targeting moieties to improve drug delivery into the tumour microenvironment. As a result, PMs have been widely used as a delivery vehicle for hydrophobic anticancer drugs in cancer treatment in the last few years. Chen *et al.* developed two kinds of paclitaxel conjugated PMs; among these, two folic acids functionalized PMs showed enhanced cell apoptosis and subsequently inhibited the CCs tumour growth than without folic acid-containing PMs [80]. Wei *et al.* have developed TMTP1 peptide-functionalized PEG-PLGA micelles. They were encapsulated in indocyanine green for imaging the primary cancer cells and metastasized cervical cancer cells in BALB/c nude mice. Authors observed that TMTP1-PEG-PLGA micelles rapidly diffused from the injection area to metastatic sentinel lymph nodes and selectively accumulated in the metastatic tumours [81]. cRGD peptide tethered polyion complex micelles were developed for E6 and E7 oncogenes coded siRNAs to immune-compromised cervical tumor-bearing mice. These micelles decreased the non-specific interactions and selectively delivered the siRNAs into the cervical tumour cells, showing tumour growth inhibition significantly in the CC tumour model [82].

ROLE OF SURFACE-ENGINEERED DENDRIMERS IN CERVICAL CANCER

Dendrimers are promising drug delivery vehicles or stabilizers for active pharmaceutical ingredients (APIs) and nanomaterials because of their highly branched three-dimensional spherical shape, interior lipophilic cores, and various functional groups in the periphery [83]. The engineered dendrimers-based nanomaterials encumbered with APIs such as hydrophobic drugs, therapeutic genes, or nanoparticles can be further customized to have selectivity and good biocompatibility. Various dendrimer-based particles were developed for CCs. However, dto low selectivity and high toxicity, they were not successfully translated from bench to bedside [84]. Recent advances in the surface functionalization of dendrimers and the application of dendrimers as versatile platforms for different treatments to CCs. Mekuria *et al.* developed a PAMAM polymer-based dendrimer nanoparticle. Their surface was functionalized with IL-2 antibody, and RGD peptide and doxorubicin were encapsulated in the respective dendrimer's core region. Among these two, IL-6 antibody functionalized dendrimers showed enhanced cellular localization, higher doxorubicin encapsulation, and higher anticancer effect in human CC cell lines than RGD functionalized dendrimers. This could possibly be due to more multivalent ligand concreteness on the exterior surface of the IL6functionalized dendrimers, which helps to higher doxorubicin delivery *via* Her receptor-mediated endocytosis [85].

CONCLUSION AND FUTURE PERSPECTIVE

Nanomaterials are promising candidates for developing systemic delivery systems in cervical cancer chemotherapy. The scientific community proved that surface-functionalized/modified nanoparticles showed great potential in CC treatment over conventional chemotherapy because of their unique biocompatibility, low toxicity, low clearance rate, target specificity, and controlled release of chemotherapeutic agents. On the other hand, the localized delivery of anticancer molecules to the cervix gives various advantages, such as enhanced therapeutic efficacy and low detrimental effects due to the evading systemic circulation of anticancer drugs. Nevertheless, the localized chemotherapeutic drug delivery strategy can not work in metastatic cancers. Still, there are many limitations in surface-modified/functionalized nanoparticles, and so much research must be done in the future.

CONSENT FOR PUBLICATION

Not applicable.

CONFLICT OF INTEREST

The authors declare no conflict of interest, financial or otherwise.

ACKNOWLEDGMENT

We are thankful to the team at Bentham Science Publishers for giving us this opportunity, the editor of this book, and everyone who supported us directly or indirectly while writing this chapter.

REFERENCES

[1] Lei J, Ploner A, Elfström KM, *et al.* HPV vaccination and the risk of invasive cervical cancer. N Engl J Med 2020; 383(14): 1340-8.
[http://dx.doi.org/10.1056/NEJMoa1917338] [PMID: 32997908]

[2] Xing B, Guo J, Sheng Y, Wu G, Zhao Y. Human Papillomavirus-Negative Cervical Cancer: A Comprehensive Review. Front Oncol 2021; 10: 606335.
[http://dx.doi.org/10.3389/fonc.2020.606335] [PMID: 33680928]

[3] Erickson BK, Alvarez RD, Huh WK. Human papillomavirus: what every provider should know. Am J Obstet Gynecol 2013; 208(3): 169-75.
[http://dx.doi.org/10.1016/j.ajog.2012.09.007] [PMID: 23021131]

[4] Rai B, Bansal A, Singh MP. Human papillomavirus-associated cancers: A growing global problem. Int J Appl Basic Med Res 2016; 6(2): 84-9.
[http://dx.doi.org/10.4103/2229-516X.179027] [PMID: 27127735]

[5] Näsman A, Du J, Dalianis T. A global epidemic increase of an HPV-induced tonsil and tongue base cancer – potential benefit from a pan-gender use of HPV vaccine. J Intern Med 2020; 287(2): 134-52.
[http://dx.doi.org/10.1111/joim.13010] [PMID: 31733108]

[6] Monie A, Hung CF, Roden R, Wu TC. Cervarix: a vaccine for the prevention of HPV 16, 18-associated cervical cancer. Biologics 2008; 2(1): 97-105.
[PMID: 19707432]

[7] Pinidis P, Tsikouras P, Iatrakis G, *et al.* Human Papilloma Virus' Life Cycle and Carcinogenesis. Maedica (Buchar) 2016; 11(1): 48-54.
[PMID: 28465751]

[8] Luvero D, Lopez S, Bogani G, Raspagliesi F, Angioli R. From the Infection to the Immunotherapy in Cervical Cancer: Can We Stop the Natural Course of the Disease? Vaccines (Basel) 2020; 8(4): 597.
[http://dx.doi.org/10.3390/vaccines8040597] [PMID: 33050484]

[9] Buskwofie A, David-West G, Clare CA. A review of cervical cancer: incidence and disparities. J Natl Med Assoc 2020; 112(2): 229-32.
[http://dx.doi.org/10.1016/j.jnma.2020.03.002] [PMID: 32278478]

[10] Kagabu M, Nagasawa T, Sato C, *et al.* Immunotherapy for uterine cervical cancer using checkpoint inhibitors: future directions. Int J Mol Sci 2020; 21(7): 2335.
[http://dx.doi.org/10.3390/ijms21072335] [PMID: 32230938]

[11] Senapati S, Mahanta AK, Kumar S, Maiti P. Controlled drug delivery vehicles for cancer treatment and their performance. Signal Transduct Target Ther 2018; 3(1): 7.

[http://dx.doi.org/10.1038/s41392-017-0004-3] [PMID: 29560283]

[12] Major I, McConville C. Vaginal drug delivery for the localised treatment of cervical cancer. Drug Deliv Transl Res 2017; 7(6): 817-28.
[http://dx.doi.org/10.1007/s13346-017-0395-2] [PMID: 28597123]

[13] Golombek SK, May JN, Theek B, *et al.* Tumor targeting *via* EPR: Strategies to enhance patient responses. Adv Drug Deliv Rev 2018; 130: 17-38.
[http://dx.doi.org/10.1016/j.addr.2018.07.007] [PMID: 30009886]

[14] Patra JK, Das G, Fraceto LF, *et al.* Nano based drug delivery systems: recent developments and future prospects. J Nanobiotechnology 2018; 16(1): 71.
[http://dx.doi.org/10.1186/s12951-018-0392-8] [PMID: 30231877]

[15] ud Din F, Aman W, Ullah I, Qureshi OS, Mustapha O, Shafique S. Effective use of nanocarriers as drug delivery systems for the treatment of selected tumors. Int J Nanomed 2017; 12: 7291.

[16] Jeevanandam J, Barhoum A, Chan YS, Dufresne A, Danquah MK. Review on nanoparticles and nanostructured materials: history, sources, toxicity and regulations. Beilstein J Nanotechnol 2018; 9(1): 1050-74.
[http://dx.doi.org/10.3762/bjnano.9.98] [PMID: 29719757]

[17] Jin C, Wang K, Oppong-Gyebi A, Hu J. Application of nanotechnology in cancer diagnosis and therapy - a mini-review. Int J Med Sci 2020; 17(18): 2964-73.
[http://dx.doi.org/10.7150/ijms.49801] [PMID: 33173417]

[18] Rosenblum D, Joshi N, Tao W, Karp JM, Peer D. Progress and challenges towards targeted delivery of cancer therapeutics 2018; 9(1): 1410.
[http://dx.doi.org/10.1038/s41467-018-03705-y]

[19] Villaverde G, Baeza A. Targeting strategies for improving the efficacy of nanomedicine in oncology. Beilstein J Nanotechnol 2019; 10: 168-81.
[http://dx.doi.org/10.3762/bjnano.10.16] [PMID: 30746311]

[20] Chenthamara D, Subramaniam S, Ramakrishnan SG, *et al.* Therapeutic efficacy of nanoparticles and routes of administration. Biomater Res 2019; 23(1): 20.
[http://dx.doi.org/10.1186/s40824-019-0166-x] [PMID: 31832232]

[21] Madamsetty VS, Mukherjee A, Mukherjee S. Recent trends of the bio-inspired nanoparticles in cancer theranostics. Front Pharmacol 2019; 10(1264): 1264.
[http://dx.doi.org/10.3389/fphar.2019.01264] [PMID: 31708785]

[22] G Lahori D, Varamini P. Nanotechnology-based platforms to improve immune checkpoint blockade efficacy in cancer therapy. Future Oncol 2021; 17(6): 711-22.
[http://dx.doi.org/10.2217/fon-2020-0720] [PMID: 33136464]

[23] Mitchell MJ, Billingsley MM, Haley RM, Wechsler ME, Peppas NA, Langer R. Engineering precision nanoparticles for drug delivery. Nat Rev Drug Discov 2021; 20(2): 101-24.
[http://dx.doi.org/10.1038/s41573-020-0090-8] [PMID: 33277608]

[24] Chenthamara D, Subramaniam S, Ramakrishnan SG, *et al.* Therapeutic efficacy of nanoparticles and routes of administration. Biomaterials research 2019; 23: 20.
[http://dx.doi.org/10.1186/s40824-019-0166-x]

[25] Riaz M, Riaz M, Zhang X, *et al.* Surface functionalization and targeting strategies of liposomes in solid tumor therapy: a review. Int J Mol Sci 2018; 19(1): 195.
[http://dx.doi.org/10.3390/ijms19010195] [PMID: 29315231]

[26] Narum SM, Le T, Le DP, *et al.* Passive targeting in nanomedicine: fundamental concepts, body interactions, and clinical potential. In: Chung EJ, Leon L, Rinaldi C, Eds. Nanoparticles for Biomedical Applications. Elsevier 2020; pp. 37-53.
[http://dx.doi.org/10.1016/B978-0-12-816662-8.00004-7]

[27] Attia MF, Anton N, Wallyn J, Omran Z, Vandamme TF. An overview of active and passive targeting strategies to improve the nanocarriers efficiency to tumour sites. J Pharm Pharmacol 2019; 71(8): 1185-98.
[http://dx.doi.org/10.1111/jphp.13098] [PMID: 31049986]

[28] Bertrand N, Wu J, Xu X, Kamaly N, Farokhzad OC. Cancer nanotechnology: The impact of passive and active targeting in the era of modern cancer biology. Adv Drug Deliv Rev 2014; 66: 2-25.
[http://dx.doi.org/10.1016/j.addr.2013.11.009] [PMID: 24270007]

[29] Sutradhar KB, Amin ML. Nanotechnology in cancer drug delivery and selective targeting. ISRN Nanotechnology 2014; 2014: 1-12.
[http://dx.doi.org/10.1155/2014/939378]

[30] Zein R, Sharrouf W, Selting K. Physical properties of nanoparticles that result in improved cancer targeting. J Oncol 2020; 2020: 1-16.
[http://dx.doi.org/10.1155/2020/5194780] [PMID: 32765604]

[31] Zhang J, Tang H, Liu Z, Chen B. Effects of major parameters of nanoparticles on their physical and chemical properties and recent application of nanodrug delivery system in targeted chemotherapy. Int J Nanomedicine 2017; 12: 8483-93.
[http://dx.doi.org/10.2147/IJN.S148359] [PMID: 29238188]

[32] Zhang M, Gao S, Yang D, *et al.* Influencing factors and strategies of enhancing nanoparticles into tumors *in vivo.* Acta Pharm Sin B 2021; 11(8): 2265-85.
[http://dx.doi.org/10.1016/j.apsb.2021.03.033] [PMID: 34522587]

[33] Jin Q, Deng Y, Chen X, Ji J. Rational design of cancer nanomedicine for simultaneous stealth surface and enhanced cellular uptake. ACS Nano 2019; 13(2): acsnano.8b07746.
[http://dx.doi.org/10.1021/acsnano.8b07746] [PMID: 30681834]

[34] Chauhan VP, Stylianopoulos T, Boucher Y, Jain RK. Delivery of molecular and nanoscale medicine to tumors: transport barriers and strategies. Annu Rev Chem Biomol Eng 2011; 2(1): 281-98.
[http://dx.doi.org/10.1146/annurev-chembioeng-061010-114300] [PMID: 22432620]

[35] Suk JS, Xu Q, Kim N, Hanes J, Ensign LM. PEGylation as a strategy for improving nanoparticle-based drug and gene delivery. Adv Drug Deliv Rev 2016; 99(Pt A): 28-51.
[http://dx.doi.org/10.1016/j.addr.2015.09.012] [PMID: 26456916]

[36] Fam SY, Chee CF, Yong CY, Ho KL, Mariatulqabtiah AR, Tan WS. Stealth coating of nanoparticles in drug-delivery systems. Nanomaterials (Basel) 2020; 10(4): 787.
[http://dx.doi.org/10.3390/nano10040787] [PMID: 32325941]

[37] Yang Q, Jones SW, Parker CL, Zamboni WC, Bear JE, Lai SK. Evading immune cell uptake and clearance requires PEG grafting at densities substantially exceeding the minimum for brush conformation. Mol Pharm 2014; 11(4): 1250-8.
[http://dx.doi.org/10.1021/mp400703d] [PMID: 24521246]

[38] Pathak YV. Surface modification of nanoparticles for targeted drug delivery. Springer 2019; p. 517.
[http://dx.doi.org/10.1007/978-3-030-06115-9]

[39] Kim CH, Lee SG, Kang MJ, Lee S, Choi YW. Surface modification of lipid-based nanocarriers for cancer cell-specific drug targeting. J Pharm Investig 2017; 47(3): 203-27.
[http://dx.doi.org/10.1007/s40005-017-0329-5]

[40] Large DE, Soucy JR, Hebert J, Auguste DT. Advances in receptor-mediated, tumor-targeted drug delivery. Adv Ther (Weinh) 2019; 2(1): 1800091.
[http://dx.doi.org/10.1002/adtp.201800091]

[41] Rosenblum D, Joshi N, Tao W, Karp JM, Peer D. Progress and challenges towards targeted delivery of cancer therapeutics. Nat Commun 2018; 9(1): 1410.
[http://dx.doi.org/10.1038/s41467-018-03705-y] [PMID: 29650952]

[42] Allen TM. Ligand-targeted therapeutics in anticancer therapy. Nat Rev Cancer 2002; 2(10): 750-63. [http://dx.doi.org/10.1038/nrc903] [PMID: 12360278]

[43] Kumar Khanna V. Targeted delivery of nanomedicines. ISRN Pharmacol 2012; 2012: 571394. [http://dx.doi.org/10.5402/2012/571394]

[44] Yoo J, Park C, Yi G, Lee D, Koo H. Active targeting strategies using biological ligands for nanoparticle drug delivery systems. Cancers (Basel) 2019; 11(5): 640. [http://dx.doi.org/10.3390/cancers11050640] [PMID: 31072061]

[45] Daniels TR, Bernabeu E, Rodríguez JA, *et al.* The transferrin receptor and the targeted delivery of therapeutic agents against cancer. Biochim Biophys Acta, Gen Subj 2012; 1820(3): 291-317. [http://dx.doi.org/10.1016/j.bbagen.2011.07.016] [PMID: 21851850]

[46] Mehra NK, Mishra V, Jain NK. Receptor-based targeting of therapeutics. Ther Deliv 2013; 4(3): 369-94. [http://dx.doi.org/10.4155/tde.13.6] [PMID: 23442082]

[47] Kumar P, Huo P, Liu B. Formulation strategies for folate-targeted liposomes and their biomedical applications. Pharmaceutics 2019; 11(8): 381. [http://dx.doi.org/10.3390/pharmaceutics11080381] [PMID: 31382369]

[48] Mahalunkar S, Yadav AS, Gorain M, *et al.* Functional design of pH-responsive folate-targeted polymer-coated gold nanoparticles for drug delivery and *in vivo* therapy in breast cancer. Int J Nanomedicine 2019; 14: 8285-302. [http://dx.doi.org/10.2147/IJN.S215142] [PMID: 31802866]

[49] Morales-Cruz M, Delgado Y, Castillo B, *et al.* Smart targeting to improve cancer therapeutics. Drug Des Devel Ther 2019; 13: 3753-72. [http://dx.doi.org/10.2147/DDDT.S219489] [PMID: 31802849]

[50] Zhao M, Sun Y, Zhu X, Chen D, Feng S, Guo S, *et al.* Antibody-Targeted Immunocarriers for Cancer Treatment. Smart Drug Delivery System 2016; p. 139.

[51] Dorjsuren B, Chaurasiya B, Ye Z, *et al.* Cetuximab-coated thermo-sensitive liposomes loaded with magnetic nanoparticles and doxorubicin for targeted egfr-expressing breast cancer combined therapy. Int J Nanomedicine 2020; 15: 8201-15. [http://dx.doi.org/10.2147/IJN.S261671] [PMID: 33122906]

[52] Shmeeda H, Tzemach D, Mak L, Gabizon A. Her2-targeted pegylated liposomal doxorubicin: Retention of target-specific binding and cytotoxicity after *in vivo* passage. J Control Release 2009; 136(2): 155-60. [http://dx.doi.org/10.1016/j.jconrel.2009.02.002] [PMID: 19331844]

[53] Navya PN, Kaphle A, Srinivas SP, Bhargava SK, Rotello VM, Daima HK. Current trends and challenges in cancer management and therapy using designer nanomaterials. Nano Converg 2019; 6(1): 23. [http://dx.doi.org/10.1186/s40580-019-0193-2] [PMID: 31304563]

[54] Ordikhani F, Erdem Arslan M, Marcelo R, *et al.* Drug delivery approaches for the treatment of cervical cancer. Pharmaceutics 2016; 8(3): 23. [http://dx.doi.org/10.3390/pharmaceutics8030023] [PMID: 27447664]

[55] Pattni BS, Chupin VV, Torchilin VP. New developments in liposomal drug delivery. Chem Rev 2015; 115(19): 10938-66. [http://dx.doi.org/10.1021/acs.chemrev.5b00046] [PMID: 26010257]

[56] Bulbake U, Doppalapudi S, Kommineni N, Khan W. Liposomal formulations in clinical use: an updated review. Pharmaceutics 2017; 9(4): 12. [http://dx.doi.org/10.3390/pharmaceutics9020012] [PMID: 28346375]

[57] Wang X, Song Y, Su Y, *et al.* Are PEGylated liposomes better than conventional liposomes? A special

case for vincristine. Drug Deliv 2016; 23(4): 1092-100.
[http://dx.doi.org/10.3109/10717544.2015.1027015] [PMID: 26024386]

[58] Yan W, Leung SSY, To KKW. Updates on the use of liposomes for active tumor targeting in cancer therapy. Nanomedicine (Lond) 2020; 15(3): 303-18.
[http://dx.doi.org/10.2217/nnm-2019-0308] [PMID: 31802702]

[59] Jahan ST, Sadat S, Walliser M, Haddadi A. Targeted therapeutic nanoparticles: an immense promise to fight against cancer. Journal of drug delivery 2017.
[http://dx.doi.org/10.1155/2017/9090325]

[60] Sriraman SK, Salzano G, Sarisozen C, Torchilin V. Anti-cancer activity of doxorubicin-loaded liposomes co-modified with transferrin and folic acid. Eur J Pharm Biopharm 2016; 105: 40-9.
[http://dx.doi.org/10.1016/j.ejpb.2016.05.023] [PMID: 27264717]

[61] Rangel-Corona R, Corona-Ortega T, del Río-Ortiz I, *et al.* Cationic liposomes bearing IL-2 on their external surface induced mice leukocytes to kill human cervical cancer cells *in vitro*, and significantly reduced tumor burden in immunodepressed mice. J Drug Target 2011; 19(2): 79-85.
[http://dx.doi.org/10.3109/10611861003733920] [PMID: 20367025]

[62] Gupta S, Gupta MK. Possible role of nanocarriers in drug delivery against cervical cancer 2017; 8(1): 1335567.
[http://dx.doi.org/10.1080/20022727.2017.1335567]

[63] Wang L, Liang TT. CD59 receptor targeted delivery of miRNA-1284 and cisplatin-loaded liposomes for effective therapeutic efficacy against cervical cancer cells. AMB Express 2020; 10(1): 54.
[http://dx.doi.org/10.1186/s13568-020-00990-z] [PMID: 32185543]

[64] Yadav SK. Nanoscale materials in targeted drug delivery, theragnosis and tissue regeneration. Springer 2016.
[http://dx.doi.org/10.1007/978-981-10-0818-4]

[65] Saifullah S, Ali I, Kawish M, El-Shabasy RM, Chen L, El-Seedi HR. Surface functionalized magnetic nanoparticles for targeted cancer therapy and diagnosis Metal Nanoparticles for Drug Delivery and Diagnostic Applications. Elsevier 2020; pp. 215-36.
[http://dx.doi.org/10.1016/B978-0-12-816960-5.00012-4]

[66] Izci M, Maksoudian C, Manshian BB, Soenen SJ. The Use of Alternative Strategies for Enhanced Nanoparticle Delivery to Solid Tumors. Chem Rev 2021; 121(3): 1746-803.
[http://dx.doi.org/10.1021/acs.chemrev.0c00779] [PMID: 33445874]

[67] Ahmad MZ, Ahmad J, Warsi MH, Abdel-Wahab BA, Akhter S. 13 - Metallic nanoparticulate delivery systems.Nanoengineered Biomaterials for Advanced Drug Delivery. Elsevier 2020; pp. 279-328.
[http://dx.doi.org/10.1016/B978-0-08-102985-5.00013-9]

[68] Ye L, Song Q. Promising potency of retinoic acid-poly(ethylene glycol)-thiol gold nanoparticle conjugates for cervical cancer treatment. Int J Clin Exp Med 2015; 8(7): 10501-7.
[PMID: 26379840]

[69] Alshatwi AA, Athinarayanan J, Vaiyapuri Subbarayan P. Green synthesis of platinum nanoparticles that induce cell death and G2/M-phase cell cycle arrest in human cervical cancer cells. J Mater Sci Mater Med 2015; 26(1): 7.
[http://dx.doi.org/10.1007/s10856-014-5330-1] [PMID: 25577212]

[70] Daduang J, Palasap A, Daduang S, Boonsiri P, Suwannalert P, Limpaiboon T. Gallic acid enhancement of gold nanoparticle anticancer activity in cervical cancer cells. Asian Pac J Cancer Prev 2015; 16(1): 169-74.
[http://dx.doi.org/10.7314/APJCP.2015.16.1.169] [PMID: 25640346]

[71] Venditti I. Morphologies and functionalities of polymeric nanocarriers as chemical tools for drug delivery: A review. J King Saud Univ Sci 2019; 31(3): 398-411.
[http://dx.doi.org/10.1016/j.jksus.2017.10.004]

[72] Shao XR, Wei XQ, Song X, *et al.* Independent effect of polymeric nanoparticle zeta potential/surface charge, on their cytotoxicity and affinity to cells. Cell Prolif 2015; 48(4): 465-74. [http://dx.doi.org/10.1111/cpr.12192] [PMID: 26017818]

[73] Song R, Murphy M, Li C, Ting K, Soo C, Zheng Z. Current development of biodegradable polymeric materials for biomedical applications. Drug Des Devel Ther 2018; 12: 3117-45. [http://dx.doi.org/10.2147/DDDT.S165440] [PMID: 30288019]

[74] Dhar P, Samarasinghe RM, Shigdar S. Antibodies, Nanobodies, or Aptamers—Which Is Best for Deciphering the Proteomes of Non-Model Species? Int J Mol Sci 2020; 21(7): 2485. [http://dx.doi.org/10.3390/ijms21072485] [PMID: 32260091]

[75] Áyen Á, Jiménez Martínez Y, Boulaiz H. Targeted gene delivery therapies for cervical cancer. Cancers (Basel) 2020; 12(5): 1301. [http://dx.doi.org/10.3390/cancers12051301] [PMID: 32455616]

[76] Ditto AJ, Shah KN, Robishaw NK, Panzner MJ, Youngs WJ, Yun YH. The Interactions between L-tyrosine based nanoparticles decorated with folic acid and cervical cancer cells under physiological flow. Mol Pharm 2012; 9(11): 3089-98. [http://dx.doi.org/10.1021/mp300221f] [PMID: 22957928]

[77] Liu J, Liang Y, Liu T, Li D, Yang X. Anti-EGFR-conjugated hollow gold nanospheres enhance radiocytotoxic targeting of cervical cancer at megavoltage radiation energies. Nanoscale Res Lett 2015; 10(1): 218. [http://dx.doi.org/10.1186/s11671-015-0923-2] [PMID: 25995714]

[78] Maiti D, Tong X, Mou X, Yang K. Carbon-based nanomaterials for biomedical applications: a recent study. Frontiers in pharmacology 2019; 9: 1401. [http://dx.doi.org/10.3389/fphar.2018.01401]

[79] Saeed LM, Mahmood M, Pyrek SJ, *et al.* Single-walled carbon nanotube and graphene nanodelivery of gambogic acid increases its cytotoxicity in breast and pancreatic cancer cells. J Appl Toxicol 2014; 34(11): 1188-99. [http://dx.doi.org/10.1002/jat.3018] [PMID: 25220893]

[80] Sulistio A, Lowenthal J, Blencowe A, *et al.* Folic acid conjugated amino acid-based star polymers for active targeting of cancer cells. Biomacromolecules 2011; 12(10): 3469-77. [http://dx.doi.org/10.1021/bm200604h] [PMID: 21854075]

[81] Wei R, Jiang G, Lv M, *et al.* TMTP1-modified indocyanine green-loaded polymeric micelles for targeted imaging of cervical cancer and metastasis sentinel lymph node *in vivo*. Theranostics 2019; 9(24): 7325-44. [http://dx.doi.org/10.7150/thno.35346] [PMID: 31695771]

[82] Nishida H, Matsumoto Y, Kawana K, *et al.* Systemic delivery of siRNA by actively targeted polyion complex micelles for silencing the E6 and E7 human papillomavirus oncogenes. J Control Release 2016; 231: 29-37. [http://dx.doi.org/10.1016/j.jconrel.2016.03.016] [PMID: 26979870]

[83] Mittal P, Saharan A, Verma R, *et al.* Dendrimers: a new race of pharmaceutical nanocarriers. Biomed Res Int 2021; 2021: 8844030. [http://dx.doi.org/10.1155/2021/8844030]

[84] Hsu HJ, Bugno J, Lee S, Hong S. Dendrimer-based nanocarriers: a versatile platform for drug delivery. Wiley Interdiscip Rev Nanomed Nanobiotechnol 2017; 9(1). [http://dx.doi.org/10.1002/wnan.1409] [PMID: 27126551]

[85] Mekuria SL, Debele TA, Chou HY, Tsai HC. IL-6 antibody and RGD peptide conjugated poly (amidoamine) dendrimer for targeted drug delivery of HeLa cells. J Phys Chem B 2016; 120(1): 123-30.
[http://dx.doi.org/10.1021/acs.jpcb.5b11125] [PMID: 26670944]

CHAPTER 8

Importance of Nanocarriers in Colon Cancer

Neha Srivastava[1,2], Yachana Mishra[3] and Vijay Mishra[2,*]

[1] *Faculty of Pharmaceutical Sciences, PCTE Group of Institutes, Ludhiana (Punjab), India*

[2] *School of Pharmaceutical Sciences, Lovely Professional University, Phagwara (Punjab), India*

[3] *Department of Zoology, School of Bioengineering and Biosciences, Lovely Professional University, Phagwara (Punjab), India*

Abstract: Colon cancer is the third most common cause of cancer globally and leads to many deaths. Conventional chemotherapy has severe side effects and toxicities, which are significant challenges for cancer treatment. Current therapy has an essential concern of target specificity. In colon cancer, the primary concern is to deliver the drug to cancer cells in the colon in a reproducible and predictable manner. The oral route has its limitations. The drug delivered through this route gets degraded or may not be subsequently absorbed to produce the effects or lessen them before reaching the colon. Nanocarriers empowered the delivery of chemotherapeutics at specific sites and enhanced cellular penetrability. Within the organism, the cytotoxic substance will quickly accumulate. The present chapter focuses on the different nanostructures designed to deliver the drugs to treat colon cancer.

Keywords: Colon cancer, Chemotherapy, Nanocarriers, Nanoparticles.

INTRODUCTION

Colon cancer starts with the change in the normal epithelium of the colon to an adenomatous polyp [1]. The study reveals that colon cancer cases are steadily increasing, and genetic mutation is responsible for cancerous cells' formation. Urbanized lifestyles and changing living patterns worldwide are responsible for increasing colon cancer cases [2]. Different conventional approaches have been used to obtain specific targeted oral drug delivery strategies for decades. Anti-cancer therapy consists of high doses of the anti-tumor drug to achieve maximum efficacy, which leads to toxicity [3]. To reduce the toxicity and effect of anti-tumor drugs on healthy cells, different dosage forms such as nanoparticles (NPs) [4], liposomes [5], carbon nanotubes (CNTs) [6], and dendrimers [7] were utilized, which provides target specificity against tumor cells. Lymphoid tissue is

* **Corresponding author Vijay Mishra:** School of Pharmaceutical Sciences, Lovely Professional University, Phagwara (Punjab), 144411, India; Tel: +91-8989154900; E-mail: vijaymishra2@gmail.com

present in large amounts in the colon. Antigen taken up by mast cells of the mucosa of the colon leads to the production of antibodies, which helps target specific delivery. The colon region is considered a region with less diversity and less activity intensity (Fig. **1**). It has a less hostile environment when compared to the stomach or intestine [8]. Age is one of the significant factors that lead to colonic cancer development. Specifically, adolescents and aged people are more susceptible to colon cancer [9]. Different approaches, such as surgery, radiation, chemotherapy, cryosurgery, and targeted drug therapy, are used to diagnose and treat colonic cancer [10]. Among the different approaches, chemotherapy is one of the most frequently used strategies to kill and reduce cancer cells. Conventional therapy includes other drugs or combinations of medicines taken by the cancerous and non-cancerous cells, causing severe adverse effects [11]. The common side effects are liver toxicity, gastrointestinal toxicity, neutropenia, hand-foot syndrome, anemia, diarrhea, nausea and vomiting, mucositis, hematologic disorders, and fatigue. Due to the risk of adverse effects and drug resistance, chemotherapy is not considered safe and successful [12].

Hence, surgery is the primary way of removing tumors for cancer treatment, which can cure approximately 50% of patients. However, in many cases, relapse or reoccurrence of disease occurs after surgery, which is a significant limitation and causes death. Different efforts are approved for early diagnosis and treatment to improve the survival of patients. Surgery may not have an excellent survival rate; radiotherapy and chemotherapy have drawbacks [13]. The side effects of anti-tumor drugs are very high; researchers are trying to identify different molecular biomarkers, improving diagnostic and therapeutic values [14].

The epigenetic and genetic factors are the connected factors that increase colon cancer incidence [15]. The cancerous cell cannot be targeted by most anti-cancer drugs by cancer therapy, resulting in serious adverse effects and various organ toxicities. Further, the drug gets distributed to different non-cancerous organs/cells, reducing the concentration of the drug reaching the tumor site [16, 17].

Nanocarriers have a large surface area and large surface/volume ratio, modify a surface functional group, bind easily with other structures, and are biodegradable. Due to these qualities, nanostructures are gaining popularity worldwide [18]. Due to the smaller nanostructure size and its ability to conjugate with different ligands, various nanostructures, such as nanoparticles, liposomes and dendrimers, are gaining attention and laying the new path for targeted drug therapy. Cancer therapy can be achieved by targeting; the nanostructure can form bioconjugation with different ligands, antibodies, and anti-cancer drugs by covalent linkage and effectively target cancer cells [19, 20].

Both passive and active targeting approaches can deliver the anti-cancer drug, increase drug efficacy, and reduce side effects [21].

EPIDEMIOLOGY OF COLON CANCER

According to the WHO GLOBOCAN database, in males, colon cancer is prevalent and the second common type of cancer in males and the third common type of cancer in females. In addition, mortality and incidence rates are comparatively more in males than in females.

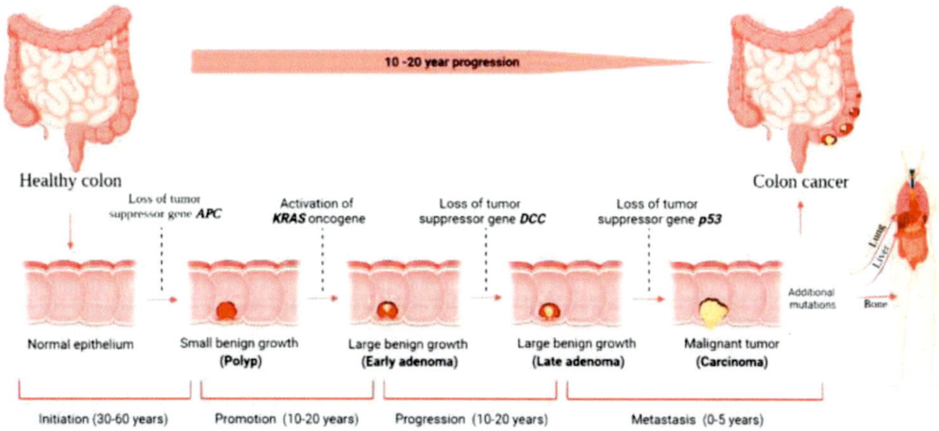

Fig. (1). Stages of colon cancer [22].

Incidence

The incidence of colon cancer globally tends to vary over ten folds. The disease is common in New Zealand, Australia, Europe, and North America, and the lowest rates are found in South-Central Asia and Africa [23]. Genetic susceptibility is the geographic differences that cause the differences in environmental factors and dietary habits. Besides geographical factors, social and economic status is also responsible for colon cancer [24]. According to the studies conducted, it is estimated that colon cancer risk is 30% more in lower socio-economical status strata than in the highest strata. The recent changes in the behavior pattern, such as unhealthy diet, physical inactivity, smoking, sedentary lifestyle, and obesity, are responsible for one-third of the proportion of the risk of newer-onset colon cancer. Other factors, such as a lower colon cancer screening rate, also contribute to colon cancer risk [25].

Mortality

In 2018, International Agency estimated that 18.1 million newer cases were detected and that deaths of 9.6 million were reported across the world. As per data, the patient seen with colon cancer is around 1.1 million, which adds up to 6.1% to the final number of new patients with cancer and leads to about 551,000 deaths contributing to 5.8% of cancer deaths [26]. Regarding CC, 1.1 million patients were diagnosed (6.1% of the total number of new cancer cases), and more than 551,000 deaths were recorded (5.8% of total deaths from cancer). The incidence and mortality will almost double as expected in 2040 compared to the cases predicted in 2018. Males are affected more as compared to females with colon cancer. Asia has the highest incidence of colon cancer, around 49.2%, contributing to 49.3% of deaths. Europe follows Asia in incidences and mortality (28.5% incidence and 28.5% mortality. The concern rises when colon cancer incidence and mortality in older adults are less compared to the young age group, less than 50 (Fig. **2**) [27].

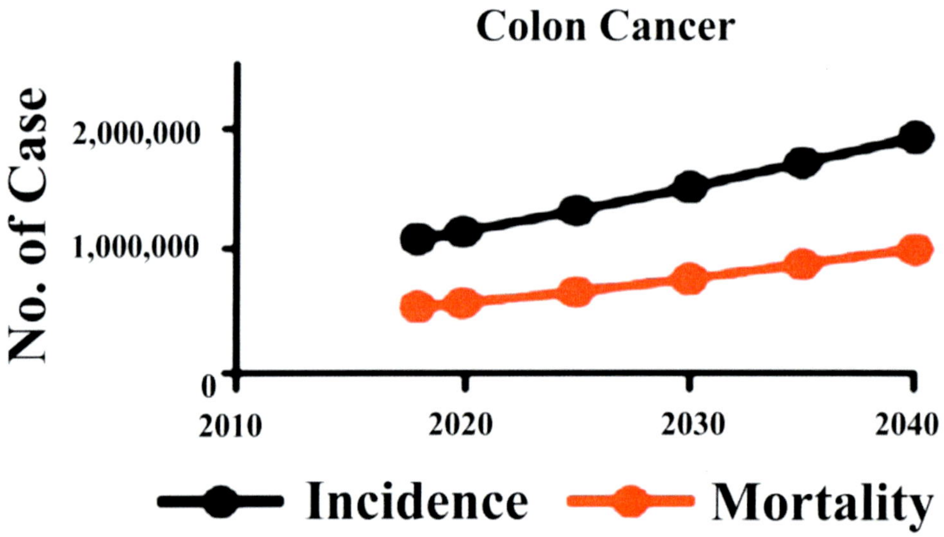

Fig. (2). Incidence and Mortality due to colon cancer.

In the United States and other western countries, death rates from colon cancer have declined since the mid-1980s [28]. The improvement in mortality was observed by early detection and removal of polyps outgrown in the colon. Early detection and effective treatments are also responsible for lower incidences and death at an early stage. In the USA, colon cancer mortality was started well before widespread screening and adjuvant therapy [29].

PATHOGENESIS

Instability in genomic and epigenomic factors is responsible for forming colorectal cancers [30].

Progression of Carcinoma Sequence

The study reveals that most colon cancer emerges from the pre-cancerous lesion and adenomatous polyps. It is a multistage development of cancer in colon cells starting from aberrant crypt focus and then transforming into adenomatous polyps and then into pre-cancerous lesions, which converts into invasive cancer [31]. Carcinogenesis occurs due to progressive development at the molecular level, leading to changes that are beneficial for tumor growth over time, which causes invasive malignancy. This is the adenoma-carcinoma sequence [32]. Firstly, APC gene mutation occurs, followed by TP53 and KRAS mutation. This alternative pathway causes colorectal cancer evolution and phenotypically presents a heterogenous outgrowth such as sessile serrated adenomas, hyperplastic polyps, or mixed hyperplastic polyps/serrated adenoma [33]. The first observed mutation is BARF mutation caused by epigenetic CpG island methylator phenotype. Combining a high degree of CIMP (CIMP-H), microsatellite stability (MSS), and BRAF mutation carries the worst prognosis. KRAS mutations and somatic copy number modifications are vital genetic causes of the adenocarcinoma series. In contrast, BRAF mutations followed by gene promoter hypermethylation drive the serrated polyp pathway [34].

Chromosomal Instability Pathway/APC Pathway

The mutation is the common cause of cancer; in colon cancer, it can be traced to two modes of genomic instability: microsatellite instability and chromosomal instability. Among 70% of colon cancer chromosomal instability cases [35]. When the *Apc* gene undergoes mutation leads to the conversion of adenoma into carcinoma through chromosomal instability due to different chromosomal changes, especially in subchromosomal aberrations, chromosome 18, and inefficient heterozygosity. Chromosomal instability has a specific feature; it causes the tumor suppressor gene's deletion. CIN's significant genes include TP53, APC, PI3KCA, KRAS, *etc.* Chromosomal instability leads to worse consequences than cancer developed by microsatellite instability [36].

Mismatch Repair Mechanism

During DNA replication, errors are common, and there are different mechanisms to control the errors. Among the various tools, one is the mismatch repair mechanism. In case of dysfunctioning of mismatch, repairing protein leads to the generation of Lynch syndrome. The other system can also be inactivated by mutation, epigenetic silencing, or heterozygosity loss [37]. DNA errors increase much fold when the cell faces MMR deficiency. Microsatellites are the region in the genome that is repeated hundreds of times. The issue with misaligned proteins causes the microsatellite area to contract and expand. Lynch syndrome causes cancer to appear at a young age. Lynch syndrome patients are more likely to develop aggressive cancer at an earlier age [38].

Hypermethylation BRAF Pathway

One of the reasons for sporadic colon cancer is V600 BRAF mutant and instability in microsatellites. The main reason is the silencing of a protein involved in mismatch repair *via* CpG sequence hypermethylation. This happens in the genomic sequence promoter region responsible for mismatch repair proteins and results in enzyme deficiency in the mismatch repair mechanism. These types of tumors are called CIMP+ tumors. BRAF mutation activation causes BRAF V600, an exclusive feature of such tumors [39].

NANOTECHNOLOGY-BASED APPROACHES FOR COLON CANCER TREATMENT

Nanotechnology in medicine is a novel and interdisciplinary approach with various diagnostics and drug delivery applications. The nanoscale structure with drug or diagnostic agents helps deliver the target sites [40]. Nanomedicine improves target specificity and reduces adverse effects produced by anti-cancer drugs or diagnostic agents used to discover cancer biomarkers, detect tumors, and develop novel treatments [41, 42]. Nanotechnology has provided an extended platform for cancer treatment, which creates the hope of designing different therapeutic strategies for cancer. Nanovectors can be surface engineered to deliver the drug at the target sites by interacting with biomolecules present inside the cell or on the outer surface [43]. Anti-cancer agents lead to severe side effects due to the delivery system's inability to differentiate cancerous and non–cancerous cells. Various nanovectors can visualize and target the cancerous cell, reducing its potential side effects [44]. Different nanovectors are available for target-specific delivery of anti-cancer drugs such as liposomes, nanoparticles (NPs), dendrimers, carbon nanotubes (CNTs), and various others to efficiently target and deliver the drug to the colon.

Liposomes

Liposomes are spherical vesicles composed of lipids that can accommodate lipophilic and hydrophilic drugs as novel and reliable carriers and cargo for anti-cancer drugs [45]. Liposomes possess several advantages, including;

biocompatibility, biodegradability, and low toxicity, making them suitable for drug-targeted delivery. Despite various benefits, liposomes show disadvantages such as disruption or leakage of drugs from vesicles, stability problems, and hydrophilic drug entrapment inefficiency [46]. The liposomal structure has significantly improved the pharmacokinetics and distributions of loaded drugs, especially lipophilic drugs. Improvement in biodistribution helps increase the selectivity of prescriptions, reduce toxicities to a normal cell, reduce adverse effects, and give prolonged drug release [47, 48].

The encapsulated drug is unavailable for binding for plasma protein, and protected from enzymatic degradation but undergoes opsonization by a reticular endothelial system, reducing liposomes' circulation time [49]. PEGylation lipidic vesicles can improve liposomes and make them safe, effective, and long-lasting against tumor cells. PEG is a neutral (non-ionic) polymer that can develop near-zero zeta potential and overcome surface charges. Coating the structure with PEG assures the reduction of non-specific interaction with macrophages and increases liposomes' circulation time in blood. The drug can be taken up by cells by active targeting or passive targeting. Passive targeting helps accumulate a large amount of drugs specifically to the solid tumor cell due to the EPR effect. Charged lipoproteins, either positive or negative, tend to attract complement proteins and be highly sequestered by RES organs. Positively charged nanostructure interacts with negatively charged proteins in plasma which causes higher RES uptake [50, 51].

PEGylation of the delivery system can help release drugs near the tumor cell but may not be uptaken by the tumor cell. Ligands can increase the internalization of anti-tumor drugs in tumor cells, allowing for faster uptake and medication retention. Liposomes can be coated with a hydrophilic and biocompatible polymeric coat that binds with specific biomolecules on the surface, imparting easy access to the tumor cell and target specificity [52, 53]. The study conducted by Maryam E Nik and coworkers prepared PEGylated liposomal using Galbanic acid (Gba) as ligand, HSPC 56.2%/, Cholesterol 38.3%, mPEG2000-DSPE) in molar ratio. Liposomes were prepared using a thin film hydration method with a remote loading method with calcium acetate. Liposomes were labeled with fluorescent material for tracing the targeting track. It was observed in *in vitro* studies that labeled liposomes were targeted, and cellular uptake is also improved by human umbilical vein in endothelial cells—the studies conducted in the chicken membrane angiogenesis model confirm the *in vivo* targeting of liposomes. The research also indicates the increased deposition of liposomes in tumor cells. When conjugated, PEGylated liposomes of doxorubicin and PLGba tend to produce synergistic and work against the anti-proliferative effect on the cell line [54].

Another research study involves developing and characterizing liposomes targeting 5-Fluorouracil (5-FU) to improve the safety and efficacy of the anti-cancer molecule. The ligand used for targeting 5-FU to cancer cells is folic acid. *In vitro* cytotoxicity of the prepared formulation was performed in different cell lines with MTT assay. *In vivo* tumor inhibition studies were conducted in animals by administrating both drug and folic acid conjugated drug liposomes. The result indicates that the cytotoxicity of targeted liposomes is much higher than the drug itself or liposomes without ligand. Liposomes directly targeted HeLa cells and HT 29 cells containing narcotic cells. It causes the activation of the apoptotic pathway by the collapse of mitochondrial membrane potential, and increases caspase and cytochrome-c activity [55].

Researchers studied the properties of chitosan to improve the characteristics of liposomes. Chitosan-coated nanovector is considered a promising carrier for effective drug delivery. Chitosan has mucoadhesive properties, which enhance the residence time of the drug at the target site. Chitosan-coated liposomes have mucoadhesive, which enhances the residence of the drug at the predetermined site [56, 57]. When liposomes are coated with chitosan extends the residence time at the tumor site and enhances the drug 5-FU. In the study, chitosan-coated liposomes are loaded with 5-FU, and the prepared nanostructure was evaluated by zeta potential, PDI index, particle size, entrapment of drug, and stability studies. Along with this, the liposomes were also evaluated for *in vitro* drug release, cytotoxicity, and hemocompatibility and compared with liposomes without coating. The newly formed chitosomes loaded with 5-FU have a more cytotoxic effect and indicate a potential drug delivery approach [58].

Xiong has formulated paclitaxel (PTX) containing liposomes which are mannosylated for targeting cancer cells in the colorectal region. Liposomes were prepared by film dispersion method using phospholipids and cholesterol. *In vitro* and *in vivo* studies were conducted to study the efficacy and safety of liposomes. Mannose conjugated liposomes indicated high cellular uptake by CT26 cells compared to non-conjugated liposomes. *In vivo* studies were conducted in mice models with tumors; mannosylated liposomes show a higher tumor-inhibiting rate with minimum organ-related toxicity [59].

In one of the studies, liposomes are coated with eudragit for the safe and effective transport of artemisinin and resveratrol for targeting the intestine *via* the gastrointestinal route. The coating layer protects the GI tract and is confirmed by determining the physical stability of the prepared liposomes in fluids imitating the gastrointestinal environment. The vesicle tends to produce pro-oxidant activity in adenocarcinoma cells in the intestine.

The adenocarcinoma cells lead to cell death by generating reactive oxygen species (ROS). An elevated effect was observed when both drugs were given together [60].

Nanoparticles

Nanoparticles (NPs) are nano-size structures considered a potential carrier for drug delivery to cancerous cells in the colon. The NPs showed good pharmacokinetics, target specificity, lower side effects, and lesser evidence of drug resistance [61, 62]. The NP can be made from noble metals, such as gold and silver; platinum plays a challenging role in preparing biosensors, which shows high precision and sensitivity in diagnosing different ailments [63]. Gold nanoparticles (AuNPs) are gaining lots of interest in the last decades, and their use in cancer diagnosis is increasing daily. The AuNPs enables imaging in near-infrared imaging systems by surface plasma resonance [47, 64].

Inorganic materials are used to synthesize nanoparticles. Commonly gold, iron, and silica are used to prepare the NPs. These nanomaterials can be formulated and structured in different sizes and geometries. These NPs possess unique electrical, physical and optical properties because of their base materials [65].

The NPs in colon cancer need to be target-specific and designed based on the type of tumors. Targeting can be achieved with ligands attached to the surface of NPs. Ligands help to localize and internalize the drug or drug complex inside the cellular structure, where the drug is released and leads to cell death [66]. The NPs also improve drug permeability, retention, and accumulation at the target tumor site [67]. Target specificity helps identify the tumor cell and hit the tumor cell without affecting normal cells. The specificity can be achieved by making biomimetic NPs using biological stimuli or alterations in tumor cells [68].

Rayan Sabra *et al.* developed NPs containing cetuximab conjugated with modified citrus pectin for targeted delivery of curcumin to treat cancer in the colon region. The prepared NPs were evaluated and found to have a spherical shape in the nano range with relatively good encapsulation efficiency and drug profile. The outer surface of NPs was covered with 61.37% of cetuximab. The prepared structure shows you improved internalization in $CaCO_2$ cells and causes a decrease in cancer cell propagation. The citrus pectin conjugated NPs cause complete cell cycle disruption, indicating that the prepared nanostructure is efficient in drug targeting [69].

Cancer needs a specific targeted treatment to inhibit the growth of the tumor cell. Targeting the drug is the major challenge for chemotherapy. To achieve the targeting effect, different ligands were tried by other researchers. In the study,

Camptothecin (CPT) was loaded in NPs, and the surface of NPs is further functionalized with chondroitin sulfate on the surface. The structure has a desirable diameter in the nm range and low PDI index, *i.e.,* 0.192, and shows a neutral charge on the surface. *In vitro* studies revealed that the functionalization on the surface with chondroitin sulfate helps NPs be delivered to colon cancer cells by targeting it to colon cells and increasing the anti-cancer activities in the colon. It also gives pro-apoptosis against cancer cells in the colon and produces low toxicity [70].

Targeting different organelles is achieved by different uptake routes. The nanostructure can be surface functionalized for targeting specific surface receptors. Apart from surface functionalization, targeting also depends on the structure's shape, size, and aggregation [64]. Inorganic nanomaterials are easily uptaken by phagocytic cells and cleared from the body. PEGylation is used to avoid NPs entrapment in the RES environment by increasing the retention period of metallic NPs. The study presents the formulation of AuNPs, which are PEGylated, to increase the circulation time of the drug system. The prepared PEGylated structure was loaded with doxorubicin (DOX) and Kaempferol by hydrogen bond by electrostatic interaction to treat cancer cells in the colon. The ready form shows a synergistic effect in targeting and killing capacity to cancer cells in the colon compared to the plain drug [71].

In the study conducted by Pan *et al.*, the NPs were formulated by complexing DOX with hyaluronic acid. The *in vitro* studies revealed that on intravenous injection, high drug complex accumulation occurs in the intestine and resides there for 24 hrs. When the hyaluronic acid- Drug complex is given intravenously, it maintains the integrity of the epithelial mucosal lining of the intestine colon cancer-induced mice model. Furthermore, the prepared complex helps decrease the inflammatory marker and apoptotic in the intestine. The results indicate that hyaluronic acid and DOX complex inhibits colorectal cancer growth and progression without affecting the normal cells (72].

The NPs also help in delivering the specific gene to the colon region. A polyelectrolyte complex was formulated, including hyaluronate, alginate, and dextran sulfate as negative parts, trimethyl chitosan, and polysaccharides as positive. The NPs were optimized by primary screening and then with the D-optimal technique. The *in vitro* study using MCF7 cell lines indicates higher uptake by cell lines and lower toxicity of prepared polyelectrolyte NPs. The NPs showed higher cellular uptake by cancer cells and lower accumulation in different organs. The formulated polyelectrolyte structure indicates safe delivery and a more efficient colon cancer system for gene delivery [73].

Self-nano Emulsifying Drug Delivery System

The self-nano emulsifying drug delivery system, commonly abbreviated as SNEDDS, comprises oil, surfactant, and co-surfactant. It is an anhydrous nanoemulsion formulation with a globule size of 300 nm. SNEDDS system can be formulated by mixing oil with water to prepare oil in the water-stable emulsion. When administered in the body, the peristaltic movement in the gastrointestinal tract causes the emulsification of the oil droplets with GI fluids [74]. In the GI tract, submicron level globules were formed, which causes increased surface area and improves the absorption of the drug, leading to better bioavailability. The system helps to formulate the delivery system for hydrophobic drug molecules. The excipients also help in the intestinal permeability of water-insoluble drugs.

SNEDDS is gaining popularity in recent times and also addresses the solubility problem of the drug. The system is becoming the system of choice to deliver peptide and protein drugs [75]. It also helps protect the water-soluble drug from the GI environment, which adds to the system's popularity [76]. High mucus penetration, smaller droplet size, and protection from protease increase the interest of researchers in this delivery system [77]. The nanoemulsion *in vitro* system was formed by adding an aqueous phase with gentle stirring. When instilled in the body, the formulation gets prepared to have a smaller droplet size, which ranges from 20-200 nm, produced by the peristaltic movement of the gastrointestinal tract [78]. SNEDDS has a significantly smaller globule size in the nano range, with a high surface area, which could improve drug absorption and enhance bioavailability by increasing drug release and membrane permeation [79].

Curcumin is a flavonoid used for decades to treat various ailments, including cancer. In the research work, SNEDDS was prepared using curcumin for colon targeting. Nanoemulsion was designed with curcumin by a SNEDDS incorporated in tablets and further coated with pectin. The prepared formulation was elevated with tests, including *in vitro* dissolution and cell lines study. Capmul MCM and Labrafac PG added as surfactant and co-surfactant show a more significant impact on the solubility of curcumin and then converted into nano-droplets. Formulations were prepared and converted into tablets and then coated with pectin. The *in vitro* release showed 80% drug release at pH 6.8. The cell line studies show that the amount of targeted drug is compared to more than plain drug [80].

In one of the studies, SNEDDS was formulated, and the drug Genkwanin was entrapped in the emulsion. The prepared formulation has high solubility and improved permeability, enhancing the drug's bioavailability. The *in vivo* study shows anti-colitis activity associated with colon cancer. SNEEDS was formulated using oil, surfactant, and co-surfactant in proper proportion. The optimized formulation was selected based on saturated solubility by constructing a pseudo-ternary phase diagram. The formulation is also optimized based on other parameters such as emulsification efficacy, thermodynamic stability, droplet size, self-nano emulsification time, drug release, transmission electron microscopy (TEM), and intestinal permeability. Mice models were used to study colon cancer-associated anti-colitis, and its mechanism was observed using a cancer-induced model. The formulation is formulated using different ratios of Labrasol ALF, Transcutol HP, and Ma Maisine CC. The optimized formulation was selected based on nano-droplet size, fast release, good stability, and high solubility and permeability. The formulation helps control the release of inflammatory cytokinin levels and reduces the chances of tumor formation by apoptosis by tumor cells in the mice model [81].

Carbon Nanotubes

Carbon nanotubes (CNTs) are allotropes of carbon and are considered one of the novel nanoparticles used to treat cancer. CNTs are available in three main types: single-walled carbon nanotubes (SWCNTs), double-walled carbon nanotubes (DWCNTs), and multi-walled carbon nanotubes (MWCNTs) [82]. CNT is considered a suitable carrier for the diagnosis and treatment of cancer. CNTs possess unique optical, physical, and mechanical characteristics that differentiate them from other nanocarriers. It includes more surfaces and leads to high drug encapsulation [83]. The newer system and unique properties attracted the focus of many researchers. Some are working on *in vitro* studies, while others, Kesharwani *et al.*, studied the efficiency of CNTs on cell lines [84]. CNTs are insoluble in water which renders them inefficient for delivering the drug. The functionalization of CNTs with different kind of molecules make them a suitable candidate for drug delivery. CNTs are produced by various chemical, physical, and other techniques [85]. CNTs possess cytotoxicities ad reported by many researchers. Apart from cytotoxicity, water insolubility is also another major problem. To improve water insolubility, functionalization with different chemical groups is done. CNTs are highly permeable to cells and even get access to the nucleus, making the targeted delivery considerable for CNTs [86].

In one of the studies, hyaluronic acid is used to tag the SWCNTs, and the structure is coated with chlorine. The prepared nanocomposite was evaluated using UV spectroscopy, Fourier transforms electron microscopy (FTIR), X-ray diffraction analysis (XRD), and particle size and zeta potential analysis. Toxicity studies and loading efficiency were determined using cell line studies. The cytotoxic assay was performed to determine the toxicity studies, and cellular changes were observed after 24 hrs by microscopy, and annexin propidium iodide was used to assess cell death. The new structure prepared helps to enhance the ability of PDT to be used as a photosensitizer carrier and causes the death of cancer cells in the colon [87].

In another study, CNTs were functionalized with DOX and fluorescein. The toxicity of newly functionalized structures was studied at the cellular and organ level. The balb2/c mice model was used to analyze the cytotoxic effect of different functionalized structures. The drug gets immobilized on the outer surface of CNTs, and its release is controlled from the surface of the nanotube structure. Cytotoxicity is also less compared to pure drugs.

CNT surface gets associated with cell structure, and breaking bonds with CNT surface leads to drug release. This increases the cytotoxic effect of DOX and CNTs in a dose-dependent manner. The synergetic cytotoxic effect was studied on tumor cells due to the release of CNTs, DOX, and trypsin. DOX-CNT showed low toxicity when compared with pure drugs by a cytotoxic study. The synergistic effect of CNTs and DOX helps achieve higher efficacy and more excellent tumor suppression action [88].

Polymeric Nanoparticles

Polymers help control the transportation and release of the drug in a controlled manner from the delivery system made up of polymeric matrix to the surrounding environment. Drug delivery can be achieved by cellular uptake, extracellular penetration, and intracellular release [89, 90]. The goal is to bring the drug component to the tumor tissue without impairing its effects. Tumor vasculature is leaky and can affect the lymphatic system, enhancing permeability and retention. The NP can be passively targeted to tumor cells [91]. Different uptake mechanisms include TAT-mediated transduction, receptor-mediated endocytosis, and tumor pH-triggered non-specific endocytosis. The drug is uptaken by the cell and released inside the cell based on the tumor cells' pH making a tumor-responsive drug release system [92]. Tumor cells have less pH and promote hypoxia inside the tumor cells, which causes an acidic environment in the tumor cell, rendering lower pH of the cell. The pH-sensitive NP comprises polymers designed by Dandekar and coworkers containing curcumin, an anti-cancer drug. The results showed that polymer gets solubilized at the pH of the colon and helps to release entrapped drugs [93]. Drug release from polymer can occur through diffusion *via* water-filled pores, through matrix formed by polymer, erosion, and osmotic release. The critical parameters for optimum efficiency are the size and shape of NPs; surface ligands govern the targeting and therapeutic efficiency. The study conducted by different researchers reveals that circulation time can be increased by hydrophilic surface, and cellular uptake can be improved by applying a positive charge on the surface of the polymeric structure [68].

Polymeric NPs can be given by systemic route and delivered specifically. These nanostructures can sustain within the bloodstream for a long time so that drugs can be diffused continuously in the blood. Bhattacharya *et al.* formulated nanoparticles with docetaxel (DTX) containing (ethylene glycol) and poly(sarcosine), and the structure is coated further with PLGA. This nanostructure can easily encapsulate hydrophobic drugs in the PEGylated nanostructure. This structure can easily bypass the RES system and bypass microphagic opsonization. The newer construction increases the bioavailability and enhances the distribution of the drug to the target tissues. The cellular uptake of DTX and loaded polymeric NPs was evaluated in different cell lines. The PEGylated NPs show the most negligible macrophage uptake and have a long-circulating time [94].

Anti-cancer therapy is ineffective and has severe side effects; the study is designed to formulate the delivery system for colon cancer. PEGylated gold nanomaterial containing DOX with Kaempferol was prepared to deliver the drug to colon cancer cells. Drug release behavior is observed at different pH. It is observed that prepared Dox nanostructure is more efficient in producing a cytotoxic effect than free drugs. The study indicates a reduced tumor cell volume without severe side effects [95].

Dendrimers

Dendrimers are a novel and promising carrier system for the delivery of the drug to cancer cells. Dendrimers are similar polymeric components with unique properties and vast structural differences. These are the spherical structure with different generations based on concentric layers on them. Dendrimers have a complex structure with the core at the center and branches starting from the core with repetitive units. The structure grows geometrically in a concentric layer known as the generation of dendrimers. The outer surface of dendrimers is engineered with different functional groups [96]. Dendrimers can be employed to target the drug to cancerous cells by doing surface modifications helping the drug accumulate at target sites, and helping in diagnostic monitoring of the cancer cells and the progression of treatment. The target specificity will reduce the severe side effects due to anti-cancer drugs [97]. Dendrimer can also be utilized for diagnostic purposes by tagging with a suitable agent. Due to the enormous advantages of dendrimer structure, these structures are gaining much attention in the field of cancer [98].

A dendrimer is a newer type of nanostructure with numerous advantages. These highly branched polymers can incorporate or conjugate different moieties or drugs in their complex structure. PAMAM dendrimers are suitable for many applications of tissue engineering, materials science, regenerative medicine, and biotechnology. It is the most popular kind of nanomaterial and gained many researchers' attention [40]. Dendrimers' control structure makes the structure ideal in biomedical and diagnostic applications. Dendrimers' major drawback is their toxicity due to peripheral charge density. The toxicity can be reduced considerably by surface modifications and easily removed from the body through the kidney [99]. The size of the nanomaterial governs the residence of the structure. Based on the study, low generation, such as 0.5G, undergoes rapid clearance and facile elimination from the kidney. Higher-generation or PEGylated dendrimers tend to increase the circulation time and uniform distribution in the body. But the study shows that it is not efficiently transported across the BB barrier. They are quickly cleared through the kidney and found to accumulate in the tubular cell of the kidney [100].

The biodistribution studies were conducted for PAMAM dendrimers labeled with D-Cy5 and studied. The prepared dendrimers were injected in healthy rabbits on the fifth day of their birth; it was observed that there was the highest accumulation of dendrimer in the kidneys and bladder; when G4 dendrimers undergo clearance, injected dose of the G4 dendrimer over 24 h from the neonates of rabbits. Dendrimers have internal space to trap the molecules of the drug and deliver the drug intracellularly. It also has a surface function group, so the structure can be conjugated on its surface [96].

PAMAM dendrimers were conjugated with a Slex antibody to bind and capture colon cancer cells. UV spectroscopy and atomic force microscopy are used to study conjugation. Flow cytometry and microscopy analyzed the cellular uptake of dendrimers coated with a Slex in HT29 cells. The cells show maximum capture efficiency with 1 hr exposure, and capture occurs dose-dependently [101]. Sixth-generation dendrimers are conjugated with a Slex, and FITC has high capture efficiency. The cell internalization study was done on HT 29 cells when the HT29 cells were diluted to a low concentration. The activity causes a reduction of cell activity in a concentration-dependent manner. The formulated dendrimers structure with a Slex coating has high potential in controlling and restraining CTC in the blood [101, 102].

Pishavar *et al.* changed PAMAM G5-cholesteryl chloroformate structure and handled it with alkyl-PEG to administer DOX and a plasmid encoding TRAIL to cancer cells in the colon. Encapsulation results revealed that the drug's high loading capacity is observed with structure and has a high anti-tumor effect when DOX is loaded on the M-PAMAM dendrimers complex with TRAIL plasmid. *In vivo* study in mice with C26 colon cancer cells shows a decrease in tumor growth rate. These modified structures efficiently deliver both the drug and the genes to the cancer cells [103].

Dendrimers are macromolecules with a high molecular weight with a high positive charge valid for the protection and condensation of a nucleic acid structure known as the proton sponge effect [104]. PAMAM dendrimers in unmodified form show toxicity, which reduces their clinical applications. The cytotoxicity can be reduced by introducing different functional groups or attaching polymer structures to their surface. It also improves biocompatibility and cytotoxicity. Additional components can be added to the structure, such as chondroitin sulfate, poly(ethylene glycol), hyaluronate, and folic acid [105]. PAMAM has a primary amine group on its surface; an approach was developed in which cholesteryl chloroformate and alkylate PEG were attached to the primary amine group of PAMAM dendrimer G generation. Different parameters such as cellular apoptosis rate, cytotoxicity, organ toxicity, and anti-tumor efficiency were studied in DOX-loaded PAMAM modified structure and TRAIL plasmid [103].

The research was done on gabapentin for colon cancer tumor cells. Cancer in the colon is induced by azoxymethane which is a cancer-causing agent. The model was used to study PAMAM dendrimers' effect loaded with capecitabine and to observe the toxicity in different organs, including the liver, bone marrow, *etc.* In addition, the structure was prepared and evaluated for other parameters, and drug encapsulation efficiency was also calculated. The capecitabine-loaded dendrimers were found to reduce tumor size and have lesser side effects than pure drugs [106].

SMART DRUG DELIVERY SYSTEMS

According to the estimation of the most common cancers expected in the United States in 2014-15, the most common cancers among men will be the prostate (about 1/4 of new diagnoses cancers), followed by respiratory organ and colorectal cancers. Common cancer in women is breast, followed by respiratory organ and colorectal [29]. Diagnosis is undoubtedly the first and most crucial step in cancer therapy. Surgery to remove cancer cells is the first therapeutic option for patients with solid tumors. Afterward, the area is irradiated to release any cancer cells' slightest remnant. Simultaneously or later, chemotherapy can help destroy cancer cells and retard metastases [107].

Conventional anti-cancer therapies are non-specifically distributed in the body and destroy cancerous and well as non-cancerous cells. This involves the use of suboptimal treatment to prevent excessive toxicities. Most drugs are hydrophobic and face problems in absorption, and in the case of soluble, it is tough to find the path and reach the target organ. Moreover, the multiple and interconnected pathways of carcinogenesis complicate drug delivery to target sites. Therefore, considerable change is needed to design therapies for specific cancer phenotypes [108]. While the search for new strategies for cancer therapy continues, it becomes increasingly evident that targeted nano-vehicles intended to achieve the particular organ are essential to formulate an effective treatment. The most significant advantage of applying nano-medicines in cancer is the delivery system's ability to create a nanostructure that can be translocated inside the call structure and increases the delivery system's efficiency. The benefits of developing nanoparticles as drug-delivery systems include enhancing pharmacological activity, delivery of one or more therapeutic agents for combination therapy, and solubility of drugs [109].

Malignancies have a characteristic change in blood flow with leaky vasculature, lower pH in cancer cells, and expression of specific enzymes. Hence, these stimuli can target the drugs to the cancerous cells. The novel stimuli-sensitive system will also help differentiate cancerous cells from no cancerous cells [110]. Every kind of tumor can generate specific stimuli, making the nanocarrier more efficient and responding to the triggered stimuli. Different stimuli, such as pH, temperature, redox, enzymes, and the proteins generated by specific tumors, can be utilized. To target individual cells and distribute medications on demand rather than in a steady supply, external stimuli such as oscillating magnetic fields, ultrasound waves, illumination, and electric fields are used [111].

The molecules can be incorporated in the particle-matrix— stability and bioavailability (designing NPs with desired surface properties and nano-size to enhance the blood circulation time. These NPs could also improve the protection from toxicity and physical and chemical degradation, sustained delivery, the feasibility of variable routes of administration, facilitation of the drug transport across cellular barriers, *etc* [112]. Engineering materials on this scale allow for novel medical therapies, which can release the loaded drug to the target tissue site in a regulated manner, improving the specificity and decreasing side effects for patients. Another objective is to overcome the development of multiple drug resistance mechanisms, making the treatment less effective in a higher percentage of cancer cases because cancer cells can bypass cytotoxicity [113].

P-glycoprotein (P-gp) is the best-known and highly investigated mechanism of drug resistance. Upon entering the cell, NPs are involved in an endosome, allowing them to gather in the cancer cells without identifying the P-gp efflux pump, resulting in a higher intracellular concentration of the drug. These receptor targeting approaches target a specific cell by receptor-mediated endocytosis and have a high potential to avoid drug resistance [114].

Thus, a folate receptor-targeted, transferring conjugated PTX-loaded nanoparticles and pH-sensitive DOX polymeric micelles showed high inhibitory activity, and reduces drug-resistant in MCF-7 cells compared to without tagged free counterparts. Anti-cancer nano-medicines require the integration of drugs into intelligent nanoparticles. Diverse platforms can deliver one or more drugs in a single approach for a synergistic effect. These platforms are submicron-sized particles (10-1000 nm in diameter), systems, or artificial devices made by different kinds of materials such as lipids, polymers, viruses, or organometallic compounds [115].

Moreover, all nanoparticles based on a ligand-based system can translocate and deliver the drug to the target site or location. They can be classified by their physical form or functional properties, which should be adapted to the drug's specific needs to be delivered and the intended therapeutic use. Although nano-medicine emerged as a new science area, many new intelligent nanoparticles have been developed over the past three decades for drug delivery. These platforms are generally classified into the following categories: polymer-based drug carriers, Liposomes, virus-containing NPs, CNTs, ceramic NPs, and metal-based NPs [116]

Stimuli-sensitive nanogels were formulated by polymerization methodology without surfactant. The PEG methacrylate and N,N′-diethylamino ethyl methacrylate were used to prepare the cationic stimuli-oriented nanogels. The nanogel is characterized by different parameters such as size, PDI index and concludes that spherical structure is formed with core-shell morphology. The structure was also confirmed by electron microscopy and dynamic light scattering. The specific cross-linker can make nanogel responsive to different tumors, such as redox, temperature, or pH. The nanogel is formulated by cross-linking bis(acryloyl)cystamine and incubated with glutathione at pH 7.4; buffer tends to degrade in 60 minutes, while divinylacetal cross-linked nanogels degrade in 10 minutes at pH 6 or less. The nanogel structure is stable under different physiological conditions and showed a synergistic effect in the human colon cancer cell [117].

Magnetic NPs were generated mimicking MamC coupled with Oxa, demonstrated to reduce the IC_{50} compared to soluble Oxa. Oxa-BMNPs nanostructures were coated with phosphatidylcholine unilamellar liposomes. PEGylated and non-PEGylated assemblies were constructed. The result indicates that lipid covering helps to increase biocompatibility and cellular uptake. PEGylation further adds to its effects. The cytotoxic effect in colon cancer is not changed while targeting efficiency [118].

CONCLUSION

Cancer is the primary concern of the newer, fast-going, and developed world. Different approaches are used to treat cancer, but none prove their efficacy or specificity. The current chemotherapy is non-specific and targets both cancerous and non-cancerous cells, and results in severe adverse effects. Nanotechnology-based drug delivery system has put forward a new path to deliver the drug at target sites without affecting the non-cancerous cell. As a consequence, multiple methods are developed to render the treatment successful and precise. Nanotechnology is the base for future medicine and diagnostics in cancer research. It has a revolutionary and ice-breaking approach to the treatment of cancer. This kind of system can improve biodistribution, and pharmacokinetics and reduce adverse effects. Targeting specific organ and tissue uptake can be upgraded entirely by the nanotechnological approach to drug delivery. The nanocarriers can upload the drug, deliver it to the target site, and reduce its adverse effects. Thus nanocarriers are considered a novel medicine system for the future.

CONSENT FOR PUBLICATION

Not applicable.

CONFLICT OF INTEREST

The authors declare no conflict of interest, financial or otherwise.

ACKNOWLEDGEMENT

The authors would like to acknowledge the support of Lovely Professional University for providing the facilities to compile this work.

REFERENCES

[1] Rawla P, Sunkara T, Barsouk A. Epidemiology of colorectal cancer: incidence, mortality, survival, and risk factors. Prz Gastroenterol 2019; 14(2): 89-103. [http://dx.doi.org/10.5114/pg.2018.81072] [PMID: 31616522]

[2] Siegel RL, Torre LA, Soerjomataram I, *et al.* Global patterns and trends in colorectal cancer incidence in young adults. Gut 2019; 68(12): 2179-85. [http://dx.doi.org/10.1136/gutjnl-2019-319511] [PMID: 31488504]

[3] Lee SH, Bajracharya R, Min JY, Han JW, Park BJ, Han HK. Strategic approaches for colon targeted drug delivery: An overview of recent advancements. Pharmaceutics 2020; 12(1): 68. [http://dx.doi.org/10.3390/pharmaceutics12010068] [PMID: 31952340]

[4] Miri A, Darroudi M, Sarani M. Biosynthesis of cerium oxide nanoparticles and its cytotoxicity survey against colon cancer cell line. Appl Organomet Chem 2020; 34(1): e5308. [http://dx.doi.org/10.1002/aoc.5308]

[5] Kateh Shamshiri M, Jaafari MR, Badiee A. Preparation of liposomes containing IFN-gamma and their

potentials in cancer immunotherapy: *In vitro* and *in vivo* studies in a colon cancer mouse model. Life Sci 2021; 264: 118605.
[http://dx.doi.org/10.1016/j.lfs.2020.118605] [PMID: 33096119]

[6] Liu X, Liu Y, Chen X, *et al.* Multi-walled carbon nanotubes exacerbate doxorubicin-induced cardiotoxicity by altering gut microbiota and pulmonary and colonic macrophage phenotype in mice. Toxicology 2020; 435: 152410.
[http://dx.doi.org/10.1016/j.tox.2020.152410] [PMID: 32068018]

[7] Ge P, Niu B, Wu Y, *et al.* Enhanced cancer therapy of celastrol *in vitro* and *in vivo* by smart dendrimers delivery with specificity and biosafety. Chem Eng J 2020; 383: 123228.
[http://dx.doi.org/10.1016/j.cej.2019.123228]

[8] Sethi S, Harikumar SL. Review on advances in colon targeted drug delivery system. Int J Pharm Sci Res 2012; 3(9): 2989.

[9] Hofseth LJ, Hebert JR, Chanda A, *et al.* Early-onset colorectal cancer: initial clues and current views. Nat Rev Gastroenterol Hepatol 2020; 17(6): 352-64.
[http://dx.doi.org/10.1038/s41575-019-0253-4] [PMID: 32086499]

[10] AbouAitah K, Hassan HA, Swiderska-Sroda A, *et al.* Targeted nano-drug delivery of colchicine against colon cancer cells by means of mesoporous silica nanoparticles. Cancers (Basel) 2020; 12(1): 144.
[http://dx.doi.org/10.3390/cancers12010144] [PMID: 31936103]

[11] Bashraheel SS, Domling A, Goda SK. Update on targeted cancer therapies, single or in combination, and their fine tuning for precision medicine. Biomed Pharmacother 2020; 125(110009): 110009.
[http://dx.doi.org/10.1016/j.biopha.2020.110009] [PMID: 32106381]

[12] Dudzisz-Śledź M, Bylina E, Teterycz P, Rutkowski P. Treatment of metastatic gastrointestinal stromal tumors (GIST): A focus on older patients. Drugs Aging 2021; 38(5): 375-96.
[http://dx.doi.org/10.1007/s40266-021-00841-x] [PMID: 33651369]

[13] Chow FCL, Chok KSH. Colorectal liver metastases: An update on multidisciplinary approach. World J Hepatol 2019; 11(2): 150-72.
[http://dx.doi.org/10.4254/wjh.v11.i2.150] [PMID: 30820266]

[14] Xie YH, Chen YX, Fang JY. Comprehensive review of targeted therapy for colorectal cancer. Signal Transduct Target Ther 2020; 5(1): 22.
[http://dx.doi.org/10.1038/s41392-020-0116-z] [PMID: 32296018]

[15] Rajalekshmi M, Shreedhara CS, Lobo R, Rao PP. The review on genetics, epigenetics, risk factors and diagnosis of colon cancer. Research Journal of Pharmacy and Technology 2018; 11(11): 5147-51.
[http://dx.doi.org/10.5958/0974-360X.2018.00940.X]

[16] Kydd J, Jadia R, Velpurisiva P, Gad A, Paliwal S, Rai P. Targeting strategies for the combination treatment of cancer using drug delivery systems. Pharmaceutics 2017; 9(4): 46.
[http://dx.doi.org/10.3390/pharmaceutics9040046] [PMID: 29036899]

[17] Thakkar S, Sharma D, Kalia K, Tekade RK. Tumor microenvironment targeted nanotherapeutics for cancer therapy and diagnosis: A review. Acta Biomater 2020; 101: 43-68.
[http://dx.doi.org/10.1016/j.actbio.2019.09.009] [PMID: 31518706]

[18] Hejmady S, Pradhan R, Alexander A, *et al.* Recent advances in targeted nanomedicine as promising antitumor therapeutics. Drug Discov Today 2020; 25(12): 2227-44.
[http://dx.doi.org/10.1016/j.drudis.2020.09.031] [PMID: 33011342]

[19] Kumar CG, Poornachandra Y, Pombala S. Therapeutic nanomaterials: from a drug delivery perspective InNanostructures for Drug Delivery. Elsevier 2017; pp. 1-61.

[20] Sun Q, Barz M, De Geest BG, *et al.* Nanomedicine and macroscale materials in immuno-oncology. Chem Soc Rev 2019; 48(1): 351-81.
[http://dx.doi.org/10.1039/C8CS00473K] [PMID: 30465669]

[21] Attia MF, Anton N, Wallyn J, Omran Z, Vandamme TF. An overview of active and passive targeting strategies to improve the nanocarriers efficiency to tumour sites. J Pharm Pharmacol 2019; 71(8): 1185-98.
[http://dx.doi.org/10.1111/jphp.13098] [PMID: 31049986]

[22] Hossain MS, Karuniawati H, Jairoun AA, *et al.* Colorectal Cancer: A Review of Carcinogenesis, Global Epidemiology, Current Challenges, Risk Factors, Preventive and Treatment Strategies. Cancers (Basel) 2022; 14(7): 1732.
[http://dx.doi.org/10.3390/cancers14071732] [PMID: 35406504]

[23] Culp MB, Soerjomataram I, Efstathiou JA, Bray F, Jemal A. Recent global patterns in prostate cancer incidence and mortality rates. Eur Urol 2020; 77(1): 38-52.
[http://dx.doi.org/10.1016/j.eururo.2019.08.005] [PMID: 31493960]

[24] Hull R, Francies FZ, Oyomno M, Dlamini Z. Colorectal cancer genetics, incidence and risk factors: in search for targeted therapies. Cancer Manag Res 2020; 12: 9869-82.
[http://dx.doi.org/10.2147/CMAR.S251223] [PMID: 33116845]

[25] Douaiher J, Ravipati A, Grams B, Chowdhury S, Alatise O, Are C. Colorectal cancer-global burden, trends, and geographical variations. J Surg Oncol 2017; 115(5): 619-30.
[http://dx.doi.org/10.1002/jso.24578] [PMID: 28194798]

[26] Ferlay J, Colombet M, Soerjomataram I, *et al.* Estimating the global cancer incidence and mortality in 2018: GLOBOCAN sources and methods. Int J Cancer 2019; 144(8): 1941-53.
[http://dx.doi.org/10.1002/ijc.31937] [PMID: 30350310]

[27] Farinha P, Pinho JO, Matias M, Gaspar MM. Nanomedicines in the treatment of colon cancer: a focus on metallodrugs. Drug Deliv Transl Res 2022; 12(1): 49-66.
[http://dx.doi.org/10.1007/s13346-021-00916-7] [PMID: 33616870]

[28] Brenner H, Chen C. The colorectal cancer epidemic: challenges and opportunities for primary, secondary and tertiary prevention. Br J Cancer 2018; 119(7): 785-92.
[http://dx.doi.org/10.1038/s41416-018-0264-x] [PMID: 30287914]

[29] Siegel RL, Jakubowski CD, Fedewa SA, Davis A, Azad NS. Colorectal cancer in the young: epidemiology, prevention, management. Am Soc Clin Oncol Educ Book 2020; 40(40): e75-88.
[http://dx.doi.org/10.1200/EDBK_279901] [PMID: 32315236]

[30] Nguyen H, Duong HQ. The molecular characteristics of colorectal cancer: Implications for diagnosis and therapy (Review). Oncol Lett 2018; 16(1): 9-18.
[http://dx.doi.org/10.3892/ol.2018.8679] [PMID: 29928381]

[31] Ydy LR, Camarço-Silva WR, Medeiros-Filho WV. A Genetic Perspective on Colorectal Cancer Progression InMultidisciplinary Approach for Colorectal Cancer. IntechOpen 2019.

[32] Kasi A, Handa S, Bhatti S, Umar S, Bansal A, Sun W. Molecular pathogenesis and classification of colorectal carcinoma. Curr Colorectal Cancer Rep 2020; 16(5): 97-106.
[http://dx.doi.org/10.1007/s11888-020-00458-z] [PMID: 32905465]

[33] De Palma F, D'Argenio V, Pol J, Kroemer G, Maiuri M, Salvatore F. The molecular hallmarks of the serrated pathway in colorectal cancer. Cancers (Basel) 2019; 11(7): 1017.
[http://dx.doi.org/10.3390/cancers11071017] [PMID: 31330830]

[34] Fischer J, Walker LC, Robinson BA, Frizelle FA, Church JM, Eglinton TW. Clinical implications of the genetics of sporadic colorectal cancer. ANZ J Surg 2019; 89(10): 1224-9.
[http://dx.doi.org/10.1111/ans.15074] [PMID: 30919552]

[35] Bolhaqueiro ACF, Ponsioen B, Bakker B, *et al.* Ongoing chromosomal instability and karyotype evolution in human colorectal cancer organoids. Nat Genet 2019; 51(5): 824-34.
[http://dx.doi.org/10.1038/s41588-019-0399-6] [PMID: 31036964]

[36] Testa U, Pelosi E, Castelli G. Colorectal cancer: genetic abnormalities, tumor progression, tumor

heterogeneity, clonal evolution and tumor-initiating cells 2018; 6(2): 1-131. [http://dx.doi.org/10.3390/medsci6020031]

[37] Alhmoud JF, Woolley JF, Al Moustafa AE, Malki MI. DNA damage/repair management in cancers. Cancers (Basel) 2020; 12(4): 1050. [http://dx.doi.org/10.3390/cancers12041050] [PMID: 32340362]

[38] Pećina-Šlaus N, Kafka A, Salamon I, Bukovac A. Mismatch repair pathway, genome stability and cancer. Front Mol Biosci 2020; 7: 122. [http://dx.doi.org/10.3389/fmolb.2020.00122] [PMID: 32671096]

[39] Verma R, Sharma PC. Molecular pathogenesis and precision medicine in gastric cancer InPrecision Medicine for Investigators, Practitioners and Providers. Academic Press 2020; pp. 153-65. [http://dx.doi.org/10.1016/B978-0-12-819178-1.00015-0]

[40] Patra JK, Das G, Fraceto LF, *et al.* Nano based drug delivery systems: recent developments and future prospects. J Nanobiotechnology 2018; 16(1): 71. [http://dx.doi.org/10.1186/s12951-018-0392-8] [PMID: 30231877]

[41] El-Sayed A, Kamel M. Advances in nanomedical applications: diagnostic, therapeutic, immunization, and vaccine production. Environ Sci Pollut Res Int 2020; 27(16): 19200-13. [http://dx.doi.org/10.1007/s11356-019-06459-2] [PMID: 31529348]

[42] Zhang Y, Li M, Gao X, Chen Y, Liu T. Nanotechnology in cancer diagnosis: progress, challenges and opportunities. J Hematol Oncol 2019; 12(1): 137. [http://dx.doi.org/10.1186/s13045-019-0833-3] [PMID: 31847897]

[43] Bamburowicz-Klimkowska M, Poplawska M, Grudzinski IP. Nanocomposites as biomolecules delivery agents in nanomedicine. J Nanobiotechnology 2019; 17(1): 48. [http://dx.doi.org/10.1186/s12951-019-0479-x] [PMID: 30943985]

[44] Colone M, Calcabrini A, Stringaro A. Drug delivery systems of natural products in oncology. Molecules 2020; 25(19): 4560. [http://dx.doi.org/10.3390/molecules25194560] [PMID: 33036240]

[45] Han NK, Shin DH, Kim JS, Weon KY, Jang CY, Kim JS. Hyaluronan-conjugated liposomes encapsulating gemcitabine for breast cancer stem cells. Int J Nanomedicine 2016; 11: 1413-25. [http://dx.doi.org/10.2147/IJN.S95850] [PMID: 27103799]

[46] Plaza-Oliver M, Santander-Ortega MJ, Lozano MV. Current approaches in lipid-based nanocarriers for oral drug delivery. Drug Deliv Transl Res 2021; 11(2): 471-97. [http://dx.doi.org/10.1007/s13346-021-00908-7] [PMID: 33528830]

[47] Barani M, Bilal M, Rahdar A, *et al.* Nanodiagnosis and nanotreatment of colorectal cancer: an overview. J Nanopart Res 2021; 23(1): 18. [http://dx.doi.org/10.1007/s11051-020-05129-6]

[48] Zeinali M, Abbaspour-Ravasjani S, Ghorbani M, *et al.* Nanovehicles for co-delivery of anticancer agents. Drug Discov Today 2020; 25(8): 1416-30. [http://dx.doi.org/10.1016/j.drudis.2020.06.027] [PMID: 32622880]

[49] Matole V, Shegaonkar A, Kumbhar S, Thorat Y, Hosmani A. Need of liposomes as a novel drug delivery system. Res J Pharm Dos Forms Technol 2020; 12(4): 285-94. [http://dx.doi.org/10.5958/0975-4377.2020.00047.6]

[50] Singh A, Neupane YR, Shafi S, Mangla B, Kohli K. PEGylated liposomes as an emerging therapeutic platform for oral nanomedicine in cancer therapy: *in vitro* and *in vivo* assessment. J Mol Liq 2020; 303: 112649. [http://dx.doi.org/10.1016/j.molliq.2020.112649]

[51] Mohamed M, Abu Lila AS, Shimizu T, *et al.* PEGylated liposomes: immunological responses. Sci Technol Adv Mater 2019; 20(1): 710-24. [http://dx.doi.org/10.1080/14686996.2019.1627174] [PMID: 31275462]

[52] Jain A, Jain SK. Stimuli-responsive smart liposomes in cancer targeting. Curr Drug Targets 2018; 19(3): 259-70.
[PMID: 26853324]

[53] Yoon HJ, Lee HS, Jung JH, Kim HK, Park JH. Photothermally amplified therapeutic liposomes for effective combination treatment of cancer. ACS Appl Mater Interfaces 2018; 10(7): 6118-23.
[http://dx.doi.org/10.1021/acsami.7b15996] [PMID: 29363943]

[54] Nik ME, Malaekeh-Nikouei B, Amin M, *et al.* Liposomal formulation of Galbanic acid improved therapeutic efficacy of pegylated liposomal Doxorubicin in mouse colon carcinoma. Sci Rep 2019; 9(1): 9527.
[http://dx.doi.org/10.1038/s41598-019-45974-7] [PMID: 31267009]

[55] Moghimipour E, Rezaei M, Ramezani Z, *et al.* Folic acid-modified liposomal drug delivery strategy for tumor targeting of 5-fluorouracil. Eur J Pharm Sci 2018; 114: 166-74.
[http://dx.doi.org/10.1016/j.ejps.2017.12.011] [PMID: 29247686]

[56] Chen H, Pan H, Li P, *et al.* The potential use of novel chitosan-coated deformable liposomes in an ocular drug delivery system. Colloids Surf B Biointerfaces 2016; 143: 455-62.
[http://dx.doi.org/10.1016/j.colsurfb.2016.03.061] [PMID: 27037783]

[57] Zhou F, Xu T, Zhao Y, *et al.* Chitosan-coated liposomes as delivery systems for improving the stability and oral bioavailability of acteoside. Food Hydrocoll 2018; 83: 17-24.
[http://dx.doi.org/10.1016/j.foodhyd.2018.04.040]

[58] Alomrani A, Badran M, Harisa GI, *et al.* The use of chitosan-coated flexible liposomes as a remarkable carrier to enhance the antitumor efficacy of 5-fluorouracil against colorectal cancer. Saudi Pharm J 2019; 27(5): 603-11.
[http://dx.doi.org/10.1016/j.jsps.2019.02.008] [PMID: 31297013]

[59] Xiong M, Lei Q, You X, *et al.* Mannosylated liposomes improve therapeutic effects of paclitaxel in colon cancer models. J Microencapsul 2017; 34(6): 513-21.
[http://dx.doi.org/10.1080/02652048.2017.1339739] [PMID: 28705043]

[60] Caddeo C, Gabriele M, Nácher A, *et al.* Resveratrol and artemisinin eudragit-coated liposomes: A strategy to tackle intestinal tumors. Int J Pharm 2021; 592: 120083.
[http://dx.doi.org/10.1016/j.ijpharm.2020.120083] [PMID: 33197563]

[61] Dadwal A, Baldi A, Kumar Narang R. Nanoparticles as carriers for drug delivery in cancer. Artificial cells, Nanomedicine, and Biotechnology 2018; 46: 295-305.
[http://dx.doi.org/10.1080/21691401.2018.1457039]

[62] Bayda S, Hadla M, Palazzolo S, *et al.* Inorganic nanoparticles for cancer therapy: a transition from lab to clinic. Curr Med Chem 2018; 25(34): 4269-303.
[http://dx.doi.org/10.2174/0929867325666171229141156] [PMID: 29284391]

[63] Sugumaran S, Jamlos MF, Ahmad MN, Bellan CS, Schreurs D. Nanostructured materials with plasmonic nanobiosensors for early cancer detection: A past and future prospect. Biosens Bioelectron 2018; 100: 361-73.
[http://dx.doi.org/10.1016/j.bios.2017.08.044] [PMID: 28946108]

[64] Elahi N, Kamali M, Baghersad MH. Recent biomedical applications of gold nanoparticles: A review. Talanta 2018; 184: 537-56.
[http://dx.doi.org/10.1016/j.talanta.2018.02.088] [PMID: 29674080]

[65] Yajan P, Yulianto N, Saba M, *et al.* Intracellular gold nanoparticles influence light scattering and facilitate amplified spontaneous emission generation. J Colloid Interface Sci 2022; 622: 914-23.
[http://dx.doi.org/10.1016/j.jcis.2022.04.149] [PMID: 35561611]

[66] Chen Y, Wu Q, Song L, *et al.* Polymeric micelles encapsulating fisetin improve the therapeutic effect in colon cancer. ACS Appl Mater Interfaces 2015; 7(1): 534-42.
[http://dx.doi.org/10.1021/am5066893] [PMID: 25495760]

[67] Kalyane D, Raval N, Maheshwari R, Tambe V, Kalia K, Tekade RK. Employment of enhanced permeability and retention effect (EPR): Nanoparticle-based precision tools for targeting of therapeutic and diagnostic agent in cancer. Mater Sci Eng C 2019; 98: 1252-76. [http://dx.doi.org/10.1016/j.msec.2019.01.066] [PMID: 30813007]

[68] You X, Kang Y, Hollett G, *et al.* Polymeric nanoparticles for colon cancer therapy: overview and perspectives. J Mater Chem B Mater Biol Med 2016; 4(48): 7779-92. [http://dx.doi.org/10.1039/C6TB01925K] [PMID: 32263770]

[69] Sabra R, Billa N, Roberts CJ. Cetuximab-conjugated chitosan-pectinate (modified) composite nanoparticles for targeting colon cancer. Int J Pharm 2019; 572: 118775. [http://dx.doi.org/10.1016/j.ijpharm.2019.118775] [PMID: 31678385]

[70] Zu M, Ma L, Zhang X, Xie D, Kang Y, Xiao B. Chondroitin sulfate-functionalized polymeric nanoparticles for colon cancer-targeted chemotherapy. Colloids Surf B Biointerfaces 2019; 177: 399-406. [http://dx.doi.org/10.1016/j.colsurfb.2019.02.031] [PMID: 30785037]

[71] Meena KS, Sonia K. Doxorubicin loaded nanoparticle consisting of chitosan and mannose modified graphene oxide for intracellular drug delivery and anti-tumor activity. International Journal of Pharmaceutical Sciences and Nanotechnology 2020; 13(5): 5155-64. [http://dx.doi.org/10.37285/ijpsn.2020.13.5.13]

[72] Pan DC, Krishnan V, Salinas AK, *et al.* Hyaluronic acid-doxorubicin nanoparticles for targeted treatment of colorectal cancer. Bioeng Transl Med 2020; 6(1): e10166. [PMID: 33532580]

[73] Baghaei M, Tekie FSM, Khoshayand MR, *et al.* Optimization of chitosan-based polyelectrolyte nanoparticles for gene delivery, using design of experiment: *in vitro* and *in vivo* study. Mater Sci Eng C 2021; 118: 111036. [http://dx.doi.org/10.1016/j.msec.2020.111036] [PMID: 33254955]

[74] Gupta S, Kesarla R, Omri A. Formulation strategies to improve the bioavailability of poorly absorbed drugs with special emphasis on self-emulsifying systems. ISRN Pharm 2013; 2013: 1-16. [http://dx.doi.org/10.1155/2013/848043] [PMID: 24459591]

[75] Park H, Ha ES, Kim MS. Current status of supersaturable self-emulsifying drug delivery systems 2020; 12(4): 365, 1-57. [http://dx.doi.org/10.3390/pharmaceutics12040365]

[76] Efiana NA, Phan TNQ, Wicaksono AJ, Bernkop- Schnürch A. Mucus permeating self-emulsifying drug delivery systems (SEDDS): About the impact of mucolytic enzymes. Colloids Surf B Biointerfaces 2018; 161: 228-35. [http://dx.doi.org/10.1016/j.colsurfb.2017.10.032] [PMID: 29080507]

[77] Kumar R, Aadil KR, Ranjan S, Kumar VB. Advances in nanotechnology and nanomaterials based strategies for neural tissue engineering. J Drug Deliv Sci Technol 2020; 57: 101617. [http://dx.doi.org/10.1016/j.jddst.2020.101617]

[78] Shaker DS, Ishak RA, Ghoneim A, Elhuoni MA. Nanoemulsion: A review on mechanisms for the transdermal delivery of hydrophobic and hydrophilic drugs. Scientia Pharmaceutica 2019; 87(3): 17, 1-34. [http://dx.doi.org/10.3390/scipharm87030017]

[79] Hua S. Physiological and pharmaceutical considerations for rectal drug formulations. Front Pharmacol 2019; 10: 1196. [http://dx.doi.org/10.3389/fphar.2019.01196] [PMID: 31680970]

[80] Karthika CH, Sureshkumar RA, Suhail AM. Formulation development and *in vitro* evaluation of curcumin-loaded solid selfnanoemulsifying drug delivery system for colon carcinoma. Asian J Pharm Clin Res 2019; 12(7): 243-7.

[http://dx.doi.org/10.22159/ajpcr.2019.v12i7.33231]

[81] Yin HF, Yin CM, Ouyang T, *et al.* Self-nanoemulsifying drug delivery system of Genkwanin: A novel approach for anti-colitis-associated colorectal cancer. Drug Des Devel Ther 2021; 15: 557-76. [http://dx.doi.org/10.2147/DDDT.S292417] [PMID: 33603345]

[82] Anzar N, Hasan R, Tyagi M, Yadav N, Narang J. Carbon nanotube - A review on Synthesis, Properties and plethora of applications in the field of biomedical science. Sensors International 2020; 1: 100003. [http://dx.doi.org/10.1016/j.sintl.2020.100003]

[83] Suttee A, Mishra V, Singh M, Nayak P, Sriram P. Carbon nanotubes as emerging nanocarriers in drug delivery: An overview. Int J Pharmaceut Clin Res 2020; 11(03): 373-8.

[84] Kesharwani P, Mishra V, Jain NK. Validating the anticancer potential of carbon nanotube-based therapeutics through cell line testing. Drug Discov Today 2015; 20(9): 1049-60. [http://dx.doi.org/10.1016/j.drudis.2015.05.004] [PMID: 25997997]

[85] Rajaram DS. Carbon nanotubes an advanced drug delivery system – A review. Int J Pharm Sci Res 2020; 11(8): 3636-44.

[86] Chen Z, Zhang A, Wang X, *et al.* The advances of carbon nanotubes in cancer diagnostics and therapeutics. J Nanomater 2017; 2017: 1-13. [http://dx.doi.org/10.1155/2017/3418932]

[87] Pandey P, Dahiya M. Carbon nanotubes: Types, methods of preparation and applications. Carbon 2016; 1(4): 15-21.

[88] Perepelytsina OM, Ugnivenko AP, Dobrydnev AV, Bakalinska ON, Marynin AI, Sydorenko MV. Influence of carbon nanotubes and its derivatives on tumor cells *in vitro* and biochemical parameters, cellular blood composition *in vivo*. Nanoscale Res Lett 2018; 13(1): 286. [http://dx.doi.org/10.1186/s11671-018-2689-9] [PMID: 30209630]

[89] Deng C, Jiang Y, Cheng R, Meng F, Zhong Z. Biodegradable polymeric micelles for targeted and controlled anticancer drug delivery: Promises, progress and prospects. Nano Today 2012; 7(5): 467-80. [http://dx.doi.org/10.1016/j.nantod.2012.08.005]

[90] Meng F, Cheng R, Deng C, Zhong Z. Intracellular drug release nanosystems. Mater Today 2012; 15(10): 436-42. [http://dx.doi.org/10.1016/S1369-7021(12)70195-5]

[91] Wang AZ, Langer R, Farokhzad OC. Nanoparticle delivery of cancer drugs. Annu Rev Med 2012; 63(1): 185-98. [http://dx.doi.org/10.1146/annurev-med-040210-162544] [PMID: 21888516]

[92] Senapati S, Mahanta AK, Kumar S, Maiti P. Controlled drug delivery vehicles for cancer treatment and their performance. Signal Transduct Target Ther 2018; 3(1): 7. [http://dx.doi.org/10.1038/s41392-017-0004-3] [PMID: 29560283]

[93] Prajakta D, Ratnesh J, Chandan K, *et al.* Curcumin loaded pH-sensitive nanoparticles for the treatment of colon cancer. J Biomed Nanotechnol 2009; 5(5): 445-55. [http://dx.doi.org/10.1166/jbn.2009.1038] [PMID: 20201417]

[94] Bhattacharya S. Fabrication of poly(sarcosine), poly (ethylene glycol), and poly (lactic-co-glycolic acid) polymeric nanoparticles for cancer drug delivery. J Drug Deliv Sci Technol 2021; 61(102194): 102194. [http://dx.doi.org/10.1016/j.jddst.2020.102194]

[95] Meena D, Vimala K, Kannan S. Combined Delivery of DOX and Kaempferol using PEGylated Gold Nanoparticles to Target Colon Cancer. J Cluster Sci 2022; 33(1): 173-87. [http://dx.doi.org/10.1007/s10876-020-01961-x]

[96] Carvalho MR, Reis RL, Oliveira JM. Dendrimer nanoparticles for colorectal cancer applications. J

Mater Chem B Mater Biol Med 2020; 8(6): 1128-38.
[http://dx.doi.org/10.1039/C9TB02289A] [PMID: 31971528]

[97] Rajani C, Borisa P, Karanwad T, *et al.* Cancer-targeted chemotherapy: Emerging role of the folate anchored dendrimer as drug delivery nanocarrier InPharmaceutical Applications of Dendrimers. Elsevier 2020; pp. 151-98.

[98] Sk UH, Kojima C. Dendrimers for theranostic applications. Biomol Concepts 2015; 6(3): 205-17.
[http://dx.doi.org/10.1515/bmc-2015-0012] [PMID: 26136305]

[99] Chis AA, Dobrea C, Morgovan C, *et al.* Applications and limitations of dendrimers in biomedicine 2020; 25(17).
[http://dx.doi.org/10.3390/molecules25173982]

[100] Barraza LF, Jiménez VA, Alderete JB. Effect of PEGylation on the structure and drug loading capacity of PAMAM-G4 dendrimers: A molecular modeling approach on the complexation of 5-fluorouracil with native and PEGylated PAMAM-G4. Macromol Chem Phys 2015; 216(16): 1689-701.
[http://dx.doi.org/10.1002/macp.201500179]

[101] Xie J, Wang J, Chen H, *et al.* Multivalent conjugation of antibody to dendrimers for the enhanced capture and regulation on colon cancer cells. Sci Rep 2015; 5(1): 9445.
[http://dx.doi.org/10.1038/srep09445] [PMID: 25819426]

[102] Xie J, Zhao R, Gu S, *et al.* The architecture and biological function of dual antibody-coated dendrimers: enhanced control of circulating tumor cells and their hetero-adhesion to endothelial cells for metastasis prevention. Theranostics 2014; 4(12): 1250-63.
[http://dx.doi.org/10.7150/thno.8775] [PMID: 25285173]

[103] Pishavar E, Attaranzadeh A, Alibolandi M, Ramezani M, Hashemi M. Modified PAMAM vehicles for effective TRAIL gene delivery to colon adenocarcinoma: in vitro and in vivo evaluation. Artificial cells, Nanomedicine, and Biotechnology 2018; 46: 503-13.

[104] Golkar N, Samani SM, Tamaddon AM. Cholesterol-conjugated supramolecular assemblies of low generations polyamidoamine dendrimers for enhanced EGFP plasmid DNA transfection. J Nanopart Res 2016; 18(5): 107.
[http://dx.doi.org/10.1007/s11051-016-3413-2]

[105] Tarach P, Janaszewska A. Recent advances in preclinical research using PAMAM dendrimers for cancer gene therapy. Int J Mol Sci 2021; 22(6): 2912.
[http://dx.doi.org/10.3390/ijms22062912] [PMID: 33805602]

[106] Nabavizadeh F, Fanaei H, Imani A, *et al.* Evaluation of nanocarrier targeted drug delivery of Capecitabine-PAMAM dendrimer complex in a mice colorectal cancer model. Acta Med Iran 2016; 54(8): 485-93.
[PMID: 27701718]

[107] Oyen WJG, Bodei L, Giammarile F, *et al.* Targeted therapy in nuclear medicine—current status and future prospects. Ann Oncol 2007; 18(11): 1782-92.
[http://dx.doi.org/10.1093/annonc/mdm111] [PMID: 17434893]

[108] Mokhtari RB, Homayouni TS, Baluch N, *et al.* Combination therapy in combating cancer. Oncotarget 2017; 8(23): 38022-43.
[http://dx.doi.org/10.18632/oncotarget.16723] [PMID: 28410237]

[109] Wu Y, Wang Z, Liu G, *et al.* Novel simvastatin-loaded nanoparticles based on cholic acid-core star-shaped PLGA for breast cancer treatment. J Biomed Nanotechnol 2015; 11(7): 1247-60.
[http://dx.doi.org/10.1166/jbn.2015.2068] [PMID: 26307847]

[110] Mi P. Stimuli-responsive nanocarriers for drug delivery, tumor imaging, therapy and theranostics. Theranostics 2020; 10(10): 4557-88.
[http://dx.doi.org/10.7150/thno.38069] [PMID: 32292515]

[111] Karimi M, Ghasemi A, Sahandi Zangabad P, *et al.* Smart micro/nanoparticles in stimulus-responsive

drug/gene delivery systems. Chem Soc Rev 2016; 45(5): 1457-501.
[http://dx.doi.org/10.1039/C5CS00798D] [PMID: 26776487]

[112] Choudhary S, Gupta L, Rani S, Dave K, Gupta U. Impact of dendrimers on solubility of hydrophobic drug molecules. Front Pharmacol 2017; 8: 261.
[http://dx.doi.org/10.3389/fphar.2017.00261] [PMID: 28559844]

[113] Din F, Aman W, Ullah I, *et al.* Effective use of nanocarriers as drug delivery systems for the treatment of selected tumors. Int J Nanomedicine 2017; 12: 7291-309.
[http://dx.doi.org/10.2147/IJN.S146315]

[114] Jaramillo AC, Al Saig F, Cloos J, Jansen G, Peters GJ. How to overcome ATP-binding cassette drug efflux transporter-mediated drug resistance? Cancer Drug Resist 2018; 1(1): 6-29.
[http://dx.doi.org/10.20517/cdr.2018.02]

[115] Soe ZC, Kwon JB, Thapa RK, *et al.* Transferrin-conjugated polymeric nanoparticle for receptor-mediated delivery of doxorubicin in doxorubicin-resistant breast cancer cells. Pharmaceutics 2019; 11(2): 63.
[http://dx.doi.org/10.3390/pharmaceutics11020063] [PMID: 30717256]

[116] Sánchez-Moreno P, de Vicente J, Nardecchia S, Marchal J, Boulaiz H. Thermo-sensitive nanomaterials: recent advance in synthesis and biomedical applications. Nanomaterials (Basel) 2018; 8(11): 935-67.
[http://dx.doi.org/10.3390/nano8110935] [PMID: 30428608]

[117] Manzanares-Guevara LA, Licea-Claverie A, Oroz-Parra I, Bernaldez-Sarabia J, Diaz-Castillo F, Licea-Navarro AF. Smart nanoformulation based on stimuli-responsive nanogels and curcumin: promising therapy against colon cancer. ACS Omega 2020; 5(16): 9171-84.
[http://dx.doi.org/10.1021/acsomega.9b04390] [PMID: 32363269]

[118] Garcia-Pinel B, Jabalera Y, Ortiz R, *et al.* Biomimetic magnetoliposomes as oxaliplatin nanocarriers: *In vitro* study for potential application in colon cancer. Pharmaceutics 2020; 12(6): 589.
[http://dx.doi.org/10.3390/pharmaceutics12060589] [PMID: 32599905]

CHAPTER 9

Nanocarriers in The Treatment of Head and Neck Cancer

Ashish Garg[1,*], **Vaibhav Kumar S. Gawali**[2], **Rupesh K. Gautam**[3], **Rajeev K. Singla**[4,5] and **Sumel Ashique**[6]

[1] *Department of P. G. Studies and Research in Chemistry and Pharmacy, Rani Durgavati University, Jabalpur (M.P.), 482001, India*

[2] *Department of Internal Medicine/Nephrology, College of Medicine, University of Cincinnati, OH, USA*

[3] *Department of Pharmacology, MM School of Pharmacy, Maharishi Markandeshwar University, Ambala-Chandigarh Highway, Sadopur- Ambala-134007 (Haryana), India*

[4] *Institutes for Systems Genetics, Frontiers Science Center for Disease-related Molecular Network, West China Hospital, Sichuan University, Chengdu, 610041, Sichuan, China*

[5] *Global Research and Publishing Foundation, New Delhi, India*

[6] *Department of Pharmaceutics, Bharat Institute of Technology (BIT), School of Pharmacy, Meerut, UP, India*

Abstract: Nowadays, Head and neck cancer is treated as a major disease worldwide. Several types of treatments are involved in this type of cancer, including immunotherapy, chemotherapy, radiation therapy, and surgery. Considering the clinical results from the past decades, these types of treatments resulted in no significant improvement in survival rates. To overcome these issues, versatile nanoparticles targeting selective tumors are considered. The targeted therapeutics based on the nanoparticle has a wide range of applications, such as photothermal therapy, radio-sensitization, chemotherapeutic drug delivery, and gene splicing. In this study, we have discussed the recent advancement in targeted therapeutics based on nanoparticles for head and neck cancer. Further, we have described the targets in Head and Neck cancer and, thus, shared future perspectives.

Keywords: Head and Neck Cancer, Nanocarriers, Nanoparticles, Liposomes, Targeting.

* **Corresponding author Ashish Garg:** Department of P. G. Studies and Research in Chemistry and Pharmacy, Rani Durgavati University, Jabalpur (M.P.) 482001, India; Tel: +91-9993624362; E-mail: ashish.garg071010@gmail.com

Neeraj Mishra, Ashish Garg and Neeraj Upmanyu (Eds.)

INTRODUCTION

Worldwide, head and neck cancer take the sixth position. The new cases of head and neck cancer are estimated at around 900,000, and then the mortality per year was obtained at 350,000, which accounts for about 5-6% of overall cancer cases [1, 2]. The results have shown that males are more affected than females [3, 4]. This cancer sets about as squamous cancer, often known as Head and Neck Squamous Cell Carcinoma (HNSCC). Cancer is formed in the areas of the larynx, pharynx, oral cavity, nasal cavity, and paranasal sinuses. The major threat factor for the HNSCC is the consumption of alcohol and Tobacco [5]. For nonsmoker youngsters, the Human Papilloma Virus (HPV) infection of types 16 and then 18 have an increased cancer of the oropharyngeal [6]. Notwithstanding the recent advancement in the recognition and treatments for patients having HNSCC, disappointment occurred in the overall results and the associated toxic treatments. The death rates are considered in the cases of 50% of newly recognized people with high levels of (3 or 4). For every stage, the 5-year average rate of survival depends upon the ~60% outcome information. Still, 50−60% of the domestic HNSCC patients advance to the territorial or far-off backslides by 2 years, having a reduction in the endurance rate starting from 80% over to 50 or otherwise 35%. The patients of intermittent or metastatic survival in the middle by under one year [7]. The HNSCC is a dangerous and distorting illness, with the tumour treatment being confounded and then consistently requiring an approach of multidisciplinary [8]. Careful resection and radiotherapy have been respected as the HSCC standard treatment, particularly at the beginning phases, when chemotherapy is added as a subordinate. Nonetheless, given that facial constructions are intricate life systems and essential capacity, the medical procedure extension is consistently restricted. Conventional medicines are awesome, with low viability or serious results [9]. Recent investigations focus on advanced radiotherapy or chemotherapy to preserve organ functions and improve quality of life. Vague circulation is a significant factor that adds to the side effects and poor clinical results in customary medicines. Therapeutics of the target focused on the ailing tissue, which has arisen as the promising option over conventional approaches, and then beat certain disadvantages, like tumor resistance and nonspecific distribution. Explicit anti-tumor impacts are accomplished by hindering the gene expression fundamental for tumorigenicity or potentially for tumor development, otherwise managing coupled medication atoms into the cells of tumor mix by an over-communicated receptor. The nanoparticles had flexible materials with 1−100 nm widths, acted as transporters to some imaging specialists, and drugs, and then focused on ligands. Different sorts of NPs are created as transporters for the agents of therapy, and for the targeted NP-based, which attracts more consideration and contains latent focusing and dynamic focusing. The particle has a Nano-size aggregate in the tumour tissues without forming any targeting tumour tissues; it is known as the Enhanced Penetrability and Maintenance (EPR) impact, which understands latent focusing [10]. These beneficial impacts are abundantly accomplished on account of broken vasculature and debilitated lymphatic waste in the tumour tissues, emerging because of superfast development and lacking supplement supply [11, 12]. Due to the nanoparticle's small size, it penetrates tumour microcapillaries or extravasates through the endothelium. Beyond the effect of passive EPR, nanoparticles give a surface to the connection of explicit atomic themes to empower encouraged disguise and then to the dynamically targeted tumour. Undoubtedly, nano-based dynamic focusing has progressively pulled the concentration from aloof focusing on frameworks. Ongoing exploration has featured numerous benefits of a focused nanomedicine approach in a common treatment for treating HNSCC, for example, improved particular tumour-murdering effectiveness and diminished harmfulness to solid tissues [13]. This audit article diagrams nanoparticle-intervened focused on head-and-neck malignancy therapeutics for distinguishing different ways for dealing with improvement in forecasting the HNSCC patients. Head and neck disease (HNC) alludes to dangerous neoplasms created in the oral route, thyroid, pharynx, and larynx. An expected new HNC expense with 842,000 emerged in 2012, representing 11.9% of tumors worldwide. Around the same time, there were 319,300 passes due to HNC, representing 4.5% of cancers [14, 15]. Patients with HNC consistently accounted for having respiratory problems, dysphagia, xerostomia, and other manifestations, which is more regrettable because of the absence of craving, weight reduction, and nourishing problems [16]. Liquor and Tobacco utilization are discovered to be the greatest guilty party of HNSCC through various examinations of epidemiology, alongside the biting of areca and mate drinking [17]. Considering the previous few decades, HPV (Human Papillomavirus) (especially HPV18 and HPV16) contamination has prompted another sort of HNC patient who will be youthful and then who doesn't smoke or drink [18, 19]. The disease HPV is regular in cervical carcinoma through contact. Due to changes in the sex, this is anticipated by 2020, the 'HPV's greater part related to the HNC patient's victims, fundamentally awe-inspiring the cervical carcinoma quantity [20, 21], while comparing negative HPV patients, positive HPV patients improved treatment results. So, for instance, the endurance of two-year paces malignancy oropharynx for negative HPV and positive HPV patients having 62% and 95%, separately, and then 46% and 79%, individually for the next five years [22, 23]. Detailed analysis and then the normalized characterization of the degree of disease was imperative for designing reasonable restorative regimens by alluding to earlier cases of comparative anticipation. Tumour Hub Metastasis (TNM) disease organizing framework is a generally utilized arrangement that considers neighbourhood development of tumour degree, spreading to local hub lymph and other organ metastases. The HNC occurs at various locales, including the depression of the lip and the oral, thyroid, ethmoid sinus, nasal pit, maxillary sinus, subglottis, glottis, supraglottis, hypopharynx, oropharynx, and nasopharynx (Fig. **1**). These have exceptional malignant growth evaluating principles as indicated through the eighth Edition of the American Joint Committee on Cancer (AJCC) Cancer Manual Staging that is distributed at participation in the International Union for Cancer Control. Through this, we can sum up the HNC arrangement from 0 stages for organizing IV [24]. At 0 Stage, tumors have distinct structures and separate unmistakably from encompassing tissues typically, with no metastasis or intrusion. Tumours of Stage I hold the shape under a breadth of 2 cm, which is not pushed up through the submucosa. In Stage II, the pushing of malignancy cells through or among adjacent cells and the distance across the tumour is around 2 cm and then 4 cm. In Stage III, malignancy cells quickly separate and duplicate, reaching out to neighbourhood hubs lymph; the tumour size is in excess of 4 cm. In Stage IV, diseased cells get into the circulatory system for different districts, bringing about metastases. As referenced above, HNC is an intricate and troublesome infection that can invade encompassing frameworks without much of a stretch and prompt metastasis. Showing the facility, it is normally treated through a medical procedure, chemotherapy, and radiotherapy. Hence, the unmanageable dangers for patients with HNC were disease repeat and metastasis. Dissipated dispersion with chemotherapeutic medications in the body extraordinarily limits the use of chemotherapy. Then the emerging usage of biomedicine nanotechnologies gives different freedoms to managing the issues of medications utilized in treatments of malignancy [25, 26]. NPs drug transporters are made out of metal oxides, carbon, dendrimers, liposomes, and polymers [27 - 29]. The 'NP's size utilized the chemotherapy regularly around 1 nm to 200 nm to guarantee the tumour cells were taken viably [30, 31]. Special take-up medication containing NPs into the cells of the tumor is exceptionally attractive to stifling foundational results, however, just on the off chance that it tends to control [32, 33]. The targeted NPs conveyance frameworks are separated by two components: latent and then dynamic focusing. Latent focusing depends on the improved porousness and maintenance (EPR) impact, in which the inadequately framed, defective tumour site vasculature causes the drug-stacked NPs to gather locally. Be that as it may, the fundamental limit of aloof focusing is lacking medication fixation at the tumour site. Interestingly, NPs designed with tumour explicit focusing on moieties partake in dynamic focusing. Explicit ligands consider the molecule to interface all the more firmly with explicit cell types, in this manner taking into account NPs for conveying payload straightforwardly for the tumor cells having negligible medication siphoning into the general flow. The transporter methodology boosts medication focus inside the tumor, implying a lower general portion for managing HNC patients when keeping up efficacy helpfully [34, 35].

The active focusing NPs showed enormous guarantees in medication conveyance frameworks and sought after the chemotherapy transporters altogether cancers types. Effectively planning and then generally utilizing the focused NPs were administered through the chosen coupling reaction [36 - 38]. Hereby, we depict the current status of the focused NPs that applied to the HNC chemotherapy to discuss the expected further clinical application.

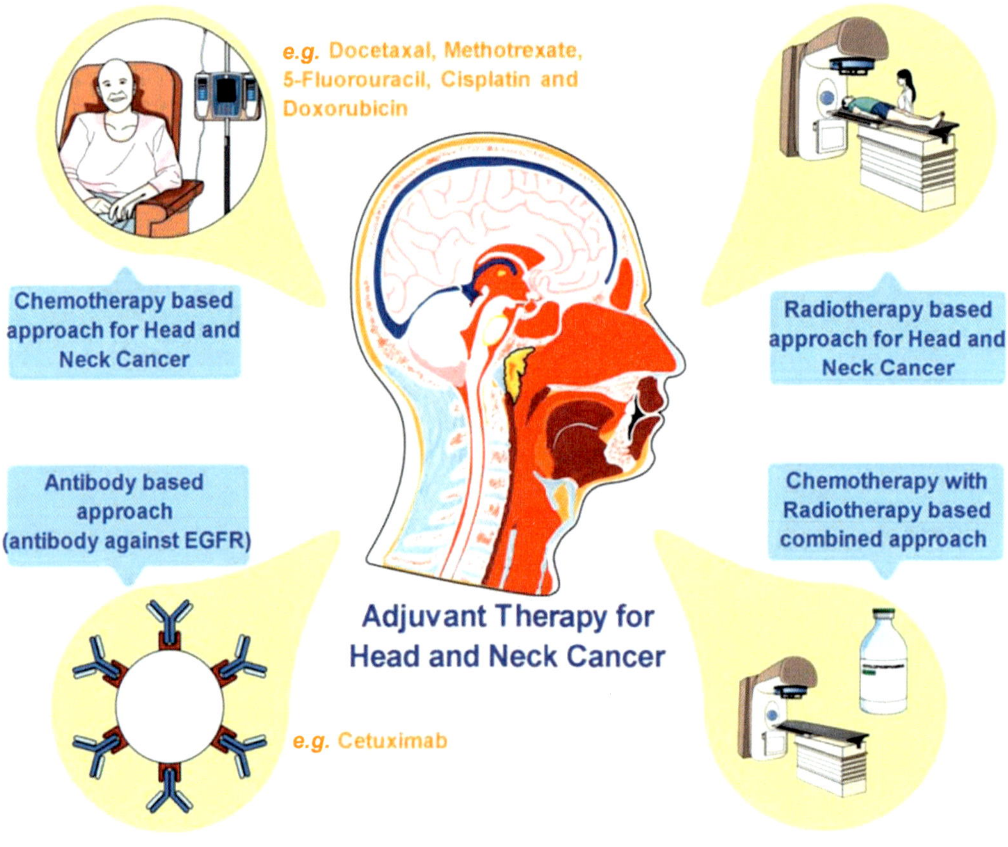

Fig. (1). Recent adjuvant therapy for Head and Neck Cancer treatment.

PRESENT ADJUVANT OF CHEMOTHERAPY AGAINST THE HNC

In the beginning phase of HNC patients, careful resection was the ideal treatment choice. However, the patients in the terminal stages, joined thorough, multimodality treatment, is supported rather than careful resection. Then the chemotherapy utilization is separated into three strategies: adjuvant chemotherapy, simultaneous chemotherapy, Induction chemotherapy, acceptance chemotherapy, and neoadjuvant chemotherapy before utilizing a medical procedure to lessen the tumour volume and improve detailed results. The coordinated chemotherapy was intended to upgrade the effectiveness of radiotherapy, at the same time diminishing the lymph hub metastasis danger. The adjuvant chemotherapy was to slaughter little sores that can't be taken out by a medical procedure or diminish repeats and improve endurance rate. As of late, the medications carboplatin, cisplatin, hydroxyurea, mitomycin C, bleomycin, methotrexate (MTX), and fluorouracil (5-FU) are utilized in the examination of restorative treatment for HNC [39]. Through current writing, chemotherapy of platinum-5-FU is viewed as the foundation of current treatment with the standard. The chemotherapy of platinum-5-FU framework was first used by Southwest Oncology Group (SWOG), which contrasted 5-FU and cisplatin viability, 5-FU carboplatin, and then single MTX specialist in the patients of HNC who are enduring deterioration and metastasis. Examination revealed total and then halfway reaction rates are 32% for the cisplatin/5-FU, 21% for the carboplatin/5-FU, and 10% for the MTX, albeit middle rate endurance has three similar treatment plans. This ought to be noticed despite the most remarkable reaction rate, with the cisplatin/5-FU bunch announcing higher rates with the fundamental side effects [40]. Simultaneously in 2004, the Radiation Therapy Oncology Group (RTOG) and the European Organization for Research and Treatment of Cancer (EORTC) distributed the path of therapy with HNC patients. The RTOG 9501 has directed an arbitrary examination of patients with HNC to treat after the medical procedure of resection. Gathering treated with the radiotherapy in addition to the cisplatin, *i.e.*, (body-surface zone of 100 mg per square meter intravenously (I.V.) on the day 1, 22, and then 43) acquired two-year high endurance rate and then sickness endurance rate free rather than radiotherapy gathering [41]. The EORTC 22931 led a practically similar path aside from some boundary contrasts and additionally showed a critical advantage of general endurance to radiotherapy with the group of cisplatin [42]. The two milestones trailed to set up a job for chemotherapy. As of now, atomically focused on the specialist, cetuximab, is additionally expected to assume a huge part later on HNC treatment from (Fig. **1**). Arising of the new helpful medications and chemotherapy created which make ready for improving the HNC treatment.

HNC NANOPARTICLES THERAPY

HNC Therapy Material Requirement

Nanotechnologies offer different pathways to biomedical applications in disease determination and therapy [43 - 46]. The NP-based conveyance vehicles, by precise size control, shape, and surface functionalization, were given different roads to convey different analytic or potentially restorative specialists for better results and fewer results. Exploiting the properties of the remarkable material at nanoscale, like enormous region surface to the volume proportion, with novel optical and attractive properties, which would be is an easy change, so the nanomaterials investigated for beating a great deal with organic obstructions for disease therapy [47]. Hence, nanomaterials were needed to achieve amazing biocompatibility, with good biodegradation and low harmfulness, before being utilized in malignant growth treatment. Moreover, the nanomaterials should stack adequate medications and precisely convey them to the tumour locales. This application's capabilities abused different materials, including metal oxides, polymers, dendrimers, liposomes, and carbon. This picking different agent guides for having an outline of nanomaterials utilization in the HNC treatment. Nearby research of HNC, the gold NPs properties with novel physicochemical for example, Localized Surface Plasmon Reverberation (LSPR), upgraded the light dispersing, and then photograph warm with properties of photograph acoustic created [48, 49], critical consideration to create indicative stages and then successful medicines in the HNC [50, 51]. By the way, nano vectors that are carbon-based, utilized for stack paclitaxel, are to be chosen by an exemplary illustration of an insoluble water medication with high remedial viability and then off-target extreme harmfulness. Simultaneously, atomically focused on specialist cetuximab, consolidated has yielded synergistic impacts, meriting future preclinical advancement for treating HNC [52, 53]. Ashwin *et al.* exhibited the decorated EGF of SWNTs explicitly the delivery system of the target squamous malignant growth for the chemotherapy of cisplatin, which brought about additional internalization of cell and then tumour development with distinct regression contrasted with a nontargeted cisplatin SWNT and shows carbon nanotube-based drug conveyance framework holding an incredible guarantee for malignancy treatment. They declare *in vivo* focused on disease therapy by connecting the anticancer specialist cisplatin alongside the Single-Walled Carbon Nanotube (SWNT) and Epidermal Development Factors (EGF) [54]. Hyperthermia induced through NPs attractive iron oxide (IO) (which is the breadth of ~15 nm) is investigated in HNC therapy utilizing a model of mouse xenograft with a cell line of HNSCC (Tu212). The 'NP's IO creates hyperthermia by substituting attractive fields for cell murdering, giving another alternative to the current treatment of HNC approaches [55]. Xie *et al.* built up folate conjugated stacked cisplatin with attractive nanomedicine (*i.e.*, CDDP-FA-A-A-MNP) and then utilized Magnetic Resonance Imaging (MRI) in the contrast specialist when at the same time conveying a chemotherapeutic medication, giving an elective stage to sedate conveyance in HNSCC patients and establishes the framework for atomic focused on cancer therapy [56]. 'NP's IO Carboxyl functionalized formed by Fibronectin-mimetic peptide (Fmp) are joined in drug (Pc) of second-age Photo-Dynamic Treatment (PDT), shows clearly restraint tumor development in the lower portion, that showed incredible potential for filling in both MRI specialist and then PDT drug at the center [57]. 'NP's of Polymeric are utilized to convey restorative medications and then bioactive particles show huge helpful worth. Matthew S. Earthy coloured utilizing the nanocapsules with sub–50-nm for conveying against the oligodeoxynucleotide CK2α/α0 shows huge concealment in the tumour development, the impacts of CK2 on the NF-κB–intervened and then TP53-interceded with signal actuation which relating quality and then protein articulation [58]. The copolymers of Diblock are utilized to adequately convey little meddling RNAs (siRNA) focusing on a proapoptotic quality and are powerful in giving radioprotection for salivary glands [59]. Colley demonstrated the pH-touchy capacity of ethyl phosphorylcholine (PMPC), poly 2-(diisopropyl-amino), poly 2-(methacryloyloxy), and then polymersomes of ethyl methacrylate (PDPA) to exemplify the chemotherapeutic specialists (paclitaxel and doxorubicin) to viable mix treatment of anticancer. Take-up and then the capacity for conveying drugs using polymersomes are estimated in the two and then three-dimensional frameworks culture [60]. Wang assessed the adequacy of the NP's poly (lactic-c--glycolic corrosive) (PLGA) which helped the 5-Aminolevulinic Acid (ALA) conveyance for the PDT, which is effective for SCC [61]. Chang *et al.* formed anticancer medication Mi-To-Xantrone (MTO) for palmitoleic corrosive, producing the two kinds with lipids Palmitoleyl MTO (Pal-MTO): dipalmitoyl MTO (di-Pal-MTO) and monopalmitoleyl MTO (mono-Pal-MTO) in molar proportion having 1:1 (md11-Pal-MTO NP's) shows most productive cell conveyance with siRNA [62]. Yu *et al.* planned the cationic nanoparticle lipids with 1,2-dioleoyl-sn-glycero-3-ethylphos-phocholine-based containing the paclitaxel and then siRNA, which showed the capability of the SSL to improve co-conveyance frameworks with lipophilic medications of anticancer and then with restorative siRNAs [63]. Another study developed cationic NPs lipid, which conveys pre-miR-107 (NPs/premier-107) [64].

The variety of nanosystems used in treating HNC is mentioned below in Table **1**.

Table 1. Nanotherapeutics for head and neck cancer treatment (Xu *et al.*, 2020).

S. No.	Nanotherapeutic System	Nanoparticle Systems with their Composition	Targeting Cancer Model/Cells	References
Nanoparticles				
1	PLGA Nanoparticles	Poly (lactic-co-glycolic acid), Nano-diamino-tetrac	Oral cancer cell lines (OEC-M1 cells)	[65]
2	-	Poly (lactic-co-glycolic acid), HPV-16 E7 peptide, ploy (I: C)	TC-1 tumour-bearing mice	[66]

(Table 1) cont.....

S. No.	Nanotherapeutic System	Nanoparticle Systems with their Composition	Targeting Cancer Model/Cells	References
3	-	Poly (lactic-co-glycolic acid), Mutated HPV-16 E7 and E6/E7 protein, R848, poly (I: C)	TC-1 tumor-bearing mice, cynomolgus monkey	[67]
4	-	PLGA NP coated with murine aCD40-mAb FGK45, HPV-16 E7, Pam3CSK4, Poly (I: C), aCD40-mAb	TC-1 tumour-bearing mice	[68]
5	-	Poly (lactic-co-glycolic acid), Cell or tumour lysate	HNSCC cell line (FaDu and FAT cells)	[69]
6	Polydopamine-coated spiky gold nanoparticles	Polydopamine-coated spiky gold nanoparticles with Doxorubicin	Mouse HNSCC, lung metastasis (TC-1 cells)	[70]
7	Co-assembled binary telodendrimers Nanoparticle	PEG5K-CA4-ICGD4 (PCI): a linear PEG block, four dendritic hydrophobic photothermal conversion agents (indocyanine green derivatives, ICGD) and four dendritic cholic acids (CA); PEG5K-Cys4-L8-CA8 (PCLC): PEG, four cysteines and eight CA. PCI: PCLC 1: 1, Doxorubicin, Imiquimod	Mouse oral cancer (OSC-3 cells)	[71]
8	Polyanhydride nanoparticle	20: 80 CPTEG: CPH. CPTEG: 1,8-bis (p-carboxyphenox-y)-3,6-dioxaoctane; CPH: 1,6-bis (p-carboxyphenoxy) hexane, IL-1α	Mouse HNSCC (SQ20B and Cal-27 cells)	[72]
9	PLGA-PEG nanoparticle	Poly (lactic-co-glycolic acid)-PEG, Doxorubicin, R848, CCL20, Poly (I: C)	TC-1 tumour-bearing mice	[73]
10	Poly (propylene sulphide) nanoparticle	Poly (propylene sulphide) nanoparticle with disulphide conjugated peptide, HPV-16 E7 peptide, CpG-B 1826 oligonucleotide	TC-1 tumor-bearing mice	[74]
11	R-DOTAP cationic lipid nanoparticle	R-1,2-dioleoyl-3-trimethyl-ammonium-propane (R-DOTAP), HPV-16 E7 and other antigens	TC-1 tumour-bearing mice	[75]
12	Hyaluronic acid-modified cationic lipid-PLGA hybrid nanoparticles	Cationic lipid (3β-[N-(N′,N′, dimethylaminoethane)-carbamoyl] cholesterol hydrochloride, DC-Chol), Hyaluronic acid, poly (lactic-co-glycolic acid), HPV-16 E7 peptide, ploy (I: C), CpG-ODN	TC-1 tumour-bearing mice	[76]

(Table 1) cont.....

S. No.	Nanotherapeutic System	Nanoparticle Systems with their Composition	Targeting Cancer Model/Cells	References
13	Heterocyclic lipid nanoparticle	Dihydroimidazole-linked lipids A2-Iso5-2DC18 and A12-Iso5-2DC18, HPV-16 E7 mRNA	TC-1 tumour-bearing mice	[77]
14	Virus-like particles	E7 inserted into Hepatitis B virus core antigen (aa. 1-149), HPV-16 E7 Epitope	-	[78]
15	PMIDA coated CoO nanoparticles	N-Phosnomethyliminodiacetic acid coated cobalt oxide nanoparticle, Human oral carcinoma (KB) cell lysate	Oral cancer cell line (KB cells)	[79]
16	Chitosan-coated selenium nanoparticle	Chitosan-coated selenium nanoparticle, *Fluc*-mRNA	Nasopharyngeal carcinoma cell line (KB cells)	[80]
Liposomes				
17	-	DOTMA: cholesterol 1: 1, Murine Interleukin 2, Murine Interleukin 12 Plasmid	Mouse HNSCC (SCCVII cells)	[81]
18	Sterically stabilized cationic liposome	DC-Chol: DOPE: PEG-PE (4: 6: 0.06), CpG-ODN	Mouse HNSCC (KCCT873 cells)	[82]
19	DOTMA/DOPE liposome	DOTMA, DOPE, HPV-16 E7 mRNA	TC-1 tumor-bearing mice	[83]
20	DOTMA/DOPE liposome	DOTMA, DOPE, Plasmid encoding HPV-16 E6, E7	TC-1 tumor-bearing mice	[84]
21	-	Cholesterol/DOPC/PEG-DSPE/maleimide-PEG-DSPE at 35/60/2.5/2.5 or 35/62.5/0/2.5 mol%, Anti-CD137, IL-2	TC-1 tumor-bearing mice	[85]
Others				
22	Multidomain peptide assembled nanofibrous matrix	K2(SL)6K2 multidomain peptide, Cyclic dinucleotides	Mouse HNSCC (MOC2-E6E7 cells)	[86]
23	Tocopherol-modified hyaluronic acid nano suspension	Tocopherol-modified hyaluronic acid (HA-Toco), TLR7/8 dual agonist resiquimod (R848)	Mouse OSCC (AT84 cells)	[87]
24	Nanoscale metal-organic framework	DBP-Hf nMOF based on 5,15-di (p-benzoato) porphyrin bridging ligand, Indoleamine 2,3-dioxygenase	Mouse HNSCC (SQ20B cells)	[88]
25	Synthetic high-density lipoprotein nanodisc	1,2-Dimyristoyl-sn-glycero-3-phosphocholine (DMPC), ApoA1 mimetic peptide 22A, HPV-16 E7 peptide, MPLA, CpG	TC-1 tumor-bearing mice	[89]

(Table 1) cont.....

S. No.	Nanotherapeutic System	Nanoparticle Systems with their Composition	Targeting Cancer Model/Cells	References
26	Mesoporous silica micro-rod	Mesoporous silica micro-rod, Polyethyleneimine, HPV-16 E7 peptide, GM-CSF, CPG-ODN	TC-1 tumor-bearing mice	[90]
27	Q11 peptide assembled nanofiber	Peptides Q11 (Ac-QQKFQFQFEQQ-Am), E7 (44-62) was appended to the N terminus of peptide Q11 through a flexible linker, Ser-Gly-Ser-Gly, HPV-16 E7 peptide	TC-1 tumor-bearing mice	[91]
28	PEG-PE micelle	Polyethylene glycol-phosphatidylethanolamine (PEG-PE) micelles, Ovalbumin peptide	TC-1 tumor-bearing mice	[92]
29	Nanosatellite	Polysiloxane-containing polymer-coated iron oxide core with inert gold satellites, E6/E7 peptide +cGAMP	Mouse HNSCC (PCI-13, UMSCC22b, UMSCC47, and FaDu cells)	[93]
30	Mesoporous silica rods	Mesoporous silica rods, GM-CSF + CpG-ODN + E7 peptide	Mouse HNSCC (MOC2-E6E7 cells)	[94]

HNC Therapy Nanostructure Requirements

An innovative nanostructure with a broad spectrum has grown to address the different HNC challenges, like albumin conjugates, dendrimers, liposomes, peptides, and polymers [95, 96]. The materials then clearly fluctuate in structures and morphologies. Considering the positive to negative charge and from the two-dimensional nanostructures to the three-dimensional nanospheres of surface, the materials introduce various properties. Hence, for treating HNC malignancy, ideal materials are wanted to be adaptable for changing the surface properties, morphologies, sizes, *etc.* Another research group enhanced HER-2 antisense oligonucleotide (HER-2 ODN) conveyance for the tumour cells through compound HER-2 ODN by the recently settled delivery system of folate-liposome, bringing about the sharpening of HNC cells to the agents of chemotherapeutic [97]. Shim *et al.* blended the Tri Lysinoyl Oleylamide (TLO)-based Liposomes (TLOL) to the foundation of siRNA with the delivery of the drug [98]. Cationic and hydrophobic polymer families can be used to develop nanoparticles that decorate the ligands of protein from the outside by conveying the helpful proteins to an inside particle. A research group has utilized G5 dendrimer polyamidoamine for targeted chemotherapy to target the moiety Folic Acid (FA) [99]. Dosio *et al.* [100], developed a paclitaxel anticancer system with the Human Serum Albumin (HSA) for shaping the drug–albumin form and then improved with the FA, which showed expanded selectivity with antitumoral action.

DELIVERY OF TARGETED NANOPARTICLES FOR THERAPY OF HNC

Strategy of Targeted Delivery for the Therapy of HNC

The principal mechanism of internalization is the passive diffusion of the free drugs into the tumour cells. However, endocytosis nanoparticles enter the cells and stay away from the drug decreases the cell's pull-out [101]. The tumour targeting strategy of nano-based systems against HNC is depicted in Fig. (**2**).

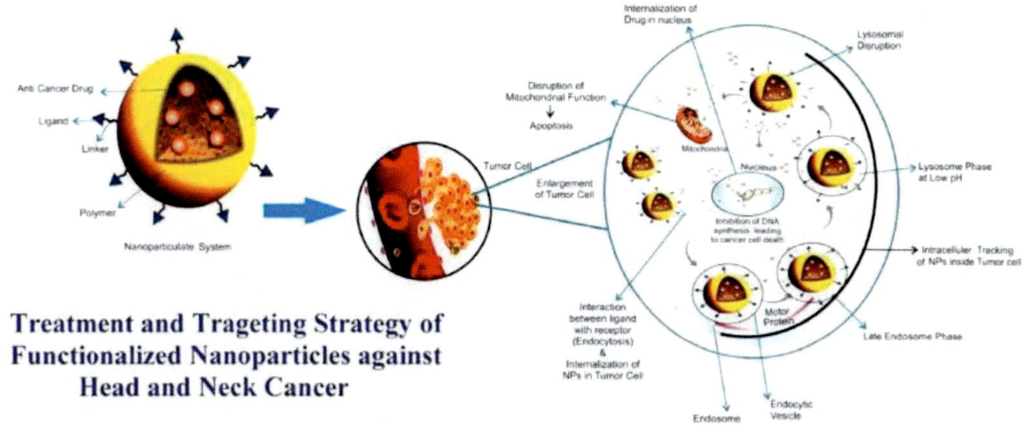

Fig. (2). Targeting strategy of nano-based system against HNC (Reproduced with permission of Elsevier; Licence No. 5064680844452) [109].

Controlling the molecule cell cooperation is perhaps the primary purpose behind the adjustment of nanoparticle, targeted ligands allowance like small molecules, peptides, nucleic acid strands, fragments and then antibodies [102, 103]. The Epidermal Growth Factor Receptor (EGFR) was then frequently more-communicated in the case of the HNSCC [104]. The EGFR expression with high levels is related to the helpless guess in an assortment of diseases, generally in the HNSCC, showing that the therapy of the receptor coordinated the valuable anticancer strategy. He *et al.* researched the transfer of intratumoral cationic liposome- antisense plasmids mediated with EGFR into the HNSCC xenografts subcutaneous by *in situ* antisense oligonucleotides articulation, which brought about expanded tumour cell apoptosis and then the hindrance of growth of the tumour [105]. A research group built up a Dextran sulfate (DEX) and Poly-L-Arginine (PLR) based polyelectrolyte nano-sized complex (nano complex) for the conveyance with EGFR-siRNA epidermal at the model of the HNSCC. The analyses showed the most elevated gene splicing EGFR effectiveness in both the FaDu and Hep-2 cell lines and then displayed brilliant tumour development restraint in a xenografted mouse tumour model [106]. Therefore, EGFR serves as an objective for drug conveyance. Berlin *et al.* consolidated poly paclitaxel-stacked (ethylene glycol) having functionalized hydrophilic carbon clusters (PEG-HCCs). Cetuximab nanoparticles targeted the monoclonal immune response, which only ties with the EGFR. The system of the targeted nano vector demonstrated the high therapeutic viability obtained as new HNSCC therapy. The Folate corrosive receptors (FRs) were the glycosylphosphatidylinositol-secured receptors cell surface has a FA which is high liking, that is overexpressed in harmful tumours, like head and neck, kidney, lung, ovarian, breast [107]. Folate corrosive is a B nutrient with water-dissolvable, fundamental for the DNA blend. The FA holds its capacity to be a tie with FRs after the formation with several different designs and then frequently increases the endocytosis by the pathway of FR-intervened. Considering, the path of FR has been concentrated widely as an objective for nanoparticle therapeutics [108]. Wang *et al.* combined focused on the polymeric nanoparticles (HFT-T) stacked with extra paclitaxel the anti-tumor's viability and then specifically perceived the positive FR of HNSCC with the cell line of KB-3-1 *in vitro* and then *in vivo*. The subsequent HFT-T NPs, and extraordinarily restrained tumour development without showing a tumour renewal development following half a month of treatment. Ward *et al.* manufactured a generation of 5 dendrimers acetylated formed to the therapeutic MTX and FA, at that point controlled to mice immunized SCID CB-17 by UM-SCC-22B, UM-SCC-17B, and then UM-SCC-1 disease cells, which shows expanded treatment.

ORGANIZATION ROUTES FOR THE THERAPY OF HNC

I.V Course is the primary and quick technique for direct chemotherapy drugs into the fundamental dissemination. To the specialists of hydrophilic chemotherapy, it is viable, guaranteeing the disease with low risk. There are additionally some disadvantages in the I.V., for instance, to self-administer is wrong for the patients, and then for the majority of drugs of the hydrophobic anticancer, it is not appropriate [110]. By latent (EPR impact) and dynamic targeting, nanomaterials are designed to send medications to tumors precisely. It is the best replacement that helpless water dissolvability drugs are stacked in the nanomaterials to improve the drugs solvency and bioavailability. Consider Wang *et al.*, who built up a stage for the targeted nanoparticle, which consolidates Pc 4, and then PDT drug of the second generation, with disease targeted ligands and then 'NP's IO. The Fmp-IO-Pc 4 was handled through the infusion of the I.V that fundamentally has high retention of tumour apart from a Pc 4 free, hence, bringing extraordinary potential at the PDT with MRI at the clinic (Wang *et al.*, 2014). Piao *et al.*, utilized cationic lipids for delivering pre-miR-107 (NPs/pre-miR-107) at the cells of HNSCC *in vitro*. Hence, NP/pre-miR-107 outcomes showed that expansion in the miR-107 delivery into HNSCC cells through above 80,000-overlay contrasting with pre-miR-107 free. The NPs/premier-107 is infused by I.V and the vein of the tail. Hence, results recommended by the nanoparticle delivery of cationic lipid of the pre-miR-107 efficiently smoothens HNSCC tumorigenesis.

Newly contemplates showing the intraperitoneal (I.P.) organization which is more legitimate than the managed I.V. to several therapies of solid tumours [111 - 113]. A study revealed a compound, Self-Amassed Nucleoside Nanoparticle (SNNP), which is an effective drug delivery system. Contrasting with 5-FU free, the SNNP stacked with the 5-Fluoro-Uracile (5-FU-SNNP) impeded remarkably by the tumor development with SNNP reduced 5-FU poisonous symptoms. In this examination, I.P. injection was utilized to assess the SNNP biosafety and then *in vivo* Antitumor Efficacy Assay. The suggested findings proposed that anti-tumor viability has better 5-FU. Then when stacked with the SNNP, the results get lower, demonstrating that the SNNP effectively provides a promising nanomaterial that evidences the wide applications in clinical later on [114]. The injection of Intratumoral is a sort of injection of local, which offers a few benefits, for example, at the site of tumour adjustment of drugs, safeguarding of anticancer action, controlled and then delayed drug discharge [115]. A research group developed a new methodology for anticancer treatment, consolidating the anticancer drug treatment and then siRNAs. The nanoparticle cationic is formed by the drug-derived anticancer lipids for the complexation of siRNA. The siGL2 or siMcl-1 is sophisticated to the to md11-Pal-MTO for the treatment of siRNA; here, NPs infused intratumorally, provides the effective siRNA cell conveyance [62]. Intra-arterial infusion is exceptionally feasible for regional chemotherapy; in the tumour site, it takes a high accumulation of the drug. Considerable advances in the technique of vascular radiology and new devices, like angiographic catheters and fluoroscopy units, have more protected and accurate intra-blood vessel chemotherapy [116, 117]. Since there are remaining infection risks and then thrombosis [118]. The infusion of an Intra-blood vessel was directed to consider paclitaxel, a novel alumni-bound nanoparticle with adequacy and security of intra-blood vessel enlistment chemotherapy. There are two to four patterns of paclitaxel of albumin-bound nanoparticle implanted into one of the branches or external carotid artery, at that point, the reaction was assessed by the actual assessment, computed multi-detector tomography, and then furthermore by the tomography of positron discharge. The tolerability and the reaction rates of intraarterial chemotherapy with the paclitaxel nanoparticle albumin-bound showed the viability and feasibility in the mix with the different specialists of advanced HNSCC [119]. Szilvia Arany utilized the injection of Retroductal. Mouse Submandibular Organs (SMG) were introduced by the siRNAs PH-responsive complexed nanoparticle; this initiated the gene splicing siRNA. In this technique, SG has protected the shields of the SG from the apoptosis of radiation-initiated.

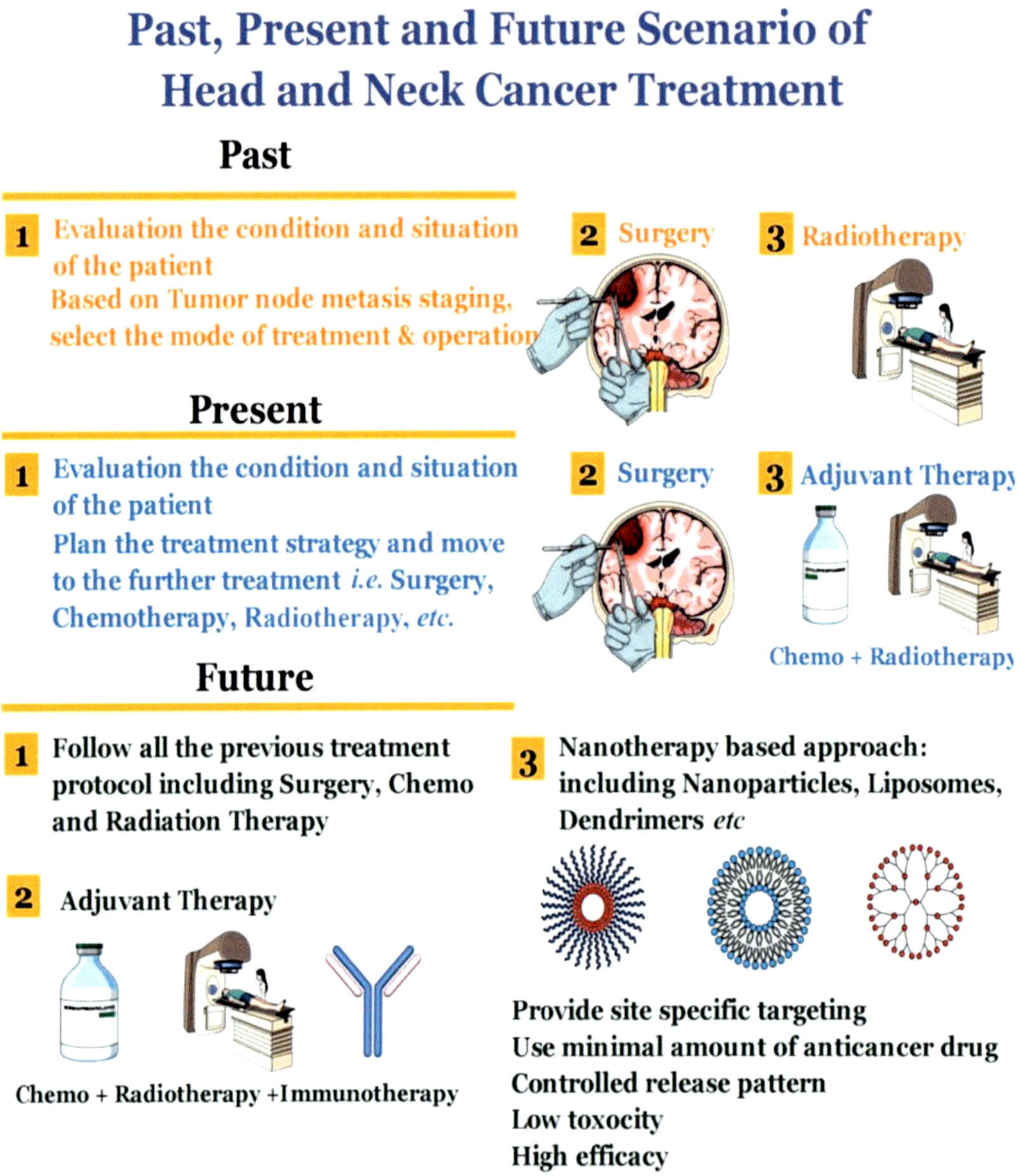

Fig. (3). Present past and future scenario of head and neck cancer therapy.

CONCLUSION

In recent times, countless features of the materials used nanotechnologies broadly. In nanomedicine, nanomaterials are engaged for the detection of cancer and therapy. Nanomaterials have high potential in the treatment of HNC to improve chemotherapy efficiency. Hence it is done without the help of maximizing the toxicities. Fig. (**3**) shows the effective treatment of HNC with the present agents of chemotherapeutic. But there are several deficiencies in the tumor site; it fails at accumulating an efficient dosage while the cytotoxic drug accumulates in the healthy tissues. The targeted nanoparticle applications show that HNC carries drugs that cover the chemotherapy treatment for alleviating the terminal patient's pain and then prolonging their entire life. A great attraction is offered towards the therapeutic authority. Many nanoscale dimension materials are exploited to utilize the targeted delivery system. For clinical, many delivery systems with nanoparticle-based targeted drugs are not translated. Here exists the brief promise for serving the HNC therapy needs. Future contexts are enhanced to the delivery system of targeted nanoparticles, which is more powerful in opposition to cancer and is lenient on the other type of tissues. Nanomaterials continuous research and then HNC therapy progress attempt, we look for the chemotherapy with nanomaterial which increases the HNC prevention, treatment and diagnosis. This will additionally bring enormous influence on human welfare, which is in the close later.

CONSENT FOR PUBLICATION

Not applicable.

CONFLICT OF INTEREST

The authors declare no conflict of interest, financial or otherwise.

ACKNOWLEGEMENT

We are thankful to the team at Bentham Science Publishers for giving us this opportunity, the editor of this book, and everyone who supported us directly or indirectly while writing this book chapter.

REFERENCES

[1] Parkin DM, Bray F, Ferlay J, Pisani P. Global cancer statistics, 2002. CA Cancer J Clin 2005; 55(2): 74-108.
[http://dx.doi.org/10.3322/canjclin.55.2.74] [PMID: 15761078]

[2] Ferlay J, Shin HR, Bray F, Forman D, Mathers C, Parkin DM. Estimates of worldwide burden of cancer in 2008: GLOBOCAN 2008. Int J Cancer 2010; 127(12): 2893-917.
[http://dx.doi.org/10.1002/ijc.25516] [PMID: 21351269]

[3] Blot WJ, McLaughlin JK, Winn DM, *et al.* Smoking and drinking in relation to oral and pharyngeal cancer. Cancer Res 1988; 48(11): 3282-7. [PMID: 3365707]

[4] Hashibe M, Brennan P, Benhamou S, *et al.* Alcohol drinking in never users of tobacco, cigarette smoking in never drinkers, and the risk of head and neck cancer: pooled analysis in the International Head and Neck Cancer Epidemiology Consortium. J Natl Cancer Inst 2007; 99(10): 777-89. [http://dx.doi.org/10.1093/jnci/djk179] [PMID: 17505073]

[5] D'Souza G, Kreimer AR, Viscidi R, *et al.* Case-control study of human papillomavirus and oropharyngeal cancer. N Engl J Med 2007; 356(19): 1944-56. [http://dx.doi.org/10.1056/NEJMoa065497] [PMID: 17494927]

[6] Carvalho AL, Nishimoto IN, Califano JA, Kowalski LP. Trends in incidence and prognosis for head and neck cancer in the United States: A site-specific analysis of the SEER database. Int J Cancer 2005; 114(5): 806-16. [http://dx.doi.org/10.1002/ijc.20740] [PMID: 15609302]

[7] Forastiere A, Koch W, Trotti A, Sidransky D. Head and neck cancer. N Engl J Med 2001; 345(26): 1890-900. [http://dx.doi.org/10.1056/NEJMra001375] [PMID: 11756581]

[8] Lango MN. Multimodal treatment for head and neck cancer. Surg Clin North Am 2009; 89(1): 43-52, viii. [http://dx.doi.org/10.1016/j.suc.2008.09.018] [PMID: 19186230]

[9] Murphy BA, Gilbert J, Ridner SH. Systemic and global toxicities of head and neck treatment. Expert Rev Anticancer Ther 2007; 7(7): 1043-53. [http://dx.doi.org/10.1586/14737140.7.7.1043] [PMID: 17627463]

[10] Maeda H. Tumor-selective delivery of macromolecular drugs *via* the EPR effect: background and future prospects. Bioconjug Chem 2010; 21(5): 797-802. [http://dx.doi.org/10.1021/bc100070g] [PMID: 20397686]

[11] Dvorak HF. Leaky tumor vessels: consequences for tumor stroma generation and for solid tumor therapy. Prog Clin Biol Res 1990; 354A: 317-30. [PMID: 2247496]

[12] Kobayashi H, Watanabe R, Choyke PL. Improving conventional enhanced permeability and retention (EPR) effects; what is the appropriate target? Theranostics 2014; 4(1): 81-9. [http://dx.doi.org/10.7150/thno.7193] [PMID: 24396516]

[13] Peer D, Karp JM, Hong S, Farokhzad OC, Margalit R, Langer R. Nanocarriers as an emerging platform for cancer therapy. Nano-Enabled Medical Applications 2020; 23: 61-91. [http://dx.doi.org/10.1201/9780429399039-2]

[14] Torre LA, Bray F, Siegel RL, Ferlay J, Lortet-Tieulent J, Jemal A. Global cancer statistics, 2012. CA Cancer J Clin 2015; 65(2): 87-108. [http://dx.doi.org/10.3322/caac.21262] [PMID: 25651787]

[15] Kang H, Kiess A, Chung CH. Emerging biomarkers in head and neck cancer in the era of genomics. Nat Rev Clin Oncol 2015; 12(1): 11-26. [http://dx.doi.org/10.1038/nrclinonc.2014.192] [PMID: 25403939]

[16] Bressan V, Stevanin S, Bianchi M, Aleo G, Bagnasco A, Sasso L. The effects of swallowing disorders, dysgeusia, oral mucositis and xerostomia on nutritional status, oral intake and weight loss in head and neck cancer patients: A systematic review. Cancer Treat Rev 2016; 45: 105-19. [http://dx.doi.org/10.1016/j.ctrv.2016.03.006] [PMID: 27010487]

[17] Goldenberg D, Lee J, Koch WM, *et al.* Habitual risk factors for head and neck cancer. Otolaryngol Head Neck Surg 2004; 131(6): 986-93. [http://dx.doi.org/10.1016/j.otohns.2004.02.035] [PMID: 15577802]

[18] Deschler DG, Richmon JD, Khariwala SS, Ferris RL, Wang MB. The "new" head and neck cancer patient-young, nonsmoker, nondrinker, and HPV positive: evaluation. Otolaryngol Head Neck Surg 2014; 151(3): 375-80.
[http://dx.doi.org/10.1177/0194599814538605] [PMID: 24925311]

[19] Young D, Xiao CC, Murphy B, Moore M, Fakhry C, Day TA. Increase in head and neck cancer in younger patients due to human papillomavirus (HPV). Oral Oncol 2015; 51(8): 727-30.
[http://dx.doi.org/10.1016/j.oraloncology.2015.03.015] [PMID: 26066977]

[20] Chaturvedi AK, Engels EA, Pfeiffer RM, *et al.* Human papillomavirus and rising oropharyngeal cancer incidence in the United States. J Clin Oncol 2011; 29(32): 4294-301.
[http://dx.doi.org/10.1200/JCO.2011.36.4596] [PMID: 21969503]

[21] Whang S, Filippova M, Duerksen-Hughes P. Recent progress in therapeutic treatments and screening strategies for the prevention and treatment of HPV-associated head and neck cancer. Viruses 2015; 7(9): 5040-65.
[http://dx.doi.org/10.3390/v7092860] [PMID: 26393639]

[22] Haughey BH, Sinha P. Prognostic factors and survival unique to surgically treated p16+ oropharyngeal cancer. Laryngoscope 2012; 122(S2) (Suppl. 2): S13-33.
[http://dx.doi.org/10.1002/lary.23493] [PMID: 22926949]

[23] Ang KK, Harris J, Wheeler R, *et al.* Human papillomavirus and survival of patients with oropharyngeal cancer. N Engl J Med 2010; 363(1): 24-35.
[http://dx.doi.org/10.1056/NEJMoa0912217] [PMID: 20530316]

[24] Edge SB, Compton CC. The American Joint Committee on Cancer: the 7th edition of the AJCC cancer staging manual and the future of TNM. Ann Surg Oncol 2010; 17(6): 1471-4.
[http://dx.doi.org/10.1245/s10434-010-0985-4] [PMID: 20180029]

[25] Caster JM, Sethi M, Kowalczyk S, *et al.* Nanoparticle delivery of chemosensitizers improve chemotherapy efficacy without incurring additional toxicity. Nanoscale 2015; 7(6): 2805-11.
[http://dx.doi.org/10.1039/C4NR07102F] [PMID: 25584654]

[26] Wang EC, Min Y, Palm RC, *et al.* Nanoparticle formulations of histone deacetylase inhibitors for effective chemoradiotherapy in solid tumors. Biomaterials 2015; 51: 208-15.
[http://dx.doi.org/10.1016/j.biomaterials.2015.02.015] [PMID: 25771011]

[27] Kamaly N, Yameen B, Wu J, Farokhzad OC. Degradable controlled-release polymers and polymeric nanoparticles: mechanisms of controlling drug release. Chem Rev 2016; 116(4): 2602-63.
[http://dx.doi.org/10.1021/acs.chemrev.5b00346] [PMID: 26854975]

[28] Yu M, Wu J, Shi J, Farokhzad OC. Nanotechnology for protein delivery: Overview and perspectives. J Control Release 2016; 240: 24-37.
[http://dx.doi.org/10.1016/j.jconrel.2015.10.012] [PMID: 26458789]

[29] Fang T, Dong Y, Zhang X, Xie K, Lin L, Wang H. Integrating a novel SN38 prodrug into the PEGylated liposomal system as a robust platform for efficient cancer therapy in solid tumors. Int J Pharm 2016; 512(1): 39-48.
[http://dx.doi.org/10.1016/j.ijpharm.2016.08.036] [PMID: 27544846]

[30] Wu J, Kamaly N, Shi J, *et al.* Development of multinuclear polymeric nanoparticles as robust protein nanocarriers. Angew Chem Int Ed 2014; 53(34): 8975-9.
[http://dx.doi.org/10.1002/anie.201404766] [PMID: 24990548]

[31] Wu J, Zhao L, Xu X, *et al.* Hydrophobic cysteine poly (disulfide)□based redox□hypersensitive nanoparticle platform for cancer theranostics. Angew Chem Int Ed 2015; 54(32): 9218-23.
[http://dx.doi.org/10.1002/anie.201503863] [PMID: 26119453]

[32] Zhao H, Lin ZY, Yildirimer L, Dhinakar A, Zhao X, Wu J. Polymer-based nanoparticles for protein delivery: design, strategies and applications. J Mater Chem B Mater Biol Med 2016; 4(23): 4060-71.
[http://dx.doi.org/10.1039/C6TB00308G] [PMID: 32264607]

[33] Tao W, Zeng X, Wu J, *et al.* Polydopamine-based surface modification of novel nanoparticle-aptamer bioconjugates for *in vivo* breast cancer targeting and enhanced therapeutic effects. Theranostics 2016; 6(4): 470-84.
[http://dx.doi.org/10.7150/thno.14184] [PMID: 26941841]

[34] Huang D, Hou YL, Yang SM, Wang RG. Advances in nanomedicine for head and neck cancer. Front Biosci 2014; 19(5): 783-8.
[http://dx.doi.org/10.2741/4245] [PMID: 24389222]

[35] Wu J, Zhao X, Wu D, Chu CC. Development of a biocompatible and biodegradable hybrid hydrogel platform for sustained release of ionic drugs. J Mater Chem B Mater Biol Med 2014; 2(38): 6660-8.
[http://dx.doi.org/10.1039/C4TB00576G] [PMID: 32261826]

[36] Hu X, Gong X. A new route to fabricate biocompatible hydrogels with controlled drug delivery behavior. J Colloid Interface Sci 2016; 470: 62-70.
[http://dx.doi.org/10.1016/j.jcis.2016.02.037] [PMID: 26930541]

[37] Wang J, Wang H, Li J, *et al.* iRGD-decorated polymeric nanoparticles for the efficient delivery of vandetanib to hepatocellular carcinoma: preparation and *in vitro* and *in vivo* evaluation. ACS Appl Mater Interfaces 2016; 8(30): 19228-37.
[http://dx.doi.org/10.1021/acsami.6b03166] [PMID: 27381493]

[38] Wang H, Xie H, Wu J, *et al.* Structure-based rational design of prodrugs to enable their combination with polymeric nanoparticle delivery platforms for enhanced antitumor efficacy. Angew Chem Int Ed 2014; 53(43): 11532-7.
[http://dx.doi.org/10.1002/anie.201406685] [PMID: 25196427]

[39] Caponigro F, Di Gennaro E, Ionna F, *et al.* Phase II clinical study of valproic acid plus cisplatin and cetuximab in recurrent and/or metastatic squamous cell carcinoma of Head and Neck-V-CHANCE trial. BMC Cancer 2016; 16(1): 918.
[http://dx.doi.org/10.1186/s12885-016-2957-y] [PMID: 27884140]

[40] Forastiere AA, Metch B, Schuller DE, *et al.* Randomized comparison of cisplatin plus fluorouracil and carboplatin plus fluorouracil *versus* methotrexate in advanced squamous-cell carcinoma of the head and neck: a Southwest Oncology Group study. J Clin Oncol 1992; 10(8): 1245-51.
[http://dx.doi.org/10.1200/JCO.1992.10.8.1245] [PMID: 1634913]

[41] Cooper JS, Pajak TF, Forastiere AA, *et al.* Postoperative concurrent radiotherapy and chemotherapy for high-risk squamous-cell carcinoma of the head and neck. N Engl J Med 2004; 350(19): 1937-44.
[http://dx.doi.org/10.1056/NEJMoa032646] [PMID: 15128893]

[42] Bernier J, Domenge C, Ozsahin M, *et al.* Postoperative irradiation with or without concomitant chemotherapy for locally advanced head and neck cancer. N Engl J Med 2004; 350(19): 1945-52.
[http://dx.doi.org/10.1056/NEJMoa032641] [PMID: 15128894]

[43] Chow EKH, Ho D. Cancer nanomedicine: from drug delivery to imaging. Sci Transl Med 2013; 5(216): 216rv4.
[http://dx.doi.org/10.1126/scitranslmed.3005872] [PMID: 24353161]

[44] Ferrari M. Cancer nanotechnology: opportunities and challenges. Nat Rev Cancer 2005; 5(3): 161-71.
[http://dx.doi.org/10.1038/nrc1566] [PMID: 15738981]

[45] Hubbell JA, Chilkoti A. Chemistry. Nanomaterials for drug delivery. Science 2012; 337(6092): 303-5.
[http://dx.doi.org/10.1126/science.1219657] [PMID: 22822138]

[46] Li Y, Huang Y, Wang Z, *et al.* Polycatechol nanoparticle MRI contrast agents. Small 2016; 12(5): 668-77.
[http://dx.doi.org/10.1002/smll.201502754] [PMID: 26681255]

[47] Di Corato R, Bigall NC, Ragusa A, *et al.* Multifunctional nanobeads based on quantum dots and magnetic nanoparticles: synthesis and cancer cell targeting and sorting. ACS Nano 2011; 5(2): 1109-21.

[http://dx.doi.org/10.1021/nn102761t] [PMID: 21218823]

[48] Eustis S, El-Sayed MA. Why gold nanoparticles are more precious than pretty gold: Noble metal surface plasmon resonance and its enhancement of the radiative and nonradiative properties of nanocrystals of different shapes. Chem Soc Rev 2006; 35(3): 209-17. [http://dx.doi.org/10.1039/B514191E] [PMID: 16505915]

[49] Huang X, Jain PK, El-Sayed IH, El-Sayed MA. Gold nanoparticles: interesting optical properties and recent applications in cancer diagnostics and therapy. Nanomedicine (Lond) 2007; 2(5): 681-93. [http://dx.doi.org/10.2217/17435889.2.5.681]

[50] Kang B, Austin LA, El-Sayed MA. Real-time molecular imaging throughout the entire cell cycle by targeted plasmonic-enhanced Rayleigh/Raman spectroscopy. Nano Lett 2012; 12(10): 5369-75. [http://dx.doi.org/10.1021/nl3027586] [PMID: 22978570]

[51] Huang X, El-Sayed IH, Qian W, El-Sayed MA. Cancer cell imaging and photothermal therapy in the near-infrared region by using gold nanorods. J Am Chem Soc 2006; 128(6): 2115-20. [http://dx.doi.org/10.1021/ja057254a] [PMID: 16464114]

[52] Sano D, Berlin JM, Pham TT, *et al.* Noncovalent assembly of targeted carbon nanovectors enables synergistic drug and radiation cancer therapy *in vivo.* ACS Nano 2012; 6(3): 2497-505. [http://dx.doi.org/10.1021/nn204885f] [PMID: 22316245]

[53] Berlin JM, Pham TT, Sano D, *et al.* Noncovalent functionalization of carbon nanovectors with an antibody enables targeted drug delivery. ACS Nano 2011; 5(8): 6643-50. [http://dx.doi.org/10.1021/nn2021293] [PMID: 21736358]

[54] Bhirde AA, Patel V, Gavard J, *et al.* Targeted killing of cancer cells *in vivo* and *in vitro* with EGF-directed carbon nanotube-based drug delivery. ACS Nano 2009; 3(2): 307-16. [http://dx.doi.org/10.1021/nn800551s] [PMID: 19236065]

[55] Zhao Q, Wang L, Cheng R, *et al.* Magnetic nanoparticle-based hyperthermia for head & neck cancer in mouse models. Theranostics 2012; 2(1): 113-21. [http://dx.doi.org/10.7150/thno.3854] [PMID: 22287991]

[56] Xie M, Liu T, Xu Y, *et al.* Expression of folate receptors in nasopharyngeal and laryngeal carcinoma and folate receptor-mediated endocytosis by molecular targeted nanomedicine. Int J Nanomedicine 2013; 8: 2443-51. [http://dx.doi.org/10.2147/IJN.S46327] [PMID: 23874095]

[57] Wang D, Fei B, Halig LV, *et al.* Targeted iron-oxide nanoparticle for photodynamic therapy and imaging of head and neck cancer. ACS Nano 2014; 8(7): 6620-32. [http://dx.doi.org/10.1021/nn501652j] [PMID: 24923902]

[58] Brown MS, Diallo OT, Hu M, *et al.* CK2 modulation of NF-kappaB, TP53, and the malignant phenotype in head and neck cancer by anti-CK2 oligonucleotides in vitro or in vivo via sub-50-nm nanocapsules. Clin Cancer Res 2010; 16(8): 2295-307. [http://dx.doi.org/10.1158/1078-0432.CCR-09-3200] [PMID: 20371694]

[59] Arany S, Benoit DSW, Dewhurst S, Ovitt CE. Nanoparticle-mediated gene silencing confers radioprotection to salivary glands *in vivo.* Mol Ther 2013; 21(6): 1182-94. [http://dx.doi.org/10.1038/mt.2013.42] [PMID: 23511246]

[60] Colley HE, Hearnden V, Avila-Olias M, *et al.* Polymersome-mediated delivery of combination anticancer therapy to head and neck cancer cells: 2D and 3D *in vitro* evaluation. Mol Pharm 2014; 11(4): 1176-88. [http://dx.doi.org/10.1021/mp400610b] [PMID: 24533501]

[61] Wang X, Shi L, Tu Q, *et al.* Treating cutaneous squamous cell carcinoma using 5-aminolevulinic acid polylactic-co-glycolic acid nanoparticle-mediated photodynamic therapy in a mouse model. Int J Nanomedicine 2015; 10: 347-55. [PMID: 25609949]

[62] Chang RS, Suh MS, Kim S, *et al.* Cationic drug-derived nanoparticles for multifunctional delivery of anticancer siRNA. Biomaterials 2011; 32(36): 9785-95. [http://dx.doi.org/10.1016/j.biomaterials.2011.09.017] [PMID: 21937102]

[63] Yu YH, Kim E, Park DE, *et al.* Cationic solid lipid nanoparticles for co-delivery of paclitaxel and siRNA. Eur J Pharm Biopharm 2012; 80(2): 268-73. [http://dx.doi.org/10.1016/j.ejpb.2011.11.002] [PMID: 22108492]

[64] Piao L, Zhang M, Datta J, *et al.* Lipid-based nanoparticle delivery of Pre-miR-107 inhibits the tumorigenicity of head and neck squamous cell carcinoma. Mol Ther 2012; 20(6): 1261-9. [http://dx.doi.org/10.1038/mt.2012.67] [PMID: 22491216]

[65] Lin SJ, Chin YT, Ho Y, *et al.* Nano-diamino-tetrac (NDAT) inhibits PD-L1 expression which is essential for proliferation in oral cancer cells. Food Chem Toxicol 2018; 120: 1-11. [http://dx.doi.org/10.1016/j.fct.2018.06.058] [PMID: 29960019]

[66] Han HD, Byeon Y, Kang TH, *et al.* Toll-like receptor 3-induced immune response by poly(D,L-lactide-co-glycolide) nanoparticles for dendritic cell-based cancer immunotherapy. Int J Nanomedicine 2016; 11: 5729-42. [http://dx.doi.org/10.2147/IJN.S109001] [PMID: 27843314]

[67] Ilyinsky PO, Kovalev GI. 'O'Neil CP, Roy CJ, Michaud AM, Drefs NM, Pechenkin MA, Fu FN, Johnston LP, Ovchinnikov DA, Kishimoto TK. Synthetic vaccine particles for durable cytolytic T lymphocyte responses and antitumor immunotherapy. PLoS One 2018; 13(6): e0197694. [http://dx.doi.org/10.1371/journal.pone.0197694] [PMID: 29856772]

[68] Rosalia RA, Cruz LJ, van Duikeren S, *et al.* CD40-targeted dendritic cell delivery of PLGA-nanoparticle vaccines induce potent anti-tumor responses. Biomaterials 2015; 40: 88-97. [http://dx.doi.org/10.1016/j.biomaterials.2014.10.053] [PMID: 25465442]

[69] Prasad S, Cody V, Saucier-Sawyer JK, *et al.* Optimization of stability, encapsulation, release, and cross-priming of tumor antigen-containing PLGA nanoparticles. Pharm Res 2012; 29(9): 2565-77. [http://dx.doi.org/10.1007/s11095-012-0787-4] [PMID: 22798259]

[70] Nam J, Son S, Ochyl LJ, Kuai R, Schwendeman A, Moon JJ. Chemo-photothermal therapy combination elicits anti-tumor immunity against advanced metastatic cancer. Nat Commun 2018; 9(1): 1074. [http://dx.doi.org/10.1038/s41467-018-03473-9] [PMID: 29317637]

[71] Zhang L, Jing D, Wang L, *et al.* Unique photo chemo-immuno-nanoplatform against orthotopic xenograft oral cancer and metastatic syngeneic breast cancer. Nano Lett 2018; 18(11): 7092-103. [http://dx.doi.org/10.1021/acs.nanolett.8b03096] [PMID: 30339018]

[72] Espinosa-Cotton M, Rodman SN III, Ross KA, *et al.* Interleukin-1 alpha increases anti-tumor efficacy of cetuximab in head and neck squamous cell carcinoma. J Immunother Cancer 2019; 7(1): 79. [http://dx.doi.org/10.1186/s40425-019-0550-z] [PMID: 30612589]

[73] Da Silva CG, Camps MGM, Li TMWY, *et al.* Effective chemoimmunotherapy by co-delivery of doxorubicin and immune adjuvants in biodegradable nanoparticles. Theranostics 2019; 9(22): 6485-500. [http://dx.doi.org/10.7150/thno.34429] [PMID: 31588231]

[74] Galliverti G, Tichet M, Domingos-Pereira S, *et al.* Nanoparticle conjugation of human papillomavirus 16 E7-long peptides enhances therapeutic vaccine efficacy against solid tumors in mice. Cancer Immunol Res 2018; 6(11): 1301-13. [http://dx.doi.org/10.1158/2326-6066.CIR-18-0166] [PMID: 30131378]

[75] Gandhapudi SK, Ward M, Bush JPC, Bedu-Addo F, Conn G, Woodward JG. Antigen priming with enantiospecific cationic lipid nanoparticles induces potent anti-tumor CTL responses through novel induction of a type I IFN response. J Immunol 2019; 202(12): 3524-36. [http://dx.doi.org/10.4049/jimmunol.1801634] [PMID: 31053626]

[76] Liu C, Chu X, Yan M, *et al.* Encapsulation of Poly I:C and the natural phosphodiester CpG ODN enhanced the efficacy of a hyaluronic acid-modified cationic lipid-PLGA hybrid nanoparticle vaccine in TC-1-grafted tumors. Int J Pharm 2018; 553(1-2): 327-37. [http://dx.doi.org/10.1016/j.ijpharm.2018.10.054] [PMID: 30393151]

[77] Miao L, Li L, Huang Y, *et al.* Delivery of mRNA vaccines with heterocyclic lipids increases anti-tumor efficacy by STING-mediated immune cell activation. Nat Biotechnol 2019; 37(10): 1174-85. [http://dx.doi.org/10.1038/s41587-019-0247-3] [PMID: 31570898]

[78] Chu X, Li Y, Long Q, *et al.* Chimeric HBcAg virus-like particles presenting a HPV 16 E7 epitope significantly suppressed tumor progression through preventive or therapeutic immunization in a TC--grafted mouse model. Int J Nanomedicine 2016; 11: 2417-29. [PMID: 27313455]

[79] Chattopadhyay S, Dash SK, Ghosh T, *et al.* Anticancer and immunostimulatory role of encapsulated tumor antigen containing cobalt oxide nanoparticles. J Biol Inorg Chem 2013; 18(8): 957-73. [http://dx.doi.org/10.1007/s00775-013-1044-y] [PMID: 24043470]

[80] Maiyo F, Singh M. Folate-targeted mRNA delivery using chitosan-functionalized selenium nanoparticles: potential in cancer immunotherapy. Pharmaceuticals (Basel) 2019; 12(4): 164. [http://dx.doi.org/10.3390/ph12040164] [PMID: 31690043]

[81] Xian J, Yang H, Lin Y, Liu S. Combination nonviral murine interleukin 2 and interleukin 12 gene therapy and radiotherapy for head and neck squamous cell carcinoma. Arch Otolaryngol Head Neck Surg 2005; 131(12): 1079-85. [http://dx.doi.org/10.1001/archotol.131.12.1079] [PMID: 16365221]

[82] Ishii KJ, Kawakami K, Gursel I, *et al.* Antitumor therapy with bacterial DNA and toxin: complete regression of established tumor induced by liposomal CpG oligodeoxynucleotides plus interleukin-13 cytotoxin. Clin Cancer Res 2003; 9(17): 6516-22. [PMID: 14695156]

[83] Grunwitz C, Salomon N, Vascotto F, *et al.* HPV16 RNA-LPX vaccine mediates complete regression of aggressively growing HPV-positive mouse tumors and establishes protective T cell memory. OncoImmunology 2019; 8(9): e1629259. [http://dx.doi.org/10.1080/2162402X.2019.1629259] [PMID: 31428528]

[84] Kranz LM, Diken M, Haas H, *et al.* Systemic RNA delivery to dendritic cells exploits antiviral defence for cancer immunotherapy. Nature 2016; 534(7607): 396-401. [http://dx.doi.org/10.1038/nature18300] [PMID: 27281205]

[85] Kwong B, Gai SA, Elkhader J, Wittrup KD, Irvine DJ. Localized immunotherapy *via* liposome-anchored Anti-CD137 + IL-2 prevents lethal toxicity and elicits local and systemic antitumor immunity. Cancer Res 2013; 73(5): 1547-58. [http://dx.doi.org/10.1158/0008-5472.CAN-12-3343] [PMID: 23436794]

[86] Leach DG, Dharmaraj N, Piotrowski SL, *et al.* STINGel: Controlled release of a cyclic dinucleotide for enhanced cancer immunotherapy. Biomaterials 2018; 163: 67-75. [http://dx.doi.org/10.1016/j.biomaterials.2018.01.035] [PMID: 29454236]

[87] Lu R, Groer C, Kleindl PA, *et al.* Formulation and preclinical evaluation of a toll-like receptor 7/8 agonist as an anti-tumoral immunomodulator. J Control Release 2019; 306: 165-76. [http://dx.doi.org/10.1016/j.jconrel.2019.06.003] [PMID: 31173789]

[88] Lu K, He C, Guo N, *et al.* Low-dose X-ray radiotherapy–radiodynamic therapy *via* nanoscale metal–organic frameworks enhances checkpoint blockade immunotherapy. Nat Biomed Eng 2018; 2(8): 600-10. [http://dx.doi.org/10.1038/s41551-018-0203-4] [PMID: 31015630]

[89] Kuai R, Sun X, Yuan W, *et al.* Dual TLR agonist nanodiscs as a strong adjuvant system for vaccines and immunotherapy. J Control Release 2018; 282: 131-9.

[http://dx.doi.org/10.1016/j.jconrel.2018.04.041] [PMID: 29702142]

[90] Li AW, Sobral MC, Badrinath S, *et al.* A facile approach to enhance antigen response for personalized cancer vaccination. Nat Mater 2018; 17(6): 528-34. [http://dx.doi.org/10.1038/s41563-018-0028-2] [PMID: 29507416]

[91] Li S, Zhang Q, Bai H, *et al.* Self-Assembled Nanofibers Elicit Potent HPV16 E7-Specific Cellular Immunity And Abolish Established TC-1 Graft Tumor. Int J Nanomedicine 2019; 14: 8209-19. [http://dx.doi.org/10.2147/IJN.S214525] [PMID: 31632028]

[92] Wang L, Wang Z, Qin Y, Liang W. Delivered antigen peptides to resident $CD8\alpha^+$ DCs in lymph node by micelle-based vaccine augment antigen-specific $CD8^+$ effector T cell response. Eur J Pharm Biopharm 2020; 147: 76-86. [http://dx.doi.org/10.1016/j.ejpb.2019.12.013] [PMID: 31887349]

[93] Tan YS, Sansanaphongpricha K, Xie Y, *et al.* Mitigating SOX2-potentiated immune escape of head and neck squamous cell carcinoma with a STING-inducing nanosatellite vaccine. Clin Cancer Res 2018; 24(17): 4242-55. [http://dx.doi.org/10.1158/1078-0432.CCR-17-2807] [PMID: 29769207]

[94] Dharmaraj N, Piotrowski SL, Huang C, *et al.* Anti-tumor immunity induced by ectopic expression of viral antigens is transient and limited by immune escape. OncoImmunology 2019; 8(4): e1568809. [http://dx.doi.org/10.1080/2162402X.2019.1568809] [PMID: 30906661]

[95] Li Y, Xie Y, Wang Z, *et al.* Structure and function of iron-loaded synthetic melanin. ACS Nano 2016; 10(11): 10186-94. [http://dx.doi.org/10.1021/acsnano.6b05502] [PMID: 27802021]

[96] Banik BL, Fattahi P, Brown JL. Polymeric nanoparticles: the future of nanomedicine. Wiley Interdiscip Rev Nanomed Nanobiotechnol 2016; 8(2): 271-99. [http://dx.doi.org/10.1002/wnan.1364] [PMID: 26314803]

[97] Rait AS, Pirollo KF, Ulick D, Cullen K, Chang EH. HER-2-targeted antisense oligonucleotide results in sensitization of head and neck cancer cells to chemotherapeutic agents. Ann N Y Acad Sci 2003; 1002(1): 78-89. [http://dx.doi.org/10.1196/annals.1281.018] [PMID: 14751825]

[98] Shim G, Han SE, Yu YH, *et al.* Trilysinoyl oleylamide-based cationic liposomes for systemic co-delivery of siRNA and an anticancer drug. J Control Release 2011; 155(1): 60-6. [http://dx.doi.org/10.1016/j.jconrel.2010.10.017] [PMID: 20971142]

[99] Ward BB, Dunham T, Majoros IJ, Baker JR Jr. Targeted dendrimer chemotherapy in an animal model for head and neck squamous cell carcinoma. J Oral Maxillofac Surg 2011; 69(9): 2452-9. [http://dx.doi.org/10.1016/j.joms.2010.12.041] [PMID: 21684654]

[100] Dosio F, Arpicco S, Stella B, Brusa P, Cattel L. Folate-mediated targeting of albumin conjugates of paclitaxel obtained through a heterogeneous phase system. Int J Pharm 2009; 382(1-2): 117-23. [http://dx.doi.org/10.1016/j.ijpharm.2009.08.018] [PMID: 19712735]

[101] Gao Z, Zhang L, Sun Y. Nanotechnology applied to overcome tumor drug resistance. J Control Release 2012; 162(1): 45-55. [http://dx.doi.org/10.1016/j.jconrel.2012.05.051] [PMID: 22698943]

[102] Kamaly N, Xiao Z, Valencia PM, Radovic-Moreno AF, Farokhzad OC. Targeted polymeric therapeutic nanoparticles: design, development and clinical translation. Chem Soc Rev 2012; 41(7): 2971-3010. [http://dx.doi.org/10.1039/c2cs15344k] [PMID: 22388185]

[103] Byrne JD, Betancourt T, Brannon-Peppas L. Active targeting schemes for nanoparticle systems in cancer therapeutics. Adv Drug Deliv Rev 2008; 60(15): 1615-26. [http://dx.doi.org/10.1016/j.addr.2008.08.005] [PMID: 18840489]

[104] Ang KK, Berkey BA, Tu X, *et al.* Impact of epidermal growth factor receptor expression on survival

and pattern of relapse in patients with advanced head and neck carcinoma. Cancer Res 2002; 62(24): 7350-6.
[PMID: 12499279]

[105] He Y, Zeng Q, Drenning SD, *et al.* Inhibition of human squamous cell carcinoma growth *in vivo* by epidermal growth factor receptor antisense RNA transcribed from the U6 promoter. J Natl Cancer Inst 1998; 90(14): 1080-7.
[http://dx.doi.org/10.1093/jnci/90.14.1080] [PMID: 9672256]

[106] Cho HJ, Chong S, Chung SJ, Shim CK, Kim DD. Poly-L-arginine and dextran sulfate-based nanocomplex for epidermal growth factor receptor (EGFR) siRNA delivery: its application for head and neck cancer treatment. Pharm Res 2012; 29(4): 1007-19.
[http://dx.doi.org/10.1007/s11095-011-0642-z] [PMID: 22169985]

[107] Elnakat H, Ratnam M. Distribution, functionality and gene regulation of folate receptor isoforms: implications in targeted therapy. Adv Drug Deliv Rev 2004; 56(8): 1067-84.
[http://dx.doi.org/10.1016/j.addr.2004.01.001] [PMID: 15094207]

[108] Leamon C, Reddy JA. Folate-targeted chemotherapy. Adv Drug Deliv Rev 2004; 56(8): 1127-41.
[http://dx.doi.org/10.1016/j.addr.2004.01.008] [PMID: 15094211]

[109] Garg A, Garg S, Sahu NK, Rani S, Gupta U, Yadav AK. Heparin appended ADH-anionic polysaccharide nanoparticles for site-specific delivery of usnic acid. Int J Pharm 2019; 557: 238-53.
[http://dx.doi.org/10.1016/j.ijpharm.2018.12.049] [PMID: 30594688]

[110] Tibbitt MW, Dahlman JE, Langer R. Emerging frontiers in drug delivery. J Am Chem Soc 2016; 138(3): 704-17.
[http://dx.doi.org/10.1021/jacs.5b09974] [PMID: 26741786]

[111] Miyagi Y, Fujiwara K, Kigawa J, *et al.* Intraperitoneal carboplatin infusion may be a pharmacologically more reasonable route than intravenous administration as a systemic chemotherapy. A comparative pharmacokinetic analysis of platinum using a new mathematical model after intraperitoneal vs. intravenous infusion of carboplatin—A Sankai Gynecology Study Group (SGSG) study. Gynecol Oncol 2005; 99(3): 591-6.
[http://dx.doi.org/10.1016/j.ygyno.2005.06.055] [PMID: 16095677]

[112] Yen MS, Juang CM, Lai CR, Chao GC, Ng HT, Yuan CC. Intraperitoneal cisplatin□based chemotherapy vs. intravenous cisplatin□based chemotherapy for stage III optimally cytoreduced epithelial ovarian cancer. (International journal of gynecology & obstetrics.)2001; 72(1): 55-60.

[113] Bristow RE, Santillan A, Salani R, *et al.* Intraperitoneal cisplatin and paclitaxel *versus* intravenous carboplatin and paclitaxel chemotherapy for Stage III ovarian cancer: A cost-effectiveness analysis. Gynecol Oncol 2007; 106(3): 476-81.
[http://dx.doi.org/10.1016/j.ygyno.2007.05.043] [PMID: 17688927]

[114] Zhao H, Feng H, Liu D, *et al.* Self-assembling monomeric nucleoside molecular nanoparticles loaded with 5-FU enhancing therapeutic efficacy against oral cancer. ACS Nano 2015; 9(10): 9638-51.
[http://dx.doi.org/10.1021/acsnano.5b04520] [PMID: 26349079]

[115] Wolinsky JB, Colson YL, Grinstaff MW. Local drug delivery strategies for cancer treatment: Gels, nanoparticles, polymeric films, rods, and wafers. J Control Release 2012; 159(1): 14-26.
[http://dx.doi.org/10.1016/j.jconrel.2011.11.031] [PMID: 22154931]

[116] Robbins KT, Storniolo AM, Kerber C, Seagren S, Berson A, Howell SB. Rapid superselective high-dose cisplatin infusion for advanced head and neck malignancies. Head Neck 1992; 14(5): 364-71.
[http://dx.doi.org/10.1002/hed.2880140505] [PMID: 1399569]

[117] Wolpert SM, Kwan ES, Heros D, Kasdon DL, Hedges TR III. Selective delivery of chemotherapeutic agents with a new catheter system. Radiology 1988; 166(2): 547-9.
[http://dx.doi.org/10.1148/radiology.166.2.3336733] [PMID: 3336733]

[118] Homma A, Onimaru R, Matsuura K, Robbins KT, Fujii M. Intra-arterial chemoradiotherapy for head

and neck cancer. Jpn J Clin Oncol 2016; 46(1): 4-12.
[http://dx.doi.org/10.1093/jjco/hyv151] [PMID: 26486825]

[119] Damascelli B, Patelli G, Tichá V, *et al.* Feasibility and efficacy of percutaneous transcatheter intraarterial chemotherapy with paclitaxel in albumin nanoparticles for advanced squamous-cell carcinoma of the oral cavity, oropharynx, and hypopharynx. J Vasc Interv Radiol 2007; 18(11): 1395-403.
[http://dx.doi.org/10.1016/j.jvir.2007.06.009] [PMID: 18003990]

CHAPTER 10

Accounts on the Nano-carrier System for Diagnosis Purposes

S.P. Pandey[1,*], P. Jangied[1], T. Shukla[2], Tripathi A.[3] and N. Upmanyu[3,4]

[1] *Department of Pharmacy, Shri G.S. Institute of Technology & Science, Indore, India*

[2] *Institute of Pharmaceutical Sciences, SAGE University, Indore, India*

[3] *School of Pharmacy and Research, Peoples University, Bhopal, India*

[4] *Sagar Institute of Research & Technology-Pharmacy, Bhopal, India, India*

Abstract: Timely diagnosis of critical diseases, such as cancer, may help in its effective management and better survival. Several techniques like magnetic resonance imaging (MRI), computed tomography scan (CT scan), positron emission tomography (PET), photoacoustic imaging (PAI), *etc.* are already being used successfully, but sometimes their high cost, spatial resolution, sensitivity, and specificity (associated with the use of contrast agent) have been questionable. The distinction between benign and malignant tumours in their early stages is also a critical issue with such methods. But the use of nano-carriers for diagnostic and theranostics purposes has opened newer dimensions and provided a better understanding and visualization of the pathophysiological condition in a specific disease. There are different nanotechnology-based systems like bio-labels containing nanoparticles, nanotechnology-based microarrays, nano-bio sensors, and nanoscale optics that can be used in molecular diagnostics. Several nano-carriers, especially after their surface functionalization, are also on the floor, showing their importance in the medical diagnosis of different diseases. The current chapter deals with the importance and significance of such different nano-carriers in the development of diagnostics and theranostics.

Keywords: Diagnosis, Imaging techniques, Nanocarriers, Surface modification, Theranostics.

INTRODUCTION

It is well evident that diagnosis of diseases, especially critical ones like cancer, at the earliest, may help to manage these diseases more effectively and achieve better survival. Currently, numbers of non-invasive techniques are there like magnetic resonance imaging (MRI), computed tomography scan (CT scan),

* **Corresponding Author S.P. Pandey:** Department of Pharmacy, Shri G. S. Institute of Technology nd Science, Indore, India; E-mail: pandesharad@gmail.com, Mob.: 9098288330

Neeraj Mishra, Ashish Garg and Neeraj Upmanyu (Eds.)

positron emission tomography (PET), photoacoustic imaging (PAI), *etc.*, are being utilized for the assessment of different pathophysiological conditions even at a molecular level too [1]. Every technique has its advantage, but at the same time, they also suffer from certain limitations in terms of sensitivity and specificity associated with the use of contrast agents, cost, spatial resolution, *etc.* At a similar time, with current techniques, it is also difficult to distinguish between benign and malignant tumors [2, 3]. Detection of cancer in its early stage is also difficult with such methods [3].

Currently, the use of nanocarriers is mainly focused on targeting medicament to specific sites due to their retention and surface behavior, leading to the increased efficiency of a therapeutic agent and reducing the associated toxicity. But, in recent years, the advancement in nanotechnology has led to the utilization of various nanocarriers for diagnostic purposes. Using such nanocarriers may provide a better understanding and visualization of the pathophysiological condition in a specific disease. But on another part, the utility of such carrier systems for diagnostic purposes is also limited due to their complex pharmacokinetic behavior and elimination. Studies show that the intrinsic property and surface behavior of nanocarrier may be better used for integration of the diagnostic and therapeutic use, and this led to the development of newer theranostics formulations which may be utilized for bio-distribution monitoring along with the accumulation of drugs at the target site, quantifying and visualizing the drug release.

A medical diagnosis of diseases has covered a long way from the conventional way of diagnosis (hematological testing, testing of biochemical parameters, microscopic testing, *etc.*) to current techniques and ways (electrochemical microarrays, lab-on-a-chip diagnostics, Nucleic Acid Amplification Tests, *etc.*) [4]. The addition of newer nanotechnology-based systems and the use of nano-carriers are giving a new dimension to the currently available techniques used for diagnosis. Detection of nucleic acid by microchip and nano-scale devices (Carbon nanotubes, nanoparticles) may be a suitable example. Some commonly used nanotechnology-based systems that can be used in molecular diagnostics include bio-labels congaing nanoparticles, nanotechnology-based microarrays, nano-biosensors, and nanoscale optics [4]. Apart from the above, several nano-carriers systems have also been developed, which have shown their importance in the medical diagnosis of the ailment, especially by various imaging techniques. Different types of nanocarriers (and ligands used for their functionalization) used for the development of newer diagnostic and theranostics are summarized in Fig. (**1**).

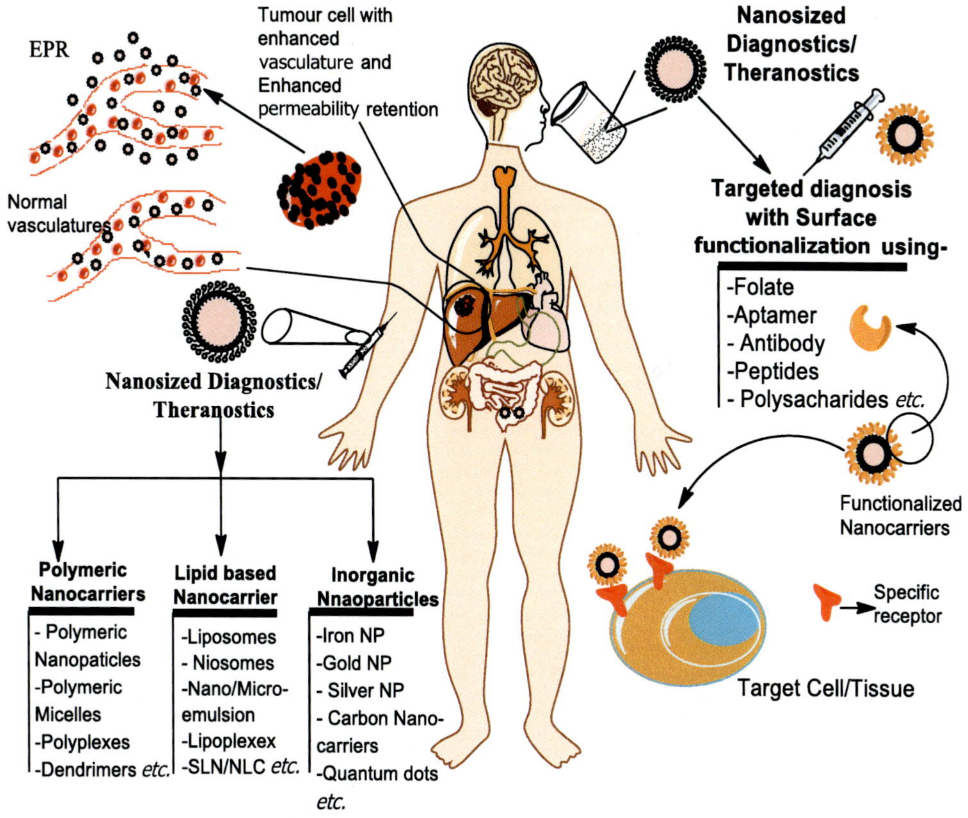

Fig. (1). Different types of nanocarriers and ligands used for the development of newer diagnostics and theranostics.

In comparison to traditional molecular-based contrast agents, these nano-carriers with a special surface characteristic and integrated design perform several functions, including cell targeting, highly sensitive imaging, and therapy as such [5]. There are a number of nano-materials that have been identified for their use in preclinical medicine, including the detection of cancer biomarkers by gold nano-particles, carbon nano-tubes, and silicon nano-wires, *in-vivo* imaging of tumors in their preliminary phase by quantum dots, and magnetic nano-particles [6].

The current chapter will cover detailed insight into different nano-carriers and their utilization, as mentioned in Fig. (**1**), for diagnostic and theranostic purposes, including lipid-based carriers, polymeric carriers, and metallic nanocarriers.

DIFFERENT NANO-CARRIERS USED FOR DIAGNOSIS

Nanocarriers used for the development of diagnostic and theranostic can be broadly classified into three major categories, *viz.* polymeric nano-carriers, Lipid-based nanocarriers, and inorganic nanoparticles. The use of these nanocarriers for drug delivery is well evident and well documented, but at a similar time, extensive research related to their use as diagnostic and theranostics is also well reported. Different uses of nanoparticles/ nanocarriers, as mentioned in Fig. (**2**), have been reported in the various literature, including their FDA-approved utility as a contrast agent for imaging and ultrasonography [7 - 9].

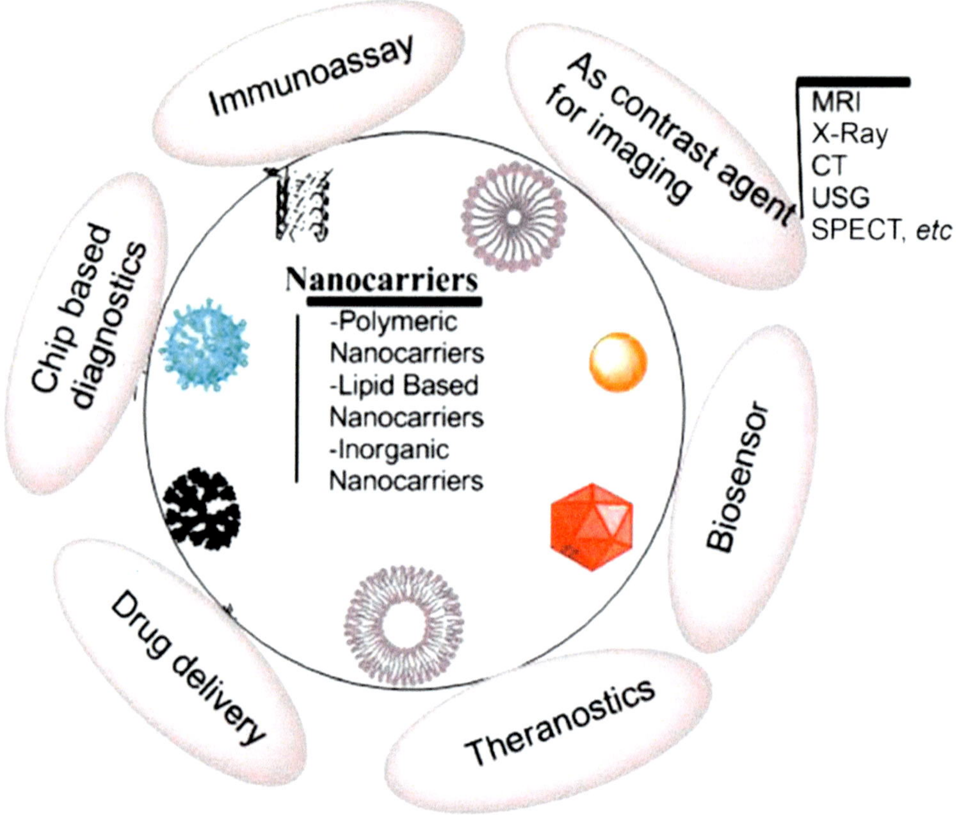

Fig. (2). Utility of different nanocarriers.

Polymeric Nano-carrier

Several polymer-based nano-carrier systems are being used for drug delivery purposes. These carriers may also be used for the development of diagnostic and theranostic agents. The major categories of this product class include polymeric nanoparticles, polymeric micelles, polyplexes, *etc.*

Polymeric Nanoparticles

The polymeric nanoparticles (PNPs) are made from biocompatible and biodegradable polymers (non-antigenic and non-toxic) with sizes ranging from 10 to 1000 nm, along with the medication dissolved, bound, encased, or linked to a nanoparticle matrix [10, 11]. Depending upon their way of formation, they can vary as nanoparticles, nanocapsules, and nanospheres [11, 12]. Both natural and artificial polymers are used in their formation [13], and their application ranges from electronics, photonics, conducting materials, sensors, healthcare, biotechnology, environmental management, and technologies [10].

Apart from the drug delivery application, polymeric nanoparticles have shown tremendous utility as diagnostic and theranostics, especially when tagged with NIR Probes [14]. These nanoparticles can be used for immunoassay [15], analysis of biomarkers [16], and as a contrast system for imaging-based and cancer diagnosis [17, 18].

The existing imaging agents utilized in clinics for diagnosis possess several drawbacks, including low target selectivity, *in vivo* instability, and compromised image quality when used in quantities. While polymeric nanoparticles can deliver a relatively higher concentration of such agents with target-specific delivery, leading to better imaging [17]. At the same time, the addition of two or more contrast agents in a single matrix may allow multimodal imaging [19]. One such attempt has been made by Teraphongphom *et al.*, where they have encapsulated quantum dots (QD), magnetic nanoparticles, and gold nanoparticles (AuNP) inside Poly lactic acid (PLA) micro-bubbles [20].

Functionalization of polymeric systems with specific ligands adds benefit during the diagnosis process by targeting a specific site and may help in targeted molecular imaging [19]. The anti-VGEF-modified gadolinium-loaded polymeric nanoparticle has also been reported as a contrast agent with improved targeting features for their use in the early diagnosis of hepato-cellular carcinoma by molecular MR imaging [21].

Despite several limitations, including low quantum yields, high plasma protein binding, lower stability against light, formation of aggregates, *etc.*, organic dyes, specifically NIR dyes including cyanins (*e.g.*, Indocyanine green), porphyrin, *etc.*, are also there, which can be used for fluorescence-based imaging of cancer [22, 23]. These shortcomings can be successfully managed with the development of several polymeric nano-carriers, such as nanoparticles, for the delivery of these dyes [24] and can be used effectively for the diagnosis as well as surgical guidance for tumor removal [25]. In a study, hyaluronic acid nanoparticles loaded with indocyanine green (NIR dye) have been reported for their utility in image-guided surgery [26]. Another polymeric nano-particle formulation composed of poly (glycerol malate co-dodecanedioate) (PGMD) loaded with IR820 (NIR dye) has also been reported for multifunctional imaging and hyperthermia-based therapy of cancer [27]. In a novel work, Pan *et al.* reported heptamethine cyanine dye (me-IR825) containing polymeric (Pluronic F127) micelle for diagnosis (fluorescence imaging of mitochondria, detection of early-stage cancer, differentiation between normal and cancerous cell) as well as mitochondria-targeted photo thermal therapy.

Surface functionalization of polymeric nano-particles loaded with the dyes has greatly impacted the stability, blood circulation time, targeting, *etc.*, of these formulations making them more useful for targeted imaging as well as therapy [28, 29].

Immunoassay is another segment where polymeric nano-particles have shown their utility due to larger surface-to-volume ratio, ease of surface functionalization, and comparatively better control of the size of nanoparticles [30]. Detection of metabolites using polymer-coated metal oxide in microarray immunoassay [31], detection of low levels of toxins by fluoroimmunoassay using surface-modified fluorescent core-shell nanoparticles [32], detection of bacteria using fluorescent polymeric nano-particles bio-conjugated with specific bacterial antibody [30], detection of different carcinomas by using ferrocene molecules loaded pH-responsive polymeric micelles having a self-assembling tendency [15], *etc.*, are some common example of the use of polymeric nano-particle in the immunoassay.

Polymeric Micelles

Polymeric micelles are self-assembled nano-scale colloidal aggregates of amphiphilic block polymers distributed in a specific medium with core-shell architecture [33, 34]. When block polymers are dispersed in the water, it starts to assemble in such a way that the hydrophobic part of the polymer forms the inner core accommodating the drug, while the hydrophilic part forms a soluble outer shell [35]. Depending on the architecture of the molecule and the interaction parameter, these micelles may have several structures such as rod, spherical, disc, *etc* [36], and apart from drug delivery purposes [37], they can also be used as a carrier for different contrast agents for different imaging modalities such as MRI, X-Ray computed tomography, scintigraphy, *etc* [35].

Hydrophobic contrast can be loaded as such in the hydrophobic core of the polymeric micelles. In this regard, Ai, Hua, *et al.* reported the magnetite-loaded polymeric micelles of a di-block copolymer of Poly-Ɛ caprolactone-b-poly (ethylene glycol) (PCL-b-PEG) as an ultrasensitive probe for MR imaging [38]. Apart from this, several other magnetite nanoparticles loaded polymeric micelles have also been reported for drug delivery and imaging [39, 40]. But, it has been noted that the majority of imaging agents, such as metal chelates showing para-magnetism (gadolinium, iron oxide, dysprosium, and magnese), which are preferred in the case of the above-mentioned modalities, are hydrophilic in nature and a limited number of methods are there for their incorporation in the polymeric micelle [35, 41, 42]. Incorporation of such chelated metals needs their conversion in amphiphilic structure like Gd-DTPA-PE (Gadolinium-diethylene triaminepentaacetyl-phosphatidylethanolamine) as mentioned in Fig. (**3**) [41]. Several other probes have also been developed for their incorporation in liposomal structure [42]. These Amphiphilic probes can be incorporated into polymeric micelles through their hydrophobic part and can be used effectively as a contrast for Gama- scintigraphy and MR imaging [43, 44].

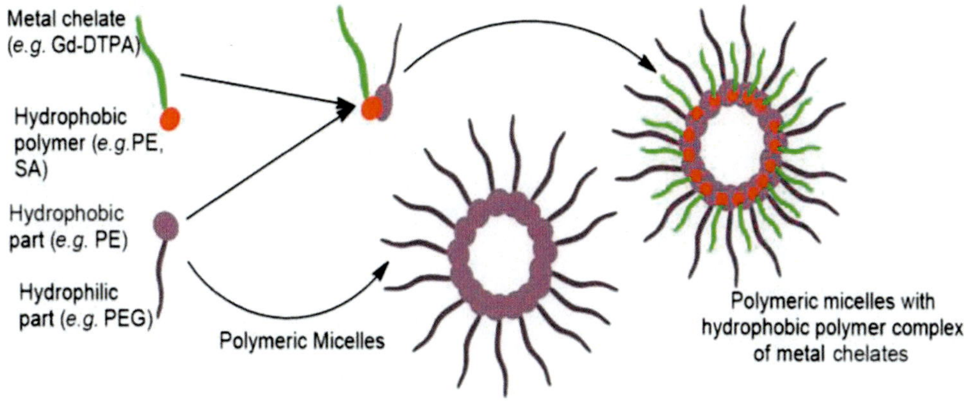

Fig. (3). Probable mechanism of hydrophilic molecule incorporation in polymeric micelles.

Torchilin has also mentioned the concept of poly-chelating amphiphilic polymers (PAP) in detail for different purposes. He mentions that amphiphilic poly L-lysin (PLL) based chelate, which carries 111In and Gd (important metal ions for diagnostic purposes), can be loaded to Poly ethylene glycol-phosphatidyl ethanolamine (PEG-PE) self-assembled polymeric micelles [45].

Polymeric micelles have also been reported for their theranostic use. In their work, Liu *et al.* reported the biotinylated alpha-fetoprotein (AFP) antibody functionalized polymeric micelles containing gadolinium (gd) and paclitaxel (PTX) for MR imaging and chemotherapy of Hepato cellular carcinoma [46].

Polyplexes

Polyplexes are regarded as a system in which cationic polymers are condensed with anionic DNA or siRNA by electrostatic interactions between the polymer's cationic groups and negatively charged nucleic acids [47, 48]. These polyplexes are mainly used to deliver viable nucleic acid to the specific site, without any nucleic acid degradation by the enzymes [49].

Gene therapy is considered to be the ultimate treatment of critical diseases, but still, there are miles to go [50]. Before that, the identification of faulty genome sequences and their analysis is of utmost importance for understanding the disease and developing diagnostic tools [51]. Several advances have taken place, but getting a correct vector for the above purposes is typical [52]. The development of polyplexes due to their smaller size may show better transfection and can be a better alternative for an effective gene delivery system [53]. It is also a known fact that the process of avoiding lysosomal degradation by preparation of polyplexes may impart cytotoxicity too [54, 55], which can be minimized by pegylation to a certain extent with increased stability [56]. At the same time, the functionalization of polyplexes with folic acid and the addition of SPION in the system increases the possibility of targeted delivery with the ability to work as a contrast agent for imaging. One such FA-PEG-SS-PEI-SPION/siRNA polyplex has been reported by Luo *et al.* for its ability to work as a probe for MR imaging of cancer as well as efficient blockade of programmed death-1 (PD-1) /Programmed death ligand-1(PD-L) after internalization [57]. In a similar work, a polyplex possessing SPION and functionalized with CD3 single-chain antibody (scAbCD3) have been reported by Guo et.al. for non-invasive and real time imaging and therapy for acute rejection of donor tissue in heart transplanted rat model [58]. Detection of tumour lesions and transfection efficiency of polyplexes can also be measured by combining the reporter gene (firefly luciferase) and infrared fluorescent protein 720 (iRFP720) with polyplexes [59].

Dendrimers

Dendrimers are complex macromolecules with a critical molecular design possessing highly branched structures with ample terminal groups, making them very suitable for drug delivery and other biomedical applications [60, 61]. Water solubility, mono-dispersibility, presence of hydrophobic and hydrophilic cavities and nanometric size are other important characteristics that make it a suitable nano-carrier [60, 62]. Dendrimers have shown their excellent utility in drug delivery, and the limitation associated with other polymeric delivery systems with regard to oral delivery can also be minimized by it [63]. PAMAM dendrimers have shown their potential for oral drug delivery with enhanced transepithelial permeability of loaded molecules [64, 65]. Apart from the use of dendrimers in drug delivery and other biomedical applications, they can also be effectively used for the generation of diagnostics and theranostics. Since the first report published in the early 90's regarding the *in-vivo* use of MRI contrast agents based on dendrimers [66, 67], several reports have been published regarding the development and use of different dendrimer-based MR imaging contrast agents [70 - 73]. In the developmental phases, it has also been noted that newer generations of dendrimers like 7 & 8 have shown their usefulness in the imaging of inner as well as outer vasculatures of a tumour [68]. Similar to the above, dendrimer-based contrast agents have been developed for x-ray computed tomography too [69, 70]. Nanoprobes, based on dendrimers for dual imaging modalities, can also be developed. With regard to it, a generation 6 PAMAM ethylenediamine dendrimer core having gadolinium chelate and NIR dye has been reported for the dual imaging modalities, *i.e.*, Magnetic resonance and fluorescence imaging [71].

The development of theranostics based on the dendrimers is another important utility, which has been reported in the various literature [78 - 81]. In general, it has been observed that gadolinium (Gd) and superparamagnetic iron oxide (SPIO) -based dendrimers are the points of interest among the research fraternity for the development of cancer theranostics [72].

Lipid-based Nanocarriers

Lipid-based nanocarriers (LNs) is a catch-all term for a variety of systems, namely Liposomes, nano/micro-emulsions solid lipid nanoparticles (SLN), nanostructured lipid carriers (NLC), lipid nanocapsules (LNC), and drug–lipid conjugates. LNs have advantages over polymeric nanoparticles (NPs) with regards to the biocompatibility and lower cost of the material used, production cost and scalability, and encapsulation efficiency of highly lipophilic actives LNs can be used for drug targeting and for delivering poorly water-soluble drugs and the cationic lipid-based formulations are also used for the gene delivery [82 - 84].

Nanoemulsions

Nanoemulsions are colloidal dispersion made up of nanometre-sized particles. They are thermodynamically metastable and kinetically stable systems composed of two immiscible liquids, *i.e.*, oily phase and aqueous phase (stabilized with the help of surfactant and cosurfactant) [73]. In the majority of conditions, they have a hydrophobic core and are composed of safe gradient excipients, which provide aid in encapsulating the poorly water-soluble drug and make it a safe option for drug delivery [74, 75]. Nano/Micro emulsion can also be used for bioavailability enhancement of hydrophilic drugs too [76]. At the same time, nano/micro emulsion can also be used for the transdermal administration of hydrophilic drugs alone [77, 78] and in combination with hydrophobic drugs [79, 80].

Traditional contrast agents used in the enhancement of the CT contrast are based on iodinated molecules, and compounds with high X-Ray absorption coefficient, which will lead to increased visibility in the body's administrated region with a disadvantage of rapidly eliminated from the blood vessels and/or lymphatic vessels uptake after intravenous injection. However, to overcome this problem, CT contrast agents are encapsulated in various nanoparticulate carriers, namely nanoemulsion and liposome [81]. Despite CT scan's advantages as a powerful diagnostic suffers from low target sensitivity due to which large doses of small iodinated agents are required for adequate contrast. While optical probes have a relatively high sensitivity, they are restricted by low tissue penetration depths. As a result, incorporating fluorescent species such as fluorescence quantum dots (QDs) into an iodine-containing nanoemulsion will result in a dual-modal contrast agent, which benefits both CT and optical imaging.

In some literature, the theranostic application of nanoemulsions in cancer has also been reported [82]. Gianella *et al.* developed and evaluated a multimodal nanoparticulate system for imaging as well as the delivery of therapeutic agents in mouse model colon cancer. They developed a "theranostic" platform centered on the oil-in-water nanoemulsions using pegylated lipid and iron oxide nanocrystals coated with soyabean oil and oleic acid [83].

It is also well evident that macrophages are one of the most prevalent cell types in inflammation and play their role in the pathogenesis of different diseases, including cancer, and show natural phagocytic activity. It can be targeted easily using a nanoparticulate system loaded with imaging and therapeutic agents. In their work, Patel *et al.* reported the theranostic application of fluorescent per-fluorocarbon nano-emulsions, which can be utilized for delivery of a therapeutic agent to macrophages with the monitoring of their movement using optical microscopy [84].

Another area, which has fascinated the researcher working in the area of diagnosis using nanomaterial is the finding the application of nanoemulsions in the diagnosis of atherosclerosis. Atherosclerosis is a chronic vascular disease that impacts medium and large-sized arteries and is characterized by the multiplication of so-called atheroma plaques, which are distinguished by an abnormal accumulation of lipid and immune cells in the artery wall. Prevot *et al.* reported the use of superparamagnetic iron oxide nanoparticles loaded nano-emulsion coupled with atheroma-specific monoclonal antibody for early diagnosis of atherosclerosis using magnetic resonance imaging (MRI) and magnetic particle imaging (MPI) [85].

Liposomes/Niosomes

Liposomes are tiny spherical vesicles (artificial) of cholesterol and non-toxic phospholipids, first described by Bengham in 1965 [86], and for a long time, it is being used as a carrier system for the delivery of therapeutic agents (for the management of diseases) [87] and contrast agents (during the diagnosis process) [88]. The liposomal delivery system has always drawn the attention of the scientific community, working for the development of an efficient delivery system for the targeting of therapeutics as well as contrast agents used for different imaging techniques and diagnosis of other diseases due to their specific properties such as their size, amphiphilic behavior, surface characteristics, ease of modification in composition, encapsulation behavior, *etc* [34, 98, 101, 102].

In recent decades, numerous studies have been reported regarding the use of liposomes, including their use as a carrier system for contrast agents for effective imaging through PET, MRI, SEPCT, *etc* [89]. Probably, Richardson was the first who utilized the Tc-99m labeled liposomes for tumor imaging to study the localization behavior of liposomes [90]. In the past 80s, another report also states the successful use of ml In-111-labeled Liposomes for the imaging of tumors [91].

Functionalization and Surface modification of liposomes also have a significant impact on the effectiveness of the diagnosis process by minimizing the issues related to the drawbacks of conventional vesicles, including instability in biological systems as such [106, 107]. Such functionalized liposomal delivery of contrast agents may facilitate the accumulation of these agents in the required zone leading to better imaging. In an exhaustive review, Torchilin has mentioned the use of such surface-modified liposomes with polychelators and polyethylene glycol for the delivery of contrast agents during imaging of various organs and pathological conditions with improved results [92]. In a comparative PET imaging using 18F-FDG (gold standard radiotracer) and Cu-labelled liposome, it has been observed that C- labeled liposome was much more sensitive in the detection of pre-neoplastic lesions [93, 94].

Apart from the above use of liposomes in different imaging techniques, it can also act as a biosensor for the detection of different other bio-molecules too, including proteins, DNA, *etc.*, and can be used for different homogenous as well as heterogeneous assays [95, 96]. Theranostic application is another dimension, where liposomes have proven their significance [5]. These theranostic formulations get designed in such a way that they could facilitate imaging as well as therapy. In this context, Sonali *et al.* developed docetaxel, and quantum dots (QDs) loaded TPGS (D-alpha-tocopheryl polyethylene glycol 1000 succinate mono-ester) liposome conjugated with transferrin, for targeted delivery of both the materials in cancer cells of the brain [97]. In another study, Prasad *et al.* performed bimodal imaging and chemotherapy of malignant tumors in mice models using gold nanoparticle and grapheme quantum dot-loaded liposomes (NFGL), which were further loaded with doxorubicin and functionalized with folate for targeted delivery [98].

Niosomes

Niosomes are non-ionic surfactant vesicles having a closed bilayer structure, formed by the self-clustering of the surfactants. Niosomes possess several advantages over the liposomes, such as low cost, having no purity issues, so they can be used as it is, and can be prepared and stored in ambient situations. Apart from that, the surfactant in niosomes is much more stable than the liposome phospholipids [99].

Similar to liposomes, this vesicular system can accommodate both hydrophilic and lipophilic molecules in the aqueous core and bilayer [100] and can be utilized for the delivery of contrast agents used for imaging as well as therapeutic agents for therapy [101]. So, it is very much clear that niosomes can be effectively used for diagnosis purposes, and supporting it, a study reports the utility of iobitridol (a diagnostic agent)-loaded niosomes in x-ray imaging [102]. Surface functionalization is another way to increase the efficacy of noisome in targeting a diagnostic agent, which makes imaging techniques more effective [103]. It has been noticed that when a paramagnetic agent (gadobenatedimeglumine) loaded niosome is functionalized with PEG and glucose conjugate, shows better targeting which can be assessed by MRI [104]. Here, Transferrin conjugated pegylated niosomes loaded with magnetic iron oxide nanoparticles (MIONs) and quantum dots (QDs) have also been reported for dual targeting and imaging of glioma [105].

These formulations have also been explored for their theranostic application too, which enables the simultaneous administration of therapeutic as well as diagnostic agents for effective therapy and précised imaging [106]. In context to this, a theranostic system based on gadolinium nanoparticles (GdNP) and protoporphyrin IX (PpIX) loaded niosomal formulation has been reported for serving as a dual imaging probe and for multimodal treatment based on radiotherapy and photo-dynamic therapy [101]. In a similar report, gold nanoparticle (AuNP) and protoporphyrin IX (PpIX) loaded folate conjugated niosome have been reported for their activity in different positive and negative folate receptor (FR) cell lines

[106]. A niosomal system containing doxorubicin and Ag2S quantum dots has also been reported for bio-imaging and therapy after intra-tumoral injection [107].

Lipoplexes

Lipoplexes are the synthetic non-viral lipid carriers of DNA, having a positive charge on the surface, which helps them to form complexes with negatively charged DNA [108]. They are formed of 3 units: cationic lipid, neutral lipid, and plasmid DNA. The inner part of the lipoplexes encloses the fused DNA. Lipoplexes are commonly produced by mixing a lipid suspension with plasmid DNA and incubating it at room temperature. The function of lipoplexes is to guard the nucleic acid against enzyme degradation and prevention of activation of the immune system through DNA. Disadvantages of it are the low gene transfer efficacy and the transient transgene expression. Lipoplexes invade cells primarily through clathrin-mediated endocytosis (CME) or merging with the cell membrane. After invading the cell, it should release the nucleic acid in its original, allowing gene expression to take place. The factors that influence the effectiveness of nucleic acid transferal are the lipid-to-DNA ratio, size of the lipoplex, and nature of the additional lipid [109]. Some studies have recently demonstrated conjugating siRNA to lipid nanoparticles, such as liposomes or lipoplexes, improves the transport of siRNA to cancer cells.

It is a well-known fact that messenger RNA (mRNA) and micro RNA (mi-RNA) have proven to be important biomarkers for the detection of cancer [126 - 128]. Although, quantitative real time-PCR (qRT-PCR) is currently being used for the detection of m-RNA and mi-RNA but proven to be time and cost-consuming in specific cases [129 - 131]. Similarly, the detection of viral infection also depends on the identification of antibodies and genetic material, which is quite a cumbersome and time-consuming process [110, 111]. In context to it, Wu *et al.* reported tethered cationic lipoplex nanoparticle(having molecular beacon) biochip, which facilitates the diagnosis of cancer and other viral diseases by virtue of low-level RNA detection after apprehending the viruses or exosomes derived from cancer cells [112]. Similarly, Wang *et al.* reported a novel tethered lipoplex nanoparticle (TLN) biochip, which contains an engineered molecular beacon for AFP and GPC-3 for the detection of Hepatocellular carcinoma HCC biomarkers [113]. Another tethered lipoplex nanoparticle (TLN) biochip has also been reported for the diagnosis of lung cancer which almost works on a similar principle [114].

Xiaofan Pu *et al.* also reported the use of TLN biochip for examining the role of different exosomal micro RNA (exmiR 21, exmiR 10b, and exmiR 212 3p) expression in pancreatic cancer (PC) and mentioned the significance of methodology, in the identification of the PC patient in an early stage of the disease [115]. Lipoplex, loaded with quantum dots (QD605) as an imaging agent and Cy5-labeled antisense oligodeoxynucleotides (Cy5-G3139) as a therapeutic agent, has been reported for their theranostic application [116].

Solid lipid Nanocarriers/Nanostructures Lipid Carriers

Solid lipid nanocarriers (SLNC) have shown considerable promise in drug delivery, particularly in terms of regulating drug release and targeting specific tissues. The main components of SLNC are neutral solid lipids like triglycerides (TG), monoglycerides (MG), and diglycerides (DG), and saturated fatty acids, with lipophilic emulsifiers such polar phospholipids (PL) [117]. SLNC are classified into two types, namely solid lipid nanoparticles (SLN), having major constituents as solid lipid at room temperature, and nano-structured lipid carriers (NLC), having both solid and lipid [118]. The lipid composition variation has a significant influence on the drug loading capacity of SLNC and the drug release profile. The therapeutic benefits of SLNC-carried drug compounds are directly linked to particle properties and drug delivery methods (route of administration) [119].

Biocompatibility, stability, ease of surface functionalization, and ability to load both hydrophilic and hydrophobic materials make SLN a good alternative to polymeric nanoparticles and other vesicular systems concerning the delivery of therapeutic agents as well as a diagnostic agent [120]. One such SLN loaded with gadolinium (Gd) diethylenetriaminepentaacetic acid (Gd-DTPA) and octadecylamine fluorescein isothiocyanate (FITC) has been reported for MRI of colorectal tumors [121]. Another MRI contrast system based on the surface loading of SLN with gadolinium complex has also been reported [122]. In this series. Peira *et al.* reported the use of super magnetic iron oxide loaded SLN as a contrast agent for MRI of the central nervous system [123]. A report also mentions the use of Technetium-99 m (99mTc) labeled curcumin-loaded SLN for imaging of the liver and spleen [124]. Two different functionalized solid lipid nanoparticles have also been exploited for their theranostic application in the case of Rheumatoid arthritis [125] and Atherosclerosis [126].

It has also been noted that similar to the drug delivery *via* the lymphatic system [127] by using SLN, may also be used for the delivery of the diagnostic agent for imaging of lymphatic system too and can be used as a tool for the diagnosis of cancer and nodal diseases [128] but still, it is needed to be explored more for such diagnostic and theranostic application [129].

Nano-structured lipid carriers are modified from solid lipid nanoparticles which show better loading capacity and stability [117, 130]. Currently, no NLC formulation is approved by any regulatory agency, yet, this platform can be used for the development of an effective platform for diagnostics and theranostics [131]. One such NLC, loaded with camptothecin and quantum dot (QD), working as a theranostic, has been reported for bio-imaging and therapy of cancer [132]. Similarly, another NLC co-loaded with CdTe/CdS/ZnS-quantum dots and paclitaxel has been reported for fluorescence optical imaging and chemotherapy [133]. For better and targeted imaging and therapy in case of tumors, surface functionalization of nano-carriers with different ligands such as folic acid [134], glucosamine derivative [135], transferrin [136], erythropoietin [137], *etc.* has been extensively studied [155, 159 - 161]. In a novel work, Lu *et al.* reported the use of an A54-SNPD nano-particle composed of A54 peptide-functionalized and super-magnetic iron oxide loaded NLC (A54-SNLC), protamine, and AFP promoter DNA as MRI contrast agents for early diagnosis of hepatic tumor [138]. In another work, they also reported using A54 peptide-functionalized and NLC loaded with super-magnetic iron oxide nano-particle (A54-SNLC) for T-2 weighed MR imaging of hepatic cancer [139].

Inorganic Nanocarriers

Metal-based Nanoparticles

Metallic or metal oxide nano-particles have specific physicochemical, electro-magnetic, optical, and electrochemical properties along with better control of size and surface behaviour, stability, and ease of surface functionalization, which are some important characteristics that make them useful for the development of diagnostics and theranostics [140, 141]. Metals and metal oxide nano-particles have shown their significance as contrast agent for imaging [142, 143], in the development of nano-chip based diagnosis kit [144, 145], immunoassay [146, 147] *etc.* Several methods based on the use of metal nano-particles, as mentioned in the Fig. (**4**), have also been reported for the detection of bacteria [140]. Some commonly used metals for the development of diagnostics and theranostics include gold, silver, iron, gadolinium, cobalt, *etc.*

With regard to diagnostics and theranostics development, cancer, neurodegenerative brain diseases [148], Immunoassay [60, 146], bacterial [140], and viral infection [149] are some important areas where maximum research is going on, and it is expected to have some good results in terms of regulatory approved products.

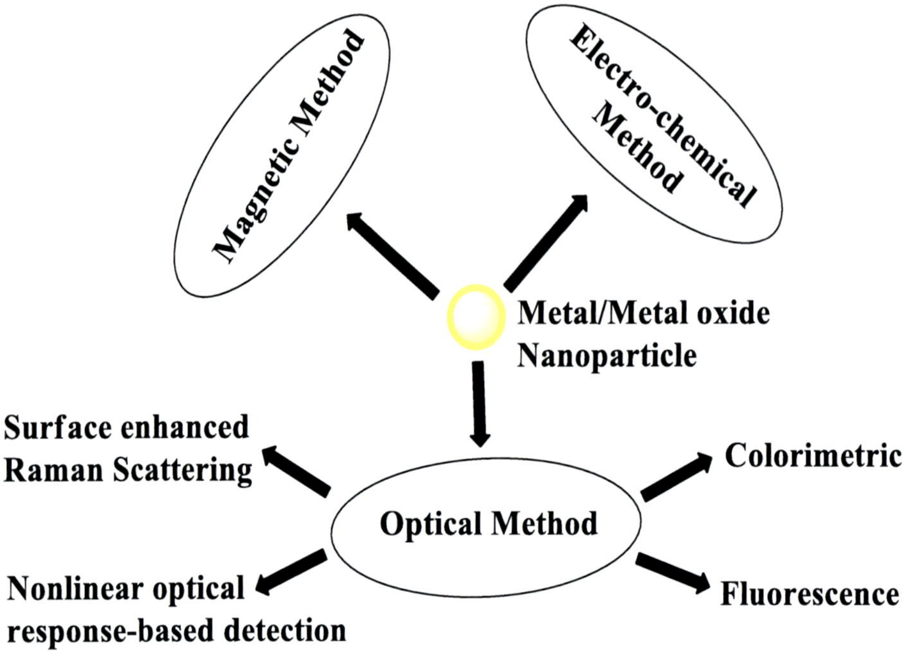

Fig. (4). Methods used for detection of bacteria involving metal/metal oxide nanoparticles.

Gold Nano-particles

Gold Nanoparticles possess numerous size and shape-dependent properties such as surface plasmon resonance, optical, electrical, and thermal, which can be utilized for better targeting, radio imaging, photoacoustic imaging, phototherapy, *etc.* and have proven to be beneficial for different applications in the medical field including diagnosis [150, 151]. Due to the presence of surface plasmon resonance and unique optical characteristics, gold nanoparticles are preferred in ultrasensitive and imaging-based therapy and diagnosis of certain fatal diseases like cancer [152]. A study shows that smaller gold nanoparticles (1.9 mm) can be utilized for the contrast imaging of tumors by X-ray. It reveals the accumulation of such smaller gold particles in the tumors as compared to the muscles, and this retention of gold nanoparticles may be utilized for the increased detection of tumors as well as therapy [153].

Broadly, we can classify the gold nanoparticle-based diagnostics in three major categories depending on different approaches: First, a diagnostic system that utilizes the color change behavior on aggregation [154, 155]. Several researchers utilized this approach for colorimetric screening of DNA- binding molecules with the help of gold nanoparticles. They observed that when a molecule of interest was introduced in a system with two different populations of gold nanoparticles functionalized with different modified oligonucleotide strands, it started to aggregate through a reversible DNA hybridization process leading to a change of color from red to blue (or purple) [180 - 182].

Second, surface-functionalized gold nanoparticle shows better targetting and provides selective nanoprobes for diagnosis [154, 155]; it has been observed that in comparison to the conventional strategies of diagnosis, AuNPs, which have a higher surface-to-volume ratio, can be used more effectively and selectively with surface functionalization which facilitates the detection of specific organs [2]. Popovtzer *et al.* reported better targeting of cancer cells by UM-A9 coated gold nanoparticles and showed better contrast during the CT with a higher attenuation coefficient [156].

A study shows that conjugation of monoclonal anti-epidermal growth factor receptor (anti-EGFR) antibodies with gold nanoparticles bind on cancerous cells with more specificity in a homogenous manner and higher affinity in comparison to the non-cancerous cells generating the sharper surface plasmon resonance (SPR) absorption band with a maximum red sift [157]. Gold nanoparticles may also be used for the early diagnosis of different diseases, such as the detection of Amyloid β oligomer in case of Alzheimer's disease [158].

Third, utilizing the electrochemical property of gold is sometimes potentiated with catalytic deposition of metals on nanoparticle surfaces [154, 155]. There are several reports which mention the development of electrochemical sensors using gold nanoparticles for the diagnosis of the different types of cancer, micro RNA, cognitive impairment, detection of the pathogen [159], *etc.* Three major ways are there by which a gold nano-particle modified electrode can be prepared and utilized for biosensors [160, 161].

I. Gold nano-particles can be coupled with self-assembled mono-layers possessing different required functional groups.

II. Gold nano-particle can be deposited on the surface of electrode as such.

III. Colloidal gold can be mixed in the component of the composite electrode matrix.

Silver Nano-particles

Silver nanoparticles (colloidal silver) are mainly prepared by reducing the silver ions in an aqueous system and are known for their antimicrobial property, but similar to the gold nanoparticles, it also possesses different perceptible features like small size, good conductivity, chemical stability, unique optical property (surface plasmon resonance), *etc* [162, 163], which makes it important in the designing of different advanced methods of diagnosis.

There are several ways and techniques which utilize silver nanoparticles for the generation of a system for the early detection of different types of cancer, including breast cancer, lung cancer, prostate cancer, cervical cancer, colorectal cancer, *etc.* The ways or techniques which involve the use of silver nanoparticles for diagnosis include the formation of biosensors, used as nanoclusters in conjunction with quantum dots, production of nanohybrids, used as a contrast agent, *etc* [191 - 194]. Several applications of a Silver nanomaterial, as reported in the literature, are mentioned below.

1) Silver nanoparticles conjugated with antibodies can be used to detect cancer biomarkers [164].

2) These nanoparticles may be used as a contrast agent in different techniques. Mondal *et al.* reported the use of AgNP as an exogenous contrast agent for optical coherence tomography [165], while in another work, it was utilized as a possible alternative to iodine for dual-energy (DE) X-ray imaging of the breast [165].

3) Biosensors can be developed using silver nanoparticles/silver nanoclusters which can be utilized for the detection of DNA [166], micro RNA, cancer cells [167], *etc.* Liang *et al.* reported the use of triangular silver nano prisms for generating a modified ELISA method for the detection of a prostate-specific antigen in a more selective manner [168].

4) Silver nanoparticles, in conjunction with reducing graphene oxide, may be utilized to fabricate an electrochemical immunosensor to detect carcinoembryonic antigen (CEA) associated with different types of cancers in their early stage [169].

5) Formation of fluorescent silver nanoclusters by utilizing DNA as an effective template can be used for the colorimetric/fluorometric estimation/detection of methylated or unmethylated DNA sequences. With the benefits of quantitative estimation of partially methylated DNA, too, the methodology can be used for early diagnosis of Cancer [170].

6) The adherence of silver nanoparticles on the surface of a pathogen like E. Coli can be utilized for their electrochemical detection [171]. In another work, Ellairaza *et al.* reported an immunoassay that utilizes pyrimidine-tagged silver nanoparticle-based nanosensors for the detection of Pseudomonas aeruginosa in different food materials, water, *etc* [172].

Iron Oxide Nano-particles

Iron oxide nano-particles are ferrimagnetic materials having wide applications in therapy and diagnosis, including cancer, diabetes, atherosclerosis, *etc* [173, 174]. These nanoparticles may contain magnetite, maghemite, and mixed ferrites [174]. Some recent literature reveals that magnetic resonance imaging is one of the unique, impressive, and robust techniques for imaging, and superoxide iron nano-particles having specific magnetic properties and better biocompatibility, can be used as a powerful contrast agent [175]. Several kinds of literature also report the surface modification of superparamagnetic iron oxide nanoparticles (SPION), which makes them more stable in the biological media, especially against possible oxidation [173, 176]. Some common polymers which are used for the functionalization of these nanoparticles include chitosan, dextran, polyethylene glycol (PEG), polyvinyl alcohol (PVA), *etc.* and these coated nanoparticles may also be suitably utilized for the targeting too by selecting a proper ligand for further functionalization [176]. Ferumoxtran and Ferumoxide (coated or covered with dextran) [177], Ferumoxsil (coated with siloxane) [177], Ferucarbotran (coated with carboxydextran) [7], Ferumoxytol (coated with polyglucose sorbitol-carboxymethylether) [178], Feruglose (coated with PEGylated modified starch) [179] are some common examples of iron oxide nanoparticles with surface modification which are either clinically approved or in their trial phase for their application in imaging of lymph node, central nervous system, microphage, liver, gastric system, tumors in the breast, *etc* [204, 211 - 213]. Apart from the above, different organic materials like amino acids (Cysteine lysine, tyrosine, *etc.*) [214, 215], Citric acid [180], oleic acid [181], proteins (Albumin, casein), *etc.* and inorganic materials like metals (gold, silver, *etc.*) [182, 183] and metal oxide (Titanium dioxide and silica) may also be used for functionalization of iron oxide nanoparticles [173, 183].

Iron nanoparticles can also be utilized for the development of biosensors and could be helpful in the detection of different biomolecules, such as proteins, nucleic acid, *etc.*, in biological samples. Literature reports the development of a chip-based diagnostic magnetic resonance (DMR) system in support of the above. This DMR system even can detect pathogens too more selectively and rapidly [184].

These nano-particles, due to their specific abilities concerning MRI, bio-catalytic activity, phototherapy, delivery of the therapeutic agent, *etc.*, can be used successfully for the development of theranostics too [185]. El- Dakdouki *et al.* reported that Doxorubicin conjugated SPION coated with hyaluronan shows better activity against CD44 expressed ovarian cancer and can be used for tracking nanoparticle delivery *via* MRI [186]. It has also been noted that using the ligands like antibodies, peptides, and aptamers attached to the surface of iron oxide nano-particles may lead to better targeting [173], but at the same time, controlling the size of nano-particles, a better targeting may be achieved due to EPR effect, especially in tumorous mass leading to proper imaging and therapeutic effect [185]. It is also very much clear that EPR effects are very much variable and its effect on the nanoparticles loaded with therapeutics is not clear, but magnetic nano-particle as a companion particle may help to predict the co-localization of therapeutic loaded nano-particles [187].

Quantum Dots

These are nearly spherical nano-crystals with zero dimension, mainly prepared by using semiconductor material (element having s and p valent electron belonging to IIB- VI B or IIIB-VB of the periodic table) and possess specific electrical and optical behavior [188, 189], which makes it very useful for its biomedical application in comparison to conventional luminescent dyes. The extraordinary photoluminescence property of Quantum dots (QD) makes it more useful for diagnosis based on bio-imaging and sensing of fluorescence. An effective system for targeted drug delivery and luminescent imaging with QD can be achieved by the modification of its surface [190]. Biocompatibility, solubility, and sensitivity towards light can be increased with surface modification of QD. The addition of different ligands at the surface of QD may sometimes reduce or even eliminates the surface defect, which is believed to be the reason for such increment or improved activity of QD. Some common techniques used for surface modification of QD include modification using multidentate ligand, sulfhydryl coupling, amphiphilic molecule, cavity chain molecules, and dendrimers [191]. An efficient biosensing system has always been required for diagnosis, and having specific properties like good stability against light, high brightness, a broad spectrum of absorption, a narrow spectrum of emission tunable due to size, *etc.*, makes QD more valuable and important in biosensor development [192, 193]. There are several reports regarding the development of QD-based biosensors, including fluorescent biosensors (probes), which show high sensitivity and capability during multiplex analysis [194]. Bhattacharya *et al.* reported CDse QD-based and carbon dot-based fluorescent sensors for the detection of biomarkers of tuberculosis [195]. In another work, CdSe/ZnS quantum dots capped with adenosine have also been reported for the selective and sensitive detection of dopamine in human samples, which is of great importance as it is very much clear that disturbance in the dopamine concentration may lead to the change in behavioral response as well as it may lead to several neurological disorders [196]. The role of QD biosensors (based on FRET) can also be utilized for the detection of DNA even in lower concentration which may be helpful in finding the pathogen [197, 198]. Apart from the above some other QD based biosensing systems have also been reported for the analysis of various biomarkers, *viz.* electro-chemiluminescence, photo-electrochemical and electrochemical [226, 235 - 237].

Quantum dot can also be used for the construction of lateral flow systems (LFA), which is a paper-based technique used to analyze a specific component in a mixture and can be used for testing different biological samples, including blood, urine, saliva, *etc* [238, 239]. and can be best understood with the example of pregnancy testing kit. Several analytes, including antigens, antibodies, specific biomarkers, pathogens, *etc.*, can be tested with the help of LFA [199]. Chen *et al.* reported the QD-based immunochromatographic test strips (ICTS) for the detection of staphylococcus aureus in food samples [200]. A cardiac biomarker NT-proBNP (predictor of acute heart failure) can also be identified and quantified by LFA, which utilizes quantum dots conjugated with monoclonal antibodies [201]. Similarly, high sensitivity cardiac troponin is one of the significant biomarkers for heart health in case of myocardial infarction and can be significantly detected more rapidly with POCT quantum dot fluorescence immunoassay rather than the conventional methods [202]. C-reactive protein, a potent marker of inflammatory response in the system and indicative of infection, trauma, or other acute inflammation condition, may be detected with the help of quantitative fluorescence point-of-care tests (QF-POCT) based on the use of quantum dots as fluorescent probes and immune-chromatographic strip with higher sensitivity [203]. These QD-based immune-chromatographic assays may also be used for the detection of hepatitis B virus surface antigen and other protein biomarkers with higher sensitivity [204].

Amidst all, quantum dots can be used for theranostics purposes. Ho and Leong have summarized various reports related to the use of QD in the development of theranostics, with special mention of cancer [205]. A recent study reports the development of large amino acid mimicking (LAAM) carbon quantum dots for delivery of therapeutics as well as imaging of tumors of different locations, including brain tumors with more specificity [206].

Carbon Nanotubes

In recent decades, the use of carbon nanotube (an allotrope of carbon belonging to the family of fullerenes) for diagnostic and theranostic purposes has increased due to their specific physicochemical properties along with their ability to absorb or conjugate with different bio-molecules, which may be necessary for certain instances where surface modification may be required to get the optimum activity [207, 208].

Carbon nanotubes have a great potential to be used for imaging-based diagnosis of disease, specifically cancer, due to their unique structural and functional characteristics [209]. But the solubility and dispersibility of carbon nanotubes in water have always been a major concern regarding their application in the biomedical field. To overcome this problem, the functionalization of carbon nanotubes can be done either by absorption or electrostatic interaction or by covalent bonding of different molecules [251-253]. In context to this, among the two major categories of carbon nanotubes, *i.e.*, single-walled carbon nanotubes (SWCNTs) and multiwalled carbon nanotubes (MWCNTs) [207], a report has been published regarding the adsorption of gadolinium (III) chelate (amphiphilic) on the MWCNT leading to its stable suspension and its utilization as a powerfully positive and negative contrast agent for MRI [210]. Servant *et al.* also reported the covalent functionalization of MWCNT by Gadolinium in the presence of a chelating agent, *i.e.*, diethylene triamine pentaacetic acid (DTPA), which can be used as a contrast agent for MRI and may act as an efficient cell probe [211]. Another report mentions the noncovalent functionalization of SWCNT (containing iron as a trace) with pegylated lipid, which shows better stability in the biological media and can be used as negative contrast in the liver [212]. Near-infrared fluorescence emitting property of SWCNT at a longer wavelength can also be used for imaging. Yudasaka *et al.* have shown the significance of poly(2-methacryloyloxyethyl phosphorylcholine-co-n-butyl methacrylate) coated SWCNT for imaging brown fat [213]. Another report states the use of gold-plated carbon nanotube conjugated with a specific antibody for lymphatic endothelial hyaluronan receptor-1 as a near-infrared contrast agent for *in-vivo* mapping of the lymphatic system using photoacoustic and photothermal imaging [214].

Dip coating is another way that can be used for preparing functionalized SWCNT with multiple functionalities, which can be used for the generation of polyvalent biosensors [215].

One important fact is that the variation in the DNA sequence may lead to serious genetic diseases [216]. At the same time detection of DNA is also of utmost importance in certain infectious diseases for their better management [217]. The studies show that CNT may be a better alternative than the conventional approach. Kuralay *et al.* have reported the use of CNT-modified, CNT-polymer-modified, and CNT-nanoparticle-modified electrodes for electrochemical detection of DNA [218]. A biosensing system comprising CNT decorated with a multifunctional binary nanoparticle (gold & iron oxide) has been reported for the detection of influenza and norovirus DNA. In this system, a thiol group functionalized probe DNA was attached to the gold nanoparticle surface in gold/iron oxide-CNT aligned on the Pt-interdigitated electrode. Changes in the electrical conductivity of gold/iron oxide-CNT can be measured due to the hybridization of target DNA (Influenza & norovirus) and probe DNA [219, 220].

Carbon nanotubes can also be used to prepare disposable electrochemical immunosensing for the detection of fibrinogen in a biological sample [221].

Theranostic application is another dimension where different carbon nanomaterial has proven their importance [222]. As mentioned earlier, carbon nanotubes, especially MWCNT, possess several properties such as larger surface area, strong near-infrared absorbance, photothermal performance, *etc.* can be utilized for the development of a better theranostic system. Zang *et al.* reported magneto-fluorescent MWCNT (GP-GdN@CQDs-MWCNTs/DOX-EGFR) for magnetic resonance and fluorescent imaging and photothermal and chemotherapy [220, 223].

Apart from the above, different carbon materials such as nanohorns, fullerenes, nanographene, nanodiamonds, and nanodots are also there, which are being used successfully for the diagnosis and theranostic purposes for different diseases, especially cancer [222].

Others

Apart from the above, several other inorganic material/metals/metal oxide nanoparticles like silica& silica-based nanoparticles [224, 225], zinc oxide nanoparticles [226], graphene-based nanocarriers [227], cobalt-containing nanoparticles [228, 229], titanium or titanium-containing nano-materials [230, 231], *etc.* are also there which are being investigated for the development of diagnostics and theranostics, and the results indicate their potential for such uses.

NANOTECHNOLOGY BASED FORMULATION AT THE CLINICAL LEVEL

Different nanotechnology-based formulations, such as liposomes, polymeric nanoparticles, micelles, inorganic nano-particles, *etc.*, have proven their significance in terms of their utility for drug delivery systems. Since the approval of Doxil, several such formulations are there, which are either FDA approved or in different clinical phases [232, 233]. But, when we look after the development of diagnostics or theranostics, it is very limited to some iron-based formulations used for imaging (Feridex®; first clinically approved contrast agent for liver imaging [8, 234], Reservist for imaging of liver lesions [7], Ferumoxtran-10 for MR imaging of lymph node metastases [235]), microsphere and microbubble formulations as contrast agents for ultrasound (Definity® and Optison® [9], SonoVue®/Lumason® [236]) and silica nanoparticles (Cornell Dots for imaging of melanoma and malignant tumor [237]) [233]. But as mentioned in the different parts of the chapter, it is observed that an exhaustive study is going on related to the development of different diagnostic and theranostic use, and on the positive side, it may be assumed that in the near future we will have some more clinically approved products.

Among the above-mentioned clinically approved iron-based formulations, feridex® (ferumoxide) and Resovist® are superparamagnetic iron oxide (SPIO) dextran colloid and carboxydextran colloid, respectively, used for MR imaging of the liver [238], whileFerumoxtran-10 possess dextran-coated superparamagnetic iron oxide particles used for MR imaging of lymph nodes [235, 239].

Definity® and Optison® are injectable suspensions of lipid and protein type-A microspheres, respectively, having perflutren, which have been developed as contrast agents for ultrasound imaging [9]. While SonoVue®/Lumason® are the same product having phospholipid shell surrounded microbubbles of stabilized sulphur hexafluoride and can be used as a contrast agent for ultrasound and electrocardiography [236, 240].

CONCLUSION

For decades, the nano-delivery system has fascinated the scientific community, and extensive work has been done and still going on, especially concerning their use for drug delivery. Literature also reveals their utility for the delivery of diagnostics and for the development of newer contrast systems for different imaging modalities used for the diagnosis of diseases, especially cancer, as it is well evident that the effective management of any critical illness always starts with its timely and effective diagnosis. With surface functionalization of these carriers containing diagnostic molecules has proven to be very significant in the case of targeted imaging and diagnosis without affecting the normal physiology and normal organs. These systems have made the diagnosis process comparatively easier, targeted, and less invasive. At the same time, the use of these carriers for the development of theranostics has opened a way for developing the therapy approaches on a personalized basis. But, on the other end, nanomaterials and nanocarriers also suffer from a lot of limitations and face challenges concerning their biological distribution, technological development, *etc.* Similarly, when we start to find out the application of different nano-materials or systems based on nano-carriers for the diagnosis with regard to clinical approval or we focus on regulatory approval of such systems, we feel a serious gap, and it is of utmost need to fill it.

But, based on rigorous studies related to the development of newer diagnostic and theranostic agents by using nano-materials built hope regarding the generation of more clinically useful and approved products. As already mentioned, to date, maximum research, including nano-material, is more focused related to the diagnosis and therapy of cancer, but at the same time, reports are available regarding the development of nano-material and nano-carrier-based diagnostics for atherosclerosis and CNS diseases too, which may be proven a milestone in development more précised, authentic, less time consuming and clinically approved newer diagnostics and theranostics products for different other diseases too along with above-mentioned disorders.

CONSENT FOR PUBLICATION

Not applicable.

CONFLICT OF INTEREST

The authors declare no conflict of interest, financial or otherwise.

ACKNOWLEDGMENT

We are thankful to the Bentham Science Publishers team for giving us this opportunity and to everyone who supported us directly or indirectly while writing this book chapter.

REFERENCES:

[1] Baetke SC, Lammers T, Kiessling F. Applications of nanoparticles for diagnosis and therapy of cancer. Br J Radiol 2015; 88(1054): 20150207.
[http://dx.doi.org/10.1259/bjr.20150207] [PMID: 25969868]

[2] Zhang Y, Li M, Gao X, Chen Y, Liu T. Nanotechnology in cancer diagnosis: progress, challenges and opportunities. J Hematol Oncol 2019; 12(1): 137.
[http://dx.doi.org/10.1186/s13045-019-0833-3] [PMID: 31847897]

[3] Choi YE, Kwak JW, Park JW. Nanotechnology for early cancer detection. Sensors (Basel) 2010; 10(1): 428-55.
[http://dx.doi.org/10.3390/s100100428] [PMID: 22315549]

[4] Bunn TW, Sikarwar AS. Diagnostics: conventional *versus* modern methods. Journal of Advances in Medical and Pharmaceutical Sciences 2016; 1-7.

[5] Sumer B, Gao J. Theranostic nanomedicine for cancer. Nanomedicine (Lond) 2008; 3(2): 137-40.
[http://dx.doi.org/10.2217/17435889.3.2.137]

[6] Lee SB. Focus on nanoparticles for cancer diagnosis and therapeutics. Future Med 2007; 2(5).
[http://dx.doi.org/10.2217/17435889.2.5.647]

[7] Reimer P, Balzer T. Ferucarbotran (Resovist): a new clinically approved RES-specific contrast agent for contrast-enhanced MRI of the liver: properties, clinical development, and applications. Eur Radiol 2003; 13(6): 1266-76.
[http://dx.doi.org/10.1007/s00330-002-1721-7] [PMID: 12764641]

[8] Clément O, Siauve N, Cuénod C-A, Frija G. Liver imaging with ferumoxides (Feridex): fundamentals, controversies, and practical aspects. Top Magn Reson Imaging 1998; 9(3): 167-82.
[http://dx.doi.org/10.1097/00002142-199806000-00003] [PMID: 9621405]

[9] Main ML, Goldman JH, Grayburn PA. Ultrasound contrast agents: balancing safety *versus* efficacy. Expert Opin Drug Saf 2009; 8(1): 49-56.
[http://dx.doi.org/10.1517/14740330802658581] [PMID: 19236217]

[10] Nagavarma B, Yadav HK, Ayaz A, Vasudha L, Shivakumar H. Different techniques for preparation of polymeric nanoparticles-a review. Asian J Pharm Clin Res 2012; 5(3): 16-23.

[11] Soppimath KS, Aminabhavi TM, Kulkarni AR, Rudzinski WE. Biodegradable polymeric nanoparticles as drug delivery devices. J Control Release 2001; 70(1-2): 1-20. [http://dx.doi.org/10.1016/S0168-3659(00)00339-4] [PMID: 11166403]

[12] El-Say KM, El-Sawy HS. Polymeric nanoparticles: Promising platform for drug delivery. Int J Pharm 2017; 528(1-2): 675-91. [http://dx.doi.org/10.1016/j.ijpharm.2017.06.052] [PMID: 28629982]

[13] Crucho CIC, Barros MT. Polymeric nanoparticles: A study on the preparation variables and characterization methods. Mater Sci Eng C 2017; 80: 771-84. [http://dx.doi.org/10.1016/j.msec.2017.06.004] [PMID: 28866227]

[14] Perumal V, Sivakumar PM, Zarrabi A, *et al.* Near infra-red polymeric nanoparticle based optical imaging in Cancer diagnosis. J Photochem Photobiol B 2019; 199: 111630. [http://dx.doi.org/10.1016/j.jphotobiol.2019.111630] [PMID: 31610429]

[15] Mouffouk F, Aouabdi S, Al-Hetlani E, Serrai H, Alrefae T, Leo Chen L. New generation of electrochemical immunoassay based on polymeric nanoparticles for early detection of breast cancer. Int J Nanomedicine 2017; 12: 3037-47. [http://dx.doi.org/10.2147/IJN.S127086] [PMID: 28450780]

[16] Pont L, Marin G, Vergara-Barberán M, *et al.* Polymeric monolithic microcartridges with gold nanoparticles for the analysis of protein biomarkers by on-line solid-phase extraction capillary electrophoresis-mass spectrometry. J Chromatogr A 2020; 1622: 461097. [http://dx.doi.org/10.1016/j.chroma.2020.461097] [PMID: 32381302]

[17] Srikar R, Upendran A, Kannan R. Polymeric nanoparticles for molecular imaging. Wiley Interdiscip Rev Nanomed Nanobiotechnol 2014; 6(3): 245-67. [http://dx.doi.org/10.1002/wnan.1259] [PMID: 24616442]

[18] Fukumori Y, Ichikawa H. Nanoparticles for cancer therapy and diagnosis. Adv Powder Technol 2006; 17(1): 1-28. [http://dx.doi.org/10.1163/156855206775123494]

[19] Payne WM, Hill TK, Svechkarev D, Holmes MB, Sajja BR, Mohs AM. Multimodal imaging nanoparticles derived from hyaluronic acid for integrated preoperative and intraoperative cancer imaging. Contrast Media Mol Imaging 2017; 9616791. [http://dx.doi.org/10.1155/2017/9616791]

[20] Teraphongphom N, Chhour P, Eisenbrey JR, *et al.* Nanoparticle loaded polymeric microbubbles as contrast agents for multimodal imaging. Langmuir 2015; 31(43): 11858-67. [http://dx.doi.org/10.1021/acs.langmuir.5b03473] [PMID: 26446176]

[21] Liu Y, Chen Z, Liu C, Yu D, Lu Z, Zhang N. Gadolinium-loaded polymeric nanoparticles modified with Anti-VEGF as multifunctional MRI contrast agents for the diagnosis of liver cancer. Biomaterials 2011; 32(22): 5167-76. [http://dx.doi.org/10.1016/j.biomaterials.2011.03.077] [PMID: 21521627]

[22] Luo S, Zhang E, Su Y, Cheng T, Shi C. A review of NIR dyes in cancer targeting and imaging. Biomaterials 2011; 32(29): 7127-38. [http://dx.doi.org/10.1016/j.biomaterials.2011.06.024] [PMID: 21724249]

[23] Resch-Genger U, Grabolle M, Cavaliere-Jaricot S, Nitschke R, Nann T. Quantum dots *versus* organic dyes as fluorescent labels. Nat Methods 2008; 5(9): 763-75. [http://dx.doi.org/10.1038/nmeth.1248] [PMID: 18756197]

[24] Canfarotta F, Whitcombe MJ, Piletsky SA. Polymeric nanoparticles for optical sensing. Biotechnol Adv 2013; 31(8): 1585-99. [http://dx.doi.org/10.1016/j.biotechadv.2013.08.010] [PMID: 23968893]

[25] Cho H, Indig GL, Weichert J, Shin HC, Kwon GS. *In vivo* cancer imaging by poly(ethylene glycol)--poly(ε-caprolactone) micelles containing a near-infrared probe. Nanomedicine 2012; 8(2): 228-36. [http://dx.doi.org/10.1016/j.nano.2011.06.009] [PMID: 21704593]

[26] Hill TK, Abdulahad A, Kelkar SS, *et al.* Indocyanine green-loaded nanoparticles for image-guided tumor surgery. Bioconjug Chem 2015; 26(2): 294-303. [http://dx.doi.org/10.1021/bc5005679] [PMID: 25565445]

[27] Lei T, Fernandez-Fernandez A, Manchanda R, Huang YC, McGoron AJ. Near-infrared dye loaded polymeric nanoparticles for cancer imaging and therapy and cellular response after laser-induced heating. Beilstein J Nanotechnol 2014; 5(1): 313-22. [http://dx.doi.org/10.3762/bjnano.5.35] [PMID: 24778954]

[28] Bahmani B, Guerrero Y, Bacon D, Kundra V, Vullev VI, Anvari B. Functionalized polymeric nanoparticles loaded with indocyanine green as theranostic materials for targeted molecular near infrared fluorescence imaging and photothermal destruction of ovarian cancer cells. Lasers Surg Med 2014; 46(7): 582-92. [http://dx.doi.org/10.1002/lsm.22269] [PMID: 24961210]

[29] Cai Y, Si W, Huang W, Chen P, Shao J, Dong X. Organic dye based nanoparticles for cancer phototheranostics. Small 2018; 14(25): 1704247. [http://dx.doi.org/10.1002/smll.201704247] [PMID: 29611290]

[30] Jain S, Chattopadhyay S, Jackeray R, Abid Z, Singh H. Detection of Salmonella typhi utilizing bioconjugated fluorescent polymeric nanoparticles. J Nanopart Res 2016; 18(5): 111. [http://dx.doi.org/10.1007/s11051-016-3414-1]

[31] Nichkova M, Dosev D, Gee SJ, Hammock BD, Kennedy IM. Microarray immunoassay for phenoxybenzoic acid using polymer encapsulated Eu:Gd2O3 nanoparticles as fluorescent labels. Anal Chem 2005; 77(21): 6864-73. [http://dx.doi.org/10.1021/ac050826p] [PMID: 16255584]

[32] Hun X, Zhang Z. A novel sensitive staphylococcal enterotoxin C1 fluoroimmunoassay based on functionalized fluorescent core-shell nanoparticle labels. Food Chem 2007; 105(4): 1623-9. [http://dx.doi.org/10.1016/j.foodchem.2007.03.068]

[33] Ding J, Cheng Y, Li M, Gref R, Chen X. Smart polymeric nanocarriers. J Nanomater 2016; 3710921. [http://dx.doi.org/10.1155/2016/3710921]

[34] Shukla T, Upmanyu N, Pandey SP, Sudheesh M. Site-specific drug delivery, targeting, and gene therapy Nanoarchitectonics in Biomedicine. Elsevier 2019; pp. 473-505.

[35] Trubetskoy V. Polymeric micelles as carriers of diagnostic agents. Adv Drug Deliv Rev 1999; 37(1-3): 81-8. [http://dx.doi.org/10.1016/S0169-409X(98)00100-8] [PMID: 10837728]

[36] Mortensen K. Structural properties of self-assembled polymeric micelles. Curr Opin Colloid Interface Sci 1998; 3(1): 12-9. [http://dx.doi.org/10.1016/S1359-0294(98)80036-8]

[37] Ahmad Z, Shah A, Siddiq M, Kraatz HB. Polymeric micelles as drug delivery vehicles. RSC Advances 2014; 4(33): 17028-38. [http://dx.doi.org/10.1039/C3RA47370H]

[38] Ai H, Flask C, Weinberg B, *et al.* Magnetite□loaded polymeric micelles as ultrasensitive magnetic□resonance probes. Adv Mater 2005; 17(16): 1949-52. [http://dx.doi.org/10.1002/adma.200401904]

[39] Ashjari M, Panahandeh F, Niazi Z, Abolhasani MM. Synthesis of PLGA–mPEG star-like block copolymer to form micelle loaded magnetite as a nanocarrier for hydrophobic anticancer drug. J Drug Deliv Sci Technol 2020; 56: 101563. [http://dx.doi.org/10.1016/j.jddst.2020.101563]

[40] Cheng D, Hong G, Wang W, *et al.* Nonclustered magnetite nanoparticle encapsulated biodegradable polymeric micelles with enhanced properties for *in vivo* tumor imaging. J Mater Chem 2011; 21(13): 4796-804.
[http://dx.doi.org/10.1039/c0jm03783d]

[41] Trubetskoy VS, Cannillo JA, Milshtein A, Wolf GL, Torchilin VP. Controlled delivery of Gd-containing liposomes to lymph nodes: surface modification may enhance MRI contrast properties. Magn Reson Imaging 1995; 13(1): 31-7.
[http://dx.doi.org/10.1016/0730-725X(94)00083-F] [PMID: 7534860]

[42] Kabalka GW, Davis MA, Moss TH, *et al.* Gadolinium-labeled liposomes containing various amphiphilic Gd-DTPA derivatives: Targeted MRI contrast enhancement agents for the liver. Magn Reson Med 1991; 19(2): 406-15.
[http://dx.doi.org/10.1002/mrm.1910190231] [PMID: 1881329]

[43] Torchilin VP. PEG-based micelles as carriers of contrast agents for different imaging modalities. Adv Drug Deliv Rev 2002; 54(2): 235-52.
[http://dx.doi.org/10.1016/S0169-409X(02)00019-4] [PMID: 11897148]

[44] Torchilin VP. Structure and design of polymeric surfactant-based drug delivery systems. J Control Release 2001; 73(2-3): 137-72.
[http://dx.doi.org/10.1016/S0168-3659(01)00299-1] [PMID: 11516494]

[45] Torchilin V. Polymeric contrast agents for medical imaging. Curr Pharm Biotechnol 2000; 1(2): 183-215.
[http://dx.doi.org/10.2174/1389201003378960] [PMID: 11467336]

[46] Liu Y, Li J, Liu F, *et al.* Theranostic polymeric micelles for the diagnosis and treatment of hepatocellular carcinoma. J Biomed Nanotechnol 2015; 11(4): 613-22.
[http://dx.doi.org/10.1166/jbn.2015.1945] [PMID: 26310068]

[47] Rehman Z, Hoekstra D, Zuhorn IS. Mechanism of polyplex- and lipoplex-mediated delivery of nucleic acids: real-time visualization of transient membrane destabilization without endosomal lysis. ACS Nano 2013; 7(5): 3767-77.
[http://dx.doi.org/10.1021/nn3049494] [PMID: 23597090]

[48] Debus H, Beck-Broichsitter M, Kissel T. Optimized preparation of pDNA/poly(ethylene imine) polyplexes using a microfluidic system. Lab Chip 2012; 12(14): 2498-506.
[http://dx.doi.org/10.1039/c2lc40176b] [PMID: 22552347]

[49] Vasile C. Polymeric nanomaterials: recent developments, properties and medical applications. Polymeric nanomaterials in nanotherapeutics 2019; 1-66.

[50] Kamimura K, Suda T, Zhang G, Liu D. Advances in gene delivery systems. Pharmaceut Med 2011; 25(5): 293-306.
[http://dx.doi.org/10.1007/BF03256872] [PMID: 22200988]

[51] Ramamoorth M, Narvekar A. Non viral vectors in gene therapy- an overview. J Clin Diagn Res 2015; 9(1): GE01-6.
[http://dx.doi.org/10.7860/JCDR/2015/10443.5394] [PMID: 25738007]

[52] Abootalebi SN, Shorafa E. The Recent advances in gene delivery using nanostructures and future prospects. Advances in Applied NanoBio-Technologies 2020; 1(2): 45-52.

[53] Zhang S, Xu Y, Wang B, Qiao W, Liu D, Li Z. Cationic compounds used in lipoplexes and polyplexes for gene delivery. J Control Release 2004; 100(2): 165-80.
[http://dx.doi.org/10.1016/j.jconrel.2004.08.019] [PMID: 15544865]

[54] Gebhart CL, Kabanov AV. Evaluation of polyplexes as gene transfer agents. J Control Release 2001; 73(2-3): 401-16.
[http://dx.doi.org/10.1016/S0168-3659(01)00357-1] [PMID: 11516515]

[55] Zintchenko A, Philipp A, Dehshahri A, Wagner E. Simple modifications of branched PEI lead to highly efficient siRNA carriers with low toxicity. Bioconjug Chem 2008; 19(7): 1448-55. [http://dx.doi.org/10.1021/bc800065f] [PMID: 18553894]

[56] Fitzsimmons REB, Uludağ H. Specific effects of PEGylation on gene delivery efficacy of polyethylenimine: Interplay between PEG substitution and N/P ratio. Acta Biomater 2012; 8(11): 3941-55. [http://dx.doi.org/10.1016/j.actbio.2012.07.015] [PMID: 22820308]

[57] Luo X, Peng X, Hou J, Wu S, Shen J, Wang L. Folic acid-functionalized polyethylenimine superparamagnetic iron oxide nanoparticles as theranostic agents for magnetic resonance imaging and PD-L1 siRNA delivery for gastric cancer. Int J Nanomedicine 2017; 12: 5331-43. [http://dx.doi.org/10.2147/IJN.S137245] [PMID: 28794626]

[58] Guo Y, Chen W, Wang W, *et al.* Simultaneous diagnosis and gene therapy of immuno-rejection in rat allogeneic heart transplantation model using a T-cell-targeted theranostic nanosystem. ACS Nano 2012; 6(12): 10646-57. [http://dx.doi.org/10.1021/nn3037573] [PMID: 23189971]

[59] Geyer A, Taschauer A, Alioglu F, *et al.* Multimodal fluorescence and bioluminescence imaging reveals transfection potential of intratracheally administered polyplexes for breast cancer lung metastases. Hum Gene Ther 2017; 28(12): 1202-13. [http://dx.doi.org/10.1089/hum.2017.137] [PMID: 28874076]

[60] Hirsch LR, Jackson JB, Lee A, Halas NJ, West JL. A whole blood immunoassay using gold nanoshells. Anal Chem 2003; 75(10): 2377-81. [http://dx.doi.org/10.1021/ac0262210] [PMID: 12918980]

[61] Tsai HC, Imae T. Fabrication of dendrimers toward biological application. Prog Mol Biol Transl Sci 2011; 104: 101-40. [http://dx.doi.org/10.1016/B978-0-12-416020-0.00003-6] [PMID: 22093218]

[62] Hawker CJ, Frechet JMJ. Preparation of polymers with controlled molecular architecture. A new convergent approach to dendritic macromolecules. J Am Chem Soc 1990; 112(21): 7638-47. [http://dx.doi.org/10.1021/ja00177a027]

[63] Noriega-Luna B, Godínez LA, Rodríguez FJ, *et al.* Applications of dendrimers in drug delivery agents, diagnosis, therapy, and detection. J Nanomater 2014; 2014: 507273. [http://dx.doi.org/10.1155/2014/507273]

[64] Kolhatkar RB, Swaan P, Ghandehari H. Potential oral delivery of 7-ethyl-10-hydroxy-camptothecin (SN-38) using poly(amidoamine) dendrimers. Pharm Res 2008; 25(7): 1723-9. [http://dx.doi.org/10.1007/s11095-008-9572-9] [PMID: 18438703]

[65] Najlah M, Freeman S, Attwood D, D'Emanuele A. *In vitro* evaluation of dendrimer prodrugs for oral drug delivery. Int J Pharm 2007; 336(1): 183-90. [http://dx.doi.org/10.1016/j.ijpharm.2006.11.047] [PMID: 17188439]

[66] Tomalia DA, Reyna L, Svenson S. Dendrimers as multi-purpose nanodevices for oncology drug delivery and diagnostic imaging. Biochem Soc Trans 2007; 35(Pt 1): 61-7. [http://dx.doi.org/10.1042/BST0350061]

[67] Wiener E, Brechbiel MW, Brothers H, *et al.* Dendrimer-based metal chelates: A new class of magnetic resonance imaging contrast agents. Magn Reson Med 1994; 31(1): 1-8. [http://dx.doi.org/10.1002/mrm.1910310102] [PMID: 8121264]

[68] Longmire M, Choyke P, Kobayashi H. Dendrimer-based contrast agents for molecular imaging. Curr Top Med Chem 2008; 8(14): 1180-6. [http://dx.doi.org/10.2174/156802608785849021] [PMID: 18855704]

[69] Kojima C, Umeda Y, Ogawa M, Harada A, Magata Y, Kono K. X-ray computed tomography contrast agents prepared by seeded growth of gold nanoparticles in PEGylated dendrimer. Nanotechnology

2010; 21(24): 245104.
[http://dx.doi.org/10.1088/0957-4484/21/24/245104] [PMID: 20498528]

[70] Wang H, Zheng L, Guo R, *et al.* Dendrimer-entrapped gold nanoparticles as potential CT contrast agents for blood pool imaging. Nanoscale Res Lett 2012; 7(1): 190.
[http://dx.doi.org/10.1186/1556-276X-7-190] [PMID: 22429280]

[71] Talanov VS, Regino CAS, Kobayashi H, Bernardo M, Choyke PL, Brechbiel MW. Dendrimer-based nanoprobe for dual modality magnetic resonance and fluorescence imaging. Nano Lett 2006; 6(7): 1459-63.
[http://dx.doi.org/10.1021/nl060765q] [PMID: 16834429]

[72] Ray S, Li Z, Hsu CH, *et al.* Dendrimer- and copolymer-based nanoparticles for magnetic resonance cancer theranostics. Theranostics 2018; 8(22): 6322-49.
[http://dx.doi.org/10.7150/thno.27828] [PMID: 30613300]

[73] Zeeshan F, Mishra DK, Kesharwani P. From the nose to the brain, nanomedicine drug delivery Theory and Applications of Nonparenteral Nanomedicines. Elsevier 2021; pp. 153-80.
[http://dx.doi.org/10.1016/B978-0-12-820466-5.00008-9]

[74] Sánchez-López E, Guerra M, Dias-Ferreira J, *et al.* Current applications of nanoemulsions in cancer therapeutics. Nanomaterials (Basel) 2019; 9(6): 821.
[http://dx.doi.org/10.3390/nano9060821] [PMID: 31159219]

[75] Shukla T, Upmanyu N, Agrawal M, Saraf S, Saraf S, Alexander A. Biomedical applications of microemulsion through dermal and transdermal route. Biomed Pharmacother 2018; 108: 1477-94.
[http://dx.doi.org/10.1016/j.biopha.2018.10.021] [PMID: 30372850]

[76] Tiwari P, Sinha VR, Kaur R. Clinical considerations on micro-and nanodrug delivery systems Drug Delivery Trends. Elsevier 2020; pp. 77-101.

[77] Lou H, Qiu N, Crill C, Helms R, Almoazen H. Development of w/o microemulsion for transdermal delivery of iodide ions. AAPS PharmSciTech 2013; 14(1): 168-76.
[http://dx.doi.org/10.1208/s12249-012-9901-5] [PMID: 23250709]

[78] Shukla T, Pandey SP, Khare P, Upmanyu N. Development of ketorolac tromethamine loaded microemulsion for topical delivery using D-optimal experimental approach: Characterization and evaluation of analgesic and anti-inflammatory efficacy. J Drug Deliv Sci Technol 2021; 64: 102632.
[http://dx.doi.org/10.1016/j.jddst.2021.102632]

[79] Lee PJ, Langer R, Shastri VP. Novel microemulsion enhancer formulation for simultaneous transdermal delivery of hydrophilic and hydrophobic drugs. Pharm Res 2003; 20(2): 264-9.
[http://dx.doi.org/10.1023/A:1022283423116] [PMID: 12636166]

[80] Hosmer J, Reed R, Bentley MVLB, Nornoo A, Lopes LB. Microemulsions containing medium-chain glycerides as transdermal delivery systems for hydrophilic and hydrophobic drugs. AAPS PharmSciTech 2009; 10(2): 589-96.
[http://dx.doi.org/10.1208/s12249-009-9251-0] [PMID: 19440842]

[81] Ding J, Wang Y, Ma M, *et al.* CT/fluorescence dual-modal nanoemulsion platform for investigating atherosclerotic plaques. Biomaterials 2013; 34(1): 209-16.
[http://dx.doi.org/10.1016/j.biomaterials.2012.09.025] [PMID: 23069709]

[82] Gorain B, Choudhury H, Nair AB, Dubey SK, Kesharwani P. Theranostic application of nanoemulsions in chemotherapy. Drug Discov Today 2020; 25(7): 1174-88.
[http://dx.doi.org/10.1016/j.drudis.2020.04.013] [PMID: 32344042]

[83] Gianella A, Jarzyna PA, Mani V, *et al.* Multifunctional nanoemulsion platform for imaging guided therapy evaluated in experimental cancer. ACS Nano 2011; 5(6): 4422-33.
[http://dx.doi.org/10.1021/nn103336a] [PMID: 21557611]

[84] Patel SK, Beaino W, Anderson CJ, Janjic JM. Theranostic nanoemulsions for macrophage COX-2 inhibition in a murine inflammation model. Clin Immunol 2015; 160(1): 59-70.

[http://dx.doi.org/10.1016/j.clim.2015.04.019] [PMID: 25959685]

[85] Prévot G, Kauss T, Lorenzato C, *et al.* Iron oxide core oil-in-water nanoemulsion as tracer for atherosclerosis MPI and MRI imaging. Int J Pharm 2017; 532(2): 669-76. [http://dx.doi.org/10.1016/j.ijpharm.2017.09.010] [PMID: 28899764]

[86] Silindir M, Erdoğan S, Özer AY, Maia S. Liposomes and their applications in molecular imaging. J Drug Target 2012; 20(5): 401-15. [http://dx.doi.org/10.3109/1061186X.2012.685477] [PMID: 22553977]

[87] Poste G, Bucana C, Raz A, Bugelski P, Kirsh R, Fidler IJ. Analysis of the fate of systemically administered liposomes and implications for their use in drug delivery. Cancer Res 1982; 42(4): 1412-22. [PMID: 7060015]

[88] Seltzer SE. The role of liposomes in diagnostic imaging. Radiology 1989; 171(1): 19-21. [http://dx.doi.org/10.1148/radiology.171.1.2648470] [PMID: 2648470]

[89] Lamichhane N, Udayakumar T, D'Souza W, *et al.* Liposomes: clinical applications and potential for image-guided drug delivery. Molecules 2018; 23(2): 288. [http://dx.doi.org/10.3390/molecules23020288] [PMID: 29385755]

[90] Richardson VJ, Jeyasingh K, Jewkes RF, Ryman BE, Tattersall MH. Possible tumor localization of Tc-99m-labeled liposomes: effects of lipid composition, charge, and liposome size. J Nucl Med 1978; 19(9): 1049-54. [PMID: 690706]

[91] Turner AF, Presant CA, Proffitt RT, Williams LE, Winsor DW, Werner JL. In-111-labeled liposomes: dosimetry and tumor depiction. Radiology 1988; 166(3): 761-5. [http://dx.doi.org/10.1148/radiology.166.3.3340774] [PMID: 3340774]

[92] Torchilin VP. Surface-modified liposomes in gamma- and MR-imaging. Adv Drug Deliv Rev 1997; 24(2-3): 301-13. [http://dx.doi.org/10.1016/S0169-409X(96)00472-3]

[93] Mahakian LM, Farwell DG, Zhang H, *et al.* Comparison of PET imaging with 64Cu-liposomes and 18F-FDG in the 7,12-dimethylbenz[a]anthracene (DMBA)-induced hamster buccal pouch model of oral dysplasia and squamous cell carcinoma. Mol Imaging Biol 2014; 16(2): 284-92. [http://dx.doi.org/10.1007/s11307-013-0676-1] [PMID: 24019092]

[94] Man F, Gawne PJ, T M de Rosales R. Nuclear imaging of liposomal drug delivery systems: A critical review of radiolabelling methods and applications in nanomedicine. Adv Drug Deliv Rev 2019; 143: 134-60. [http://dx.doi.org/10.1016/j.addr.2019.05.012] [PMID: 31170428]

[95] Bally M, Vörös J. Nanoscale labels: nanoparticles and liposomes in the development of high-performance biosensors. Nanomedicine (Lond) 2009; 4(4): 447-67. [http://dx.doi.org/10.2217/nnm.09.16] [PMID: 19505247]

[96] Xing H, Hwang K, Lu Y. Recent developments of liposomes as nanocarriers for theranostic applications. Theranostics 2016; 6(9): 1336-52. [http://dx.doi.org/10.7150/thno.15464] [PMID: 27375783]

[97] Transferrin liposomes of docetaxel for brain-targeted cancer applications: formulation and brain theranostics. Drug delivery 2016; 23(4): 1261-71.

[98] Prasad R, Jain NK, Yadav AS, *et al.* Liposomal nanotheranostics for multimode targeted *in vivo* bioimaging and near□infrared light mediated cancer therapy. Commun Biol 2020; 3(1): 284. [http://dx.doi.org/10.1038/s42003-020-1016-z] [PMID: 32504032]

[99] Singh TG, Sharma N. Nanobiomaterials in cosmetics: current status and future prospects. In: Grumezescu A, (Ed.) Nanobiomaterials in Galenic Formulations and Cosmetics. Elsevier 2016; pp. 149-74.

[http://dx.doi.org/10.1016/B978-0-323-42868-2.00007-3]

[100] Sankhyan A, Pawar P. Recent trends in niosome as vesicular drug delivery system. J Appl Pharm Sci 2012; 2(6): 20-32.

[101] Barlas FB, Demir B, Guler E, *et al.* Multimodal theranostic assemblies: double encapsulation of protoporphyrine-IX/Gd $^{3+}$ in niosomes. RSC Advances 2016; 6(36): 30217-25. [http://dx.doi.org/10.1039/C5RA26737D]

[102] Muller D, Foulon M, Bonnemain B, Vandamme TF. D. Muller, M. Foulon, B. Bonnemain. Niosomes as carriers of radiopaque contrast agents for X-ray imaging. J Microencapsul 2000; 17(2): 227-43. [http://dx.doi.org/10.1080/026520400288463] [PMID: 10738698]

[103] De A, Venkatesh N, Senthil M, Sanapalli BKR, Shanmugham R, Karri VVSR. Smart niosomes of temozolomide for enhancement of brain targeting. Nanobiomedicine (Rij) 2018; 5. [http://dx.doi.org/10.1177/1849543518805355] [PMID: 30344765]

[104] Luciani A, Olivier JC, Clement O, *et al.* Glucose-receptor MR imaging of tumors: study in mice with PEGylated paramagnetic niosomes. Radiology 2004; 231(1): 135-42. [http://dx.doi.org/10.1148/radiol.2311021559] [PMID: 15068944]

[105] Ag Seleci D, Maurer V, Barlas FB, *et al.* Transferrin-decorated niosomes with integrated INP/ZNS quantum dots and magnetic iron oxide nanoparticles: dual targeting and imaging of glioma. Int J Mol Sci 2021; 22(9): 4556. [http://dx.doi.org/10.3390/ijms22094556] [PMID: 33925347]

[106] Demir B, Barlas FB, Gumus ZP, Unak P, Timur S. Theranostic niosomes as a promising tool for combined therapy and diagnosis:"all-in-one" approach. ACS Appl Nano Mater 2018; 1(6): 2827-35. [http://dx.doi.org/10.1021/acsanm.8b00468]

[107] Nowroozi F, Dadashzadeh S, Soleimanjahi H, *et al.* Theranostic niosomes for direct intratumoral injection: marked enhancement in tumor retention and anticancer efficacy. Nanomedicine (Lond) 2018; 13(17): 2201-19. [http://dx.doi.org/10.2217/nnm-2018-0091] [PMID: 29993311]

[108] Bansal SK, Rajpoot K, Sreeharsha N, Youngren-Ortiz SR, Anup N, Tekade RK. Endosomal escape tendency of drug delivery systems to mediate cytosolic delivery of therapeutics The Future of Pharmaceutical Product Development and Research. Elsevier 2020; pp. 227-58.

[109] Ostróżka-Cieślik A, Sarecka-Hujar B. The use of nanotechnology in modern pharmacotherapy Multifunctional Systems for Combined Delivery, Biosensing and Diagnostics. Elsevier 2017; pp. 139-58. [http://dx.doi.org/10.1016/B978-0-323-52725-5.00007-1]

[110] Mustafa MA, AL-Samarraie MQ, Ahmed MT. Molecular techniques of viral diagnosis. Science Archives 2020; 1(3): 89-92. [http://dx.doi.org/10.47587/SA.2020.1304]

[111] Chaibun T, Puenpa J, Ngamdee T, *et al.* Rapid electrochemical detection of coronavirus SARS-CoV-2. Nat Commun 2021; 12(1): 802. [http://dx.doi.org/10.1038/s41467-021-21121-7] [PMID: 33547323]

[112] Wu Y, Kwak KJ, Agarwal K, *et al.* Detection of extracellular RNAs in cancer and viral infection *via* tethered cationic lipoplex nanoparticles containing molecular beacons. Anal Chem 2013; 85(23): 11265-74. [http://dx.doi.org/10.1021/ac401983w] [PMID: 24102152]

[113] Wang X, Kwak KJ, Yang Z, *et al.* Extracellular mRNA detected by molecular beacons in tethered lipoplex nanoparticles for diagnosis of human hepatocellular carcinoma. PLoS One 2018; 13(6): e0198552. [http://dx.doi.org/10.1371/journal.pone.0198552] [PMID: 29879168]

[114] Lee LJ, Yang Z, Rahman M, *et al.* Extracellular mRNA detected by tethered lipoplex nanoparticle

biochip for lung adenocarcinoma detection. Am J Respir Crit Care Med 2016; 193(12): 1431-3. [http://dx.doi.org/10.1164/rccm.201511-2129LE] [PMID: 27304243]

[115] Pu X, Ding G, Wu M, Zhou S, Jia S, Cao L. Elevated expression of exosomal microRNA-21 as a potential biomarker for the early diagnosis of pancreatic cancer using a tethered cationic lipoplex nanoparticle biochip. Oncol Lett 2020; 19(3): 2062-70. [http://dx.doi.org/10.3892/ol.2020.11302] [PMID: 32194703]

[116] Wu Y, Li L, Mao Y, Lee LJ. Static micromixer-coaxial electrospray synthesis of theranostic lipoplexes. ACS Nano 2012; 6(3): 2245-52. [http://dx.doi.org/10.1021/nn204300s] [PMID: 22320282]

[117] Naseri N, Valizadeh H, Zakeri-Milani P. Solid lipid nanoparticles and nanostructured lipid carriers: structure, preparation and application. Adv Pharm Bull 2015; 5(3): 305-13. [http://dx.doi.org/10.15171/apb.2015.043] [PMID: 26504751]

[118] Tamjidi F, Shahedi M, Varshosaz J, Nasirpour A. Nanostructured lipid carriers (NLC): A potential delivery system for bioactive food molecules. Innov Food Sci Emerg Technol 2013; 19: 29-43. [http://dx.doi.org/10.1016/j.ifset.2013.03.002]

[119] Mu H, Holm R. Solid lipid nanocarriers in drug delivery: characterization and design. Expert Opin Drug Deliv 2018; 15(8): 771-85. [http://dx.doi.org/10.1080/17425247.2018.1504018] [PMID: 30064267]

[120] Sussman EM, Jayagopal A, Haselton FR, Shastri VP. Engineering of solid lipid nanoparticles for biomedical applications. In: Parris N, Liu L, Cunxian Song C, Shastri P, Eds. New Delivery Systems for Controlled Drug Release from Naturally Occurring Materials. ACS Publications 2008; pp. 139-52. [http://dx.doi.org/10.1021/bk-2008-0992.ch008]

[121] Sun J, Zhang S, Jiang S, *et al.* Gadolinium-loaded solid lipid nanoparticles as a tumor-absorbable contrast agent for early diagnosis of colorectal tumors using magnetic resonance colonography. J Biomed Nanotechnol 2016; 12(9): 1709-23. [http://dx.doi.org/10.1166/jbn.2016.2285] [PMID: 29345451]

[122] Rolla GA, Botta M, Tei L, *et al.* Paramagnetic solid lipid nanoparticles as a novel platform for the development of molecular MRI probes. Chemistry 2013; 19(34): 11189-93. [http://dx.doi.org/10.1002/chem.201301837] [PMID: 23843364]

[123] Peira E, Marzola P, Podio V, Aime S, Sbarbati A, Gasco MR. *In vitro* and *in vivo* study of solid lipid nanoparticles loaded with superparamagnetic iron oxide. J Drug Target 2003; 11(1): 19-24. [http://dx.doi.org/10.1080/1061186031000086108] [PMID: 12852437]

[124] Ayan AK, Yenilmez A, Eroglu H. Evaluation of radiolabeled curcumin-loaded solid lipid nanoparticles usage as an imaging agent in liver-spleen scintigraphy. Mater Sci Eng C 2017; 75: 663-70. [http://dx.doi.org/10.1016/j.msec.2017.02.114] [PMID: 28415513]

[125] Oumzil K, Ramin MA, Lorenzato C, *et al.* Solid lipid nanoparticles for image-guided therapy of atherosclerosis. Bioconjug Chem 2016; 27(3): 569-75. [http://dx.doi.org/10.1021/acs.bioconjchem.5b00590] [PMID: 26751997]

[126] Albuquerque J, Moura C, Sarmento B, Reis S. Solid lipid nanoparticles: a potential multifunctional approach towards rheumatoid arthritis theranostics. Molecules 2015; 20(6): 11103-18. [http://dx.doi.org/10.3390/molecules200611103] [PMID: 26087258]

[127] Singh I, Swami R, Khan W, Sistla R. Lymphatic system: a prospective area for advanced targeting of particulate drug carriers. Expert Opin Drug Deliv 2016; 11(2): 211-9. [http://dx.doi.org/10.5005/jp/books/12847_29]

[128] Cai S, Yang Q, Bagby TR, Forrest ML. Lymphatic drug delivery using engineered liposomes and solid lipid nanoparticles. Adv Drug Deliv Rev 2011; 63(10-11): 901-8. [http://dx.doi.org/10.1016/j.addr.2011.05.017] [PMID: 21712055]

[129] Truzzi E, Bongio C, Sacchetti F, *et al.* Self-assembled lipid nanoparticles for oral delivery of heparin-coated iron oxide nanoparticles for theranostic purposes. Molecules 2017; 22(6): 963. [http://dx.doi.org/10.3390/molecules22060963] [PMID: 28598368]

[130] Chauhan I, Yasir M, Verma M, Singh AP. Nanostructured lipid carriers: A groundbreaking approach for transdermal drug delivery. Adv Pharm Bull 2020; 10(2): 150-65. [http://dx.doi.org/10.34172/apb.2020.021] [PMID: 32373485]

[131] Khosa A, Reddi S, Saha RN. Nanostructured lipid carriers for site-specific drug delivery. Biomed Pharmacother 2018; 103: 598-613. [http://dx.doi.org/10.1016/j.biopha.2018.04.055] [PMID: 29677547]

[132] Hsu SH, Wen CJ, Al-Suwayeh SA, Huang YJ, Fang JY. Formulation design and evaluation of quantum dot-loaded nanostructured lipid carriers for integrating bioimaging and anticancer therapy. Nanomedicine (Lond) 2013; 8(8): 1253-69. [http://dx.doi.org/10.2217/nnm.12.170] [PMID: 23384703]

[133] Olerile LD, Liu Y, Zhang B, *et al.* Near-infrared mediated quantum dots and paclitaxel co-loaded nanostructured lipid carriers for cancer theragnostic. Colloids Surf B Biointerfaces 2017; 150: 121-30. [http://dx.doi.org/10.1016/j.colsurfb.2016.11.032] [PMID: 27907859]

[134] Ucar E, Teksoz S, Ichedef C, *et al.* Synthesis, characterization and radiolabeling of folic acid modified nanostructured lipid carriers as a contrast agent and drug delivery system. Appl Radiat Isot 2017; 119: 72-9. [http://dx.doi.org/10.1016/j.apradiso.2016.11.002] [PMID: 27866122]

[135] Chen J, Chen H, Cui S, *et al.* Glucosamine derivative modified nanostructured lipid carriers for targeted tumor delivery. J Mater Chem 2012; 22(12): 5770-83. [http://dx.doi.org/10.1039/c2jm15830b]

[136] Shao Z, Shao J, Tan B, *et al.* Targeted lung cancer therapy: preparation and optimization of transferrin-decorated nanostructured lipid carriers as novel nanomedicine for co-delivery of anticancer drugs and DNA. Int J Nanomedicine 2015; 10: 1223-33. [http://dx.doi.org/10.2147/IJN.S77837] [PMID: 25709444]

[137] Beh CY, How CW, Foo JB, Foong JN, Selvarajah GT, Rasedee A. Development of erythropoietin receptor-targeted drug delivery system against breast cancer using tamoxifen-loaded nanostructured lipid carriers. Drug Des Devel Ther 2017; 11: 771-82. [http://dx.doi.org/10.2147/DDDT.S123939] [PMID: 28352153]

[138] Lu C, Ji J, Zhu X. T2-weighted magnetic resonance imaging of hepatic tumor guided by SPIO-loaded nanostructured lipid carriers and ferritin reporter genes. ACS Appl Mater Interfaces 2017; 9(41): 35548-61. [http://dx.doi.org/10.1021/acsami.7b09879] [PMID: 28944659]

[139] Lu C-y, Zhang N-N, Shu G-f, *et al.* SPIO-Loaded Nanostructured Lipid Carriers for T2-weighted Magnetic Resonance Imaging of Hepatocarcinoma 2020. [http://dx.doi.org/10.21203/rs.3.rs-23465/v1]

[140] Yuan P, Ding X, Yang YY, Xu QH. Metal nanoparticles for diagnosis and therapy of bacterial infection. Adv Healthc Mater 2018; 7(13): 1701392. [http://dx.doi.org/10.1002/adhm.201701392] [PMID: 29582578]

[141] Brainina K, Stozhko N, Bukharinova M, Vikulova E. 6 Nanomaterials: Electrochemical Properties and Application in Sensors. Nanoanalytics 2018; pp. 165-222.

[142] Braz AKS, de Araujo RE, Ohulchanskyy TY, *et al. In situ* gold nanoparticles formation: contrast agent for dental optical coherence tomography. J Biomed Opt 2012; 17(6): 066003. [http://dx.doi.org/10.1117/1.JBO.17.6.066003] [PMID: 22734759]

[143] Bautista MC, Bomati-Miguel O, Zhao X, *et al.* Comparative study of ferrofluids based on dextran-coated iron oxide and metal nanoparticles for contrast agents in magnetic resonance imaging.

Nanotechnology 2004; 15(4): S154-9.
[http://dx.doi.org/10.1088/0957-4484/15/4/008]

[144] Jackson TC, Patani BO, Ekpa DE. Nanotechnology in diagnosis: a review. Adv Nanopart 2017; 6(3): 93-102.
[http://dx.doi.org/10.4236/anp.2017.63008]

[145] Wu X, Xiao T, Luo Z, *et al.* A micro-/nano-chip and quantum dots-based 3D cytosensor for quantitative analysis of circulating tumor cells. J Nanobiotechnology 2018; 16(1): 1-9.
[http://dx.doi.org/10.1186/s12951-017-0328-8] [PMID: 29321058]

[146] Tang J, Tang D. Non-enzymatic electrochemical immunoassay using noble metal nanoparticles: a review. Mikrochim Acta 2015; 182(13-14): 2077-89.
[http://dx.doi.org/10.1007/s00604-015-1567-8]

[147] Zhang H, Song D, Gao S, Zhang J, Zhang H, Sun Y. Novel SPR biosensors based on metal nanoparticles decorated with graphene for immunoassay. Sens Actuators B Chem 2013; 188: 548-54.
[http://dx.doi.org/10.1016/j.snb.2013.07.055]

[148] Vio V, Marchant MJ, Araya E, Kogan MK. J Kogan M. Metal nanoparticles for the treatment and diagnosis of neurodegenerative brain diseases. Curr Pharm Des 2017; 23(13): 1916-26.
[http://dx.doi.org/10.2174/1381612823666170105152948] [PMID: 28056734]

[149] Chu HW, Lai CS, Ko JY, *et al.* Nanoparticle-based LDI-MS immunoassay for the multiple diagnosis of viral infections. ACS Sens 2019; 4(6): 1543-51.
[http://dx.doi.org/10.1021/acssensors.9b00054] [PMID: 31066548]

[150] Gao Q, Zhang J, Gao J, Zhang Z, Zhu H, Wang D. Gold nanoparticles in cancer theranostics. Front Bioeng Biotechnol 2021; 9: 647905.
[http://dx.doi.org/10.3389/fbioe.2021.647905] [PMID: 33928072]

[151] Hu X, Zhang Y, Ding T, Liu J, Zhao H. Multifunctional gold nanoparticles: a novel nanomaterial for various medical applications and biological activities. Front Bioeng Biotechnol 2020; 8: 990.
[http://dx.doi.org/10.3389/fbioe.2020.00990] [PMID: 32903562]

[152] Singh P, Pandit S, Mokkapati VRSS, Garg A, Ravikumar V, Mijakovic I. Gold nanoparticles in diagnostics and therapeutics for human cancer. Int J Mol Sci 2018; 19(7): 1979.
[http://dx.doi.org/10.3390/ijms19071979] [PMID: 29986450]

[153] Hainfeld JF, Slatkin DN, Focella TM, Smilowitz HM. Gold nanoparticles: a new X-ray contrast agent. Br J Radiol 2006; 79(939): 248-53.
[http://dx.doi.org/10.1259/bjr/13169882] [PMID: 16498039]

[154] Kumar A, Mazinder Boruah B, Liang X-J. Gold nanoparticles: promising nanomaterials for the diagnosis of cancer and HIV/AIDS. J Nanomater 2011; 2011: 202187.

[155] Baptista P, Pereira E, Eaton P, *et al.* Gold nanoparticles for the development of clinical diagnosis methods. Anal Bioanal Chem 2008; 391(3): 943-50.
[http://dx.doi.org/10.1007/s00216-007-1768-z] [PMID: 18157524]

[156] Popovtzer R, Agrawal A, Kotov NA, *et al.* Targeted gold nanoparticles enable molecular CT imaging of cancer. Nano Lett 2008; 8(12): 4593-6.
[http://dx.doi.org/10.1021/nl8029114] [PMID: 19367807]

[157] El-Sayed IH, Huang X, El-Sayed MA. Surface plasmon resonance scattering and absorption of anti-EGFR antibody conjugated gold nanoparticles in cancer diagnostics: applications in oral cancer. Nano Lett 2005; 5(5): 829-34.
[http://dx.doi.org/10.1021/nl050074e] [PMID: 15884879]

[158] Elbassal EA, Morris C, Kent TW, *et al.* Gold nanoparticles as a probe for amyloid-β oligomer and amyloid formation. J Phys Chem C 2017; 121(36): 20007-15.
[http://dx.doi.org/10.1021/acs.jpcc.7b05169] [PMID: 29276551]

[159] Ma X, Jiang Y, Jia F, Yu Y, Chen J, Wang Z. An aptamer-based electrochemical biosensor for the detection of Salmonella. J Microbiol Methods 2014; 98: 94-8. [http://dx.doi.org/10.1016/j.mimet.2014.01.003] [PMID: 24445115]

[160] Yáñez-Sedeño P, Pingarrón JM. Gold nanoparticle-based electrochemical biosensors. Anal Bioanal Chem 2005; 382(4): 884-6. [http://dx.doi.org/10.1007/s00216-005-3221-5] [PMID: 15864491]

[161] Sivanesan A, John SA. Gold nanoparticles modified electrodes for biosensors. Nanostructured materials for electrochemical biosensors 2009; 97-128.

[162] Schultz S, Smith DR, Mock JJ, Schultz DA. Single-target molecule detection with nonbleaching multicolor optical immunolabels. Proc Natl Acad Sci USA 2000; 97(3): 996-1001. [http://dx.doi.org/10.1073/pnas.97.3.996] [PMID: 10655473]

[163] Tran QH, Nguyen VQ, Le A-T. Silver nanoparticles: synthesis, properties, toxicology, applications and perspectives. Advances in Natural Sciences: Nanoscience and Nanotechnology 2013; 4(3): 033001. [http://dx.doi.org/10.1088/2043-6262/4/3/033001]

[164] Poon CY, Chan HM, Li HW. Direct detection of prostate specific antigen by darkfield microscopy using single immunotargeting silver nanoparticle. Sens Actuators B Chem 2014; 190: 737-44. [http://dx.doi.org/10.1016/j.snb.2013.09.057]

[165] Karunamuni R, Tsourkas A, Maidment ADA. Exploring silver as a contrast agent for contrast-enhanced dual-energy X-ray breast imaging. Br J Radiol 2014; 87(1041): 20140081. [http://dx.doi.org/10.1259/bjr.20140081] [PMID: 24998157]

[166] Borghei YS, Hosseini M, Ganjali MR, Ju H. A unique FRET approach toward detection of single-base mismatch DNA in BRCA1 gene. Mater Sci Eng C 2019; 97: 406-11. [http://dx.doi.org/10.1016/j.msec.2018.12.049] [PMID: 30678926]

[167] Liu R, Wang Q, Li Q, Yang X, Wang K, Nie W. Surface plasmon resonance biosensor for sensitive detection of microRNA and cancer cell using multiple signal amplification strategy. Biosens Bioelectron 2017; 87: 433-8. [http://dx.doi.org/10.1016/j.bios.2016.08.090] [PMID: 27589408]

[168] Liang J, Yao C, Li X, *et al.* Silver nanoprism etching-based plasmonic ELISA for the high sensitive detection of prostate-specific antigen. Biosens Bioelectron 2015; 69: 128-34. [http://dx.doi.org/10.1016/j.bios.2015.02.026] [PMID: 25721976]

[169] Lee SX, Lim HN, Ibrahim I, Jamil A, Pandikumar A, Huang NM. Horseradish peroxidase-labeled silver/reduced graphene oxide thin film-modified screen-printed electrode for detection of carcinoembryonic antigen. Biosens Bioelectron 2017; 89(Pt 1): 673-80. [http://dx.doi.org/10.1016/j.bios.2015.12.030] [PMID: 26718548]

[170] Dadmehr M, Hosseini M, Hosseinkhani S, Reza Ganjali M, Sheikhnejad R. Label free colorimetric and fluorimetric direct detection of methylated DNA based on silver nanoclusters for cancer early diagnosis. Biosens Bioelectron 2015; 73: 108-13. [http://dx.doi.org/10.1016/j.bios.2015.05.062] [PMID: 26056954]

[171] Sepunaru L, Tschulik K, Batchelor-McAuley C, Gavish R, Compton RG. Electrochemical detection of single E. coli bacteria labeled with silver nanoparticles. Biomater Sci 2015; 3(6): 816-20. [http://dx.doi.org/10.1039/C5BM00114E] [PMID: 26221841]

[172] Ellairaja S, Krithiga N, Ponmariappan S, Vasantha VS. Novel pyrimidine tagged silver nanoparticle based fluorescent immunoassay for the detection of Pseudomonas aeruginosa. J Agric Food Chem 2017; 65(8): 1802-12. [http://dx.doi.org/10.1021/acs.jafc.6b04790] [PMID: 28161944]

[173] Dadfar SM, Roemhild K, Drude NI, *et al.* Iron oxide nanoparticles: Diagnostic, therapeutic and theranostic applications. Adv Drug Deliv Rev 2019; 138: 302-25.

[http://dx.doi.org/10.1016/j.addr.2019.01.005] [PMID: 30639256]

[174] McCarthy J, Weissleder R. Multifunctional magnetic nanoparticles for targeted imaging and therapy. Adv Drug Deliv Rev 2008; 60(11): 1241-51.
[http://dx.doi.org/10.1016/j.addr.2008.03.014] [PMID: 18508157]

[175] Jin R, Lin B, Li D, Ai H. Superparamagnetic iron oxide nanoparticles for MR imaging and therapy: design considerations and clinical applications. Curr Opin Pharmacol 2014; 18: 18-27.
[http://dx.doi.org/10.1016/j.coph.2014.08.002] [PMID: 25173782]

[176] Muthiah M, Park IK, Cho CS. Surface modification of iron oxide nanoparticles by biocompatible polymers for tissue imaging and targeting. Biotechnol Adv 2013; 31(8): 1224-36.
[http://dx.doi.org/10.1016/j.biotechadv.2013.03.005] [PMID: 23528431]

[177] Jung CW, Jacobs P. Physical and chemical properties of superparamagnetic iron oxide MR contrast agents: Ferumoxides, ferumoxtran, ferumoxsil. Magn Reson Imaging 1995; 13(5): 661-74.
[http://dx.doi.org/10.1016/0730-725X(95)00024-B] [PMID: 8569441]

[178] McCormack PL. Ferumoxytol. Drugs 2012; 72(15): 2013-22.
[http://dx.doi.org/10.2165/11209880-000000000-00000] [PMID: 22994536]

[179] Cole AJ, David AE, Wang J, Galbán CJ, Hill HL, Yang VC. Polyethylene glycol modified, cross-linked starch-coated iron oxide nanoparticles for enhanced magnetic tumor targeting. Biomaterials 2011; 32(8): 2183-93.
[http://dx.doi.org/10.1016/j.biomaterials.2010.11.040] [PMID: 21176955]

[180] Răcuciu M, Creangă DE, Airinei A. Citric-acid-coated magnetite nanoparticles for biological applications. Eur Phys J E 2006; 21(2): 117-21.
[http://dx.doi.org/10.1140/epje/i2006-10051-y] [PMID: 17180642]

[181] Bloemen M, Brullot W, Luong TT, Geukens N, Gils A, Verbiest T. Improved functionalization of oleic acid-coated iron oxide nanoparticles for biomedical applications. J Nanopart Res 2012; 14(9): 1100.
[http://dx.doi.org/10.1007/s11051-012-1100-5] [PMID: 23024598]

[182] Moraes Silva S, Tavallaie R, Sandiford L, Tilley RD, Gooding JJ. Gold coated magnetic nanoparticles: from preparation to surface modification for analytical and biomedical applications. Chem Commun (Camb) 2016; 52(48): 7528-40.
[http://dx.doi.org/10.1039/C6CC03225G] [PMID: 27182032]

[183] Hajba L, Guttman A. The use of magnetic nanoparticles in cancer theranostics: Toward handheld diagnostic devices. Biotechnol Adv 2016; 34(4): 354-61.
[http://dx.doi.org/10.1016/j.biotechadv.2016.02.001] [PMID: 26853617]

[184] Lee H, Sun E, Ham D, Weissleder R. Chip–NMR biosensor for detection and molecular analysis of cells. Nat Med 2008; 14(8): 869-74.
[http://dx.doi.org/10.1038/nm.1711] [PMID: 18607350]

[185] Zhao S, Yu X, Qian Y, Chen W, Shen J. Multifunctional magnetic iron oxide nanoparticles: an advanced platform for cancer theranostics. Theranostics 2020; 10(14): 6278-309.
[http://dx.doi.org/10.7150/thno.42564] [PMID: 32483453]

[186] El-Dakdouki MH, Xia J, Zhu DC, *et al.* Assessing the *in vivo* efficacy of doxorubicin loaded hyaluronan nanoparticles. ACS Appl Mater Interfaces 2014; 6(1): 697-705.
[http://dx.doi.org/10.1021/am404946v] [PMID: 24308364]

[187] Miller MA, Gadde S, Pfirschke C, Engblom C, Sprachman MM, Kohler RH, *et al.* Predicting therapeutic nanomedicine efficacy using a companion magnetic resonance imaging nanoparticle. Science translational medicine 2015; 7(314): 314ra183-.
[http://dx.doi.org/10.1126/scitranslmed.aac6522]

[188] Pisanic TR II, Zhang Y, Wang TH. Quantum dots in diagnostics and detection: principles and paradigms. Analyst (Lond) 2014; 139(12): 2968-81.

[http://dx.doi.org/10.1039/C4AN00294F] [PMID: 24770716]

[189] Tripathi S, Kaur G, Khurana RK, Kapoor S, Singh B. Quantum dots and their potential role in cancer theranostics. Critical Reviews™ in Therapeutic Drug Carrier Systems 2015; 32(6). [http://dx.doi.org/10.1615/CritRevTherDrugCarrierSyst.2015012360]

[190] Díaz-González M, de la Escosura-Muñiz A, Fernandez-Argüelles MT, Alonso FJG, Costa-Fernandez JM. Quantum dot bioconjugates for diagnostic applications. Surface-modified Nanobiomaterials for Electrochemical and Biomedicine Applications 2020; pp. 133-76.

[191] Liu X, Luo Y. Surface modifications technology of quantum dots based biosensors and their medical applications. Chin J Anal Chem 2014; 42(7): 1061-9. [http://dx.doi.org/10.1016/S1872-2040(14)60753-2]

[192] Ma F, Li C, Zhang C. Development of quantum dot-based biosensors: principles and applications. J Mater Chem B Mater Biol Med 2018; 6(39): 6173-90. [http://dx.doi.org/10.1039/C8TB01869C] [PMID: 32254608]

[193] Montanarella F, Altantzis T, Zanaga D, *et al.* Composite supraparticles with tunable light emission. ACS Nano 2017; 11(9): 9136-42. [http://dx.doi.org/10.1021/acsnano.7b03975] [PMID: 28787121]

[194] Wegner KD, Hildebrandt N. Quantum dots: bright and versatile *in vitro* and *in vivo* fluorescence imaging biosensors. Chem Soc Rev 2015; 44(14): 4792-834. [http://dx.doi.org/10.1039/C4CS00532E] [PMID: 25777768]

[195] Bhattacharyya D, Sarswat PK, Free ML. Quantum dots and carbon dots based fluorescent sensors for TB biomarkers detection. Vacuum 2017; 146: 606-13. [http://dx.doi.org/10.1016/j.vacuum.2017.02.003]

[196] Mu Q, Xu H, Li Y, Ma S, Zhong X. Adenosine capped QDs based fluorescent sensor for detection of dopamine with high selectivity and sensitivity. Analyst (Lond) 2014; 139(1): 93-8. [http://dx.doi.org/10.1039/C3AN01592K] [PMID: 24153190]

[197] Datta M, Desai D, Kumar A. Gene specific DNA sensors for diagnosis of pathogenic infections. Indian J Microbiol 2017; 57(2): 139-47. [http://dx.doi.org/10.1007/s12088-017-0650-8] [PMID: 28611490]

[198] Liang SS, Qi L, Zhang RL, Jin M, Zhang ZQ. Ratiometric fluorescence biosensor based on CdTe quantum and carbon dots for double strand DNA detection. Sens Actuators B Chem 2017; 244: 585-90. [http://dx.doi.org/10.1016/j.snb.2017.01.032]

[199] Yang H, Li D, He R, *et al.* A novel quantum dots-based point of care test for syphilis. Nanoscale Res Lett 2010; 5(5): 875-81. [http://dx.doi.org/10.1007/s11671-010-9578-1] [PMID: 20672123]

[200] Chen X, Gan M, Xu H, *et al.* Development of a rapid and sensitive quantum dot-based immunochromatographic strip by double labeling PCR products for detection of Staphylococcus aureus in food. Food Control 2014; 46: 225-32. [http://dx.doi.org/10.1016/j.foodcont.2014.04.044]

[201] Wilkins MD, Turner BL, Rivera KR, Menegatti S, Daniele M. Quantum dot enabled lateral flow immunoassay for detection of cardiac biomarker NT-proBNP. Sens Biosensing Res 2018; 21: 46-53. [http://dx.doi.org/10.1016/j.sbsr.2018.10.002]

[202] Zhou P, Liu H, Gong L, *et al.* A faster detection method for high-sensitivity cardiac troponin—POCT quantum dot fluorescence immunoassay. J Thorac Dis 2019; 11(4): 1506-13. [http://dx.doi.org/10.21037/jtd.2019.03.25] [PMID: 31179093]

[203] Cheng X, Pu X, Jun P, Zhu X, Zhu D, Chen M. Rapid and quantitative detection of C-reactive protein using quantum dots and immunochromatographic test strips. Int J Nanomedicine 2014; 9: 5619-26. [PMID: 25506215]

[204] Shen J, Zhou Y, Fu F, *et al.* Immunochromatographic assay for quantitative and sensitive detection of hepatitis B virus surface antigen using highly luminescent quantum dot-beads. Talanta 2015; 142: 145-9.
[http://dx.doi.org/10.1016/j.talanta.2015.04.058] [PMID: 26003704]

[205] Ho YP, Leong KW. Quantum dot-based theranostics. Nanoscale 2010; 2(1): 60-8.
[http://dx.doi.org/10.1039/B9NR00178F] [PMID: 20648364]

[206] Li S, Su W, Wu H, *et al.* Targeted tumour theranostics in mice *via* carbon quantum dots structurally mimicking large amino acids. Nat Biomed Eng 2020; 4(7): 704-16.
[http://dx.doi.org/10.1038/s41551-020-0540-y] [PMID: 32231314]

[207] Ji S-r, Liu C, Zhang B, Yang F, Xu J, Long J, *et al.* Carbon nanotubes in cancer diagnosis and therapy. Biochimica et Biophysica Acta (BBA)-. Rev Can 2010; 1806(1): 29-35.

[208] He H, Pham-Huy LA, Dramou P, Xiao D, Zuo P, Pham-Huy C. Carbon nanotubes: applications in pharmacy and medicine. Biomed Res Int 2013; 2013: 578290.
[http://dx.doi.org/10.1155/2013/578290]

[209] Gong H, Peng R, Liu Z. Carbon nanotubes for biomedical imaging: The recent advances. Adv Drug Deliv Rev 2013; 65(15): 1951-63.
[http://dx.doi.org/10.1016/j.addr.2013.10.002] [PMID: 24184130]

[210] Richard C, Doan BT, Beloeil JC, Bessodes M, Tóth É, Scherman D. Noncovalent functionalization of carbon nanotubes with amphiphilic gd3+ chelates: toward powerful t1 and t2 MRI contrast agents. Nano Lett 2008; 8(1): 232-6.
[http://dx.doi.org/10.1021/nl072509z] [PMID: 18088153]

[211] Servant A, Jacobs I, Bussy C, *et al.* Gadolinium-functionalised multi-walled carbon nanotubes as a T 1 contrast agent for MRI cell labelling and tracking. Carbon 2016; 97: 126-33.
[http://dx.doi.org/10.1016/j.carbon.2015.08.051]

[212] Doan BT, Seguin J, Breton M, *et al.* Functionalized single-walled carbon nanotubes containing traces of iron as new negative MRI contrast agents for *in vivo* imaging. Contrast Media Mol Imaging 2012; 7(2): 153-9.
[http://dx.doi.org/10.1002/cmmi.474] [PMID: 22434627]

[213] Yudasaka M, Yomogida Y, Zhang M, *et al.* Near-infrared photoluminescent carbon nanotubes for imaging of brown fat. Sci Rep 2017; 7(1): 44760.
[http://dx.doi.org/10.1038/srep44760] [PMID: 28317858]

[214] Kim JW, Galanzha EI, Shashkov EV, Moon HM, Zharov VP. Golden carbon nanotubes as multimodal photoacoustic and photothermal high-contrast molecular agents. Nat Nanotechnol 2009; 4(10): 688-94.
[http://dx.doi.org/10.1038/nnano.2009.231] [PMID: 19809462]

[215] Holzinger M, Baur J, Haddad R, Wang X, Cosnier S. Multiple functionalization of single-walled carbon nanotubes by dip coating. Chem Commun (Camb) 2011; 47(8): 2450-2.
[http://dx.doi.org/10.1039/C0CC03928D] [PMID: 21173960]

[216] Wei F, Lillehoj PB, Ho CM. DNA diagnostics: nanotechnology-enhanced electrochemical detection of nucleic acids. Pediatr Res 2010; 67(5): 458-68.
[http://dx.doi.org/10.1203/PDR.0b013e3181d361c3] [PMID: 20075759]

[217] Yang S, Rothman RE. PCR-based diagnostics for infectious diseases: uses, limitations, and future applications in acute-care settings. Lancet Infect Dis 2004; 4(6): 337-48.
[http://dx.doi.org/10.1016/S1473-3099(04)01044-8] [PMID: 15172342]

[218] Kuralay F, Karadeniz H, Muti M, Erdem A. Electrochemical DNA detection using carbon nanotubes. Curr Phys Chem 2011; 1(4): 325-33.
[http://dx.doi.org/10.2174/1877946811101040325]

[219] Lee J, Morita M, Takemura K, Park EY. A multi-functional gold/iron-oxide nanoparticle-CNT hybrid

nanomaterial as virus DNA sensing platform. Biosens Bioelectron 2018; 102: 425-31. [http://dx.doi.org/10.1016/j.bios.2017.11.052] [PMID: 29175218]

[220] Negri V, Pacheco-Torres J, Calle D, López-Larrubia P. Carbon nanotubes in biomedicine. Surface-modified Nanobiomaterials for Electrochemical and Biomedicine Applications 2020; pp. 177-217.

[221] Ojeda I, Garcinuño B, Moreno-Guzmán M, *et al.* Carbon nanohorns as a scaffold for the construction of disposable electrochemical immunosensing platforms. Application to the determination of fibrinogen in human plasma and urine. Anal Chem 2014; 86(15): 7749-56. [http://dx.doi.org/10.1021/ac501681n] [PMID: 25001594]

[222] Chen D, Dougherty CA, Zhu K, Hong H. Theranostic applications of carbon nanomaterials in cancer: Focus on imaging and cargo delivery. J Control Release 2015; 210: 230-45. [http://dx.doi.org/10.1016/j.jconrel.2015.04.021] [PMID: 25910580]

[223] Zhang M, Wang W, Wu F, Yuan P, Chi C, Zhou N. Magnetic and fluorescent carbon nanotubes for dual modal imaging and photothermal and chemo-therapy of cancer cells in living mice. Carbon 2017; 123: 70-83. [http://dx.doi.org/10.1016/j.carbon.2017.07.032]

[224] Arap W, Pasqualini R, Montalti M, *et al.* Luminescent silica nanoparticles for cancer diagnosis. Curr Med Chem 2013; 20(17): 2195-211. [http://dx.doi.org/10.2174/09298673113201700005] [PMID: 23458621]

[225] Jafari S, Derakhshankhah H, Alaei L, Fattahi A, Varnamkhasti BS, Saboury AA. Mesoporous silica nanoparticles for therapeutic/diagnostic applications. Biomed Pharmacother 2019; 109: 1100-11. [http://dx.doi.org/10.1016/j.biopha.2018.10.167] [PMID: 30551360]

[226] Barui AK, Kotcherlakota R, Patra CR. Biomedical applications of zinc oxide nanoparticles Inorganic frameworks as smart nanomedicines. Elsevier 2018; pp. 239-78. [http://dx.doi.org/10.1016/B978-0-12-813661-4.00006-7]

[227] Eskiizmir G, Baskın Y, Yapıcı K. Graphene-based nanomaterials in cancer treatment and diagnosis Fullerens, graphenes and nanotubes. Elsevier 2018; pp. 331-74. [http://dx.doi.org/10.1016/B978-0-12-813691-1.00009-9]

[228] Parkes LM, Hodgson R, Lu LT, *et al.* Cobalt nanoparticles as a novel magnetic resonance contrast agent-relaxivities at 1.5 and 3 Tesla. Contrast Media Mol Imaging 2008; 3(4): 150-6. [http://dx.doi.org/10.1002/cmmi.241] [PMID: 18756588]

[229] Hatamie S, Ahadian MM, Ghiass MA, *et al.* Graphene/cobalt nanocarrier for hyperthermia therapy and MRI diagnosis. Colloids Surf B Biointerfaces 2016; 146: 271-9. [http://dx.doi.org/10.1016/j.colsurfb.2016.06.018] [PMID: 27351138]

[230] Sherin S, Balachandran S, Abraham A. Curcumin incorporated titanium dioxide nanoparticles as MRI contrasting agent for early diagnosis of atherosclerosis- rat model. Vet Anim Sci 2020; 10: 100090. [http://dx.doi.org/10.1016/j.vas.2020.100090] [PMID: 32734023]

[231] Řehoř I, Vilímová V, Jendelová P, *et al.* Phosphonate-titanium dioxide assemblies: platform for multimodal diagnostic-therapeutic nanoprobes. J Med Chem 2011; 54(14): 5185-94. [http://dx.doi.org/10.1021/jm200449y] [PMID: 21662977]

[232] Anselmo AC, Mitragotri S. Nanoparticles in the clinic. Bioeng Transl Med 2016; 1(1): 10-29. [http://dx.doi.org/10.1002/btm2.10003] [PMID: 29313004]

[233] Anselmo AC, Mitragotri S. Nanoparticles in the clinic: An update. Bioeng Transl Med 2019; 4(3): e10143. [http://dx.doi.org/10.1002/btm2.10143] [PMID: 31572799]

[234] Sakamoto JH, van de Ven AL, Godin B, *et al.* Enabling individualized therapy through nanotechnology. Pharmacol Res 2010; 62(2): 57-89. [http://dx.doi.org/10.1016/j.phrs.2009.12.011] [PMID: 20045055]

[235] Anzai Y, Piccoli CW, Outwater EK, *et al.* Group. Evaluation of neck and body metastases to nodes with ferumoxtran 10-enhanced MR imaging: phase III safety and efficacy study. Radiology 2003; 228(3): 777-88.
[http://dx.doi.org/10.1148/radiol.2283020872] [PMID: 12954896]

[236] Ntoulia A, Anupindi SA, Darge K, Back SJ. Applications of contrast-enhanced ultrasound in the pediatric abdomen. Abdom Radiol (NY) 2018; 43(4): 948-59.
[http://dx.doi.org/10.1007/s00261-017-1315-0] [PMID: 28980061]

[237] Phillips E, Penate-Medina O, Zanzonico PB, Carvajal RD, Mohan P, Ye Y, *et al.* Clinical translation of an ultrasmall inorganic optical-PET imaging nanoparticle probe. Science translational medicine 2014; 6(260): 260ra149.
[http://dx.doi.org/10.1126/scitranslmed.3009524]

[238] Wang YX, Xuan S, Port M, Idee JM. Recent advances in superparamagnetic iron oxide nanoparticles for cellular imaging and targeted therapy research. Curr Pharm Des 2013; 19(37): 6575-93.
[http://dx.doi.org/10.2174/1381612811319370003] [PMID: 23621536]

[239] PROFILE AR. Ferumoxtran-10 2003.

[240] Galema TW, Geleijnse ML, Vletter WB, de Laat L, Michels M, Cate FJ. Clinical usefulness of SonoVue contrast echocardiography: the Thoraxcentre experience. Neth Heart J 2007; 15(2): 55-60.
[http://dx.doi.org/10.1007/BF03085955] [PMID: 17612661]

CHAPTER 11

Toxicology Related to Nanoparticles – Challenges and Future Prospects

Sweta Garg[1,*], **Prakash Pandey**[2], **Sumel Ashique**[3] and **Neeraj Mishra**[4]

[1] *Shri Ram Institute of Pharmacy, Jabalpur, M.P., India*

[2] *RKDF College of Pharmacy, Sarvepalli Radhakrishnan University, Bhopal, M.P., India*

[3] *Department of Pharmaceutics, Bharat Institute of Technology (BIT), School of Pharmacy, Meerut, UP, India*

[4] *Amity Institute of Pharmacy, Amity University, Gwalior, M.P., India*

Abstract: As the nano-world continues to evolve, nanotechnology offers tremendous potential in everyday goods and creating future, environmentally friendly technologies. The advantages of nanotechnology are being realized in various areas, including engineering, medicine, biology, the environment, and communication. However, nanomaterials production is expected to increase exponentially in the next few years, resulting in significant difficulties linked to their potentially harmful impacts on human health and the environment. Furthermore, the detrimental effect of the toxicity of nanomaterials on human health is one of the industry's most critical problems as it works to exhaust its supply of nano-products. The use of nanomaterials in biological applications is the scenario with the most significant risk. Therefore, the investigation of nanotoxicity and its interaction with biomolecules continues, as are many other projects.

On the other hand, assessing and validating nanotoxicity in a biological system are complex tasks. This chapter aims to examine the difficulties associated with evaluating the toxicity of nanomaterials. The evaluation of toxicity and the problems encountered in assessing the effect on biological systems are historic. The findings of in-vitro, in-vivo, and in-silico investigations on the toxicity of engineered nanomaterials are described in this chapter. The various toxicity evaluation methods each have challenges that researchers must overcome when evaluating nanomaterials in powder form, solution-based approaches, and when interacting with biological systems. The evaluation tools and characterization methods are critical in overcoming the difficulties, while the cytotoxic tests consider nanoparticle form, morphology, and size.

Keywords: Nanotechnology, Nanoparticles, Nanotoxicity, *In-vitro*, *In-vivo*.

---

* **Corresponding author Sweta Garg:** Shri Ram Institute of Pharmacy, Jabalpur, M.P. India; Tel: +91-79740 13484; E-mail: swetagarg2@gmail.com

Neeraj Mishra, Ashish Garg and Neeraj Upmanyu (Eds.)

INTRODUCTION

In recent years, the word "Nanotechnology" has been exaggerated to the point that it has virtually become synonymous with new and promising things [1 - 3]. Using nanotechnology, we may design and build valuable materials, devices, and systems by manipulating matter on atomic and molecular sizes and harnessing new characteristics and phenomena that occur at the nanoscale. For example, sensor design will witness significant reductions in size and weight, as well as reductions in power consumption. We will also see increases in sensitivity and specificity, to name a few of the enhancements.

As a result of the production of high-volume commercial nanomaterials (NMs), such as fullerenes, quantum dots (QDs), carbon nanotubes (CNs), and metal-oxide nanoparticles, the field of nanotechnology has grown to become a multibillion-dollar business globally (NPs). A wide range of nanotechnology applications continues to be developed and implemented in all sectors of human activity (including health, food and nutrition, water treatment, manufacturing, and engineering) and our everyday lives. As a result of its positive impacts on key problems like energy generation, application to technical equipment and the addition of new features to consumer items, it is gaining in importance. The widespread usage of this ingredient in healthcare and personal care products is due to its possible advantages for diagnosis and treatment. Approximately 6214 entities from 32 countries utilized nanomaterials in 1814 consumer goods as of 2014. Most of them (42%) were in the area of health [4]. According to the statistics from this inventory, the most often used category is the health category (almost 2000 items), with more than 900 items being cosmetics and personal care items. For these reasons, silver is the most frequently utilized nanomaterial, followed by titanium and silicon [5]. Parallel to these rapid advancements in nanotechnology, the question of whether nanomaterials have harmful consequences has risen to the top of the public's priority list. As a result of the interaction of nanomaterials, which are very tiny in comparison to the size of biological creatures, with tissues, cells, and the microenvironment, potentially detrimental consequences may be revealed that cannot be produced by their chemically similar and bigger counterparts. The topic of nanotechnology is addressed in this study because it is both a significant challenge and a double-edged sword that will face the field of medicine in the future. Nanoparticles have advantageous properties such as a direct band gap, a high optical absorption coefficient, a layered structure, and adjustable band edges, which allow them to be used for improved catalysis [6]. Integrating synergistically diverse components in a regulated manner is required to convert single-component nanomaterials to hybrid materials, which may be used to create nanocomposites [7]. Compared to single-component nanomaterials, hybrid nanostructures offer many benefits, including multi-functionality, extremely efficient charge separation at the interface, and the ability to tune the band gap [8]. Because of the employment of nanoparticles for photocatalytic degradation, the quantity of pesticide present in the water will be reduced by an impressive amount [9]. Using nanoparticles in conjunction with bio-adsorbents to create nanocomposites, it is anticipated that enhanced performance in terms of high efficiency of photoinduced charge separation and photostability would result [10]. The surface modification of the nanoparticles will enhance the interaction of heavy metal ions with the particle's surface, resulting in increased adsorption and performance of the photocatalyst because of modification [11]. It is also anticipated that using hybrid nanostructures would be beneficial over using single-component and pure systems. It is anticipated that the new systems will outperform the current systems in terms of material stability, efficiency, and cost [12]. The recent development in the nanotechnology sector has shown a spectacular transformation over the past several decades, which is expected to continue gradually and optimistically. Nanotechnology has shown that it can significantly contribute to the future of health research and medical treatment [13]. Ideal nanomaterials for gene delivery, immunotherapy, and drug delivery systems have biocompatibility, high payload, low immunogenicity, effective penetration, and selective targeting, allowing them to reach target tissues promptly [14]. The continuous exponential development of nanotechnology has prompted the consideration of new problems in managing, predicting, and understanding the possible negative health consequences that may result from exposure [15]. Varying nanomaterials with different surface topographies, sizes, and compositions, as well as a variety of other characteristics, must be thoroughly investigated to determine their safety and effectiveness for usage in the human population [16]. Nanotoxicology is primarily concerned with determining the toxic nature of nanoparticles and determining the hazardous impact of nanoparticles on biological systems [17]. Most inert elements become increasingly active when scaled down to the nanoscale. Most nanoparticles are non-toxic, but they may spread throughout the body and cause inflammation, oxidative stress, and other severe side effects [18]. High doses of nanoparticles reflect actual exposure and should be evaluated with care, as they may result in changes in toxicokinetic and exposure estimation [19].

Occupational exposure to nanomaterials (NMs) is rising as the usage and manufacturing of nanomaterials (NMs) continues to increase. Another source of worry is the state of the environment and the disruption of ecosystems. Certain aspects of these concerns have compelled scientists to study and better understand the possible harmful impacts of engineered nanomaterials on human health and the environment while also exploring the difficulties associated with determining the level of toxicity of these materials—several publications on the toxicity of NMs published in the past few decades. However, investigating the interactions of nanoparticles (NPs) with biological systems continues to be a difficult job. One of the reasons for this is possibly related to experimental techniques and detailed characterization, including toxicological evaluation of NMs [20].

NANOMATERIAL

Nanotechnology is a multidisciplinary area of research in which unique phenomena allow the development of novel applications, the design and synthesis of goods and applications based on the synthesis of nanometer (10-9 meters) molecules, and the study of the interactions between these molecules. Furthermore, because of the reduction in particle size at the nanoscale, it is well known that the physical properties of the particles may be changed, resulting in the development of characteristics such as resistance, conductivity, toughness, lightness, reactivity, lifespan, and vast surface areas. Thus, it may be utilized to develop innovative goods and biomedical and software-based applications [21].

Properties and application of Nanomaterials

A wide range of characteristics is shown by nanomaterials, including those electrical, chemical, magnetic, optical, physical, thermal, and elastic properties. Because of their small size and physicochemical properties (size, shape, sizing, and so on), nanoparticles have found applications in a variety of fields, including the medical field for drug delivery *in vivo* and *in vitro* [22, 23], agriculture and wastewater treatment, pesticide degradation [24 - 26].

Nanomaterials have found a wide range of uses in various areas, including nanoscale transporters, nano-herbicides, nano-fertilizers, nano-pesticides, nanosensors, veterinary care, and other fields [27]. Clay nanotubes (Halloysite) were created to decrease the concentration of pesticides by more than 70%, thus decreasing the efficacy of pesticides and their impact on water streams [28, 29]. The researchers created poly(d,l-lactide-co-glycolide) (PLGA) nanoparticles for the localized/targeted delivery of various agents, including peptides, plasmid DNA, and proteins [30]. There have recently been discoveries of titanium-based nanomaterials with a wide range of uses, including water splitting, degradation of organic molecules, and solar sensitizers. Various characteristics distinguish titanium dioxide (TiO_2), including polymorphism, cheap cost, excellent stability, ecologically benign, and strong optical and electrical properties. Li *et al.* [31] examined whether core–shell-structured TiO_2 composites have adjustable optical and electrical properties and the ability to perform novel tasks derived from the core-shell structures' distinctive characteristics. Because of the tiny size of nanoparticles, their magnetic characteristics are changed from paramagnetic to ferromagnetic and superparamagnetic, and they are employed as contrast agents in intravenously injected T2 MRI procedures [32]. TiO_2 nanoparticles are an efficient photocatalyst for the photocatalytic destruction of pesticides containing the triazine ring, such as atrazine, in the laboratory [33]. According to the manufacturer, chitosan-based zinc oxide nanoparticles (CZNP) have a spherical form and are utilized in the therapy of cervical cancer cells [34]. The utilization of gold nanoparticles (GNPs) in conjunction with TiO_2 nanoparticles is used in the fabrication of conformal nanocomposite (NC) films of TiO_2–Au in this study [35]. According to Yuan *et al.* [36], the production of ZnO quantum dots (QDs) coupled with chitosan (N-acetylglucosamine) was studied for its efficacy in tumour-targeted medication delivery against tumour cells. Because of the cationic charge and hydrophilicity of chitosan, it has been discovered that the stability of ZnO quantum dots is reliant on the presence of chitosan. Qiu *et al.* [37] have created a composite with a core-shell structure made of a ZnO interlayer and a magnetic Fe_3O_4 core, which has a core-shell structure. As a result of its characteristics, it has been proven effective in delivering anticancer medicines to cancer patients.

Routes for Nanoparticle Administration

It is unavoidable that the human person, as a social entity, will come into touch with the nanoparticles that surround them in some way. A great deal of study has been done on nanoparticles, which have been shown to cause harm to many areas of the body. Nanomaterials are most often introduced into the body *via* the respiratory system, where they come into close contact with the lungs. The introduction of nanomaterials into the body is also widespread, mainly *via* skin contact and the gastrointestinal system. Furthermore, nanomaterials may enter the body *via* implants and injections [38].

Inhalation Exposure

The size of the nanoparticles, their resistance to gravity, and their distribution pattern all influence the region in which they will settle in the respiratory system when they enter. Affiliations with nanoparticles include inhalation of nanoparticles that have been cleansed in various sections of the respiratory system by the mucociliary layer and macrophages, as well as clustering in the lungs and spread to other regions of one's body *via* blood circulation [39]. According to Sajid *et al.* [40], the respiratory tract's defence mechanism can remove 33% of the nanoparticles breathed into the body and eliminate them from the body. Carbon nanotubes have been shown in animal experiments to induce fibrosis, inflammation, and granuloma in the lungs. These toxic effects in the lungs have been linked to systemic cardiovascular diseases [41]. Aside from that, it was claimed that inhaled nanoparticles may reach many organs of the body, including the brain, and an investigation into the possibility of a connection with prostate cancer was carried out [42, 43].

Dermal Exposure

The physicochemical characteristics of nanoparticles, the physicochemical properties of the instrument used to disperse the penetrating molecule, and the location and skin conditions are the three most important variables in the absorption of nanoparticles from the skin, according to the research. Cosmetic products such as creams, lotions, and toothpaste include nanoparticles and are often utilized in skin exposure. Nanoparticles tend to concentrate in the stratum corneum and dermis, where they may irritate [44, 45]. It has also been suggested that some of the nanoparticles absorbed *via* the skin may seep into the circulation, according to the research.

Ingestion

It is possible to absorb nanoparticles efficiently either directly from the gastrointestinal system or indirectly *via* the inhalation of inhaled particles. Essential to notice are nanoparticles that have a high likelihood of being accidentally consumed, such as metal compounds and insecticides. In many cases, this may be overlooked since it is assumed to occur solely on purpose or because of severe carelessness. The inability of nanoparticles to be absorbed from the intestines and processed by the liver also adds to this scenario [46, 47].

Medical use of Nanoparticles

A relatively recent branch of medical sciences, nanomedicine, is taking place in the context of emerging disciplines developing in tandem with nanotechnology advancements. Nanoparticles have various uses due to their ability to be modified in terms of their physical properties. As a result, a variety of nanoparticles are currently being used or studied in a variety of medical fields, including the treatment of diseases or malignancies, surgery, medical implants, intelligent drug delivery systems, gene delivery, diagnosis/imaging, tissue engineering, regenerative medicine, antimicrobial resistance, and other areas.

Cancer Diagnosis and Treatment

The use of nanoparticles in cancer detection and therapy, particularly in imaging, is becoming more prevalent daily. When used with magnetic resonance imaging, quantum dots may be used to detect tumor locations and determine their location more precisely. On the other hand, cancer biomarkers may be detected by nanoparticle-based test chips, such as lab on a chip, which can be used for non-invasive cancer detection at the earliest possible stage [48]. Carbon nanotubes are utilized for various purposes, including exposing DNA abnormalities and detecting biomarkers. Dendrimers and nanoparticles may be used as contrast agents in imaging studies and in the administration of drugs in innovative (targeted or controlled release) delivery systems [49]. In vivo applications of lanthanide (Gd3+ and Yb3+) functionalized gold nanoparticles include imaging (MRI and CT) and therapeutic (photothermal) applications. Aside from that, ion-doped nanomaterials are utilized in the medical field of bio-imaging [50].

Gene Therapy

Gene therapy is a highly researched field devoted to the prevention and treatment of genetic diseases *via* the repair of faulty genes. This may be accomplished *via* the delivery or replacement of the repaired or corrected gene using various techniques. This technique can potentially be used in treating some kinds of cancer, infections, cardiovascular illnesses, autoimmune diseases, and monogenic diseases such as haemophilia, among other conditions.

Treatment of Neural Degeneration

Treatment of degenerative illnesses or posttraumatic pathologies is like other treatment methods in that it focuses on the regeneration and protection of brain tissue and directed axon development. Consequently, nanomedical applications have great promise for the treatment of Parkinson's and Alzheimer's illnesses, as well as the regeneration of axonal damage. For example, using nanoparticles with a high affinity for circulating amyloid-beta (A-beta) subtypes may be effective in alleviating the symptoms of Alzheimer's disease [51].

Tissue Engineering

This is a subject that is well-known among experts in the fields of regenerative medicine, nanomedicine, and biomedical engineering. It has applications in the healing or regeneration of injured tissues by using different forms and compositions of biocompatible, biodegradable nanomaterial-based bioscaffolds with the least amount of adverse effects.

Antimicrobial Activity

It is recognized that various metallic nanoparticles possess antibacterial action, and these particles may be utilized in conjunction with other medicines to decrease antibiotic resistance. Nanoparticles of gold, silver, zinc oxide and other metals and oxides are found amid these agents. These nanoparticles are also used in producing various surgical and implantable devices for use in the body, including [52].

Orthopaedic Implants

In orthopaedic surgery, various implants are used, including bone tissue engineering materials, nanostructured implantable materials, and implants created by surface modification or coating. Synthetic and natural polymers are the most often encountered nanomaterials in bone and cartilage tissue engineering. Collagen, hyaluronic acid, chitosan, titanium alloys, ceramic-coated metal-oxides (alumina, zirconia, and titania), hydroxyapatites, and carbon nanomaterials such as graphene and diamond are examples of such materials [53]. In addition, it is necessary to utilize carbon nanocomposites, including a ceramic or polymer matrix, to obtain more bioactivity, improved mechanical characteristics, and increased osteoconductivity to facilitate a quicker and more effective healing process [54].

Dental Application

Most nanomaterials used in dentistry are antibacterial, medicinal, and reinforcing materials, among other things. They are also used in the polishing of the enamel surface, the placement of dental fillings, and the placement of dental implants. Carbon nanotubes, graphene, hydroxyapatite, iron oxide Zirconia, silica-based nanomaterials, and titanium and silver nanoparticles are examples of composites [55, 56]. Composites may be made from a variety of materials.

Cardiovascular Applications

Natural and manufactured nanoparticles are also used in the bioengineering of cardiac tissue. For example, alginate and collagen are often utilized for biocompatibility. In contrast, synthetic polyesters such as poly-L-lactic and poly (lactic-co-glycolic) acids are regularly employed for strength and durability. Carbon nanotubes are also used for covering stents and cardiac implants, among other things [57].

Dermal Applications

Skin implants, which help to speed up the healing process by enhancing tissue restoration, are often utilized in wound healing. However, although its frequency changes according to therapeutic necessity, it is mainly composed of poly (lactic-co-glycolic acid)/chitin indicators that resemble human keratinocytes and fibroblasts when used as autologous skin grafts [58].

NANOTOXICITY

The field of nanotoxicology is concerned with identifying the harmful effects of nanomaterials on human health and the environment. To establish and identify the harms caused by engineered nanomaterials, a multidisciplinary team approach is required, with members from various disciplines such as toxicology, biology, chemistry, physics, material science, geology, exposure assessment, pharmacokinetics, and medicine all contributing to the effort [59]. As a result, although almost everything may be hazardous if consumed in large quantities, the more pertinent issue is: how dangerous are nanomaterials when consumed at the amounts they may be used? Any harmful consequences of nanoparticles will be unique to the kind of base material used, as well as its size, shape, and any coatings applied to it. Nonetheless, to accurately assess and comprehend the harmful consequences of nanomaterials, methods and data interpretation must be carried out with care, and assumptions must be taken into account. Various research organizations employed different cell lines, culturing settings, and incubation periods in their toxicity investigations of nanoparticles. The results were compared by considering our current knowledge of the nature of nanoparticles during toxicity testing; it is difficult to compare findings from various research groups and establish whether the cytotoxicity seen is physiologically meaningful [60]. The harmful consequences of such particles are currently being studied, with regulatory concerns shifting away from the conventional particles having an aerodynamic diameter of fewer than 10 m and lower. The findings of the experiments show that finer-sized particles are more hazardous than larger-sized ones.

Nonetheless, to accurately assess and comprehend the harmful consequences of nanomaterials, methods and data interpretation must be carried out with care, and assumptions must be considered. It is possible to categorize nanotechnology products into many distinct chemical classes, which include metals (including metal oxides), carbon (including carbon nanotubes), and semiconductor nanomaterials (including semiconductor nanomaterials). Engineered nanomaterials are used in a variety of fields, such as the automotive and aerospace industries (car tires, glass, and fuel cells), agriculture (food processing, production, packaging, and storage), construction (cement-based material for insulation, exterior, self-cleaning glass, and paint, among other things), energy (thermoelectric, solar cells, long-life batteries, fossil fuel, nuclear energy), health and medicine (diagnosis, treatment, and prevention), and many others [61]. However, although it is widely employed in diagnosing and treating illnesses around biomedicine, on the one hand, concerns have started to be raised that it may be a cause of disease on the other. In addition, the unpleasant experience humans have had with carcinogenic goods like cigarettes and asbestos, which they initially believed to be harmless, has also raised concerns among NPs. Because specific nanoparticles (NPs) have a long, thin, fibrous structure asbestos-like, and exhibit fibrogenic and toxic effects, the question "Can nanoparticles be the asbestos of the future?" was posed as a result [62].

TOXICITY OF NANOMATERIALS

The harmful consequences of such particles are currently being studied, with regulatory concerns shifting away from the conventional particles having an aerodynamic diameter of fewer than 10 m and lower. The findings of the experiments show that finer-sized particles are more hazardous than larger-sized ones. Nonetheless, to accurately assess and comprehend the harmful consequences of nanomaterials, methods and data interpretation must be carried out with care, and assumptions must be taken into account. The range of nanotechnology products is extensive, and they can be divided into several different compound classes, including metals, metal oxides, carbon, and semiconductor nanomaterials. Metals, metal oxides, carbon, and semiconductor nanomaterials are among the most common types of nanotechnology products. The following talks will be organized around different types of nanomaterials.

Metal Nanomaterials

Even though metallic nanoparticles are among the most frequently utilized kinds of manufactured nanomaterials, little is known about their destiny and impacts on the natural environment. While bulk gold has long been considered harmless, many research groups have investigated the absorption and toxicity of gold nanoparticles in living cells owing to the remarkable characteristics of gold nanoparticles. They have discovered that gold nanoparticles are harmful to cells [63]. Chithrani *et al.* [64] have studied the intracellular absorption of colloidal gold nanoparticles of various sizes and shapes in the laboratory. Because of their findings concluded that the kinetics and saturation concentrations of gold nanoparticles strongly depend on their physical dimensions, with the uptake half-lives of 14 nm, 50 nm, and 74 nm gold nanoparticles being 2.10, 1.90, and 2.24 hr, respectively. They could determine the absolute gold amounts present in cells through digestion and subsequent inductively coupled plasma atomic emission spectroscopy investigations. Spheres with dimensions in the 10–100 nm range were taken up more quickly by cells than smaller and larger spheres in the 10–100 nm range. They also discovered that spheres were taken up more efficiently than nanorods with dimensions in the 10–100 nm range, which had dimensions in the 10–100 nm range. Researchers at the University of California, Los Angeles (UCLA) have investigated the absorption and possible toxicity of various gold nanoparticles in human leukaemia cells. The findings indicate that spherical gold nanoparticles coated with a range of surface modifiers are not intrinsically harmful to human cells, even though they are taken up by cells in large quantities [65]. On human skin keratinocytes (HaCaT), Wang and his colleagues studied the cellular absorption and cytotoxicity of gold nanoparticles in terms of shape and size dependence [66].

Metal Oxide Nanomaterials

Metal oxide nanoparticles are significant industrial materials extensively utilized as additives in various products, including cosmetics, medicines, and food colouring. Solid nanoparticles are often introduced to the skin *via* sunscreen lotions or creams containing nano-TiO_2 or ZnO as a sunscreen component or using fibrous materials coated with nanoscale compounds to provide water or stain-resistant qualities to the skin. Because the production and usage of nanoparticles are growing, people are increasingly likely to be exposed to them in the workplace, *via* consumer goods, or the environment. Several research groups have investigated the environment's absorption and toxicity of metal oxide nanoparticles. Grassian *et al.* published inhalation exposure research utilizing TiO_2 nanoparticles with sizes ranging from 2–5 nm. According to the findings, nanoparticles aggregate to produce aerosol particles in the exposure chamber, with the geometric mean of the mobility diameter ranging between 120 and 130 nm. Animals necropsied at weeks 0, 1, or 2 following their final exposure to these aggregates revealed a substantial but moderate inflammatory response, with recovery occurring at week three post-exposure [67]. To determine the cytotoxicity of various concentrations of homogeneous and weakly aggregated TiO_2 nanoparticles in an aqueous solution, Jin *et al.* utilized murine fibroblast (L929) cells. The researchers' findings indicate that greater TiO_2 nanoparticle concentrations (>60 g/mL) result in a substantial increase in oxidative stress in the body [68]. Increasing the concentration of TiO_2 nanoparticles in the culture medium resulted in increased amounts of reactive oxygen species and lactate dehydrogenase in the culture media. Park *et al.* [69] demonstrated that TiO_2 nanoparticles were lethal in cultured BEAS-2B cells by inducing reactive oxygen species (ROS). Scientists have discovered that nanoparticles have pierced the plasma membrane and are situated in the peri-region of nuclear membranes, suggesting that nanoparticles may have direct interactions with cellular molecules and therefore induce undesirable biological reactions in living organisms. The researchers' findings indicate that the production of ROS enhanced the expression of oxidative stress-related genes such as heme oxygenase-1 and inflammation-related genes such as IL-8.

Carbon Nanomaterials

Carbon nanotubes, known for their unique one-dimensional hollow nanostructure and their peculiar characteristics, are emerging as a significant new class of multifunctional building blocks for the advancement of nanotechnology. Due to the fast rise of nanotechnology in recent years, there is a renewed need for large-scale manufacturing of carbon nanotubes (CNTs) for use in commercial goods. A significant increase in the number of industrial-scale facilities for the relatively low-cost production of multi-walled carbon nanotubes (MWCNTs) is expected to occur in the coming years as the number of MWCNTs produced at these facilities grows. As a result, exposure to MWCNTs by professionals and the public is expected to increase significantly in the coming years. Several research groups have investigated the absorption and possible dangers of carbon nanotubes (CNTs), especially multi-walled carbon nanotubes (MWCNTs), in humans and other biological systems. The ability of carbon nanotubes to elicit inflammatory and apoptotic responses in human T cells, for example, has been shown [70, 71]. According to their findings, Ding *et al.* found that MWCNTs induced the expression of genes involved in cellular transport, metabolism, cell cycle control, and stress response in human skin fibroblasts. In their study, Magrez *et al.* discovered cytotoxicity for carbon-based nanomaterials. Still, MWCNTs were among the least hazardous of the several carbon nanotubes, nanofibers, and nanoparticles examined [72]. In a slightly similar article, the findings of Dumortier *et al.* showed that water-soluble CNTs functionalized with polyethene glycol chains did not have harmful effects when tested in a broad range of immune system cells [73].

Quantum Dots

When Quantum Dots are formed, they show unique "quantum effects" such as extended fluorescence. Quantum Dots are nanocrystals comprising 1000 to 100,000 atoms that exhibit remarkable "quantum effects" such as prolonged fluorescence. QDs are presently used in biological imaging and the electronics industry because of their unique optical and electrical characteristics. In particular, the fluorescence spectrum of QDs makes them ideal fluorophores for biomedical imaging applications. For example, fluorescent QDs can be conjugated with bioactive moieties to target specific biologic events and cellular structures, such as labelling neoplastic cells, DNA, and cell membrane receptors to detect cancerous tumours [74 - 77]. However, each type of QD has unique physicochemical properties, which determine its potential toxicity. As a result, there are discrepancies in the current literature regarding the toxicity of QDs, which can be attributed to several factors, including a lack of toxicology-based studies, a wide range of QD dosage/exposure concentrations reported in the literature, and a lack of consistent data. The importance of this point is that QD toxicity is determined by several factors derived from both individual QD physicochemical properties and environmental conditions: size, charge, concentration, outer coating bioactivity, as well as oxidative and photolytic stability, have all been demonstrated to be essential factors in determining QD toxicity [78, 79].

TOXIC EFFECTS OF NANOPARTICLES ON SYSTEMS

As a result of the fact that nanoparticles enter the body in three distinct routes, it has been shown *via* experimental investigations that they have harmful effects in various systems. This section discusses the detrimental effects of nanomaterials on multiple systems, mainly *via* animal studies.

Circulatory System

Nemmar *et al.* discovered cardiac oxidative stress and DNA damage in mice after administering iron oxide nanoparticles intravenously to the animals [80]. When Ni nanoparticles were administered intravenously to rats, Magaye *et al.* [81] found heart toxicity and arrhythmia. They also noticed toxic effects in organs such as the liver, spleen and lungs.

Digestive System

According to Arefian *et al.* [82], zirconia oxide nanoparticles at a concentration of 100 parts per million (ppm) induce liver damage in rats. In addition, iron oxide nanoparticles have been shown to cause liver damage in mice [83].

Endocrine System

Another study found that the oral form of iron oxide nanoparticles caused abnormalities in thyroid hormones in rats, according to another study [84].

Immune System

According to Xu *et al.*, exposure to TiO_2 nanoparticles in mice significantly increased the number of white blood cells [85]. As a result of the presence of iron oxide nanoparticles, the number of white blood cells is seen, with the liver and spleen being the most adversely impacted organs immunologically [86].

Respiratory System

It has been observed that metal nanoparticles (Cobalt oxide, nickel oxide, titanium oxide) administered *via* oropharyngeal aspiration induce toxicity in the lung tissue of those who receive them [87]. Biomedical applications of iron oxide magnetic nanoparticles are more comprehensive than others due to biocompatibility, high stability and ease of use. Therefore, magnetic nanoparticles such as Fe_3O_4 and Fe_2O_3 have more applications in drug delivery. Similarly, Sadeghi *et al.* discovered that iron oxide nanoparticles are harmful to the lungs of rats in their study [88].

Urinary System

According to Saranya *et al.* [89], zinc oxide, iron oxide, and copper nanoparticles had harmful effects on kidney cells in various monkey, pig, and bovine models of renal disease. Furthermore, Fartkhooni *et al.* found that TiO_2 nanoparticles administered intraperitoneally induce degeneration in rat kidneys, which is consistent with previous findings [90].

Nervous System

Studies on animal ears and eyes were conducted to see whether or not there was any toxicity to vision and hearing. In most cases, little or no toxicity was found [91].

Reproductive System

A group of researchers discovered that injecting zinc oxide nanoparticles intraperitoneally into mice reduced the number of seminiferous tubule cells and their loss [92, 93]. Furthermore, according to Kong *et al.* [94], nickel nanoparticles induce a reduction in FSH and LH hormone levels in rats and alterations in sperm motility in these animals.

Hazardous Effect of Nanomaterials

The nanoparticles are tiny, *i.e.*, a few nanometers or less, and have a high reactivity when interacting with living beings. When discharged directly into the environment and coming into contact with water, air, or soil, they may threaten human health and the environment [95]. When dust and air pollution include ultrafine particles of less than 100 nm, it suggests the possibility of long-term harmful consequences of manufactured nanoparticles on humans and other animals. They may enter the body in various ways, including the oral, pulmonary (lungs), nasal, intraocular, and other channels. As a result of runoff, nanomaterials are present in aquatic and terrestrial ecosystems. These nanomaterials ultimately make their way into the food chain, where they accumulate in the body and other metabolic pathways. Many different species, including invertebrates and algae, bacteria, crustaceans and nematodes, as well as mammals, fishes and rats, are poisoned by them in one way or another [96]. In a study conducted in rats, Warheit *et al.* [97] investigated the potential dangers of several fine or nanoparticle kinds, including carbonyl iron, amorphous silica, crystalline silica, and nano zinc oxide. They discovered that silica nanoparticles are capable of sustaining cytotoxic and inflammatory responses. As corrosion, Karimi *et al.* [98] utilized colloidal nanoparticles of fumed silica (f-SiO_2), silica (c-SiO_2), alumina (Al_2O_3), and cerium (CeO_2) in chemical and mechanical planarization (CMP) procedures. When exposed to water bodies over an extended period, the CMP slurries of CeO_2 and Al_2O_3 decreased reproduction in Daphnia Magna, which has detrimental implications for water bodies. In 2006, Jeng and Swanson investigated the effects of metal oxide nanoparticles ZnO, Al_2O_3, Fe_3O_4, TiO_2, and CrO_3 on apoptosis, cell morphology, membrane leakage of lactate dehydrogenase (LDH mitochondrial function), and permeability of the plasma membrane. They discovered that ZnO nanoparticles were highly toxic, Al_2O_3 nanoparticles were moderately toxic, and TiO_2 and Fe_3 It also reduced mitochondrial activity in cells treated with ZnO nanoparticles at concentrations ranging from 50 to 100 g/L. A study conducted by Ghodake *et al.* [99] investigated the phytotoxicity of zinc and cobalt oxide nanoparticles (NPs) in the Allium cepa plant, which was used as an indicator organism to examine the impacts on cell morphology, root elongation, adsorption potential, and root shape of a plant. Zinc oxide nanoparticles (NPs) accumulate in plants' chromosomes and cellular modules, resulting in phytotoxic effects. Landa *et al.* (2012) investigated the impact of titanium dioxide (TiO_2) and zinc oxide (ZnO) nanoparticles on gene expression in Arabidopsis thaliana roots using microarrays to determine the effect of the nanoparticles on the plant's roots. A. thaliana exhibits a stress response in terms of phenotypic and gene expression when exposed to ZnO nanoparticles. "Another research group demonstrate the toxic effect of Iron oxide nanoparticles (magnetic nanoparticles) which have a widespread application in MRI and heat therapy of cancer as contrast elements. They are also used effectively for drug and gene delivery because they penetrate the cells and tissues effectively. However, these features cause Fe_2O_3 nanoparticles to have toxic effects that are not completely understood yet. This study studied the effects of iron oxide nanoparticles on lung tissue in adult male Wistar rats. They used the pulmonary inhalation method for nanoparticle administration. They were used either as a helper, and the results showed that administered nanoparticles penetrated the circulation and rapidly reached the liver, creating serious inflammation in lung and liver tissues. This study used two nanoparticle doses (20 and 40 mg/kg) and two exposing numbers (7 and 14 times). Results showed significant enhancement of free radicals and reduced GSH in lung tissue. Histological studies showed nanoparticle treatment in rats caused pulmonary emphysema, interstitial hyperemia and lung inflammation. By increasing the dose, lung tissue showed all of the mentioned symptoms with increased intensity. Nanoparticle exposition causes the presence of neutrophils, lymphocytes and eosinophils in the lung tissue, confirming a serious pathologic condition" [88].

THE TOXICITY MECHANISM OF NANOPARTICLES

Recent research has shown that the reactivity of nanoparticles causes the production of ROS (particularly hydroxyl radicals and superoxide radical anions) due to the activation of oxidative enzymes, resulting in the development of oxidative stress [100].

The initiation of oxidative stress can be caused by several factors, including (1) nanoparticles having the ability to trigger ROS production as a cellular response, (2) transition metal-based nanoparticles serving as catalysts during the formation of nonmetal nanoparticles, (3) the formation of reactive molecules on the surface of nanoparticles, and (4) the induction or activation of redox groups on nanoparticle surfaces [101]. Furthermore, particle size is believed to play a role in the cytotoxicity of particles in living cells. Because tiny particles have a high surface area, the interaction of nanoparticles with biological common [102]; on the other hand, nanosized particles offer additional advantages since they may easily penetrate the cell and cause cellular damage [103]. Aside from this, the surface charge of a particle contributes to cytotoxicity by controlling the cellular absorption of particles and the interaction between biomolecules and cell organelles.

The toxicity of nanoparticles is caused by mechanical impacts caused by the physicochemical characteristics of the particles. The production of reactive oxygen species (ROS), either directly or indirectly, is the fundamental process of producing harmful effects. *In vitro*, ROS production is dangerous due to various processes occurring inside the cell [104]. At the molecular level, the reduction of molecular oxygen to water is responsible for the production of ATP in mitochondria. Superoxide anions and radicals with various oxygen isotopes are produced as a result of this reaction. The revolutionaries had to include hydroxyl, single oxygen, hydrogen peroxide, and superoxide anion radical [105]. The overproduction of free radicals, which play a role in the mitogenic response and cellular signalling, results in the disruption of physiological processes in cells and is associated with cancer [106 - 108] found that since nanomaterials have tiny dimensions, they produce more ROS as a result of their large specific surface area and high surface reactivity.

It has been discovered *via* research in live tissues such as human erythrocytes and skin fibroblasts that various kinds of nanomaterials induce toxicity through the activation of reactive oxygen species (ROS) in different ways [109]. Winnik and

Maysinger discovered that quantum dots induce cytotoxicity by boosting the formation of reactive oxygen species (ROS) [110]. It has been shown that nano-ZnO has a lethal impact on human bronchial epithelial cells by increasing the generation of ROS [111]. Nano-FeO was shown to hurt hepatocyte cells by increasing ROS production and apoptosis. When comparing the cytotoxic effects of nano-TiO_2, nano-Co3O4, nano-ZnO, and nano-CuO on hepatocyte cells, it was discovered that nano-CuO had the most significant cytotoxic effect [112, 113]. The toxicity of nanomaterials is influenced by various variables, including surface area, surface coating, molecular size, shape, oxygenation status, solubility, and the materials' degree of aggregation and agglomeration [114]. According to the findings, the increase in the harmful impact of nanoparticles is precisely proportional to the reduction in their size. According to their results, researchers Yoshida and colleagues discovered that amorphous nano silica is detrimental to human cells by boosting ROS production and destroying DNA [115 - 117]. As a result, it has become critical to understand the cellular and molecular mechanisms of nanoparticle toxicity and their impact on the biological system to create a safe and accurate test for manufactured nanoparticles for risk assessment.

TOXICITY TESTING

It is more common to do *in vitro*studies than it is to conduct *in vivo* research. Therefore issues regarding dosing are essential to answer when trying to determine toxicity. The *in vitro*sedimentation diffusion and dosimeter model is one of the models that was utilized in the toxicity test. In this model, the difference between exposure (concentration in the cell surroundings), dose collected on the cell surface, and cellular dosage is very apparent. We may assess the dosage rate as a predictor of response when we have information about the time it takes for a particular dose to be released [118]. Given the widespread use of *in vitro*techniques to assess cell viability and proliferation in toxicity assessment, gene expression analysis, genotoxicity detection, and *in vitro*hemolysis are also commonly used. Additional microscopic and spectroscopic methods for the evaluation of cell physicochemical structure include scanning electron microscopy/energy dispersive X-ray spectroscopy (SEM-EDX), transmission electron microscopy (TEM), atomic force microscopy (AFM), video-enhanced differential interference contrast (VEDIC) microscopy, and fluorescence spectroscopy, among others. Using all of these tests in conjunction makes it simpler to identify nanotoxicity in the environment [119]. Table **1** presents a condensed list of previously performed research about presently utilized toxicity tests, the aim of the testing, and the nanomaterials being tested. The list is intended to be brief [120]. The inhalation of nanoparticles *via* the respiratory system often results in negative consequences on the lung. Much research has been conducted to determine the detection of lung toxicity, and organ-on-a-chip investigations have become more relevant in recent years. According to Zhang *et al.*, nanotoxicity was assessed by better mimicking human reactions using the chip in a 3D human lung model that was comparable to that seen in vivo. Additionally, this research demonstrated the significance of organ-based toxicity using realistic models [121]. Researchers discovered that nanoparticles penetrate through the placenta of mice and have a harmful impact on the unborn children. According to their findings, Yin *et al.* [122], revealed that chip and TiO_2 nanoparticle exposure-related research in the 3D human placenta model might have comparable harmful consequences. Additional nanotoxicity experiments were carried out using the integration of a cell-on-a-chip (CoC) with a microfluidic system, as previously mentioned [123].

CONCLUSION AND FUTURE PROSPECTIVE

Briefly, we have examined the destiny, behaviour, and toxicity of several classes of nanomaterials in the environment with a critical eye. Even though many research groups have discovered harmful consequences of nanomaterials, the underlying reasons for the toxic effects are still poorly understood. There are still significant gaps in our understanding of nanoparticle interactions with the environment and the environment's response. To properly assess the potential for human exposure to nanoscale components of currently existing goods and future products, a large number of further studies are required to evaluate the stability of these matrices in a range of test settings. Toxicology studies of nanoparticles conducted on various cell lines and incubation times are becoming increasingly common. However, because of the wide range of nanoparticle concentrations, the variety of cell lines used as well as the culturing conditions, and a lack of understanding of the mechanism, it is challenging to determine whether the toxicity observed is physiologically relevant. Importantly, analytical methods that allow for real-time, in-situ monitoring of production processes are required to improve production processes while reducing waste and energy costs and giving mechanistic information. Despite the advancements highlighted in this study, significant research difficulties in this area still need to be solved to make further progress. We don't yet know which characteristics of nanomaterials should be assessed, such as their number, surface area, or mass concentration, or whether a mixture of these characteristics or something else should be used. Is there anything new that we've learnt about biological toxicity mechanisms due to these toxicological studies? With a few notable exceptions, the answer is no, not really. It is anticipated that new knowledge about the functioning of cells and organs, internally and externally with other organisms, will be gained once the biomedical community embraces nanoparticles as new tools for *in vivo* imaging over a longer time scale. Studies dealing with the toxic effects of nanomaterials on human health have also changed in response to technological advancement.

Nanotoxicology research, such as in vivo-like experiments on 3D human organs and cells and sophisticated genetic studies, is starting to take the role of traditional *in vitro*analytical techniques [124, 125]. *In vitro* testing techniques may need the evaluation of several complex processes, such as the physicochemical characteristics of nanomaterials, the environment-targeted cell interaction, cellular uptake, and epigenetic interaction, among others [126]. Omic approaches, such as next-generation sequencing, transcriptomics, and proteomics, have provided a significant amount of additional information about the toxicity of the complex cellular processes triggered by the interaction of nanomaterials with their surrounding environments, compared to previous research [127, 128].

Another essential thing to mention is the field of customized toxicology. The possibility of genetic vulnerability to the toxicity of nanomaterials should also be further investigated within this subject [129]. In recent years, data acquired *via* new technology advancements and nanotoxicological research has become more challenging to analyze. In light of the previously mentioned problems, the remarkable rise in the usage of nanomaterial-based medicinal treatments and technologies presents a future challenge for the field of medicine. Nanomaterials are a double-edged sword for future therapy because of their nanotoxicity and harmful consequences on those exposed to them, including manufacturers, industry employees, and patients. To regulate and mitigate the dangers associated with nanotechnology, regulations and laws must be put in place, and researchers must collaborate on interdisciplinary studies in various areas, including medical sciences, nanotechnology, nanomedicine, and biomedical engineering.

CONSENT FOR PUBLICATION

Not applicable.

CONFLICT OF INTEREST

The authors declare no conflict of interest, financial or otherwise.

ACKNOWLEGEMENT

We are thankful to the team Bentham Science Publishers for giving this opportunity, the editor of this book and everyone who supported us directly or indirectly during the course of writing this book chapter.

REFERENCES

[1] Hatchett DW, Josowicz M. Composites of intrinsically conducting polymers as sensing nanomaterials. Chem Rev 2008; 108(2): 746-69.
[http://dx.doi.org/10.1021/cr068112h] [PMID: 18171087]

[2] Aslan K, Huang J, Wilson GM, Geddes CD. Metal-enhanced fluorescence-based RNA sensing. J Am Chem Soc 2006; 128(13): 4206-7.
[http://dx.doi.org/10.1021/ja0601179] [PMID: 16568977]

[3] Bagalkot V, Zhang L, Levy-Nissenbaum E, *et al.* Quantum dot-aptamer conjugates for synchronous cancer imaging, therapy, and sensing of drug delivery based on bi-fluorescence resonance energy transfer. Nano Lett 2007; 7(10): 3065-70.
[http://dx.doi.org/10.1021/nl071546n] [PMID: 17854227]

[4] Vance ME, Kuiken T, Vejerano EP, *et al.* Nanotechnology in the real world: Redeveloping the nanomaterial consumer products inventory. Beilstein J Nanotechnol 2015; 6: 1769-80.
[http://dx.doi.org/10.3762/bjnano.6.181] [PMID: 26425429]

[5] DTU environment, the Danish ecological council and Danish consumer council (2020) 2020. http://nanodb.dk/en/

[6] Khan I, Saeed K, Khan I. Nanoparticles: Properties, applications and toxicities. Arab J Chem 2019; 12(7): 908-31.
[http://dx.doi.org/10.1016/j.arabjc.2017.05.011]

[7] Camargo PHC, Satyanarayana KG, Wypych F. Nanocomposites: synthesis, structure, properties and new application opportunities. Mater Res 2009; 12(1): 1-39.
[http://dx.doi.org/10.1590/S1516-14392009000100002]

[8] Li X, Zhu J, Wei B. Hybrid nanostructures of metal/two-dimensional nanomaterials for plasmon-enhanced applications. Chem Soc Rev 2016; 45(11): 3145-87.
[http://dx.doi.org/10.1039/C6CS00195E] [PMID: 27048993]

[9] Das R, Vecitis CD, Schulze A, *et al.* Recent advances in nanomaterials for water protection and monitoring. Chem Soc Rev 2017; 46(22): 6946-7020.
[http://dx.doi.org/10.1039/C6CS00921B] [PMID: 28959815]

[10] Hasija V, Raizada P, Sudhaik A, *et al.* Recent advances in noble metal free doped graphitic carbon nitride based nanohybrids for photocatalysis of organic contaminants in water: A review. Appl Mater Today 2019; 15: 494-524.
[http://dx.doi.org/10.1016/j.apmt.2019.04.003]

[11] Upadhyay RK, Soin N, Roy SS. Role of graphene/metal oxide composites as photocatalysts, adsorbents and disinfectants in water treatment: a review. RSC Advances 2014; 4(8): 3823-51.
[http://dx.doi.org/10.1039/C3RA45013A]

[12] Sanchez C, Belleville P, Popall M, Nicole L. Applications of advanced hybrid organic–inorganic nanomaterials: from laboratory to market. Chem Soc Rev 2011; 40(2): 696-753.
[http://dx.doi.org/10.1039/c0cs00136h] [PMID: 21229132]

[13] Fakruddin M, Hossain Z, Afroz H. Prospects and applications of nanobiotechnology: a medical perspective. J Nanobiotechnology 2012; 10(1): 31.
[http://dx.doi.org/10.1186/1477-3155-10-31] [PMID: 22817658]

[14] Singh R, Lillard JW Jr. Nanoparticle-based targeted drug delivery. Exp Mol Pathol 2009; 86(3): 215-23.
[http://dx.doi.org/10.1016/j.yexmp.2008.12.004] [PMID: 19186176]

[15] Setyawati MI, Tay CY, Docter D, Stauber RH, Leong DT. Understanding and exploiting nanoparticles' intimacy with the blood vessel and blood. Chem Soc Rev 2015; 44(22): 8174-99.
[http://dx.doi.org/10.1039/C5CS00499C] [PMID: 26239875]

[16] Jeevanandam J, Barhoum A, Chan YS, Dufresne A, Danquah MK. Review on nanoparticles and nanostructured materials: history, sources, toxicity and regulations. Beilstein J Nanotechnol 2018; 9(1): 1050-74.
[http://dx.doi.org/10.3762/bjnano.9.98] [PMID: 29719757]

[17] Taghavi SM, Momenpour M, Azarian M, *et al.* Effects of nanoparticles on the environment and outdoor workplaces. Electron Physician 2013; 5(4): 706-12.
[PMID: 26120406]

[18] Buzea C, Pacheco II, Robbie K. Nanomaterials and nanoparticles: Sources and toxicity. Biointerphases 2007; 2(4): MR17-71.
[http://dx.doi.org/10.1116/1.2815690] [PMID: 20419892]

[19] Laux P, Tentschert J, Riebeling C, *et al.* Nanomaterials: certain aspects of application, risk assessment and risk communication. Arch Toxicol 2018; 92(1): 121-41.
[http://dx.doi.org/10.1007/s00204-017-2144-1] [PMID: 29273819]

[20] Gupta A, Kumar S, Kumar V. Challenges for assessing toxicity of nanomaterials. In: Ince M, Ince OK, Ondrasek G, Eds. Biochemical Toxicology - Heavy Metals and Nanomaterials [Internet]. London: IntechOpen 2019. Available from: https://www.intechopen.com/chapters/70500
[http://dx.doi.org/10.5772/intechopen.89601]

[21] Colvin VL. The potential environmental impact of engineered nanomaterials. Nat Biotechnol 2003; 21(10): 1166-70.
[http://dx.doi.org/10.1038/nbt875] [PMID: 14520401]

[22] Singh S, Kumar V, Singh J. Kinetic study of the biodegradation of glyphosate by indigenous soil bacterial isolates in presence of humic acid, Fe(III) and Cu(II) ions. J Environ Chem Eng 2019; 7(3): 103098.
[http://dx.doi.org/10.1016/j.jece.2019.103098]

[23] Kumar V, Singh S, Srivastava B, Bhadouria R, Singh R. Green synthesis of silver nanoparticles using leaf extract of Holoptelea integrifolia and preliminary investigation of its antioxidant, anti-inflammatory, antidiabetic and antibacterial activities. J Environ Chem Eng 2019; 7(3): 103094. [http://dx.doi.org/10.1016/j.jece.2019.103094]

[24] Bhati S, Kumar V, Singh S, Singh J. Synthesis, biological activities and docking studies of piperazine incorporated 1, 3, 4-oxadiazole derivatives. J Mol Struct 2019; 1191: 197-205.
[http://dx.doi.org/10.1016/j.molstruc.2019.04.106]

[25] Kapoor D, Singh S, Kumar V, Romero R, Prasad R, Singh J. Antioxidant enzymes regulation in plants in reference to reactive oxygen species (ROS) and reactive nitrogen species (RNS). Plant Gene 2019; 19: 100182.
[http://dx.doi.org/10.1016/j.plgene.2019.100182]

[26] Sidhu GK, Singh S, Kumar V, Dhanjal DS, Datta S, Singh J. Toxicity, monitoring and biodegradation of organophosphate pesticides: A review. Crit Rev Environ Sci Technol 2019; 49(13): 1135-87.
[http://dx.doi.org/10.1080/10643389.2019.1565554]

[27] Kumar V, Singh S, Singh A, Subhose V, Prakash O. Assessment of heavy metal ions, essential metal ions, and antioxidant properties of the most common herbal drugs in Indian Ayurvedic hospital: For ensuring quality assurance of certain Ayurvedic drugs. Biocatal Agric Biotechnol 2019; 18: 101018.
[http://dx.doi.org/10.1016/j.bcab.2019.01.056]

[28] Murphy K. Nanotechnology: agriculture's next industrial revolution Financial Partner, Yankee Farm Credit. ACA, Williston 2008; pp. 3-5.

[29] Tarafdar JC, Indira R. Nanonutrient from fungal protein: future prospects on crop production. Emerging Trends in Agri-nanotechnology In: Singh HB, Mishra S, Fraceto LF, Lima R de, Eds. Fundamental and Applied Aspects. 2018.
[http://dx.doi.org/10.1079/9781786391445.0037]

[30] Panyam J, Labhasetwar V. Biodegradable nanoparticles for drug and gene delivery to cells and tissue. Adv Drug Deliv Rev 2003; 55(3): 329-47.
[http://dx.doi.org/10.1016/S0169-409X(02)00228-4] [PMID: 12628320]

[31] Li W, Elzatahry A, Aldhayan D, Zhao D. Core–shell structured titanium dioxide nanomaterials for

solar energy utilization. Chem Soc Rev 2018; 47(22): 8203-37.
[http://dx.doi.org/10.1039/C8CS00443A] [PMID: 30137079]

[32] Lee JH, Ju JE, Kim BI, *et al.* Rod-shaped iron oxide nanoparticles are more toxic than sphere-shaped nanoparticles to murine macrophage cells. Environ Toxicol Chem 2014; 33(12): 2759-66.
[http://dx.doi.org/10.1002/etc.2735] [PMID: 25176020]

[33] Yola ML, Eren T, Atar N. A novel efficient photocatalyst based on TiO_2 nanoparticles involved boron enrichment waste for photocatalytic degradation of atrazine. Chem Eng J 2014; 250: 288-94.
[http://dx.doi.org/10.1016/j.cej.2014.03.116]

[34] Wu H, Zhang J. Chitosan-based zinc oxide nanoparticle for enhanced anticancer effect in cervical cancer: A physicochemical and biological perspective. Saudi Pharm J 2018; 26(2): 205-10.
[http://dx.doi.org/10.1016/j.jsps.2017.12.010] [PMID: 30166917]

[35] Chander N, Khan AF, Thouti E, *et al.* Size and concentration effects of gold nanoparticles on optical and electrical properties of plasmonic dye sensitized solar cells. Sol Energy 2014; 109: 11-23.
[http://dx.doi.org/10.1016/j.solener.2014.08.011]

[36] Yuan Q, Hein S, Misra RDK. New generation of chitosan-encapsulated ZnO quantum dots loaded with drug: Synthesis, characterization and *in vitro*drug delivery response. Acta Biomater 2010; 6(7): 2732-9.
[http://dx.doi.org/10.1016/j.actbio.2010.01.025] [PMID: 20100604]

[37] Qiu H, Cui B, Li G, *et al.* Novel Fe_3O_4@ ZnO@ $mSiO_2$ nanocarrier for targeted drug delivery and controllable release with microwave irradiation. J Phys Chem C 2014; 118(27): 14929-37.
[http://dx.doi.org/10.1021/jp502820r]

[38] De Matteis V. Exposure to inorganic nanoparticles: routes of entry, immune response, biodistribution and *in vitro*/*in vivo* toxicity evaluation. Toxics 2017; 5(4): 29.
[http://dx.doi.org/10.3390/toxics5040029] [PMID: 29051461]

[39] Sharifi S, Behzadi S, Laurent S, Laird Forrest M, Stroeve P, Mahmoudi M. Toxicity of nanomaterials. Chem Soc Rev 2012; 41(6): 2323-43.
[http://dx.doi.org/10.1039/C1CS15188F] [PMID: 22170510]

[40] Sajid M, Ilyas M, Basheer C, *et al.* Impact of nanoparticles on human and environment: review of toxicity factors, exposures, control strategies, and future prospects. Environ Sci Pollut Res Int 2015; 22(6): 4122-43.
[http://dx.doi.org/10.1007/s11356-014-3994-1] [PMID: 25548015]

[41] DTU environment, the Danish ecological council and Danish consumer council (2020) 2020. http://nanodb.dk/en/

[42] Mar NY. Approaches and Concerns in Myanmar. Prospects 2005; 35(3): 331-42.
[http://dx.doi.org/10.1007/s11125-005-4273-1]

[43] Weichenthal S, Lavigne E, Valois MF, *et al.* Spatial variations in ambient ultrafine particle concentrations and the risk of incident prostate cancer: A case-control study. Environ Res 2017; 156: 374-80.
[http://dx.doi.org/10.1016/j.envres.2017.03.035] [PMID: 28395241]

[44] Senzui M, Tamura T, Miura K, Ikarashi Y, Watanabe Y, Fujii M. Study on penetration of titanium dioxide (TiO_2) nanoparticles into intact and damaged skin *in vitro*. J Toxicol Sci 2010; 35(1): 107-13.
[http://dx.doi.org/10.2131/jts.35.107] [PMID: 20118631]

[45] Desai P, Patlolla RR, Singh M. Interaction of nanoparticles and cell-penetrating peptides with skin for transdermal drug delivery. Mol Membr Biol 2010; 27(7): 247-59.
[http://dx.doi.org/10.3109/09687688.2010.522203] [PMID: 21028936]

[46] Bouwmeester H, van der Zande M, Jepson MA. Effects of food-borne nanomaterials on gastrointestinal tissues and microbiota. Wiley Interdiscip Rev Nanomed Nanobiotechnol 2018; 10(1): e1481.

[http://dx.doi.org/10.1002/wnan.1481] [PMID: 28548289]

[47] Cherrie JW, Semple S, Christopher Y, Saleem A, Hughson GW, Philips A. How important is inadvertent ingestion of hazardous substances at work? Ann Occup Hyg 2006; 50(7): 693-704. [PMID: 16840437]

[48] Gengfeng Z, Fernando P, Yi C, Wang Wayne U, Lieber Charles M. Nat Biotechnol 2005; 23: 1294. [http://dx.doi.org/10.1038/nbt1138] [PMID: 16170313]

[49] Nahar M, Dutta T, Murugesan S, *et al.* Functional polymeric nanoparticles: an efficient and promising tool for active delivery of bioactives. Critical Reviews™ in Therapeutic Drug Carrier Systems 2006; 23(4).
[http://dx.doi.org/10.1615/CritRevTherDrugCarrierSyst.v23.i4.10]

[50] Qiao Y, Li S, Liu W, Ran M, Lu H, Yang Y. Recent advances of rare-earth ion doped luminescent nanomaterials in perovskite solar cells. Nanomaterials (Basel) 2018; 8(1): 43.
[http://dx.doi.org/10.3390/nano8010043] [PMID: 29342950]

[51] Brambilla D, Le Droumaguet B, Nicolas J, *et al.* Nanotechnologies for Alzheimer's disease: diagnosis, therapy, and safety issues. Nanomedicine 2011; 7(5): 521-40.
[http://dx.doi.org/10.1016/j.nano.2011.03.008] [PMID: 21477665]

[52] Banoee M, Seif S, Nazari ZE, *et al.* ZnO nanoparticles enhanced antibacterial activity of ciprofloxacin against *Staphylococcus aureus* and *Escherichia coli*. J Biomed Mater Res B Appl Biomater 2010; 93B(2): 557-61.
[http://dx.doi.org/10.1002/jbm.b.31615] [PMID: 20225250]

[53] Zhou C, Deng C, Chen X, *et al.* Mechanical and biological properties of the micro-/nano-grain functionally graded hydroxyapatite bioceramics for bone tissue engineering. Journal of the mechanical behavior of biomedical materials 2015; 48: 1-1.

[54] Tamjid E, Bagheri R, Vossoughi M, Simchi A. Effect of TiO_2 morphology on *in vitro*bioactivity of polycaprolactone/TiO_2 nanocomposites. Mater Lett 2011; 65(15-16): 2530-3.
[http://dx.doi.org/10.1016/j.matlet.2011.05.037]

[55] Priyadarsini S, Mukherjee S, Mishra M. Nanoparticles used in dentistry: A review. J Oral Biol Craniofac Res 2018; 8(1): 58-67.
[http://dx.doi.org/10.1016/j.jobcr.2017.12.004] [PMID: 29556466]

[56] García-Contreras R, Argueta-Figueroa L, Mejía-Rubalcava C, *et al.* Perspectives for the use of silver nanoparticles in dental practice. Int Dent J 2011; 61(6): 297-301.
[http://dx.doi.org/10.1111/j.1875-595X.2011.00072.x] [PMID: 22117785]

[57] Reis LA, Chiu LLY, Feric N, Fu L, Radisic M. Biomaterials in myocardial tissue engineering. J Tissue Eng Regen Med 2016; 10(1): 11-28.
[http://dx.doi.org/10.1002/term.1944] [PMID: 25066525]

[58] AS A, N Gade W, Vats T, Lenardi C, Milani P. Nanomaterials: New generation therapeutics in wound healing and tissue repair. Curr Nanosci 2010; 6(6): 577-86.
[http://dx.doi.org/10.2174/157341310793348632]

[59] Klaassen CD, Watkins JB III. Fundamentos em Toxicologia de Casarett e Doull (Lange). AMGH Editora 2009.

[60] Ray PC, Yu H, Fu PP. Toxicity and environmental risks of nanomaterials: challenges and future needs. J Environ Sci Health Part C Environ Carcinog Ecotoxicol Rev 2009; 27(1): 1-35.
[http://dx.doi.org/10.1080/10590500802708267] [PMID: 19204862]

[61] Nowack B, Brouwer C, Geertsma RE, *et al.* Analysis of the occupational, consumer and environmental exposure to engineered nanomaterials used in 10 technology sectors. Nanotoxicology 2012; 7(6): 1152-6.
[http://dx.doi.org/10.3109/17435390.2012.711863] [PMID: 22783888]

[62] Berk S, Akkurt İ. Nanoparticle: a nightmare for the future. Tuberk Toraks 2012; 60(2): 180-4. [http://dx.doi.org/10.5578/tt.3557] [PMID: 22779942]

[63] Shukla R, Bansal V, Chaudhary M, Basu A, Bhonde RR, Sastry M. Biocompatibility of gold nanoparticles and their endocytotic fate inside the cellular compartment: a microscopic overview. Langmuir 2005; 21(23): 10644-54. [http://dx.doi.org/10.1021/la0513712] [PMID: 16262332]

[64] Chithrani BD, Ghazani AA, Chan WCW. Determining the size and shape dependence of gold nanoparticle uptake into mammalian cells. Nano Lett 2006; 6(4): 662-8. [http://dx.doi.org/10.1021/nl052396o] [PMID: 16608261]

[65] Connor EE, Mwamuka J, Gole A, Murphy CJ, Wyatt MD. Gold nanoparticles are taken up by human cells but do not cause acute cytotoxicity. Small 2005; 1(3): 325-7. [http://dx.doi.org/10.1002/smll.200400093] [PMID: 17193451]

[66] Wang S, Lu W, Tovmachenko O, Rai US, Yu H, Ray PC. Challenge in understanding size and shape dependent toxicity of gold nanomaterials in human skin keratinocytes. Chem Phys Lett 2008; 463(1-3): 145-9. [http://dx.doi.org/10.1016/j.cplett.2008.08.039] [PMID: 24068836]

[67] Grassian VH, O'Shaughnessy PT, Adamcakova-Dodd A, Pettibone JM, Thorne PS. Inhalation exposure study of titanium dioxide nanoparticles with a primary particle size of 2 to 5 nm. Environ Health Perspect 2007; 115(3): 397-402. [http://dx.doi.org/10.1289/ehp.9469] [PMID: 17431489]

[68] Jin CY, Zhu BS, Wang XF, Lu QH. Cytotoxicity of titanium dioxide nanoparticles in mouse fibroblast cells. Chem Res Toxicol 2008; 21(9): 1871-7. [http://dx.doi.org/10.1021/tx800179f] [PMID: 18680314]

[69] Park EJ, Yi J, Chung KH, Ryu DY, Choi J, Park K. Oxidative stress and apoptosis induced by titanium dioxide nanoparticles in cultured BEAS-2B cells. Toxicol Lett 2008; 180(3): 222-9. [http://dx.doi.org/10.1016/j.toxlet.2008.06.869] [PMID: 18662754]

[70] Ding L, Stilwell J, Zhang T, *et al.* Molecular characterization of the cytotoxic mechanism of multiwall carbon nanotubes and nano-onions on human skin fibroblast. Nano Lett 2005; 5(12): 2448-64. [http://dx.doi.org/10.1021/nl051748o] [PMID: 16351195]

[71] Peters K, Unger RE, Kirkpatrick CJ, Gatti AM, Monari E. Effects of nano-scaled particles on endothelial cell function *in vitro*: Studies on viability, proliferation and inflammation. J Mater Sci Mater Med 2004; 15(4): 321-5. [http://dx.doi.org/10.1023/B:JMSM.0000021095.36878.1b] [PMID: 15332593]

[72] Magrez A, Kasas S, Salicio V, *et al.* Cellular toxicity of carbon-based nanomaterials. Nano Lett 2006; 6(6): 1121-5. [http://dx.doi.org/10.1021/nl060162e] [PMID: 16771565]

[73] Dumortier H, Lacotte S, Pastorin G, *et al.* Functionalized carbon nanotubes are non-cytotoxic and preserve the functionality of primary immune cells. Nano Lett 2006; 6(7): 1522-8. [http://dx.doi.org/10.1021/nl061160x] [PMID: 16834443]

[74] Alivisatos P. The use of nanocrystals in biological detection. Nat Biotechnol 2004; 22(1): 47-52. [http://dx.doi.org/10.1038/nbt927] [PMID: 14704706]

[75] Gao X, Cui Y, Levenson RM, Chung LWK, Nie S. In vivo cancer targeting and imaging with semiconductor quantum dots. Nat Biotechnol 2004; 22(8): 969-76. [http://dx.doi.org/10.1038/nbt994] [PMID: 15258594]

[76] Michalet X, Pinaud FF, Bentolila LA, *et al.* Quantum dots for live cells, in vivo imaging, and diagnostics 2005; 307(5709): 538-44.

[77] Lovrić J, Bazzi HS, Cuie Y, Fortin GRA, Winnik FM, Maysinger D. Differences in subcellular

distribution and toxicity of green and red emitting CdTe quantum dots. J Mol Med (Berl) 2005; 83(5): 377-85.
[http://dx.doi.org/10.1007/s00109-004-0629-x] [PMID: 15688234]

[78] Zhang LW, Monteiro-Riviere NA. Assessment of quantum dot penetration into intact, tape-stripped, abraded and flexed rat skin. Skin Pharmacol Physiol 2008; 21(3): 166-80.
[http://dx.doi.org/10.1159/000131080] [PMID: 18523414]

[79] Gopee NV, Roberts DW, Webb P, *et al.* Migration of intradermally injected quantum dots to sentinel organs in mice. Toxicol Sci 2007; 98(1): 249-57.
[http://dx.doi.org/10.1093/toxsci/kfm074] [PMID: 17404394]

[80] Nemmar A, Beegam S, Yuvaraju P, *et al.* Ultrasmall superparamagnetic iron oxide nanoparticles acutely promote thrombosis and cardiac oxidative stress and DNA damage in mice. Part Fibre Toxicol 2015; 13(1): 22.
[http://dx.doi.org/10.1186/s12989-016-0132-x] [PMID: 27138375]

[81] Magaye RR, Yue X, Zou B, *et al.* Acute toxicity of nickel nanoparticles in rats after intravenous injection. Int J Nanomedicine 2014; 9: 1393-402.
[PMID: 24648736]

[82] Arefian Z, Pishbin F, Negahdary M, Ajdary M. Potential toxic effects of Zirconia Oxide nanoparticles on liver and kidney factors 2015; 26(1).

[83] Bellusci M, La Barbera A, Padella F, *et al.* Biodistribution and acute toxicity of a nanofluid containing manganese iron oxide nanoparticles produced by a mechanochemical process. Int J Nanomedicine 2014; 9: 1919-29.
[PMID: 24790434]

[84] Yousefi Babadi V, Amraeai E, Salehh H, Sadeghi L, Najafi L, Fazilati M. Evaluation of iron oxide nanoparticles effects on tissue and enzymes of thyroid in rats. Int Res J Biol Sci 2013; 2(7): 67-9.

[85] Xu J, Shi H, Ruth M, *et al.* Acute toxicity of intravenously administered titanium dioxide nanoparticles in mice. PLoS One 2013; 8(8): e70618.
[http://dx.doi.org/10.1371/journal.pone.0070618] [PMID: 23950972]

[86] Awaad A. Histopathological and immunological changes induced by magnetite nanoparticles in the spleen, liver and genital tract of mice following intravaginal instillation. J Basic Appl Zool 2015; 71: 32-47.
[http://dx.doi.org/10.1016/j.jobaz.2015.03.003]

[87] Cai X, Lee A, Ji Z, *et al.* Reduction of pulmonary toxicity of metal oxide nanoparticles by phosphonate-based surface passivation. Part Fibre Toxicol 2017; 14(1): 13.
[http://dx.doi.org/10.1186/s12989-017-0193-5] [PMID: 28069023]

[88] Sadeghi L, Babadi VY, Espanani HR. Toxic effects of the Fe_2O_3 nanoparticles on the liver and lung tissue. Bratisl Med J 2015; 116(6): 373-8.
[http://dx.doi.org/10.4149/BLL_2015_071] [PMID: 26084739]

[89] S S, K V, S P, N R, K K. *In vitro* cytotoxicity of zinc oxide, iron oxide and copper nanopowders prepared by green synthesis. Toxicol Rep 2017; 4: 427-30.
[http://dx.doi.org/10.1016/j.toxrep.2017.07.005] [PMID: 28959669]

[90] Fartkhooni FM, Noori A, Mohammadi A. Effects of titanium dioxide nanoparticles toxicity on the kidney of male rats. Int J Life Sci (Kathmandu) 2016; 10(1): 65-9.
[http://dx.doi.org/10.3126/ijls.v10i1.14513]

[91] Raju HB, Hu Y, Vedula A, Dubovy SR, Goldberg JL. Evaluation of magnetic micro- and nanoparticle toxicity to ocular tissues. PLoS One 2011; 6(5): e17452.
[http://dx.doi.org/10.1371/journal.pone.0017452] [PMID: 21637340]

[92] Kim DK. Nanomedicine for inner ear diseases: a review of recent *in vivo* studies. BioMed Res Int 2017; 2017: 1-6.

[http://dx.doi.org/10.1155/2017/3098230] [PMID: 29130038]

[93] Ibrahim AI, Amira FA, Manal MM, Hanan MM, Hanan EM. Effect of zinc oxide nanoparticles on the structure of testis of adult albino rats and the possible protective role of naringenin. Med J Cairo Univ 2019; 87(September): 3469-83. [http://dx.doi.org/10.21608/mjcu.2019.65644]

[94] Kong L, Tang M, Zhang T, *et al.* Nickel nanoparticles exposure and reproductive toxicity in healthy adult rats. Int J Mol Sci 2014; 15(11): 21253-69. [http://dx.doi.org/10.3390/ijms151121253] [PMID: 25407529]

[95] Elsaesser A, Howard CV. Toxicology of nanoparticles. Adv Drug Deliv Rev 2012; 64(2): 129-37. [http://dx.doi.org/10.1016/j.addr.2011.09.001] [PMID: 21925220]

[96] Landa P, Vankova R, Andrlova J, *et al.* Nanoparticle-specific changes in Arabidopsis thaliana gene expression after exposure to ZnO, TiO_2, and fullerene soot. J Hazard Mater 2012; 241-242: 55-62. [http://dx.doi.org/10.1016/j.jhazmat.2012.08.059] [PMID: 23036700]

[97] Warheit DB, Sayes CM, Reed KL, Swain KA. Health effects related to nanoparticle exposures: Environmental, health and safety considerations for assessing hazards and risks. Pharmacol Ther 2008; 120(1): 35-42. [http://dx.doi.org/10.1016/j.pharmthera.2008.07.001] [PMID: 18703086]

[98] Karimi S, Troeung M, Wang R, *et al.* Acute and chronic toxicity to Daphnia magna of colloidal silica nanoparticles in a chemical mechanical planarization slurry after polishing a gallium arsenide wafer. NanoImpact 2019; 13: 56-65. [http://dx.doi.org/10.1016/j.impact.2018.12.004]

[99] Ghodake G, Seo YD, Lee DS. Hazardous phytotoxic nature of cobalt and zinc oxide nanoparticles assessed using Allium cepa. J Hazard Mater 2011; 186(1): 952-5. [http://dx.doi.org/10.1016/j.jhazmat.2010.11.018] [PMID: 21122986]

[100] Kim KS, Lee D, Song CG, Kang PM. Reactive oxygen species-activated nanomaterials as theranostic agents. Nanomedicine (Lond) 2015; 10(17): 2709-23. [http://dx.doi.org/10.2217/nnm.15.108] [PMID: 26328770]

[101] Fu PP, Xia Q, Hwang HM, Ray PC, Yu H. Mechanisms of nanotoxicity: generation of reactive oxygen species. Yao Wu Shi Pin Fen Xi 2014; 22(1): 64-75. [PMID: 24673904]

[102] Wang L, Hu C, Shao L. The antimicrobial activity of nanoparticles: present situation and prospects for the future. Int J Nanomedicine 2017; 12: 1227-49. [http://dx.doi.org/10.2147/IJN.S121956] [PMID: 28243086]

[103] Wang EC, Wang AZ. Nanoparticles and their applications in cell and molecular biology. Integr Biol 2014; 6(1): 9-26. [http://dx.doi.org/10.1039/c3ib40165k] [PMID: 24104563]

[104] Gonzalez L, Lison D, Kirsch-Volders M. Genotoxicity of engineered nanomaterials: A critical review. Nanotoxicology 2008; 2(4): 252-73. [http://dx.doi.org/10.1080/17435390802464986]

[105] Yin JJ, Liu J, Ehrenshaft M, *et al.* Phototoxicity of nano titanium dioxides in HaCaT keratinocytes—Generation of reactive oxygen species and cell damage. Toxicol Appl Pharmacol 2012; 263(1): 81-8. [http://dx.doi.org/10.1016/j.taap.2012.06.001] [PMID: 22705594]

[106] Valko M, Leibfritz D, Moncol J, Cronin MTD, Mazur M, Telser J. Free radicals and antioxidants in normal physiological functions and human disease. Int J Biochem Cell Biol 2007; 39(1): 44-84. [http://dx.doi.org/10.1016/j.biocel.2006.07.001] [PMID: 16978905]

[107] Meng H, Xia T, George S, Nel AE. A predictive toxicological paradigm for the safety assessment of nanomaterials. ACS Nano 2009; 3(7): 1620-7.

[http://dx.doi.org/10.1021/nn9005973] [PMID: 21452863]

[108] Oberdorster G, Maynard A, Donaldson K, *et al.* A report from the ILSI Research Foundation/Risk Science Institute Nanomaterial Toxicity Screening Working Group Principles for Characterizing the Potential Human Health Effects from Exposure to Nanomaterials: elements of a screening strategy. Part Fibre Toxicol 2005; 6: 2-8.

[109] Li Y, Yu S, Wu Q, Tang M, Pu Y, Wang D. Chronic Al_2O_3-nanoparticle exposure causes neurotoxic effects on locomotion behaviors by inducing severe ROS production and disruption of ROS defense mechanisms in nematode Caenorhabditis elegans. J Hazard Mater 2012; 219-220: 221-30. [http://dx.doi.org/10.1016/j.jhazmat.2012.03.083] [PMID: 22521136]

[110] Winnik FM, Maysinger D. Quantum dot cytotoxicity and ways to reduce it. Acc Chem Res 2013; 46(3): 672-80. [http://dx.doi.org/10.1021/ar3000585] [PMID: 22775328]

[111] Fan Z, Lu JG. Zinc oxide nanostructures: synthesis and properties. J Nanosci Nanotechnol 2005; 5(10): 1561-73. [http://dx.doi.org/10.1166/jnn.2005.182] [PMID: 16245516]

[112] Liu Y, Li X, Bao S, Lu Z, Li Q, Li CM. Plastic protein microarray to investigate the molecular pathways of magnetic nanoparticle-induced nanotoxicity. Nanotechnology 2013; 24(17): 175501. [http://dx.doi.org/10.1088/0957-4484/24/17/175501] [PMID: 23558511]

[113] Wang Y, Aker WG, Hwang H, Yedjou CG, Yu H, Tchounwou PB. A study of the mechanism of *in vitro*cytotoxicity of metal oxide nanoparticles using catfish primary hepatocytes and human HepG2 cells. Sci Total Environ 2011; 409(22): 4753-62. [http://dx.doi.org/10.1016/j.scitotenv.2011.07.039] [PMID: 21851965]

[114] Nel A, Xia T, Mädler L, Li N. Toxic potential of materials at the nanolevel science 2006; 311(5761): 622-7.

[115] Auffan M, Rose J, Wiesner MR, Bottero JY. Chemical stability of metallic nanoparticles: A parameter controlling their potential cellular toxicity *in vitro*. Environ Pollut 2009; 157(4): 1127-33. [http://dx.doi.org/10.1016/j.envpol.2008.10.002] [PMID: 19013699]

[116] Yoshida T, Yoshikawa T, Nabeshi H, Tsutsumi Y. [Relation analysis between intracellular distribution of nanomateriarls, ROS generation and DNA damage]. Yakugaku Zasshi 2012; 132(3): 295-300. [http://dx.doi.org/10.1248/yakushi.132.295] [PMID: 22382833]

[117] Boyoglu C, He Q, Willing G. Microscopic studies of various sizes of gold nanoparticles and their cellular localizations. ISRN Nanotechnol 2013. [http://dx.doi.org/10.1155/2013/123838]

[118] Thomas DG, Smith JN, Thrall BD, *et al.* ISD3: a particokinetic model for predicting the combined effects of particle sedimentation, diffusion and dissolution on cellular dosimetry for *in vitro*systems. Part Fibre Toxicol 2018; 15(1): 6. [http://dx.doi.org/10.1186/s12989-018-0243-7] [PMID: 29368623]

[119] Arora S, Rajwade JM, Paknikar KM. Nanotoxicology and *in vitro*studies: The need of the hour. Toxicol Appl Pharmacol 2012; 258(2): 151-65. [http://dx.doi.org/10.1016/j.taap.2011.11.010] [PMID: 22178382]

[120] Shukla RK, Sharma V, Pandey AK, Singh S, Sultana S, Dhawan A. ROS-mediated genotoxicity induced by titanium dioxide nanoparticles in human epidermal cells. Toxicol In Vitro 2011; 25(1): 231-41. [http://dx.doi.org/10.1016/j.tiv.2010.11.008] [PMID: 21092754]

[121] Zhang M, Xu C, Jiang L, Qin J. A 3D human lung-on-a-chip model for nanotoxicity testing. Toxicol Res (Camb) 2018; 7(6): 1048-60. [http://dx.doi.org/10.1039/C8TX00156A] [PMID: 30510678]

[122] Yin F, Zhu Y, Zhang M, Yu H, Chen W, Qin J. A 3D human placenta-on-a-chip model to probe

nanoparticle exposure at the placental barrier. Toxicol In Vitro 2019; 54: 105-13. [http://dx.doi.org/10.1016/j.tiv.2018.08.014] [PMID: 30248392]

[123] Shah P, Kaushik A, Zhu X, Zhang C, Li CZ. Chip based single cell analysis for nanotoxicity assessment. Analyst (Lond) 2014; 139(9): 2088-98. [http://dx.doi.org/10.1039/C3AN02280C] [PMID: 24567949]

[124] Dusinska M, Boland S, Saunders M, *et al.* Towards an alternative testing strategy for nanomaterials used in nanomedicine: lessons from NanoTEST 2015; 9(sup1): 118-32. [http://dx.doi.org/10.3109/17435390.2014.991431]

[125] Lan J, Gou N, Gao C, He M, Gu AZ. Comparative and mechanistic genotoxicity assessment of nanomaterials *via* a quantitative toxicogenomics approach across multiple species. Environ Sci Technol 2014; 48(21): 12937-45. [http://dx.doi.org/10.1021/es503065q] [PMID: 25338269]

[126] Smolkova B, Dusinska M, Gabelova A. Nanomedicine and epigenome. Possible health risks. Food Chem Toxicol 2017; 109(Pt 1): 780-96. [http://dx.doi.org/10.1016/j.fct.2017.07.020] [PMID: 28705729]

[127] Paunovska K, Loughrey D, Sago CD, Langer R, Dahlman JE. Using large datasets to understand nanotechnology. Adv Mater 2019; 31(43): 1902798. [http://dx.doi.org/10.1002/adma.201902798] [PMID: 31429126]

[128] Gallud A, Klöditz K, Ytterberg J, *et al.* Cationic gold nanoparticles elicit mitochondrial dysfunction: a multi-omics study. Sci Rep 2019; 9(1): 4366. [http://dx.doi.org/10.1038/s41598-019-40579-6] [PMID: 30867451]

[129] Scoville DK, Botta D, Galdanes K, *et al.* Genetic determinants of susceptibility to silver nanoparticle-induced acute lung inflammation in mice. FASEB J 2017; 31(10): 4600-11. [http://dx.doi.org/10.1096/fj.201700187R] [PMID: 28716969]

CHAPTER 12

Cancer Drug Products Containing Nano-materials: Key Regulatory Issues

Jinu Mathew[1], **Pallav Namdeo**[1] and **Ashish Garg**[1,*]

[1] *Department of P.G. Studies and Research in Chemistry and Pharmacy, Rani Durgavati University Jabalpur, M.P.482001, India*

Abstract: Nanoparticles are expected to have a broad array of applications, ranging from delivery of therapeutic agents to bio-imaging and, quite lately, personalized treatments, due to their diameter ranging (1-100 nm), which coincides with fundamental biomolecules, such as Genetic material (DNA), significantly increased surface area (1000 m2/g), and remarkable mechanical, electrical, magnetic and photonic characteristics. The capacity to deliver targeted anti-cancer drugs to tumors, cancer detection, their capability to contain hundreds of pharmaceutical units, and their ability to resist dispersion, stability, and tolerance difficulties are all significant benefits of employing nanoparticles as a transporter for chemotherapeutics. Numerous nano-materials and therapeutic & diagnostic compounds are now conducting clinical tests, and a couple has already received regulatory approval. The "Enhanced Permeation and Retention Effect", a distinguishing trait of tumor cells, is used to promote controlled administration of chemotherapeutic agents. In contrast to passive targeting, depending on size, the surface of the nano-materials may be changed with a range of ligands that bind with particular receptors highly expressed on the membrane of tumor cells, resulting in precise active targeting. Yet a novel technique for site-specific delivery is using environmental stimulation like heat to a thermo-responsive apparatus to deliver a medicine encapsulated in a nanosized structure at a specified location. This chapter offers information on accepted tumour nanoparticles, such as Oncaspar, Daunoxome, Doxil, Abraxane, and DepoCyt, as well as nanoplatforms utilizing albumin nanospheres, lipoplexes, lipid nanoparticles, liposomes, micelles and gold nanoparticles, which have attained an advanced level of clinical testing.

Keywords: Cancer, Clinical trials, Drug delivery, FDA, Nanoparticles, Regulatory approval.

INTRODUCTION

Nanomedicine, which combines nanotechnology with biological and pharmaceutical fields of science, would be a relatively emerging and highly

* **Corresponding Author Ashish Garg:** Department of P. G. Studies and Research in Chemistry and Pharmacy, Rani Durgavati University, Jabalpur (M.P.), 482001, India; Tel: +91-9993624362; E-mail: ashish.garg071010@gmail.com

Neeraj Mishra, Ashish Garg and Neeraj Upmanyu (Eds.)

developing field [1 - 3]. When nanoparticles (NPs) are used in medicated formulations, they could provide numerous pharmacokinetic, performance, security, and therapeutic advantages. Several nano drugs were approved for human usage, and more have been tested in clinical studies for several reasons [2]. On the other hand, nanopharmaceuticals encounter hurdles like the demand for improved classification, potential toxicity concerns, the shortage of defined regulatory requirements, price considerations, and decreasing excitement among certain medical professionals [4, 5]. As a result, expectations for nano-based drugs in the initial phases of development and clinical studies must remain realistic [4].

Nano-materials have become more common in therapeutic products on the market, and the US "Food and Drug Administration (FDA)" has accepted hundreds of applications from organizations interested in bringing nanomedicine/nano-material to the marketplace [6]. Such medication and services were frequently sophisticated, and the applications of this technology are numerous [6]. Cancer treatment is the most popularly claimed diagnosis in these nanotechnology-related applications. Nano-materials could enhance cancer treatments resulting in improved drug solubility, drug possession, and focused delivery methods like active & passive, which could vastly enhance drug accumulation at the specific site of the tumour whereas lowering negative impacts [7 - 9]. During 2011 and 2016, the FDA has seen an 8% rise in applications for cancer medicines, including nano-materials, demonstrating both potential of such materials and the significant risk threshold for innovative treatments between cancer sufferers and clinicians [9, 10]. "The FDA's Center for Drug Evaluation and Research (FDA/CDER)" examines the efficacy and then safety of those drug products with drug substances when they are presented for approval in the United States. The range of development and diversity in drug products utilizing nano-materials was wide, and the FDA had created analytical and conceptual approaches that uniformly address the hazards posed by novel treatment strategies. The FDA evaluates its entire product when examining drug product submissions, from clinical efficacy data through biochemistry, manufacturing, preservation, and delivery systems. These four areas were grouped as a medicine's quality characteristics, and FDA has concluded that they are significant for drug products that include nano-materials. Following with a summary of immunotherapies of nano-materials among products prescribed to remove cancer and even regulatory framework description wherein applications of cancer therapies were examined, some relevant quality characteristics were reviewed in detail in this section [11].

CHARACTERISTICS OF NANO-MATERIALS

Nano-materials have several characteristics, making them useful in various clinical settings. Nanoparticles with a standard/ideal size of 10–200 nm allow particles to circulate throughout the body without interrupting blood circulation and avoiding removal by renal and immune mechanisms [12]. The increasing size of therapeutically employed nano-materials is significant in cancer treatments since it was previously considered that increased viscosity and persistence had been one of the methods of nanoparticles that might effectively reach tumour cells [13]. Furthermore, this theory has been highlighted in the research world, with new evidence indicating that active transport pathways dominate nanoparticle transport, leading to tumour accumulation [14]. Many people in the community are still divided on this, but more attention is being paid to the tumour microenvironment. It has become evident that regionalized stress inside the tumour cells would not be conducive to passive targeting through EPR. It, therefore, is possibly the most significant determining factor towards this occurrence. Another critical aspect of nanoparticles is their optical and electrical characteristics, particularly in metal nanoparticles. Such characteristics are based mostly on the surface plasmon resonance concept, which states that free electrons in metallic nanoparticles fluctuate [15]. Specific metal oxide nanoparticles were therefore magnetized, enabling particles just to be employed for scanning, cell imaging, focusing, and drug delivery, among many other purposes. Nanomedicines often become straightforward and inexpensive to make on such a microscopic level, but scaling up and maintaining stability on such a massive scale has proven difficult [16].

Once manufactured, nano-materials are relatively simple to sterilize before clinical use, with the majority being syringes filtered below the molecular cut-off for biological contaminants such as bacteria.

ANTI-CANCER DRUG COMPOUNDS AND PRODUCTS CONTAINING NANO-MATERIALS

Cancer was the second most prevalent source of death in the United States, according to "the Centers for Disease Control and Prevention" [17], and then as a category of disorders, this is a target of government-funded development projects [18].

The disease's course and propensity for causing death make it an excellent target for the production of new therapeutic ingredients. On the other hand, most anti-cancer medication ingredients have low water solubility and poisoning concerns [19], reducing their overall safety and effectiveness. Since a molecule's physicochemical properties could alter particle size, incorporating nano-materials inside the therapeutic product was the potential option for overcoming these challenges. For instance, by simply decreasing a therapeutic substance's particle size to just the nanoscale, the total beneficial surface area could be raised several folds, allowing surface-related properties like apparent disintegration efficiency to be altered [20, 21]. In addition, however, the features of nanoscale drug delivery systems could be "taken" for enhancing the efficacy of a low soluble and poorly tolerated therapeutic material by allowing for extended in-vivo circulation or focused delivery (active/passive) [22]. As a result, medication developers are turning to nano-materials to increase drug accumulation only at cancer sites and lower the side effects associated with traditional preparations [23]. Fig. (**1**) depicts numerous nanocarriers used in cancer treatment.

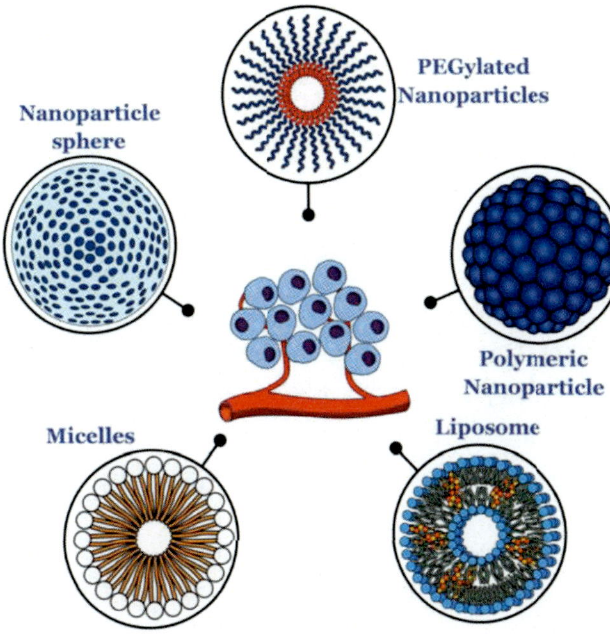

Fig. (1). Various nano-materials are utilized in the treatment and drug delivery device for cancer.

TRENDS IN APPROVAL AND DEVELOPMENT

Anti-cancer medications frequently have poor physicochemical qualities, like low water solubility and substantial systemic toxicity after administration, owing to their strength. As a result, significant effort has gone into forming such molecules, which has consumed most of the nanomedicine research for over 30 years. "A liposome-based doxorubicin hydrochloride" composition (Doxil®) for the Kaposi's sarcoma therapy among patients having "human immunodeficiency virus (HIV)" received FDA approval by the year 1995 [24]. Several lipid-based compositions, like Daunorubicin® [25] and then Myocet® [26], have been approved. Protein drug nanoparticles, like Abraxane®, which was licensed throughout the United States by the year 2005 [27], are another big success in cancer nanomedicine. Abraxane® is a nanoparticle made up of albumin and paclitaxel that has been approved to treat a variety of malignancies, especially pancreatic and then metastatic breast tumours. In certain countries, virosomes were often approved to be used in therapeutic settings; for instance, Rexin-G® for solid tumours was already utilized within the Philippines until 2007 because of its capacity to precisely target unprotected collagen, which is typically seen in metastatic cancers [28]. FDA has recently approved Rexin-G against pancreatic tumors [29]. Establishing therapeutic agents inside a nano platform is a new focus under chemotherapy-driven nanocarriers. Combination therapy was shown to improve effectiveness against such a variety of malignancies. The introduction of combination medicines has brought great hope to cancer patients, especially those with complicated tumours. Vyxeos®, specifically, has shown to be particularly effective in the "adult acute myeloid leukemia" treatment [30]. Vyxeos® contains cytarabine and daunorubicin liposomal composition. In the third clinical trials, patients who received Vyxeos® had a better overall lifespan and a lower chance of mortality than those who received the two medications in such a combination regimen without nanotechnology. More emphasis on combination therapy is expected to result in a higher amount of certain drugs undergoing clinical studies and seeking regulatory approval. Unwell patients could scarcely withstand chemotherapy regimens with only one medicine, thus, nanotechnology holds significant promise in this field. The safety against systemic toxicity of such strong drugs provided by nanotechnology and site-specificity are critical to the domain's success.

In 1995, the FDA approved 50 nanopharmaceuticals, which is now utilized for clinical application [1, 2, 31, 32]. Nano drugs were usually given orally or by injection, with transdermal administration less common [2]. Among authorized nano drugs, polymeric, nanocrystal, and liposomal formulations were extensively featured [33]. Other NP-based drug discovery systems, like micelles or artificial NPs (metalloid oxides and other artificial nano-materials), are also used for authorized nano drugs. Nano drugs were approved for several uses, notably cancer treatment. The FDA approved the most nano drugs from 2001 to 2005, then saw a considerable reduction in 2006, probably due to reduced cost following the global financial crisis in 2008 [4]. Fig. (**2**) summarises a list of authorized nano drugs. Compared to traditional preparations, most nano drugs licensed recently demonstrated reduced toxicity instead of enhanced efficacy. Several nano drugs have failed to make it through clinical trials since they failed to show considerable effectiveness and because increased toxicity might be produced with the other medicines and nanoformulations [2]. Nanoformulated formulations of medical therapies in clinical trials, on the other hand, have demonstrated encouraging results in terms of increased effectiveness and, as a result, appear to be important for successful regulatory approval [2].

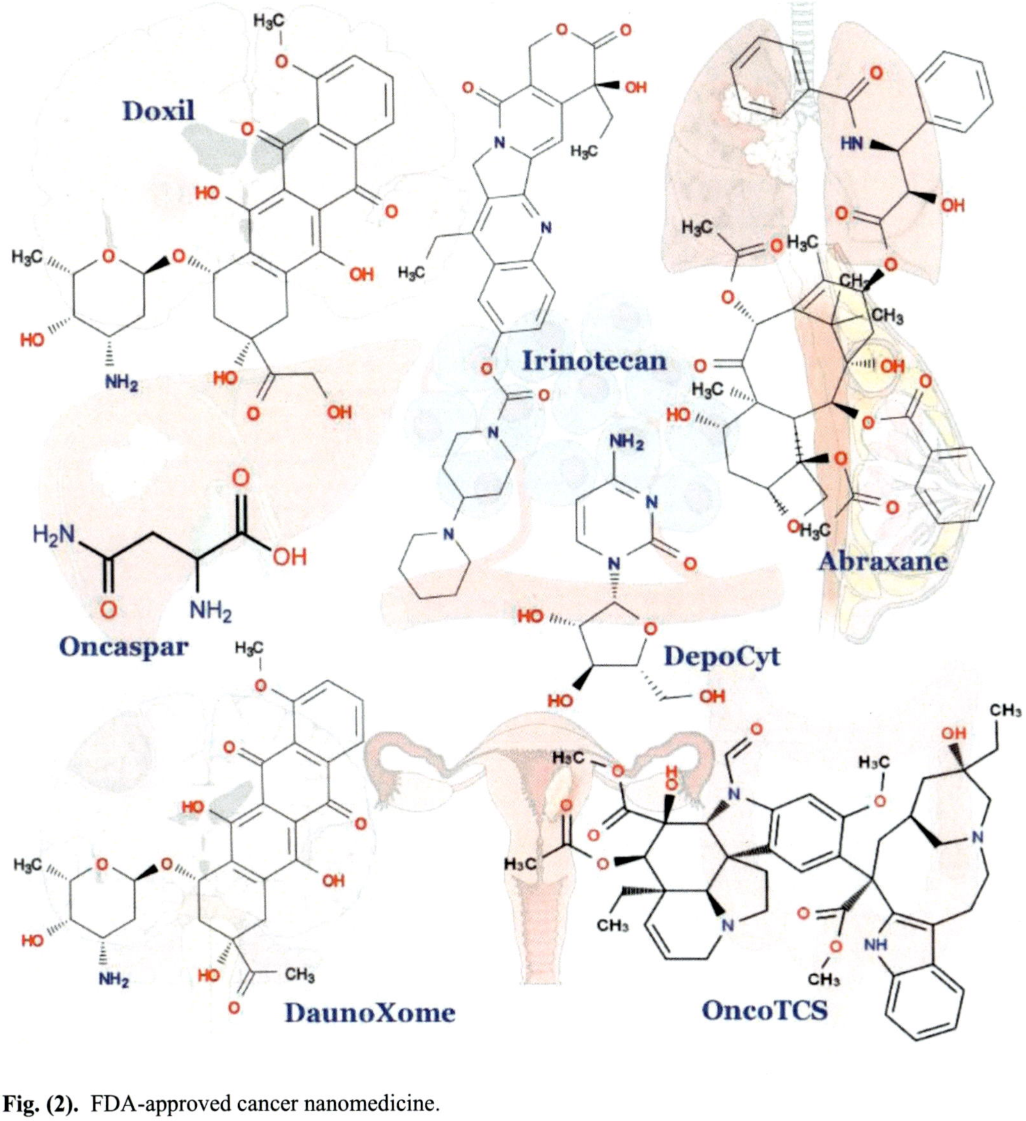

Fig. (2). FDA-approved cancer nanomedicine.

NANO-MATERIALS FOR CANCER TREATMENT

Many nanotechnology-based system innovations were aimed at taking advantage of nano-materials' characteristics that transport therapeutic compounds to malignant tissue, including nanoparticles, liposomes, drug conjugates, and micelles. They've been enough to help with the new formulation of existing cancer treatments and the innovation of quality medicines (Table **1**) to decrease tumours and major cancer occurrences without harming normal tissue. Such materials come in various shapes and sizes and can be included metallic, lipidic, proteinic, or polymeric. They could be used to enhance cellular uptake and/or facilitate drug solubilization or enzymatic stabilization *via* complexing and covalently translating with medication. In several instances, such materials were also designed to target cells ("*e.g.*, Doxil®, Genexol, Marqibo®, Taxotere®, DaunoXome®,") and positively ("*e.g.*, MCC-465 & Tf-LPN-G3139") through exploiting the unique characteristics of such cancer's microenvironment ("namely the Enhanced Permeability and Retention (EPR effect) and the surface enzymatic activities of tumour cells") [34 - 45].

Table 1. Various nano-materials approved from FDA for cancer management.

S. No.	Nanotechnology Plateform	Drug Product	Active Ingredient	Types of Cancer Targeting	Manufacturer	Approved year/ Clinical Trials Status
1	Drug-polymer conjugate	Oncaspar	L-asparaginase	Acute Lymphocytic Leukemia	Enzon	FDA (1994)
	Liposome	Doxil	Doxorubicin	Breast cancer, Kaposi's sarcoma	Janssen Products, LP	EMA (1996); FDA (1995)
2	Liposome	Myocet	Non-PEGylate-DOX	Breast cancer	Teva UK	EMA (2000)
3	Liposome	DaunoXome	Non-PEGylated -DOX	Kaposi's sarcoma	Galen	FDA (1996)
4	Nanoparticles (protein-bound particles)	Abraxane	Paclitaxel	Pancreatic, lung and breast cancer	Celgene	FDA (2005) EMA (2008)
5	Liposome	Marqibo	Vincristine	Acute lymphoblastic leukemia and Philadelphia (Ph) chromosome	Spectrum	FDA (2012)
6	Liposome	Onivyde MM-398	Irinotecan hydrochloride	Pancreatic cancer	Merrimack	FDA (2015)
7	Liposome	MEPACT	Mifamurtide	Treatment for osteosarcoma	Millennium	EMA (2009)

(Table 1) cont.....

S. No.	Nanotechnology Plateform	Drug Product	Active Ingredient	Types of Cancer Targeting	Manufacturer	Approved year/ Clinical Trials Status
8	Micelles	Taxoter	Docetaxel	NSLCS, Prostate, Gastric cancer and Breast cancer	-	ANDA (1996)
9	Liposme	VYXEOS CPX-351	Cytarabin:daunorubicin (5:1M ratio)	Acute myeloid leukemia	Jazz Pharmaceuticals	FDA (2017) EMA (2018)
10	Lipid Nanoparticles	ONPATTRO Patisiran ALN-TTR02	Lipid nanoparticle RNAi for the knockdown of disease-causing TTR protein	Transthyretin (TTR)-mediated amyloidosis	Alnylam Pharmaceuticals	FDA (2018) EMA (2018
11	Nanoparticles	NBTXR3 Hensify	Hafnium oxide nanoparticles	Locally advanced squamous cell carcinoma	Nanobiotix	CE Market (2019)

The use of twin chemotherapeutic medications combined into a single brand was one of two new ideas in nanoparticle cancer therapy that is, "CPX-1, CPX-351 & ALN-VSP" and also two components that require the use of such environmental stimulation that engages its item. The second generation of pharmaceuticals, which employ "SMART" manufacturing techniques, were developed to activate when subjected to heat, ultrasound, radiofrequency, and even other resource signals. Such product can then alternate (that is, Thermodox®) and allow the nanoparticle that directly influences each cell, for instance, selectively raising the temperature within such a cell, which could alter permeability and induce direct cell damage (*i.e.*, Auroshell and NanoTherm™) [34, 46 - 48]. Various nano-materials approved by FDA for cancer management are depicted in Table **1**.

Liposomal Doxorubicin (Doxil)

Doxil ("pegylated liposomal doxorubicin") was the first FDA-approved nano-drug in 1995, and it is used for treating diseases like metastatic ovarian tumours and Kaposi's sarcoma, which is linked to AIDS. The drug was created to balance doxorubicin's therapeutic toxicity and efficacy better. This contains anthracycline doxorubicin (Adriamycin) encapsulated in such a unilamellar liposome of 80-90 nm covered by PEG, which permits the medicine to stay within that bloodstream and reaches the cancer cell more effectively [49 - 52]. The chances of chronic cardiac problems differ depending on the total dose and circumstances. This has fewer adverse effects upon healthy cells when delivered as liposomes than conventional doxorubicin [53 - 55]. "Llipodox from Sun Pharma, Evacet from Liposome business INC., Caelyx from Janssen-Cilag, Europe, and Doxil from Johnson & Johnson, USA," are all names for liposomal doxorubicin. PEG surface coating sterically stabilizes liposomes. "Distearoyl-phosphatidyl-ethanolami-e-PEG (DSPE-PEG)" is linked to phospholipid bilayers, formed of ""cholesterol and hydrogenated soy phosphatidylcholine" to achieve surface coating of PEG [56]. The FDA has placed doxorubicin hydrochloride liposome shot on its medication shortage list. To alleviate medicine shortages, "the US Food and Drug Administration (FDA)" licensed "Sun Pharma Global FZE", the subsidiary of India's "Sun Pharmaceutical Industries Ltd", to produce the very first common form of Doxil. Lipodox [57] would be a second-generation "pegylated liposomal doxorubicin" made out (up) of "cholesterol and distearoyl phosphatidylcholine (DSPC)" with a cholesterol PEG surface coating. By such a passive targeting method, lipodox and Doxil (each pegylated) aggregate at tumour cells.

Myocet

Enzon Pharmaceuticals manufactures Myocet, "the non-pegylated liposomal doxorubicin citrate" for Cephalon throughout Europe, and Spherion Therapies throughout Canada and US. On December 21, 2001, Myocet was authorized in Canada as the very first metastatic tumor medication in association with cyclophosphamide. Myocet was also legal in Europe, although not in the U.S. It is being tested in conjunction (combination) with Taxol (paclitaxel) and Herceptin (trastuzumab) to treat HER2-positive metastatic breast tumors [58].

The Myocet liposome comprises cholesterol and egg phosphatidylcholine within a 55:45 molar ratio and includes 50 mg doxorubicin hydrochloride. The liposome's diameter is roughly 180 nm. One syringe contains doxorubicin HCl lyophilized red powder, the other has a liposome solution in sodium chloride and citric acid, and the third vial has a sodium carbonate solution. Myocet (60-75 mg/m2) is prescribed at first (as the first line of action), followed by cyclophosphamide (600 mg/m2) every three weeks. The elimination of doxorubicin was 5-9 times lower in patients with breast cancer getting Myocet [59, 60]. While Doxil and Myocet use the same API within liposomes (While the same API within liposomes is used in Doxil and Myocet), their lipid content, shape, loaded mechanism, plasma, and cell dispersion characteristics, and also dosing and toxicity characteristics are all different. They are not bio-equivalent in any way.

ThermoDox

To maximize medication distribution just (particularly) at the pathological region, a method was developed to lead revolutionary nanoformulations concentrates upon nanosystems that may be triggered to discharge their contents when subjected to external stimuli like light, ultrasound, heat, and magnetic fields. "ThermoDox" was made up of 90:10:4 molar ratios of "dipalmitoylphosphatidylcholine (DPPC), monostearoyl phosphatidylcholine, and PEG2000 DSPE (distearoyl phosphatidylethanolamine)". Because DPPC does have a 41.5°C transition temperature, it is suitable for temperature-stimulated innovation [61, 62].

Liposomal Daunorubicin (DaunoXome)

Anthracycline antibiotic daunorubicin has antineoplastic action. A glycosidic relationship connects the anthracycline molecule to a daunosamine, amino-sugar. The daunorubicin citrate solution is encapsulated in liposomes composed of "di-stearoyl phosphatidylcholine, cholesterol, and daunorubicin in a molar ratio of 10:5:1", including that (that includes) 45 nm mean diameter and a total lipid with the 18.7:1 daunorubicin ratio. The liposome shot does have a pH of 4.9 to 6 and even a red, transparent dispersion. In 1996, the FDA approved this for "HIV-associated Kaposi sarcoma" [63].

Paclitaxel protein-bound, Albumin-bound Paclitaxel (Abraxane)

Paclitaxel (Taxol, Bristol-Myers Squibb) is a member of a class of anti-cancer drugs known as taxanes. Paclitaxel would be a semisynthetic diterpenoid taxane compound used to treat several cancers, particularly breast cancer, lung disease, anti-cell lung disease, and ovarian tumor. Taxanes were cell cycle-specific drugs that will bind to microtubules with a high affinity, preventing mitosis and the death of cells.

Paclitaxel: Taxanes are extremely hydrophobic compounds with such low water solubility. To increase the solubility of paclitaxel, a castor oil compound termed "polyethoxylated castor oil," and ethanol 50:50 is employed. The polyethoxylated castor oil is called cremophore EL, a non-ionic surfactant [64]. Abraxane, albumin-bound paclitaxel, does not have a chromophore. As a result, there is no need for premedication and unique apparatus to give Abraxane. "Abraxane (Abraxis Bioscience/ Celgene)" has been FDA approved for the advanced anti-small cell lung tumor treatment in carboplatin of patients who have not been eligible for therapeutic surgery. Abraxane, however, has shown promise in the treatment of pancreatic tumors [65], and then the FDA extended its approval in 2013 to cover metastatic pancreatic cancer. To obtain increased intra-tumoral levels, albumin-bound paclitaxel would be the first biological therapeutic compound using "gp60 receptors (albondin)-mediated" route within endothelial cell membranes of cancer microvessels. Due to albumin-receptor (gp60) induced endothelium transcytosis, Abraxane composition boosted paclitaxel bioavailability and led to higher intra-tumor levels [66 - 68].

Cell therapies are working on a new paclitaxel nanocarrier named "Paclitaxel poliglumex (PPX)." "Xyotax, Opaxio, and CT 2103" are all brand names for this product. This is a massive macromolecular combination of paclitaxel with poly-L-Glutamic acid soluble and includes 37% paclitaxel. Poly-L glutamic acid would be a biodegradable polymer. Paclitaxel was rendered inactive when attached towards (to/with) the polymer, possibly protecting normal tissue from the harmful effects of high concentrations of paclitaxel. PPX develops (spread/grows) in cancer cells due to its enormous size, taking advantage of the increasing susceptibility of damaged tissue as well as the absence of lymphatic outflow. The intrinsic lysosomal enzyme cathepsin B and protease, which have been linked to an increase in numerous forms of cancer, are responsible for initially releasing the drug from the polymeric backbone [69]. Clinical trials with animal tumor analysis show that PPX seems more beneficial than harmful paclitaxel and is linked to longer usable drug exposure in the tumor, thus decreasing therapeutic efficacy. Compared to typical taxanes, stage 1 & 2 medical studies using PPX revealed promising results, including decreased neutropenia or alopecia [69].

EndoTAG-1

Since May 2012, "Medigene AG (a Munich-based biotechnology business)" has received a US patent on EndoTag®-1 (previously known as lipo pack) for such therapy of triple-negative breast tumor. There are no HER2 receptors and estrogen or progesterone hormone receptors in triple-negative breast tumors. As traditional antihormonal medication and therapies addressing HER2 were ineffective in this tumor, several (other) treatment choices exist. Endotag®-1 would be a paclitaxel-containing cationic liposome. The liposome was made up of "12 dioleoyl-3-trimethylammonium-propane (DOTAP), 12 dioleoyl-sn-glycero-3-phosphocho line (DOPC), and paclitaxel" in a 50:45:5 molar ratio with only a diameter of 220 nm. Endotag®-1 addresses the cancer cells while leaving healthy tissue's endothelial cells unaffected. This inhibits tumor growth by preventing the production of a new cancer vascular system, enhancing cancer vascular permeability [70].

Liposomal Cisplatin (Lipoplatin)

Lipoplatin is a pharmacological product of the FDA-approved toxic agent cisplatin that is liposomal encapsulated, having a diameter of around 110 nm.

Nephrotoxicity is a serious issue when cisplatin or other platinum drugs are used. "Cisplatin (cis-diamino dichloro-platinum)" is enclosed inside a liposome coat made up of "dipalmitoyl phosphatidylglycerol, soy phosphatidylcholine, cholesterol, and a lipid conjugate of methoxy-polyethylene glycol-distearoyl phosphatidyl-ethanolamine". A cisplatin to lipids ratio is 8.9%: 91.1% & (8.9:91.1 w/w) [71, 72]. As first-line therapy for pancreatic cancer, lipoplatine was combined with gemcitabine. "For non-small cell lung cancer (NSCLC) adenocarcinomas", it outperformed cisplatin in conjunction with paclitaxel as a chemotherapy treatment. Lipoplatin grows in tumor cells due to nanoparticle extravasation through the tumor tissue's faulty vasculature throughout neoangiogenesis. Total platinum has a half-life of 60-117 hours in human plasma, compared to 6 hours with cisplatin [73]. The European Medicines Agency (EMA) approved Lipoplatin, also known as Nanoplatin, in 2009 and has been evaluated as the first treatment for non-squamous NSCLC, which is mostly made up of adenocarcinomas.

Onco TCS: Vincristine

The alkaloids vincristine (VCR) and vinblastine (VLB) are derived from the seedling of the*Catharanthus roseus,* also known as Madagascar periwinkle. Each has potent anti-cancer properties. "Vincristine sulphate liposome injection (Marqibo®), produced by Talon Therapeutics, Inc.)" for the management of "Philadelphia chromosome-negative (Ph) acute lymphoblastic leukaemia (ALL)" has been granted accelerated approval by the FDA on August 9, 2012 [74, 75]. For such therapy of recurrent severe "non-lymphoma Hodgkin's (NHL)" and other cancers, INEX Pharmaceuticals are producing the liposomal preparation with vincristine-like Vincristine sulfate liposomes for injection (VSLI), vincamine, and Onco TCS". Vincristine has been created by employing INEX's patented "transmembrane carrier systems (TCS)" medication technology platform.

Vinorelbine

Vinorelbine, the microtubule regulator, would be a semi-synthetic vinca alkaloid that has been demonstrated to be effective in treating small-cell lung cancer, heart disease, uterine cancer, Kaposi sarcoma, cervical cancer, and head and neck cancer. Allocrest would be a new vinorelbine composition that contains vinorelbine tartrate enclosed within the hydrophilic portion of the liposome. Such a composition was designed to meet focused medication delivery at large levels throughout cancer and long-term release. In managing elderly malignancy patients and individuals with consistently low condition, the possibility of offering increased (high) anti-cancer effectiveness without increased toxicity was significant. Nanovinorelbine (nanovnb) is effective in human breast tumors and lung tumor xenografts [76].

DepoCyt (Liposomal Cytarabine)

DepoCyt has become a cytarabine-prolonged liposomal compound (prolonged cytarabine liposomal compound/ sustained-release form of liposomal cytarabine compound) made (formulated/synthesized) with a proprietary termed DepoFoam (formulation). The DepoFoam is often a multivesicular system with hundreds of liquid divisions divided by a bilayer membrane, unlike the standard unilamellar and significant unilamellar liposomes. This structure enables the absorption of vast amounts of pharmaceuticals while ensuring long-term release [77 - 79].

The FDA gave full approval to cytarabine liposome shot (DepoCyt, Enzon Pharmaceuticals") in April 2007, and for lymphomatous meningitis treatment, the existence of lymphoma complications. It became approved under accelerated approval rules in April 1999, depending on a higher success rate than the unencapsulated medication. Cytarabine is an antineoplastic drug that affects cells only during the cell division of the s-phase. Depocyt was widely dispersed in the cerebrospinal fluid, allowing tumor cells to be continuously subjected to cytarabine. "Dioleoyl phosphatidylcholine, dipalmitoyl phosphatidylglycerol, cholesterol, and triolein" are all found in the liposome. This is a protectant, long-acting formula. This formulation had a pharmacokinetic benefit: the final half-life is 40 times bigger than usual cytarabine [80, 81].

Annamycin

Annamycin, a chemically synthesized doxorubicin analog, was developed at the M.D. Anderson Cancer Center in Houston, Texas. Annamycin was first studied as an anti-cancer medication without the antibiotic resistance associated with p-glycoprotein [82]. Annamycin, unlike doxorubicin, will not have an amino group throughout the sugar moiety. Annamycin is a DNA intercalator that suppresses topoisomerase II. As a result, DNA replication, repairing, and protein synthesis with RNA are all inhibited. Compared to annamycin, liposomal annamycin becomes less toxic and has better anti-cancer activity and is used to treat breast cancer [83, 84].

Oncaspar (Asparaginase)

Leading to a shortage of asparagine synthesis, leukemic cells are often unable to manufacture asparagine and must rely upon an external phase of asparagine to survive. The enzyme asparaginase reduces the amino acid asparagine. Asparagine depletion (malnutrition of leukemic cells) results in leukemic cell damage.

Because normal cells can produce asparagine, they have become less harmed. L-asparaginase was used to treat acute lymphoblastic leukemia (ALL) for many years [85, 86]. Oncaspar is a modified version of the enzyme L-asparaginase. The tetrameric protein is covalently conjugated by monomethoxy polyethylene glycol and is produced by E.coli (MPEG). L-Asparaginase is related to approximately 69-82 molecules in MPEG. Each MPEG molecule does have a molecular weight of 5 kDa (KDa). The FDA approved PEG asparaginase (Enzon) for treating acute lymphoblastic leukemia (ALL) in July 1994. Throughout the 20-week treatment, fewer pharmaceutical injections were needed when Oncaspar was used instead of L-asparaginase, with 21 shots of Elspar (L-asparaginase) and three injections of Oncaspar [87]. Compared to native L-asparaginase (non-pegylated version), Oncaspar includes treatment having all of the benefits of asparaginase treatment while also being more convenient [87].

Camptothecins

Lurtotecan

Lurtotecanis is a potent semi-synthetic derivative of Camptothecin. It is a water-soluble analog. Topoisomerase inhibitor, utilized for cancer, occurs in the epithelial ovary. Lurtotecan devise in the liposomes is called unilamellar [88, 89].

Irinotecan (NKTR-102)

There is another substance (drug) called irinotecan which is added in the group called fluorouracil, and its result presented in the first main development in frequent ages inside the action of colorectal tumor which amalgamation of application of a quantity of medicine develop into the good care [90]. Nektar has developed Irinotecan. Most of the therapeutics have pegylated the formulation of liposomal to cure colorectal cancer. A new therapeutic choice also improved for breast cancer is called NKTR-102, which acts as a topoisomerase I inhibitor. This NKTR-102 has been considered to get into the vasculature tumor and its surroundings readily compared with common vasculature; it enhances the focus on active medication in the cancer tissue, improving the anti-cancer potency. Approval of irinotecan was received in 1996, and in 1998, it received complete approval. It is called CPT-11 while it is being improved in the process.

REGULATORY GUIDELINES FOR NANO-MATERIAL-BASED FORMULATION

The FDA's prescription review approach is the same regardless of the substance that incorporates nanoparticles; nevertheless, certain agencies have not authorized the use of nano-materials [91]. However, it helped some industries to discover the utilization of nanoformulations techniques in the production of nano-materials and the authorities provided an approval file of FDA- activated materials that involve the utilization of nanotechnology [92]. Direction files are the method/guidelines by which an organization interacts with the public and industry, and they lead 'FDA's recent recognition of the topic. It does not produce the correct function of FDA [93]. According to the guidance of nanotechnology [92], FDA sponsors value and submits the applications of medication products:

1. A material or final product is designed to get one internal or external dimension of surface structure in the nanoscale range.

2. A material or final product is designed to exhibit the characteristics /phenomena, which consist of chemical and physical properties and biological effects characteristic to its size, even though the dimension drops out of the nanoscale range (1000 nm).

The acting guidelines medication of nanotechnology characteristics particular guidances, *e.g.*, Product-specific bioequivalence for classes of materials, *e.g.*, Liposome guidance. Nanoparticle expertise is an example of the materials of a particular direction of bioequivalence of lanreotide acetate direction [94] injection based on polymer [95]. The FDA accepts some primarily consisting of active focusing and various nanotechnologies, and supplementary advice may be specified to speed up the application evaluation and submission process. This must be mentioned in the FDA's detailed analysis of the capitulation of pharmaceutical materials that contain nano-materials. As per the review, the approval rate of medication items containing nano-materials was compared to biologics and small molecules [96].

THE APPLICATION REVIEW PROCESS

In the review process, Fig. (**3**) explains the medication improvement process and methods of application that the FDA sponsor presents. Once CDER/FDA receives a medication application, it is given to a proper division for feedback, depending on the 'material's indication for new medication or some dosage from generic medications. Once the new medication successfully passes preclinical trials, it is tested with the help of animals for studies to ensure the sponsor decides whether the materials are safe to be used on human beings.

A fee to submit an (IND) Investigational New Drug Application to the US FDA is necessary for the first medication testing of a human being. There are various kinds of Investigational new drugs that have been deliberated under [97]:

• An investigator IND is filed by a professional who begins and supervises a study and is directly responsible for the administration or dispensing of the experimental medicine. In addition, a specialist may file a clinical IND to examine an investigational medicine or an established medication for a new drug or in a different patient group.

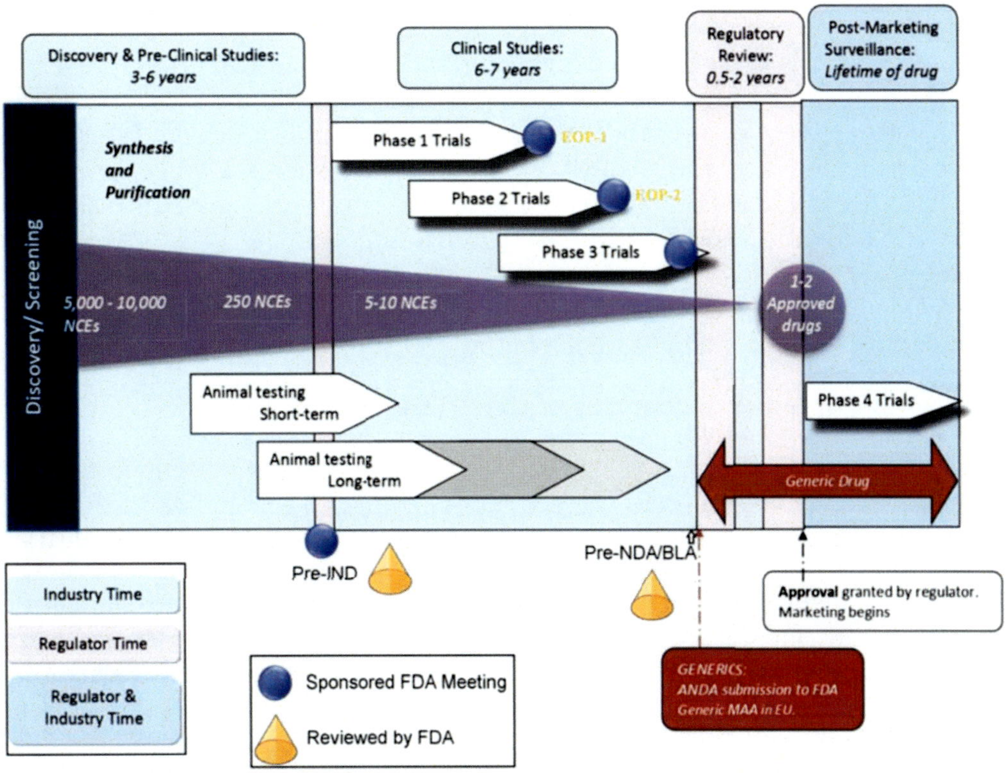

Fig. (3). Representation of the guideline for drug formulation. EOP-2: End of Phase II; ; EOP-1: End of Phase I; NDA: New Drug Application; BLA: Biologics License Application; IND: Investigational New Drug [138].

• Uses in an emergency In compliance with 21 CFR 312 Section 312.23 & Section 312.20 of the Federal regulations code, an IND authorizes the FDA to approve the use of an investigational medicine in an emergency that would not require longer for the filing of an IND. It is also utilized for individuals who would not satisfy the requirements of an established research process or who do not have access to an authorized research design.

• A treatment IND is filed for investigational treatments that have shown potential in clinical studies for severe or urgently life-threatening illnesses. In contrast, the clinical construction is finished, and the FDA evaluation is underway.

An IND mainly consists of details and qualifications of the researcher and the researched medication, producing information about animal toxicology and pharmacology studies, and medical study actions [97, 98]. The sponsor should wait 30 days before initiating medical (clinical) trials, once the Investigational New Drug is presented. Meanwhile, the FDA gets to screen the Investigational New Drug for safety (safeness) to guarantee that researched patients are not exposed to unnecessary risks). An investigational new drug has been authorized, and medical trains have started evaluating Phase I clinical trials utilizing a selected population of healthy individuals to determine the dose and tolerance of health effects [99]. As a result, if the Phase I test demonstrates the safety of the healthy patient/person, the medication will then be tested in a bigger population *via* Phase II and Phase III trials of the researched compound to assess medication safety, toxicity and efficacy in the diseased subject/patient [40]. The sponsors submit/present New Drug Application (NDA) to the FDA by summarizing the clinical studies obtained from early Phase III or end of Phase II, which determine the medication efficacy and its toxicity [100].

Types of NDA, as per Section 505 of the FD&C Act

***505(b)(1)*:** The application is being used for a unique medication containing active materials that have not been agreed upon before. The application contains complete investigation information on effectiveness/efficacy and safety [101].

***505(b)(2)*:** This submission is specifically for a novel drug molecule that depends on the last part, and the applicant has not developed information. The application has entire reports of research of effective and secure, some of the information is needed to get approval for studies and is not organized, or the applicant does not get a correct reference [102]. The applications 505 (b)(2) consist of changes in the form of dosage and strength administration route compared to agreeing on the product or other production with the good ingredient in an agreed combination material [103]. This application 505(b) (2) is always utilized for materials that consist of nano-materials, particularly the nano-material used to take previously agreed medication substances. *E.g.*, Taxol® got approved in the year 1998, and it utilized paclitaxel as an active material [104]. The next product is Abraxane® which consists of paclitaxel and was approved by FDA in the year 2005 under section 505 (b)(2) in the normal pathway [105].

Application 505(b)(1) and 505(b)(2) needs investigational new drugs and applications of NDA presented for review by FDA. Other side regulatory needs for investigational new drug applications are discussed in the chapter. The expected NDA comprises (CMC) chemistry, manufacturing, control of the data and medication substance and medication product and the data are availability, packaging information, labeling, analytical data for every form of dosage, and the sponsor propose the extra toxicological study, and it reports that are not mentioned in the application of IND [106].

Biologics License Application (BLA)

For biological, new medicine application items have been developed. The Public Health Service Act (PHS) requirements have been agreed upon for the sale of these biological products. The proposal request is the same as NDA, which consists of other data on manufacturing processes, pharmacology, chemistry, clinical pharmacology, and the medical effects of biological materials [107]. BLA requests are submitted to the Center for Biologics Evaluation and Research (CBER), which evaluates and researches biological materials. CDER and CBER attain BLA reference [108].

505(j) (Generics)

Fresh medication while developing some years the post has approved and it always secured control of patent to provide the sponsor and the time is precious to sell the medication and recover improvement amount. When the patent expires, the further companies also apply to the FDA to sell the generic versions of medication materials by using the ANDA [109, 110].

This application consists of data to discover the proposed materials in the same ingredient, strength, dosage form, quality, labeling, performance characteristic, intended use, route of administration, and other things the product agreed upon previously. Those applications are called ANDA applications; it does commonly not need to mention clinical and non-clinical information to give competence and security. Instead, the generic applicants are scientifically shown the bioequivalent products [110].

FDA supports timely in all cases, which transparent, effective interaction sponsor during medication improvement method. This result is highly efficient improvement programs that considering *via* FDA-sponsor interactions, the main issues are addressed in the initial stages of medication improvement. Meetings of FDA, while medication improvement particularly in a challenging time: end of the first phase, end of the second phase, pre- IND and pre-NDA/BLA meetings mentioned in Fig. (**3**) [111].

Suppose the medication is generic or new appreciation for the agreed stage, and the FDA needs to submit extra information of medication to assure the security and efficacy of period medication in the market. In that case, these are called phase IV, and in phase IV, the needs are mostly submitted in the post-approval.

For example, the post-marketing clinical test/studies have shown the secure power of medication support under the approval needs in phase IV.

SPECIAL REGULATORY PROVISION FOR CANCER PRODUCTS

For treatment, the address is unmet in clinical requirements for the treatment of severe conditions like cancer, and the FDA permits sponsors to allow the quick feedback method *via* four programs of FDA "fast track designation, breakthrough therapy designation, accelerated approval, and priority review designation" [112]. Many applications are approved in the programs expedited, which is undergoing the review of accelerated and thereby the facilitating of the initial product of new treatment to patients are quick shows the benefits of the risks. For new cancer, expedites available are crucial, particularly in some cases where no satisfactory treatments exist. Early in the development process, proponents of new chemotherapy drugs seek for development and revolutionary treatment categories, resulting in significant improvements in labels during BLA or NDA filing and expedited clearance accreditations throughout BLA or NDA review [113].

The FDA has designated CPX-351 as a groundbreaking therapy for managing myeloid leukaemia [114], as well as Doxil® for managing Kaposi's sarcoma [115] and Merrimack Pharmaceuticals' product Onivyde® for the management of severe pancreatic cancer [116]. These altered timelines have approached the feedback designed to develop the numerous novel treatment available for patients, according to the FDA, to enrich and promote public health.

REGULATORY CHALLENGES FOR NANOMEDICINES

The biggest problem for the maintenance of nanomedicines is real; the bodies of regulations like the FDA utilize secure information depending on the enormous materials that are not shown in the same pharmacokinetic and pharmacodynamic of nanomedicines methods [117]. This is called the information gathered on secure and powerful. It is not at all higher that nanomedicine is utilized in medical conditions when it is achieved in the marketing of authorization. These issues lead to maintaining the regulations of secure and powerful parameters of non-nano medicines versions that can correct the standards of nanomedicine [118]. The next big challenge has been practiced in the classification of nanomedicine. It can be divided into medicines, or the clinical devices are inconsistent across the world supervisor. This is called nanomedicine, and it can be classified in the medicine of one country and clinical device. Therefore the regulations should be adhered to change the basic divisions. For particular secure and robust standards, this should pass one market, and it will differ. Few countries will use nanomedicine that is not passed in the standards regulatory of another country [119]. In the year 2009, Owen and Rannard warned that one size does not correct in all times of nanomedicines, and it depends on their medical requirements and applications of physiology and route [120]; this is largely deleted in the recent frameworks. The complexity, size, form and medical application of nanomedicines challenge the regulatory bodies to categorize and characterize nanomedicines.

Frequently scale and producing methods are hit for nano-material and stability of nanomedicine [121]. Therefore the stringent procedure ensures the need for support [121]. There is a requirement to discover and manage producing methods in difficult points and basics to innovate the (CQA) critical quality attributes to improve the comprehensive of non-medicine producing ideas [122]. To highly difficult structures, materials are very critical to find a strong and steady manufacturing process that defines the nanomedicine's efficacy, quality, stability, and safety [123]. For a detailed explanation of critical quality, attributes would mean recognition and examination of properties of nanomedicine in the small-scale process of manufacturing which facilitates the comprehensive process of large-scale production [124].

Nanotoxicology and cellular response are other challenges faced by regulators [125]. There have been a large number of proposals on the possible ways of nanotoxicity measures. Measures of traditional toxicity of the main example of large-scale animal testing in the past of small medication molecules, it has been decreased and unethical deemed, and it is too precious and impractical that apply nanotoxicity of measurement [126].

While improving the nanomedicines for medical utilization, the device and act of medication delivery need to consider safety information before agreement, which includes adverse effects. The toxic effects are high medication dope of nano shape of the toxicity of specific cells or organs or appearance of antibiotic conflict. Additionally, the particle size of the pose gives a treat to 'patients' assigned better counterparts, which allows crossing the (BBC) blood-brain barrier, possibly compromising the functions of the brain in the long term of edema causing [127]. Factors are possibly, and it is important of enough information to convince the fresh form of drugs for safety method, which lead to agreement and later it may be canceled. All difficult challenges are mentioned, and it is highly warning of further nanomedicine to hindering the method of production insecure manner, and it is good quality products of nanomedicine, leading to an ineffective executive of nanoparticles to insufficient of nanomedicine of particular secure actions. Clear and consistent directions are coming from the agencies of governing, which are extremely unlikely, the success of small and understand of filled potential.

GLOBAL STRATEGIES FOR THE REGULATION OF NANO-MATERIALS FOR DRUG DELIVERY AND TARGETING FOR ANTI-CANCER SUBSTANCES

European Medicines Agency has applied legislation to regulate nanomedicines. Simultaneously, it creates exclusive multidisciplinary expertise to determine nanomedicines using the current risk and benefit-analysis concept. A detailed explanation of nanomedicine and a list of specific guidelines regarding nanomedicine have been constructed, which can be searched on the website. The European Nanomedicines Expert Group was set up by the EMA in the year 2009 to meet the increasing demand for 'nanomedicine's therapeutic assessment from stakeholders. Established academics and regulatory science professionals from the Expert Group have been in touch with regulatory professionals from other regulatory agencies like FDA [128].

USA

Till the present time, FDA has to regulate the products of nanotechnology, which includes nanomedicines, by utilizing the recent regulatory and statutory authorities and also the product-specific standards under the authority. FDA created draft guidelines for medication products in the year 2017, that consist of biological materials as well as nano-materials. The FDA has never permitted nanotechnology to be classified as secure/safe or hazardous, yet every nanotechnology has been evaluated/determined based on case-by-case [129]. It must be noted that the FDA discovered various attributes regarding their regulatory/agency approach. Various organizations also participate in the nanomedicines regulations like NCL-NCI (Nanotechnology Characterization Laboratory of National Cancer Institute); they (which) have been participating for nearly 10 years. The FDA formed the Nanotechnology Task Force and Nanotechnology Interest Group comprised of representatives from many regulatory centers to tackle the issue of regulating nanotechnology worldwide. Despite this, the FDA is yet to produce a clear set of guidelines, rather, the Task Force has concluded that pre-existing regulations are comprehensive enough to ensure the safe production of nanomedicines as these products undergo premarket testing and approval under the New Drug Application process.

UK

Medicines and Healthcare products Regulatory Agency (MHRA) regulates nano-materials and their related products in the UK. No clear/apparent/salient direction/guideline has been given for the approval of nanomedicine, similar to the FDA, which reviews on a case-by-case basis. Researchers developing nanomedicines are encouraged to liaise with the MHRA Innovation Office for guidance and steering through the process. In common with the US, other organizations, such as the European Nanomedicine Characterization Laboratory (EU-NCL), which is based across the UK and EU, provide and constantly refine knowledge on preclinical characterization assays of nanomedicine [130].

EU

The development in the EU is the consequence of (from the) difficult task force and collaboration that join together to establish the formal meaning of nano-material in various accounts and visiting from food touch, health, and the environment. Various initiatives, including REFINE and EU-NCL proposals, have been launched, and the government has established projects to participate in the development of the field [131 - 133]. Not like the UK, the body of regulation in EU (European Medicines Agency-EMA) has established a particular range and direction of the preparation of nanomedicine values [134]. The informal regulatory direction has taken a leading place in the public discussion stage. The EU-NCL has worked closely with regulatory organizations to inform and influence decision-making on potentially hazardous materials regulation of such nano-materials.

Canada & Japan

Health Portfolio Nanotechnology Working Group is established in Canada for the gathering and discussion of issues related to nanotechnology, which consists of representatives from regulatory bodies like Health Canada and the Canadian Institutes of Health Research (CIHR). Basic Japanese medication is controlled by the MHLW (Ministry of Health, Labor, Welfare) and also PMDA (Pharmaceuticals and Medical Devices Agency). The Japanese regulatory bodies have yet to come up with a definition as well as nanomedicine-specific regulations for nanomedicines [135]. Directions for the improvement of liposome medication materials are issued in the year 2016. Nanomedicines are controlled by the pharmaceutical framework that is common in the product of medicinal legislation. It must be mentioned the reviewer and controller are gathering and analyzing the information of nanomedicine. PMDA and MHLW had combined with EMA to issue reflection papers and mentioned the development of the medication materials like nucleic acids (siRNA) based nano-materials and also medication products based on nanotechnology.

Others

While there is a small guideline concerning the field of nanotechnology in Asia, other countries like China, India, Thailand, and Japan are recently settling on a governing structure to meet the emerging challenge in nanotechnology's position.

Department of Science and Technology (DST-India), Government of India has created a team to control nanotechnology, and a list of guidance was drafted in making of the three-tiered framework of governance that has been applied to manage the policies to improve the way of nanomedicine regulation in India.

FUTURE PERSPECTIVE

At this time, the Agency anticipates continued interest in developing products utilizing a variety of nanotechnology platforms, some familiar and some novel. In particular, there will likely be an expansion of nanotechnology in cancer therapeutics designed to improve passive and active (triggered) targeting capabilities. Numerous drug-development medications employ multipurpose nanocomposites for tumour localization with or without a targeted delivery in the hopes of improving potency over current treatments. Technology is also looking into using nanoscale materials delivery strategies to deliver natural chemotherapeutic medications, which might add to the total intricacy of the goods. Such techniques might potentially be used to develop treatments that target numerous organs or operative locations. Whenever confronted with all these novel tactics, the FDA seems to have a number of choices for responding. The established guidelines apply as applicable to any new device based on a unique system or innovation. When additional features or CQAs emerge pertinent, they will be addressed in a particular manner, perhaps leading to the production of commodity guidelines that can subsequently be expanded to cover a group of goods. FDA may make use of similar technology as well. The Organization, for instance, has reviewed specific antibodies that may transport a chemical or radioactivity element to a specific location. Tailored biomaterials and pharmacological formulations utilizing nanoparticles have significant similarities, and analogies can be established between both types of products. Resemblances have indeed been discussed before [136]. In certain circumstances, the sponsor may be required to build an advanced production method in order to manufacture the new technology platform. The FDA designed the Innovative Technology Plan to contribute to the progress and assessment of modern production methodologies. This program allows promoters to review the method with administration specialists before submitting a legislative application. These meetings are intended to uncover possible sponsor issues and raise FDA knowledge of the novel method before the evaluation period starts, benefiting both organizations. FDA predicts that though these techniques advance, additional generic manufacturers of the drugs will emerge. This seems to be crucial to examine since complicated compositions and production methods may influence the formation of generic brands of medicinal goods, and a paucity of generic brands of drugs can contribute to higher consumer prices and a greater risk of adverse drug events.

Nanotechnology's influence on the generic drug development phase has indeed been thoroughly examined [137].

CONCLUSION

It is anticipated that drug products will become more complicated in order to meet unmet medical needs. Such complexity spans all indications and routes of administration and includes both drug products containing nano-materials and those taking advantage of other technologies. With the increased incorporation of nano-materials in cancer therapeutics, industry and regulatory authorities should strive for product understanding that involves adequate characterization of the nano-material, understanding of its intended use and application, and how it relates to product quality, patient safety, and efficacy. Nanodrug development has advanced significantly during the past decade. Dozens of nano drugs have received FDA approval, and many more are in the early stages of development or in clinical trials. Most of the currently approved nanodrugs are based on conventional drugs that had already been approved and are composed of simple NPs. However, nanodrug platforms are incorporating a broadening range of NP types and becoming more complex. Even though few nanodrugs in the early stages of development will ultimately receive regulatory approval, the amount of work in this field predicts that many new nanodrugs will eventually be available for clinical use.

CONSENT FOR PUBLICATION

Not applicable.

CONFLICT OF INTEREST

The authors declare no conflict of interest, financial or otherwise.

ACKNOWLEDGEMENT

We are thankful to the team at Bentham Science Publishers for giving us this opportunity, Dr. Neeraj Mishra, the editor of this book, and everyone who supported us directly or indirectly while writing this chapter.

REFERENCES

[1] Bobo D, Robinson KJ, Islam J, Thurecht KJ, Corrie SR. Nanoparticle-based medicines: A review of FDA-approved materials and clinical trials to date. Pharm Res 2016; 33(10): 2373-87. [http://dx.doi.org/10.1007/s11095-016-1958-5] [PMID: 27299311]

[2] Caster JM, Patel AN, Zhang T, Wang A. Investigational nanomedicines in 2016: a review of nanotherapeutics currently undergoing clinical trials. Wiley Interdiscip Rev Nanomed Nanobiotechnol 2017; 9(1). [http://dx.doi.org/10.1002/wnan.1416] [PMID: 27312983]

[3] Ventola CL. The nanomedicine revolution: part 1: emerging concepts. P&T 2012; 37(9): 512-25. [PMID: 23066345]

[4] Havel HA. Where are the nanodrugs? An industry perspective on development of drug products containing nano-materials. AAPS J 2016; 18(6): 1351-3. [http://dx.doi.org/10.1208/s12248-016-9970-6] [PMID: 27520380]

[5] Havel H, Finch G, Strode P, *et al.* Nanomedicines: From bench to bedside and beyond. AAPS J 2016; 18(6): 1373-8. [http://dx.doi.org/10.1208/s12248-016-9961-7] [PMID: 27480318]

[6] James K, Highsmith J, Evers P. Nanotechnology market-nanotechnology markets in healthcare & medicine. Drug Des Deliv 2014; 14(9): 43-5.

[7] Chidambaram M, Manavalan R, Kathiresan K. Nanotherapeutics to overcome conventional cancer chemotherapy limitations. J Pharm Pharm Sci 2011; 14(1): 67-77. [http://dx.doi.org/10.18433/J30C7D] [PMID: 21501554]

[8] Suzuki R, Omata D, Oda Y, Unga J, Negishi Y, Maruyama K. Cancer therapy with nanotechnology-based drug delivery systems: Applications and challenges of liposome technologies for advanced cancer therapy. Nano-materials in Pharmacology 2016; pp. 457-82.

[9] Thakor AS, Gambhir SS. Nanooncology: The future of cancer diagnosis and therapy. CA Cancer J Clin 2013; 63(6): 395-418. [http://dx.doi.org/10.3322/caac.21199] [PMID: 24114523]

[10] Blanco E, Hsiao A, Mann AP, Landry MG, Meric-Bernstam F, Ferrari M. Nanomedicine in cancer therapy: Innovative trends and prospects. Cancer Sci 2011; 102(7): 1247-52. [http://dx.doi.org/10.1111/j.1349-7006.2011.01941.x] [PMID: 21447010]

[11] Sumer B, Gao J. Theranostic nanomedicine for cancer. Nanomedicine (Lond) 2008; 3(2): 137-40. [http://dx.doi.org/10.2217/17435889.3.2.137] [PMID: 18373419]

[12] 'D'Mello SR, Cruz CN, Chen M-L, Kapoor M, Lee SL, Tyner KM. The evolving landscape of drug products containing nano-materials in the United States. Nat Nanotechnol 2017; 12(6): 523-9. [http://dx.doi.org/10.1038/nnano.2017.67] [PMID: 28436961]

[13] Hoshyar N, Gray S, Han H, Bao G. The effect of nanoparticle size on *in vivo* pharmacokinetics and cellular interaction. Nanomedicine (Lond) 2016; 11(6): 673-92. [http://dx.doi.org/10.2217/nnm.16.5] [PMID: 27003448]

[14] Golombek SK, May JN, Theek B, *et al.* Tumor targeting *via* EPR: Strategies to enhance patient responses. Adv Drug Deliv Rev 2018; 130: 17-38. [http://dx.doi.org/10.1016/j.addr.2018.07.007] [PMID: 30009886]

[15] Sindhwani S, Syed AM, Ngai J, *et al.* The entry of nanoparticles into solid tumours. Nat Mater 2020; 19(5): 566-75. [http://dx.doi.org/10.1038/s41563-019-0566-2] [PMID: 31932672]

[16] Xia Y, Halas NJ. Shape-Controlled Synthesis and Surface Plasmonic Properties of Metallic Nanostructures. MRS Bull 2005; 30(5): 338-48. [http://dx.doi.org/10.1557/mrs2005.96]

[17] Paliwal R, Babu RJ, Palakurthi S. Nanomedicine scale-up technologies: feasibilities and challenges. AAPS PharmSciTech 2014; 15(6): 1527-34. [http://dx.doi.org/10.1208/s12249-014-0177-9] [PMID: 25047256]

[18] Cancer data statistics. Centers for Disease Control and Prevention https://www.cdc.gov/cancer/dcpc/data/

[19] National Cancer Institute. Cancer Moonshot https://www.cancer.gov/research/key-initiatives/moonshot-cancer-initiative

[20] Gewirtz DA, Bristol ML, Yalowich JC. Toxicity issues in cancer drug development. Curr Opin Investig Drugs 2010; 11(6): 612-4.
[PMID: 20496255]

[21] Liversidge GG, Cundy KC. Particle size reduction for improvement of oral bioavailability of hydrophobic drugs: I. Absolute oral bioavailability of nanocrystalline danazol in beagle dogs. Int J Pharm 1995; 125(1): 91-7.
[http://dx.doi.org/10.1016/0378-5173(95)00122-Y]

[22] Jinno J, Kamada N, Miyake M, *et al.* Effect of particle size reduction on dissolution and oral absorption of a poorly water-soluble drug, cilostazol, in beagle dogs. J Control Release 2006; 111(1-2): 56-64.
[http://dx.doi.org/10.1016/j.jconrel.2005.11.013] [PMID: 16410029]

[23] Pillai G. Nanomedicines for cancer therapy: An update of FDA approved and those under various stages of development. SOJ Pharm Pharm Sci 2014; 1(2): 13.
[http://dx.doi.org/10.15226/2374-6866/1/1/00109]

[24] Cooley T, Henry D, Tonda M, Sun S, O'Connell M, Rackoff W. A randomized, double-blind study of pegylated liposomal doxorubicin for the treatment of AIDS-related Kaposi's sarcoma. Oncologist 2007; 12(1): 114-23.
[http://dx.doi.org/10.1634/theoncologist.12-1-114] [PMID: 17227906]

[25] https://drugs.ncats.io/drug/ZS7284E0ZP

[26] https://www.ema.europa.eu/en/medicines/human/EPAR/myocet-liposomal-previously-myocet

[27] https://www.drugs.com/history/abraxane.html

[28] Weissig V, Pettinger T, Murdock N. Nanopharmaceuticals (part 1): products on the market. Int J Nanomedicine 2014; 9: 4357-73.
[http://dx.doi.org/10.2147/IJN.S46900] [PMID: 25258527]

[29] Chawla SP, Chua VS, Fernandez L, *et al.* Advanced phase I/II studies of targeted gene delivery *in vivo*: intravenous Rexin-G for gemcitabine-resistant metastatic pancreatic cancer. Mol Ther 2010; 18(2): 435-41.
[http://dx.doi.org/10.1038/mt.2009.228] [PMID: 19826403]

[30] Chen KTJ, Gilabert-Oriol R, Bally MB, Leung AWY. Recent treatment advances and the role of nanotechnology, combination products, and immunotherapy in changing the therapeutic landscape of acute myeloid leukemia. Pharm Res 2019; 36(9): 125.
[http://dx.doi.org/10.1007/s11095-019-2654-z] [PMID: 31236772]

[31] https://vyxeospro.com/clinical-data/efficacy/

[32] Centerwatch. FDA approved drugs https://www.centerwatch.com/directories/1067-fda-approved-drugs

[33] Food and Drug Administration. Novel drug approvals for 2019.https://www.fda.gov/drugs/new-drug--fda-cders-new-molecular-entities-and-new-therapeutic-biological-products/novel-dr-g-approvals-2019

[34] Sainz V, Conniot J, Matos AI, *et al.* Regulatory aspects on nanomedicines. Biochem Biophys Res Commun 2015; 468(3): 504-10.
[http://dx.doi.org/10.1016/j.bbrc.2015.08.023] [PMID: 26260323]

[35] Peer D, Karp JM, Hong S, Farokhzad OC, Margalit R, Langer R. Nanocarriers as an emerging platform for cancer therapy. Nat Nanotechnol 2007; 2(12): 751-60.
[http://dx.doi.org/10.1038/nnano.2007.387] [PMID: 18654426]

[36] Brown JM, Giaccia AJ. The unique physiology of solid tumors: opportunities (and problems) for cancer therapy. Cancer Res 1998; 58(7): 1408-16.
[PMID: 9537241]

[37] Hobbs SK, Monsky WL, Yuan F, *et al.* Regulation of transport pathways in tumor vessels: Role of tumor type and microenvironment. Proc Natl Acad Sci USA 1998; 95(8): 4607-12. [http://dx.doi.org/10.1073/pnas.95.8.4607] [PMID: 9539785]

[38] Maeda H. The enhanced permeability and retention (EPR) effect in tumor vasculature: the key role of tumor-selective macromolecular drug targeting. Adv Enzyme Regul 2001; 41(1): 189-207. [http://dx.doi.org/10.1016/S0065-2571(00)00013-3] [PMID: 11384745]

[39] Maeda H, Nakamura H, Fang J. The EPR effect for macromolecular drug delivery to solid tumors: Improvement of tumor uptake, lowering of systemic toxicity, and distinct tumor imaging *in vivo*. Adv Drug Deliv Rev 2013; 65(1): 71-9. [http://dx.doi.org/10.1016/j.addr.2012.10.002] [PMID: 23088862]

[40] Yuan Y, Zhang L, Cao H, Yang Y, Zheng Y, Yang X. A polyethylenimine-containing and transferrin-conjugated lipid nanoparticle system for antisense oligonucleotide delivery to AML. BioMed Res Int 2016; 2016: 1-8. [http://dx.doi.org/10.1155/2016/1287128] [PMID: 27034925]

[41] Hamaguchi T, Matsumura Y, Nakanishi Y, *et al.* Antitumor effect of MCC-465, pegylated liposomal doxorubicin tagged with newly developed monoclonal antibody GAH, in colorectal cancer xenografts. Cancer Sci 2004; 95(7): 608-13. [http://dx.doi.org/10.1111/j.1349-7006.2004.tb02495.x] [PMID: 15245599]

[42] Clinical Trials Worldwide. www.clinicaltrials.gov

[43] Davis ME, Chen Z, Shin DM. Nanoparticle therapeutics: an emerging treatment modality for cancer. Nat Rev Drug Discov 2008; 7(9): 771-82. [http://dx.doi.org/10.1038/nrd2614] [PMID: 18758474]

[44] Thanki K, Kushwah V, Jain S. Recent advances in tumor targeting approaches.Targeted Drug Delivery: Concepts and Design. Springer 2015; pp. 41-112. [http://dx.doi.org/10.1007/978-3-319-11355-5_2]

[45] Byrne JD, Betancourt T, Brannon-Peppas L. Active targeting schemes for nanoparticle systems in cancer therapeutics. Adv Drug Deliv Rev 2008; 60(15): 1615-26. [http://dx.doi.org/10.1016/j.addr.2008.08.005] [PMID: 18840489]

[46] Morton JG, Day ES, Halas NJ, West JL. Nanoshells for photothermal cancer therapy. Methods Mol Biol 2010; 624: 101-17. [http://dx.doi.org/10.1007/978-1-60761-609-2_7] [PMID: 20217591]

[47] Stern JM, Stanfield J, Kabbani W, Hsieh JT, Cadeddu JA. Selective prostate cancer thermal ablation with laser activated gold nanoshells. J Urol 2008; 179(2): 748-53. [http://dx.doi.org/10.1016/j.juro.2007.09.018] [PMID: 18082199]

[48] MagForce AG Announces Treatment of Recurrent Glioblastoma Patient with NanoTherm® Therapy https://www.fiercebiotech.com/biotech/magforce-ag-announces-treatment-of-recurrent-gliobl-stoma-patient-nanotherm%C2%AE-therapy

[49] Pillai G, Ceballos-Coronel ML. Science and technology of the emerging nanomedicines in cancer therapy: A primer for physicians and pharmacists. SAGE Open Med 2013; 1. [http://dx.doi.org/10.1177/2050312113513759] [PMID: 26770691]

[50] Gewirtz D. A critical evaluation of the mechanisms of action proposed for the antitumor effects of the anthracycline antibiotics adriamycin and daunorubicin. Biochem Pharmacol 1999; 57(7): 727-41. [http://dx.doi.org/10.1016/S0006-2952(98)00307-4] [PMID: 10075079]

[51] Park JW. Liposome-based drug delivery in breast cancer treatment. Breast Cancer Res 2002; 4(3): 95-9. [http://dx.doi.org/10.1186/bcr432] [PMID: 12052251]

[52] Gordon AN, Granai CO, Rose PG, *et al.* Phase II study of liposomal doxorubicin in platinum- and

paclitaxel-refractory epithelial ovarian cancer. J Clin Oncol 2000; 18(17): 3093-100. [http://dx.doi.org/10.1200/JCO.2000.18.17.3093] [PMID: 10963637]

[53] Gordon AN, Fleagle JT, Guthrie D, Parkin DE, Gore ME, Lacave AJ. Recurrent epithelial ovarian carcinoma: a randomized phase III study of pegylated liposomal doxorubicin *versus* topotecan. J Clin Oncol 2001; 19(14): 3312-22. [http://dx.doi.org/10.1200/JCO.2001.19.14.3312] [PMID: 11454878]

[54] Rahman AM, Yusuf SW, Ewer MS. Anthracycline-induced cardiotoxicity and the cardiac-sparing effect of liposomal formulation. Int J Nanomedicine 2007; 2(4): 567-83. [PMID: 18203425]

[55] O'Brien MER, Wigler N, Inbar M, *et al.* CAELYX Breast Cancer Study Group. Reduced cardiotoxicity and comparable efficacy in a phase IIItrial of pegylated liposomal doxorubicin HCl(CAELYX™/Doxil®) versus conventional doxorubicin forfirst-line treatment of metastatic breast cancer. Ann Oncol 2004; 15(3): 440-9. [http://dx.doi.org/10.1093/annonc/mdh097] [PMID: 14998846]

[56] Hong RL. Liposomal anti-cancer drug researches the myth of long circulation. J Chinese Oncol Soc 2004; 20(2): 10-21.

[57] Johnston SRD, Gore ME. Caelyx®. Eur J Cancer 2001; 37 (Suppl. 9): 8-14. [http://dx.doi.org/10.1016/S0959-8049(01)00329-X] [PMID: 11741768]

[58] Leonard RCF, Williams S, Tulpule A, Levine AM, Oliveros S. Improving the therapeutic index of anthracycline chemotherapy: Focus on liposomal doxorubicin (Myocet™). Breast 2009; 18(4): 218-24. [http://dx.doi.org/10.1016/j.breast.2009.05.004] [PMID: 19656681]

[59] Gabizon A, Shmeeda H, Barenholz Y. Pharmacokinetics of pegylated liposomal Doxorubicin: review of animal and human studies. Clin Pharmacokinet 2003; 42(5): 419-36. [http://dx.doi.org/10.2165/00003088-200342050-00002] [PMID: 12739982]

[60] Lao J, Madani J, Puértolas T, *et al.* Liposomal Doxorubicin in the treatment of breast cancer patients: a review. J Drug Deliv 2013; 2013: 1-12. [http://dx.doi.org/10.1155/2013/456409] [PMID: 23634302]

[61] Swenson CE, Bolcsak LE, Batist G, *et al.* Pharmacokinetics of doxorubicin administered i.v. as Myocet (TLC D-99; liposome-encapsulated doxorubicin citrate) compared with conventional doxorubicin when given in combination with cyclophosphamide in patients with metastatic breast cancer. Anticancer Drugs 2003; 14(3): 239-46. [http://dx.doi.org/10.1097/00001813-200303000-00008] [PMID: 12634619]

[62] Slingerland M, Guchelaar HJ, Gelderblom H. Liposomal drug formulations in cancer therapy: 15 years along the road. Drug Discov Today 2012; 17(3-4): 160-6. [http://dx.doi.org/10.1016/j.drudis.2011.09.015] [PMID: 21983329]

[63] Yarmolenko PS, Zhao Y, Landon C, *et al.* Comparative effects of thermosensitive doxorubicin-containing liposomes and hyperthermia in human and murine tumours. Int J Hyperthermia 2010; 26(5): 485-98. [http://dx.doi.org/10.3109/02656731003789284] [PMID: 20597627]

[64] Gill PS, Espina BM, Muggia F, *et al.* Phase I/II clinical and pharmacokinetic evaluation of liposomal daunorubicin. J Clin Oncol 1995; 13(4): 996-1003. [http://dx.doi.org/10.1200/JCO.1995.13.4.996] [PMID: 7707129]

[65] Guarneri V, Dieci MV, Conte P. Enhancing intracellular taxane delivery: current role and perspectives of nanoparticle albumin-bound paclitaxel in the treatment of advanced breast cancer. Expert Opin Pharmacother 2012; 13(3): 395-406. [http://dx.doi.org/10.1517/14656566.2012.651127] [PMID: 22263900]

[66] Von Hoff DD, Ramanathan RK, Borad MJ, *et al.* Gemcitabine plus nab-paclitaxel is an active regimen

in patients with advanced pancreatic cancer: a phase I/II trial. J Clin Oncol 2011; 29(34): 4548-54. [http://dx.doi.org/10.1200/JCO.2011.36.5742] [PMID: 21969517]

[67] Desai N, Trieu V, Yao Z, *et al.* Increased antitumor activity, intratumor paclitaxel concentrations, and endothelial cell transport of cremophor-free, albumin-bound paclitaxel, ABI-007, compared with cremophor-based paclitaxel. Clin Cancer Res 2006; 12(4): 1317-24. [http://dx.doi.org/10.1158/1078-0432.CCR-05-1634] [PMID: 16489089]

[68] Desai N, Trieu V, Yao R, Labao E, Soon-Shiong P. Increased endothelial transcytosis of nanoparticle albumin-bound paclitaxel (ABI-007) by gp60-receptors: a pathway inhibited by taxol. *SABCS.* 2004 Abstract No. 1071 San Antonio Breast Cancer Symposium. 1071.

[69] Gradishar WJ. Albumin-bound paclitaxel: a next-generation taxane. Expert Opin Pharmacother 2006; 7(8): 1041-53. [http://dx.doi.org/10.1517/14656566.7.8.1041] [PMID: 16722814]

[70] Stathopoulos GP, Boulikas T. Lipoplatin formulation review article. J Drug Deliv 2012; 2012: 1-10. [http://dx.doi.org/10.1155/2012/581363] [PMID: 21904682]

[71] Boulikas T, Stathopoulos GP, Volakakis N, Vougiouka M. Systemic Lipoplatin infusion results in preferential tumor uptake in human studies. Anticancer Res 2005; 25(4): 3031-9. [PMID: 16080562]

[72] Boulikas T. Clinical overview on Lipoplatin ™ : a successful liposomal formulation of cisplatin. Expert Opin Investig Drugs 2009; 18(8): 1197-218. [http://dx.doi.org/10.1517/13543780903114168] [PMID: 19604121]

[73] Mayer LD, Bally MB, Loughrey H, Masin D, Cullis PR. Liposomal vincristine preparations which exhibit decreased drug toxicity and increased activity against murine L1210 and P388 tumors. Cancer Res 1990; 50(3): 575-9. [PMID: 2297698]

[74] Zhigaltsev IV, Maurer N, Akhong QF, *et al.* Liposome-encapsulated vincristine, vinblastine and vinorelbine: A comparative study of drug loading and retention. J Control Release 2005; 104(1): 103-11. [http://dx.doi.org/10.1016/j.jconrel.2005.01.010] [PMID: 15866338]

[75] Yang SH, Lin CC, Lin ZZ, Tseng YL, Hong RL. A phase I and pharmacokinetic study of liposomal vinorelbine in patients with advanced solid tumor. Invest New Drugs 2012; 30(1): 282-9. [http://dx.doi.org/10.1007/s10637-010-9522-3] [PMID: 20809205]

[76] Mantripragada S. A lipid based depot (DepoFoam® technology) for sustained release drug delivery. Prog Lipid Res 2002; 41(5): 392-406. [http://dx.doi.org/10.1016/S0163-7827(02)00004-8] [PMID: 12121719]

[77] Angst MS, Drover DR. Pharmacology of drugs formulated with DepoFoam: a sustained release drug delivery system for parenteral administration using multivesicular liposome technology. Clin Pharmacokinet 2006; 45(12): 1153-76. [http://dx.doi.org/10.2165/00003088-200645120-00002] [PMID: 17112293]

[78] Benesch M, Urban C. Liposomal cytarabine for leukemic and lymphomatous meningitis: recent developments. Expert Opin Pharmacother 2008; 9(2): 301-9. [http://dx.doi.org/10.1517/14656566.9.2.301] [PMID: 18201152]

[79] Chamberlain MC, Kormanik P, Howell SB, Kim S. Pharmacokinetics of intralumbar DTC-101 for the treatment of leptomeningeal metastases. Arch Neurol 1995; 52(9): 912-7. [http://dx.doi.org/10.1001/archneur.1995.00540330094020] [PMID: 7661730]

[80] Kim S, Chatelut E, Kim JC, *et al.* Extended CSF cytarabine exposure following intrathecal administration of DTC 101. J Clin Oncol 1993; 11(11): 2186-93. [http://dx.doi.org/10.1200/JCO.1993.11.11.2186] [PMID: 8229133]

[81] Pearce HL, Winter MA, Beck WT. Structural characteristics of compounds that modulate P-

glycoprotein-associated multidrug resistance. Adv Enzyme Regul 1990; 30: 357-73. [http://dx.doi.org/10.1016/0065-2571(90)90026-X] [PMID: 1976291]

[82] Booser D, Esteva F, Rivera E, *et al.* Phase II study of liposomal annamycin in the treatment of doxorubicin-resistant breast cancer. Cancer Chemother Pharmacol 2002; 50(1): 6-8. [http://dx.doi.org/10.1007/s00280-002-0464-0] [PMID: 12111105]

[83] Immordino ML, Dosio F, Cattel L. Stealth liposomes: review of the basic science, rationale, and clinical applications, existing and potential. Int J Nanomedicine 2006; 1(3): 297-315. [PMID: 17717971]

[84] Alfieri DR. Pegaspargase. Pediatr Nurs 1995; 21(5): 471-474, 490. [PMID: 8684851]

[85] Avramis VI, Tiwari PN. Asparaginase (native ASNase or pegylated ASNase) in the treatment of acute lymphoblastic leukemia. Int J Nanomedicine 2006; 1(3): 241-54. [PMID: 17717965]

[86] Zeidan A, Wang ES, Wetzler M. Pegasparaginase: where do we stand? Expert Opin Biol Ther 2009; 9(1): 111-9. [http://dx.doi.org/10.1517/14712590802586058] [PMID: 19063697]

[87] Emerson DL, Bendele R, Brown E, *et al.* Antitumor efficacy, pharmacokinetics, and biodistribution of NX 211: a low-clearance liposomal formulation of lurtotecan. Clin Cancer Res 2000; 6(7): 2903-12. [PMID: 10914740]

[88] Dark GG, Calvert AH, Grimshaw R, *et al.* Randomized trial of two intravenous schedules of the topoisomerase I inhibitor liposomal lurtotecan in women with relapsed epithelial ovarian cancer: a trial of the national cancer institute of Canada clinical trials group. J Clin Oncol 2005; 23(9): 1859-66. [http://dx.doi.org/10.1200/JCO.2005.02.028] [PMID: 15699482]

[89] Saltz LB, Cox JV, Blanke C, *et al.* Irinotecan Study Group. Irinotecan plus fluorouracil and leucovorin for metastatic colorectal cancer. N Engl J Med 2000; 343(13): 905-14. [http://dx.doi.org/10.1056/NEJM200009283431302] [PMID: 11006366]

[90] Douillard JY, Cunningham D, Roth AD, *et al.* Irinotecan combined with fluorouracil compared with fluorouracil alone as first-line treatment for metastatic colorectal cancer: a multicentre randomised trial. Lancet 2000; 355(9209): 1041-7. [http://dx.doi.org/10.1016/S0140-6736(00)02034-1] [PMID: 10744089]

[91] Hamburg MA. Science and regulation. FDA's approach to regulation of products of nanotechnology. Science 2012; 336(6079): 299-300. [http://dx.doi.org/10.1126/science.1205441] [PMID: 22517845]

[92] Guidance for Industry: Considering whether an FDA-regulated product involves the application of nanotechnology (2014) U.S. Food and Drug Administration Guidance for Industry. Considering whether an FDA-regulated product involves the application of nanotechnology 2014. https://www.fda.gov/regulatory-information/search-fda-guida-ce-documents/considering-whether-fda-regulated-product-involves-application-nanotechnology

[93] Guidances (Drugs). U.S. Food and Drug Administration https://www.fda.gov/industry/fda-basic--industry/guidances

[94] Draft Guidance on Lanreotide Acetate (2014). U.S. Food and Drug Administration 2014. https://www.accessdata.fda.gov/drugsatfda_docs/psg/Lanreotide%20Acetate_draft_Subcutaneous%20injection_RLD%2022074_RC07-14.pdf

[95] D'Souza SS, DeLuca PP. Methods to assess *in vitro* drug release from injectable polymeric particulate systems. Pharm Res 2006; 23(3): 460-74. [http://dx.doi.org/10.1007/s11095-005-9397-8] [PMID: 16400516]

[96] Foulkes R, Man E, Thind J, Yeung S, Joy A, Hoskins C. The regulation of nanomaterials and nanomedicines for clinical application: current and future perspectives. Biomater Sci 2020; 8(17):

4653-64.
[http://dx.doi.org/10.1039/D0BM00558D] [PMID: 32672255]

[97] Investigational New Drug (IND) Application, U.S. Food and drug https://www.fda.gov/drugs/types-applications/investigational-new-drug-ind-application

[98] Maeda H. Macromolecular therapeutics in cancer treatment: The EPR effect and beyond. J Control Release 2012; 164(2): 138-44.
[http://dx.doi.org/10.1016/j.jconrel.2012.04.038] [PMID: 22595146]

[99] Ozcan G, Ozpolat B, Coleman RL, Sood AK, Lopez-Berestein G. Preclinical and clinical development of siRNA-based therapeutics. Adv Drug Deliv Rev 2015; 87: 108-19.
[http://dx.doi.org/10.1016/j.addr.2015.01.007] [PMID: 25666164]

[100] Step 3: Clinical Research, U.S. Food and Drug Administration. https://www.fda.gov/patients/drug-development-process/step-3-clinical-research

[101] Applications covered by NDA 505(b)(1) of the FD&;C Act, U.S. Food and Drug Administration https://www.fda.gov/regulatory-information/search-fda-guidance-documents/applications-co-ered-section-505b2

[102] What is 505(b)(2)? Camargo Pharmaceutical Services (2016). The Global 505(b)(2) Experts 2016.http://camargopharma.com/what-is-505b2/

[103] Draft Guidance for Industry: Applications Covered by Section 505(b)(2) (1999) U.S. Food and Drug Administration 1999. http://www.fda.gov/downloads/Drugs/.../Guidances/ucm079345 .pdf https://www.fda.gov/regulatory-information/search-fda-guidance-documents/ applications-covere--section-505b2

[104] NDA 20–2062/S-024.Drug approval package for Taxol Injection, Center for Drug Evaluation and Research, U.S. Food and Drug. https://www.accessdata.fda.gov/drugsatfda_docs /nda/98/20262s024.cfm2021.

[105] Abraxane paclitaxel protein-bound particles for injectable suspension, Oncologic. Drugs Advisory Committee Meeting Abraxis Bioscience 2006. https://www.accessdata.fda.gov /drugsatfda_docs/nda/2012/021660Orig1s031.pdf

[106] New Drug Application (NDA), U.S. Food and Drug Administration. https://www.fda.gov/drugs/ development-approval-process-drugs/how-drugs-are-developed-and-approved

[107] Drugs@FDA Glossary of Terms, U.S. Food and Drug Administration. http://www.fda.gov/Drugs/InformationOnDrugs/ucm079436.htm#B

[108] Drug approval package for Taxol Injection, Center for Drug Evaluation and Research, U.S. Food and Drug 2003. fda.gov/combination-products/jurisdictional-information

[109] Guidance for Industry ANDA Submissions — Content and Format of Abbreviated New Drug Applications (2014) U.S. Food and Drug Administration 2014. http://www.fda.gov/downloads /drugs/guidancecomplianceregulatoryinformation/guidances/ucm400630.pdf

[110] Abbreviated New Drug Application (ANDA): Generic Drug Development, U.S. Food and Drug Administration. https://www.fda.gov/drugs/abbreviated-new-drug-application-anda/generic-drug-development

[111] Draft Guidance on best practices for communication between IND sponsors and FDA during drug development guidance for industry and review staff (2015) U.S. Food and Drug Administration 2015. http://www.fda.gov/downloads
/drugs/guidancecomplianceregulatoryinformation/guidances/ucm475586.pdf

[112] Guidance for Industry: Expedited Programs for Serious Conditions – Drugs and Biologics 2014. https://www.federalregister.gov/documents/2014/05/30/2014-12534/guidance-for-industr--on-expedited-programs-for-serious-conditions-drugs-and-biologics-availability

[113] Cerulean Receives FDA Fast Track Designation for CRLX101. Treatment of Platinum-Resistant

Ovarian Cancer (2016) Business Wire- A Berkshire Hathaway company 2016. http://www.businesswire.com/news/home/20160719005765 /en/Cerulean-Receives-FDA-Fast-T-ack-Designation-CRLX101

[114] Lancet. Final results of a phase III randomized trial of CPX-351 versus 7+3 in older patients with newly diagnosed high risk (secondary) AML J Clin Oncol 2016; 34.

[115] Johnson JR, Ning YM, Farrell A, Justice R, Keegan P, Pazdur R. Accelerated approval of oncology products: the food and drug administration experience. J Natl Cancer Inst 2011; 103(8): 636-44. [http://dx.doi.org/10.1093/jnci/djr062] [PMID: 21422403]

[116] FDA approves Onivyde for advanced pancreatic cancer (2015) American Cancer Society, Inc 2015. http://www.cancer.org/cancer/news/news/fda-approves-onivyde-for-advanced-pancreaticcancer

[117] Bawa R, Audette GF, Reece B. Handbook of Clinical Nanomedicine: Law, Business, Regulation, Safety, and Risk, Pan Stamford Series on Nanomedicine. Boca Raton, Florida, USA: CRC Press, Taylor and Francis 2016; Vol. 2.

[118] Bawa R. Regulating nanomedicine - can the FDA handle it? Curr Drug Deliv 2011; 8(3): 227-34. [http://dx.doi.org/10.2174/156720111795256156] [PMID: 21291376]

[119] Kelly B. Nanomedicines: regulatory challenges and risks ahead 2010. https://www.cov.com/-/media/files/corporate/publications/2010/10/nanomedicinesregulatory.pdf

[120] Rannard S, Owen A. Nanomedicine: Not a case of "One size fits all". Nano Today 2009; 4(5): 382-4. [http://dx.doi.org/10.1016/j.nantod.2009.07.002]

[121] Muthu MS, Wilson B. Challenges posed by the scale-up of nanomedicines. Nanomedicine (Lond) 2012; 7(3): 307-9. [http://dx.doi.org/10.2217/nnm.12.3] [PMID: 22385192]

[122] Soares S, Sousa J, Pais A, Vitorino C. Nanomedicine. Front Chem 2018; 6: 360. [http://dx.doi.org/10.3389/fchem.2018.00360] [PMID: 30177965]

[123] Mühlebach S. Regulatory challenges of nanomedicines and their follow-on versions: A generic or similar approach? Adv Drug Deliv Rev 2018; 131: 122-31. [http://dx.doi.org/10.1016/j.addr.2018.06.024] [PMID: 29966685]

[124] Sainz V, Conniot J, Matos AI, *et al.* Regulatory aspects on nanomedicines. Biochem Biophys Res Commun 2015; 468(3): 504-10. [http://dx.doi.org/10.1016/j.bbrc.2015.08.023] [PMID: 26260323]

[125] Paradise J. Regulating Nanomedicine at the Food and Drug Administration. AMA J Ethics 2019; 21(4): E347-55. [http://dx.doi.org/10.1001/amajethics.2019.347] [PMID: 31012422]

[126] Kroll A, Pillukat MH, Hahn D, Schnekenburger J. Current *in vitro* methods in nanoparticle risk assessment: Limitations and challenges. Eur J Pharm Biopharm 2009; 72(2): 370-7. [http://dx.doi.org/10.1016/j.ejpb.2008.08.009] [PMID: 18775492]

[127] Sharma HS, Hussain S, Schlager J, Ali SF, Sharma A. Influence of Nanoparticles on Blood–Brain Barrier Permeability and Brain Edema Formation in Rats. Acta Neurochir Suppl (Wien) 2010; 106: 359-64. [http://dx.doi.org/10.1007/978-3-211-98811-4_65]

[128] Pita R, Ehmann F, Papaluca M. Nanomedicines in the EU—Regulatory Overview. AAPS J 2016; 18(6): 1576-82. [http://dx.doi.org/10.1208/s12248-016-9967-1] [PMID: 27527889]

[129] FDA. Nanotechnology Fact Sheet. https://www.fda.gov/science-research/nanotechnology-progra-s-fda/nanotechnology-fact-sheet

[130] Bremer-Hoffmann S, Halamoda-Kenzaoui B, Borgos SE. Identification of regulatory needs for nanomedicines. J Interdiscip Nanomed 2018; 3(1): 4-15.

[http://dx.doi.org/10.1002/jin2.34]

[131] Rauscher H, Roebben G, Amenta V, *et al.* Sintes,Sokull-Klüttgen and H. Stamm, Towards a review of the EC Recommendation for a definition of the term "nano-material" Part 1: Compilation of information concerning the experience with the definition, JRC Scientific Quality ReportPublications office of the European Union. Luxemburg 2014.https://euagenda.eu/upload/publications/untitled-60207-ea.pdf

[132] Roebben G, Rauscher H, Amenta V, *et al.* Towards a review of the EC Recommendation for a definition of the term "nano-material". Part 2: Assessment of collected information concerning the experience with the definition, JRC Scientific Quality Report, Publications office of the European Union. Luxemburg 2014.

[133] Rauscher H, Roebben G, Sanfeliu AB, *et al.* Towards a review of the EC Recommendation for a definition of the term ""nano-material"" Part 3: Scientific-technical evaluation of options to clarify the definition and to facilitate its implementation, JRC Scientific Quality Report, Publications office of the European Union. Luxemburg 2015.

[134] Multidisciplinary: Nanomedicine.. https://www.ema.europa.eu/en/human-regulatory/researc--development/scientific-guidelines/multidisciplinary/multidisciplinary-nanomedicines

[135] MHLW/PMDA, Current Initiative in Japan for nanomedicines. 2010. https://www.ema.europa.eu/en/documents/presentation/presentation-nanomedicines-current-initiatives-japan-kumiko-sakai-k-to-toru-kawanishi-national/mhlw_en.pdf

[136] Sapsford KE, Lauritsen K, Tyner KM. Current perspectives on the US Food and Drug 'Administration's regulatory framework for intelligent drug delivery systems. Ther Deliv 2012; 3(12): 1383-94.
[http://dx.doi.org/10.4155/tde.12.119] [PMID: 23323557]

[137] Zheng N, Sun DD, Zou P, Jiang W. Zou, Jiang W. Scientific and regulatory considerations for generic complex drug products containing Nano-materials. AAPS J 2017; 19(3): 619-31.
[http://dx.doi.org/10.1208/s12248-017-0044-1] [PMID: 28116676]

[138] Dunne S, Shannon B, Dunne C, Cullen W. A review of the differences and similarities between generic drugs and their originator counterparts, including economic benefits associated with usage of generic medicines, using Ireland as a case study. BMC Pharmacol Toxicol 2013; 14(1): 1.
[http://dx.doi.org/10.1186/2050-6511-14-1] [PMID: 23289757]

CHAPTER 13

Future Prospective and Challenges in the Treatment of Cancer

Aakriti Garg[1], Santanu Kaity[2], Manisha Thakur[3], Ashok Kumar Datusalia[3] and Anoop Kumar[4,*]

[1] *School of Pharmaceutical Sciences, Apeejay Stya University, Gurgaon, India*

[2] *Mylan Laboratories Limited, R&D Center, Bollaram (V), Hyderabad, India*

[3] *Department of Pharmacology and Toxicology, National Institute of Pharmaceutical Education and Research (NIPER), Raebareli, Lucknow, India*

[4] *Department of Pharmacology, Delhi Pharmaceutical Sciences & Research University (DPSRU), New Delhi, India*

Abstract: Cancer is responsible for millions of deaths worldwide yearly. Many miles have been crossed towards the treatment of this deadly disease, however, there are still many more to explore about the occurrence, consequences, and, specifically, the accurate therapy to win over this deadly disease. Complex areas like cancer initiation, pathogenesis and the progression of cancer in the human body should be explored with better understanding to discover specific treatments against it. Currently, cancer treatments include radiation therapy, targeted therapy, surgery, chemotherapy, radiation therapy, immunotherapy, and some existing symptomatic treatments. However, the specific treatments of cancer are still a big puzzle to solve. The challenges faced in the treatment of cancer are mainly the heterogenicity of some cancers, drug resistance, late diagnosis, few treatment advances for early-stage cancer, non-selectivity of drugs towards cancer cells leading to side effects, and many more, which are still in the dark. Exploring the solution to this challenge, we need to understand the disease in totality, and understand the existing lacunas of the existing treatments too. Thus, in this chapter, we have discussed the current challenges faced in cancer therapy, followed by the future perspectives in the treatment of a wide variety of cancer.

Keywords: Cancer, Challenges, Future perspectives, Treatment.

INTRODUCTION

The disease "Cancer" is a pathophysiologic condition of a living body in which cells start to divide in an uncontrolled manner, and further, the cells start to invade other healthy tissues, which are expressed as a tumor mass. The mass starts to

* **Corresponding author Anoop Kumar:** Department of Pharmacology, Delhi Pharmaceutical Sciences & Research University (DPSRU), New Delhi 110017, India; Tel: +91-011-29552039; E-mail: abitmesra@gmail.com

Neeraj Mishra, Ashish Garg and Neeraj Upmanyu (Eds.)

achieve its vesicles for blood supply and further spreads to other body parts. The great Greek physician Hippocrates coined the term “Cancer”. The terms introduced by him were “carcinos” and “carcinoma,” which were used to explain non-ulcerous and ulcerous tumors, respectively.

The major types of cancer leading to overall cancer mortality are lung cancer, GIT cancer, liver cancer, breast cancer, prostate cancer, *etc.* According to WHO [https://www.who.int/news-room/fact-sheets/detail/cancer], the second leading cause of death globally is cancer which claims nearly 10 million lives yearly. To date, statistics say, this disease is responsible for 1 in 6 deaths worldwide. Even though various approaches have been undertaken for the mitigation of cancer-related risk factors, in spite, the prevalence of this life-threatening disease is increasing in an almost exponential ratio. Current cancer treatment includes various therapies, including radiotherapy, surgery, chemotherapy, targeted therapy, and immunotherapy [1]. The choice of therapy is greatly influenced by the location, grade, stage, and size of the tumor, and the condition of the patient. However, the traditional treatment has various side effects, especially due to the non-selectivity of treatment against dividing cells, whether cancerous or not, making disease management more critical. Hence, there is an urgent need to explore new pave to successfully address the complications associated with this deadly disease. To do so, we need to understand the challenges faced during the diagnosis, categorization and exploring specific treatment for this disease. Thus, in this chapter, we explored the challenges faced in various types of cancer treatment and the treatment perspectives of this disease in the near future.

CURRENT CHALLENGES FOR CANCER TREATMENT

The treatment fails to elicit its desired response majorly because of the non-selectivity of the therapy and multi-drug resistance characteristic of a cancer cell. Even, chemotherapy, too, faced similar challenges for the same reason. Cancer cells accrue drug resistance due to their properties like poor vascularization of tumor region, acidic environment in the tumor which causes ionization of basic drugs, inactivation of the drug in such a complex environment, alteration in drug metabolism, or repelling of drugs from the cell due to P-glycoprotein [2 - 4]. Rapid blood clearance by the reticuloendothelial system (RES) is also a problem in cancer therapeutics [5]. Additionally, late diagnosis and few treatment advances for early cancer are also challenging cancer treatment. The sole reason or the combination of before said reasons makes the system more complex to explore a specific arsenal to break this vindication. A tabulated detail of the challenges faced in cancer treatment is presented in Table **1**.

Table 1. Challenges and future prospects in the treatment of cancer.

S. No.	Types of Cancer	Current Challenges	Future Prospective
1	Breast cancer	1. Management and minimization of post-effect of surgery like pain, smell, swelling, and risk of post-surgery infection. 2. Recurrence of cancer after radiation therapy leads to reduced quality of life and distant metastasis. 3. Minimizing side effects due to chemotherapy such as hair loss, heart damage, bone thinning, fertility issues, increased risk of leukemia, neuropathy, *etc.* 4. Tumor dormancy and relapses.	1. Advancement in surgery, targeted therapy, and diagnostic tools. 2. Understanding individual molecular patterns for individualized therapy. 3. Advancement in combination of anti-cancer drugs with nanoparticles in the treatment of breast cancer as it enhances the stability of hydrophobic drugs, reduces toxicity by using biocompatible nanomaterials and improves the pharmacokinetics of drug.
2	Lung cancer	1. Late diagnosis leads to difficulty in prognosis. 2. Minimizing post-effect of radiation therapy such as fatigue, loss of appetite, sore throat, and difficulty in swallowing. In some cases, inflammation due to radiation therapy may develop cough, fever, or shortness of breath. 3. Minimizing effects of chemotherapy such as fatigue, low numbers of blood cells, risk of infection, mouth sores, nausea and vomiting, loss of appetite, diarrhea, numbness and tingling in the hands and feet, and hair loss.	1. Understanding barriers to detection of early-lung cancer. 2. Improvement of diagnostic tools. 3. Improvement in targeted therapy. 4. Better understanding of molecular biology of lung cancer for rational drug designing.
3	GIT cancer	1. Reduced quality of life after therapy. 2. Eradication of early-stage cancer. 3. Maximization of tumor response in late-stage disease. 4. Limited advancement in the treatment of gastric cancer due to heterogenicity and genetic complexity. 5. Treatment of older patients due to physiologic changes with age.	1. Detailed understanding of the molecular pathogenesis and individual character of gastric cancer will contribute to providing personalized cancer care. 2. Development in therapy for patients with both early or advanced cancer. 3. Detailed understanding of Molecular analysis of GIT cancerous cells to learn genetic alteration leading to cancer. 4. Development in targeted drug therapy. 5. Development in minimally invasive procedure or robotic surgery
4	Hepatic cancer	Late diagnosis leads to difficulty in treatment.	1. Improvement in diagnostic tools for early detection of cancer. 2. Identification of phytochemicals for improving current therapy.

(Table 1) cont.....

S. No.	Types of Cancer	Current Challenges	Future Prospective
5	Prostate cancer	1. Minimizing post-effect of radiation therapy such as sexual dysfunction, urinary incontinence, bowel dysfunction 2. Management of side effects due to androgen deficient therapy such as Loss of sexual activity, breast swelling, hot flashes, anemia, and osteoporosis. 3. Defining progression in tumor. 4. Assessing man's risk of developing prostate cancer during his lifetime. 5. Diagnosis and prognosis of aggressive *versus* non-aggressive cancer. 6. Development of new treatments for advanced disease. 7. Best utilization of existing therapies for a favorable outcome.	1. Measures need to be taken to understand the factors influencing the management of prostate cancer and developing the techniques to minimize the side effects of current therapies. 2. Identify new biomarkers that provide prognostic estimates of prostate cancer severity and predict treatment response.
6	Blood cancer	1. Identification of the subgroup of blood cancer patients with the most detrimental genetic makeup. 2. Individualized therapy	1. Improvement in targeted drug therapy. 2. Understanding the molecular alteration in cancer. 3. Targeting iron metabolism may provide new insights for approaches to the treatment of leukemia.
7	Skin cancer	1. Variation in patient response to immunotherapy. 2. Drug resistance	1. Detailed knowledge of protein structures and the understanding of their role in key signaling pathways in melanoma development lead to the designation of new targets for the treatment of melanoma.
8	Pancreatic cancer	Microenvironment of pancreatic cancer makes the prognosis difficult.	1. Identification of new targets for improving target therapy. 2. Development in diagnostic tools for early detection of cancer.

Breast Cancer, Treatments, and Challenges

Among various cancer types, breast cancer is one of the most common types in women. This is considered the most common reason for death among women. In the global scenario, the prevalence of this disease in western countries is about 89% which may be because of lifestyle or environmental conditions. However, it is observed that, on average, women remain alive almost up to 5 years after diagnosis because of early detection and quality treatment [6]. The available solutions for breast cancer treatment are majorly like surgery, such as lumpectomy by which the affected portion along with some thin line of healthy tissues surrounding the affected region is surgically removed, and mastectomy (whole breast is removed); radiation therapy by high-energy charged beam of particles like x-ray by which the affected cells are targeted and destroyed or radiation therapy by external-beams of charged particles (radiation treatment that is given externally using specialized equipments), intra-operative radiation therapy (specialized probe guided radiation therapy), brachytherapy (radioactive source is directly placed into affected area); chemotherapy (drug induced therapy, mainly combination of drugs to fight against the malfunctioning cell clusters) such as docetaxel, paclitaxel, doxorubicin, cisplatin, fluorouracil, methotrexate, *etc.*; hormonal therapy (recommended for estrogen or progesterone receptors mediated tumor growths) such as tamoxifen, aromatase inhibitors, *etc.*; targeted therapy (prime focus is given on specific genes responsible for cancer, and other biochemical agents like proteins, and peptides, tissue extrudes which nourish the affected area for growth and survival) such as HER2-targeted therapy (Trastuzumab, Pertuzumab, Neratinib), bone modifying drugs (bisphosphonates, denosumab), CDK4/6 protein (Lapatinib, Tucatinib, Talazoparib); immunotherapy (to give synergistic impact along with the body's very own defense mechanaism) such as Atezolizumab, Pembrolizumab, *etc* [7].

The challenges faced in lumpectomy and mastectomy are the aftereffects of surgery, such as pain, smell, swelling, and risk of post-surgery infection [8]. The challenges faced after radiation therapy include a high risk of locoregional recurrence [9] associated with severe symptoms, reduced quality of life, and distant metastasis [10]. Chemotherapy for breast cancer is followed by various side effects such as hair loss, heart damage, bone thinning, fertility issues, increased risk of leukemia, neuropathy, *etc* [11]. The current challenge faced in the management of breast cancer is tumor dormancy and last relapses as exact mechanism of dormancy of tumor is not yet fully understood [12].

Lung Cancer, Treatments, and Challenges

Current therapy for lung cancer includes surgery (the affected region of lung and connected lymph nodes are completely removed) including lobectomy (the affected lobe of the lung is removed), wedge resection (the tumor part along with surrounding healthy tissues are removed), segmentectomy (affected portion of lung where cancer has developed is removed), pneumonectomy (whole lung is removed if tumor is nearer to the central part of the chest); radiation therapy; chemotherapy (cisplatin, paclitaxel, docetaxel, *etc.*); targeted therapy include EGFR inhibitors (epidermal growth factor receptor) (Osimertinib, Afatinib, Dacomitinib, etc), Anaplastic lymphoma kinase (ALK) inhibitors (alectinib, ceritinib, lorlatinib, etc), Drugs targeting ROS1 genetic changes (Crizotinib, Entrectinib), Drugs targeting NTRK fusion (Larotrectinib), Drugs targeting BRAF V600E mutations (dabrafenib and tremetinib), active ingredients which targets MET Exon 14 Skipping (Capmatinib and tepotinib), Drugs targeting RET fusion

(Selpercatinib), Anti-angiogenesis therapy (Bevacizumab, Ramucirumab, Ramucirumab); and immunotherapy (Atezolizumab, Durvalumab, *etc.*) [13, 14].

The major limitation in the treatment of lung cancer is that majority of patients have metastatic disease at the time of diagnosis, thus making prognosis difficult [15]. The most preferred treatment for lung cancer is radiation therapy. However, individuals treated with radiation therapy may experience a number of adverse events like loss of appetite and exhaustion. If the affected region is near the neck or central region of the chest and the condition is treated with radiation therapy, the patient may experience difficulty in swelling and severe sore throat. The radiation-exposed region may initiate sunburn or severe skin irritation-type feeling. However, maximum adverse events subsided within a few days of treatment. In certain circumstances, depending on the severity of radiation-exposed, the treatment may induce lung inflammation which can express as severe cough, fever, or shortness of breath even after a long time, like months or years. This situation is called radiation pneumonitis; a maximum of 15%-40% of radiation-treated patients experience such adverse events [16]. In mild radiation pneumonitis, special treatments are not advised. However, severe radiation pneumonitis requires special attention and treatments with steroids like prednisone. The extent of radiation applied to the affected area of the lung may sometime damage the healthy tissues of the surrounding area and cause scarring. Depending on the severity, the scarring can lead to shortness of breath and cough.

In spite of being the best choice for lung cancer therapy, chemotherapy itself causes a number of unwanted effects in individuals depending on the severity of the radiation dose and the number of times exposed. Radiation therapy induces various adverse effects, such as severe anemia, diarrhea, nausea, vomiting, and, most commonly, alopecia. However, radiation therapy is the best ray of hope for most lung cancer-affected patients globally.

GIT Cancer, Treatments, and Challenges

The available therapies for gastric cancer are radiation therapy, surgery, chemotherapy, immunotherapy, and targeted therapy. The major challenge in the treatment of GIT cancer is the post-effects of therapy after gastrectomy, and the patient can eat only a small amount of meals at a time. Dumping syndrome is observed in patients including a group of symptoms like diarrhea, vomiting, and severe stomach cramps. However, the severity of the symptoms gradually decreased over time. Cases where the whole stomach is removed, require a regular injection of essential vitamins, mostly vitamin B12. The major challenge in upcoming years will be tumor eradication in early-stage gastrointestinal stromal tumor (GIST) patients and maximization of tumor response in late-stage diseases

[17]. Apart from this, the genetic complexity and the heterogeneity of gastric cancer have made the treatment process more complicated. Additionally, the treatment of older patients poses a challenge due to various age-related physiological changes related to pharmacokinetic, pharmacodynamic, and organ functions. Thus, it requires a more individualized approach to treatment decisions to provide the same benefits of the therapy as that of younger patients [18].

Hepatic Cancer, Treatments, and Challenges

Carcinoma in the Hepatocellular region originates in the liver, and it accounts for almost 80%–90% of all reported primary cancer of the liver. Current treatment of liver cancer includes surgery *i.e.*, either removal of the tumor or liver transplantation in which the affected liver is removed which is replaced, and support is given by a healthy liver from a suitable donor; localized treatment (different modes directly treat affected cells and the surrounding areas) including heating cancer cells (electric current induced cell ablation by radiofrequency waves), freezing cancer cells (extreme cold-induced cell destruction named as cryoablation), injecting alcohol in tumor cell which destroys tumor cells; Chemoembolization (injecting chemotherapy drugs directly inside the tumor cells); placing spheres containing radiation inside the tumor; targeted therapy (bevacizumab with atezolizumab, lenvatinib, ramucirumab); radiation therapy; immunotherapy (nivolumab, nivolumab with ipilimumab, atezolizumab with bevacizumab); and chemotherapy [19 - 21].

The major challenge faced in hepatic cancer is that most patients with hepatic cancer are diagnosed in the advanced stage, thus making prognosis difficult.

Prostate Cancer, Treatments, and Challenges

Prostate cancer is very common in men, and it accounts for almost 29% of all reported cancer cases in men. Primarily, surgery, cryotherapy, and radiation therapy (External-beam radiotherapy and brachytherapy) are very commonly used options for prostate cancer therapy. Recently, proton beam therapy has also been introduced as a very effective option for prostate cancer therapy. However, chemotherapy (docetaxel, doxorubicin, mitoxantrone, vinblastine, paclitaxel, *etc.*), hormonal therapy (estrogens, agonist of gonadotropin-releasing hormone (GnRH), GnRH antagonist, 5-alpha reductase inhibitors, androgen receptor blockers, adrenal androgen inhibitors) are widely used treatment options in prostate cancer. Besides those, other options like high-intensity focused ultrasound (HIFU) and cryosurgery are also a few treatment options that are selected depending on the severity of the condition [22].

Patients with over-treatment may experience multiple complex adverse effects, especially in the case of radical prostatectomy and/or treatment by radiation. The most common side effects include urinary incontinence and sexual dysfunction. Radiation therapy by electron beam leads to erectile dysfunction, urinary dysfunction, and bowel dysfunction. Loss of sexual activity, breast swelling, hot flashes, anaemia, and osteoporosis are the common side effect of androgen deprivation therapy. The post-effect of brachytherapy includes distressing urinary symptoms, decreased erectile function, diarrhea, and persistent rectal bleeding [23]. Thus, the major hurdles faced in the management of prostate cancer is to prevent on minimize the adverse effects such as decreased potency and urinary incontinence after cancer therapy.

Moreover, the major difficulty faced in prostate cancer is proper sampling for biopsy. Most of the time, it remains unidentified whether, the increase in grade or volume on subsequent analysis is a result of further progression of the original tumor or the result of accurate sampling. Others challenges include to evaluate the risk whether there is a chance of developing prostate cancer and the major associated factors which can enhance the risks during his lifetime. There is not that much progress in the diagnosis and treatment of this disease however, extensive research is going on to optimize the existing options for the treatment of prostate cancer [24].

Blood Cancer, Treatments, and Challenges

The current treatment of blood cancer includes stem cell transplantation (infusion of healthy stem cells helps in blood formation, which is obtained either from the umbilical cord or bone marrow), chemotherapy, targeted therapy (monoclonal antibodies, interferons, tyrosine kinase inhibitors), and radiation therapy.

The challenges faced in blood cancer management include the identification of the blood cancer subgroup. The affected individuals with the most detrimental genetic arrays focus on the personalized approach while continuing to balance the treatment and financial toxicity and improving patient outcomes [25].

Skin Cancer, Treatments, and Challenges

Current treatment of skin cancer is surgery; targeted therapy including targeting BRAF and MEK (vemurafenib and dabrafenib), Type III transmembrane Receptor Tyrosine Kinase (nilotinib); immunotherapy (interleukin 2, interferon, Cytotoxic T-Lymphocyte-Associated Protein 4 blockers, programmed Death 1 blocking antibodies) [26]; radiation therapy, chemotherapy, photodynamic therapy; biological therapy.

At present, for the treatment of melanoma and other types of cancers, immunotherapy is considered one of the most innovative ways. However, despite its novel features, the different extent of patient response is the mostly faced rate-limiting factor of this treatment model. Improving patient response is the most challenging aspect of immunotherapy. Another high obstacle in immunotherapy is the development of resistance in subsequent therapies. It is observed that the mitogen-activated protein kinase (MAPK) pathway reactivation is the key factor for this resistance development.

Pancreatic Cancer, Treatments, and Challenges

Present treatment modes for pancreatic cancer are radiation therapy, surgery, and chemotherapy. Among various anti-cancer agents widely used chemotherapeutic agents used for the treatment of pancreatic cancer are Nab-paclitaxel, Capecitabine, Nanoliposomal irinotecan, Fluorouracil (5-FU), Leucovorin, Gemcitabine, Irinotecan, *etc.* The targeted therapies widely used in pancreatic cancer are (Erlotinib, Olaparib, Larotrectinib) and immunotherapy (pembrolizumab).

The components of the tumor microenvironment include tumor-associated macrophages and cytokines, which promote an immunosuppressive environment, thus, affecting the efficacy of treatment. The microenvironmental conditions of the tumor and the surrounding regions play a major role in response to immunotherapy. This environmental condition helps to trigger the reactivation of the immune system and helps in invading the tumor cells. In pancreatic cancer, it is observed that an inflammation-driven desmoplasia is developed in the pancreas, which forms a thick stromal microenvironment. This layer is the most challenging part to invade for the various active ingredients intended to cross this barrier and need to enter tumor cells to elicit their action. Moreover, knowledge of the molecular behavior of pancreatic cancer is limited, which is the major challenge in the management of pancreatic cancer.

FUTURE PERSPECTIVES

The current challenges discussed above can be overcome using advanced and novel techniques in cancer treatment. Many researchers across the globe are working on the development of new diagnostic, preventive, and treatment measures against all types of cancer. However, more research is required to develop early diagnostic methods and specific treatments for all types of cancer. In the case of breast surgery also, more advancement is required to produce the most favorable outcome in patients. Prescribing the drugs as per the genetic makeup of the individuals is one of the future. However, the cost is one of the biggest challenges regarding this, particularly in developing countries. We hope that in the future, personalized medicines going to be affordable to everyone. Most anti-cancer drugs are associated with major adverse drug reactions (ADRs). Thus, further studies are required to produce safe anti-cancer molecules. Nanomedicine plays a significant role in this regard by developing targeted medicines [27]. Molecularly targeted therapies, which inhibit specific growth factor receptors and their downstream signaling cascades, seem to be a favorable approach for the management of cancer. Besides monotherapy, combination therapy, either with multiple targeted agents or targeted therapy, along with traditional chemotherapy, might be a more effective modality to treat cancer [28].

In the future, identifying the specific antigen presented more readily on cancerous cells than on normal cells would be a great advantage for the development of immunotherapy for the management of cancer. The immune cell could recognize the cancer cells and can do the destruction to these cells by activating various immune signaling pathways. Surgery through robotics is also the upcoming future not only in cancer but against other diseases also [29].

Herbals can also play a significant role in the treatment of various disorders. The problems related to herbal formulations, like standardization, stability, content uniformity, *etc.*, could be solved in the future to a greater extent using upcoming advanced instruments.

Various ongoing and published studies regarding innovative approaches in the diagnosis and treatment of cancers. Current studies show that the dysregulation in iron metabolism and excess accumulation is associated with the occurrence of cancer due to its pro-oxidative nature and damaging effects on DNA. Moreover, leukemia cell utilizes surplus iron to maintain rapid growth and proliferation. Thus, targeting iron metabolism may provide new insights for approaches to the treatment of leukemia [30].

More conserved biomarkers that are expressed on the surface of tumor cells need to be discovered so that immunotherapies can be applied to a broader demographic of patients. Detailed knowledge of protein structures and the understanding of their role in key signaling pathways in melanoma development led to the designation of new targets for the treatment of melanoma. In the future, it is necessary to conduct further clinical trials and collect more data about overall survival, response rates, appropriate timing, and sequence of combination therapy to manage the complexity of skin treatment. We hope that one day we will be able to detect and treat cancer patients at an early stage.

CONCLUSION

In conclusion, although, the development of traditional therapy for cancer helps in decreasing the mortality rate. However, there are still various challenges in the management of cancer. However, understanding the pathogenesis of different types of cancers and the development of target-specific formulations will be of great help for its precise treatment.

CONSENT FOR PUBLICATION

Not applicable.

CONFLICT OF INTEREST

The authors declare no conflict of interest, financial or otherwise.

ACKNOWLEDGEMENTS

The authors are thankful to Vice-Chancellor, Prof. R.K. Goyal, Delhi Pharmaceutical Sciences & Research University (DPSRU), New Delhi, and Director, National Institute of Pharmaceutical Education and Research (NIPER), Raebareli, India, for their continuous support and motivation.

REFERENCES

[1] Arruebo M, Vilaboa N, Sáez-Gutierrez B, *et al.* Assessment of the evolution of cancer treatment therapies. Cancers (Basel) 2011; 3(3): 3279-330.
[http://dx.doi.org/10.3390/cancers3033279] [PMID: 24212956]

[2] Mansoori B, Mohammadi A, Davudian S, Shirjang S, Baradaran B. The different mechanisms of cancer drug resistance: a brief review. Adv Pharm Bull 2017; 7(3): 339-48.
[http://dx.doi.org/10.15171/apb.2017.041] [PMID: 29071215]

[3] Trédan O, Galmarini CM, Patel K, Tannock IF. Drug resistance and the solid tumor microenvironment. J Natl Cancer Inst 2007; 99(19): 1441-54.
[http://dx.doi.org/10.1093/jnci/djm135] [PMID: 17895480]

[4] Alfarouk KO, Stock CM, Taylor S, *et al.* Resistance to cancer chemotherapy: failure in drug response from ADME to P-gp. Cancer Cell Int 2015; 15(1): 71.
[http://dx.doi.org/10.1186/s12935-015-0221-1] [PMID: 26180516]

[5] Tran S, DeGiovanni PJ, Piel B, Rai P. Cancer nanomedicine: a review of recent success in drug delivery. Clin Transl Med 2017; 6(1): 44.
[http://dx.doi.org/10.1186/s40169-017-0175-0] [PMID: 29230567]

[6] Momenimovahed Z, Salehiniya H. Epidemiological characteristics of and risk factors for breast cancer in the world. Breast Cancer (Dove Med Press) 2019; 11: 151-64.
[http://dx.doi.org/10.2147/BCTT.S176070] [PMID: 31040712]

[7] Moo TA, Sanford R, Dang C, Morrow M. Overview of breast cancer therapy. PET Clin 2018; 13(3): 339-54.
[http://dx.doi.org/10.1016/j.cpet.2018.02.006] [PMID: 30100074]

[8] Collins KK, Liu Y, Schootman M, *et al.* Effects of breast cancer surgery and surgical side effects on

body image over time. Breast Cancer Res Treat 2011; 126(1): 167-76. [http://dx.doi.org/10.1007/s10549-010-1077-7] [PMID: 20686836]

[9] Bhattacharyya GS, Doval DC, Desai CJ, Chaturvedi H, Sharma S, Somashekhar SP. Overview of breast cancer and implications of overtreatment of early-stage breast cancer: an indian perspective. JCO Glob Oncol 2020; 6(6): 789-98. [http://dx.doi.org/10.1200/GO.20.00033] [PMID: 32511068]

[10] Ghiam AF, Spayne J, Lee J. Current challenges and future perspectives of radiotherapy for locally advanced breast cancer. Curr Opin Support Palliat Care 2014; 8(1): 46-52. [http://dx.doi.org/10.1097/SPC.0000000000000032] [PMID: 24441684]

[11] Kayl AE, Meyers CA. Side-effects of chemotherapy and quality of life in ovarian and breast cancer patients. Curr Opin Obstet Gynecol 2006; 18(1): 24-8. [http://dx.doi.org/10.1097/01.gco.0000192996.20040.24] [PMID: 16493256]

[12] Brackstone M, Townson JL, Chambers AF. Tumour dormancy in breast cancer: an update. Breast Cancer Res 2007; 9(3): 208. [http://dx.doi.org/10.1186/bcr1677] [PMID: 17561992]

[13] Zappa C, Mousa SA. Non-small cell lung cancer: current treatment and future advances. Transl Lung Cancer Res 2016; 5(3): 288-300. [http://dx.doi.org/10.21037/tlcr.2016.06.07] [PMID: 27413711]

[14] Hirsch FR, Scagliotti GV, Mulshine JL, *et al.* Lung cancer: current therapies and new targeted treatments. Lancet 2017; 389(10066): 299-311. [http://dx.doi.org/10.1016/S0140-6736(16)30958-8] [PMID: 27574741]

[15] Bunn PA Jr. The treatment of non-small cell lung cancer: current perspectives and controversies, future directions. Semin Oncol 1994; 21(3) (Suppl. 6): 49-59. [PMID: 8052874]

[16] Jain V, Berman A. Radiation pneumonitis: old problem, new tricks. Cancers (Basel) 2018; 10(7): 222. [http://dx.doi.org/10.3390/cancers10070222] [PMID: 29970850]

[17] Serrano C, George S. Gastrointestinal stromal tumor: challenges and opportunities for a new decade. Clin Cancer Res 2020; 26(19): 5078-85. [http://dx.doi.org/10.1158/1078-0432.CCR-20-1706] [PMID: 32601076]

[18] Joharatnam-Hogan N, Shiu KK, Khan K. Challenges in the treatment of gastric cancer in the older patient. Cancer Treat Rev 2020; 85: 101980. [http://dx.doi.org/10.1016/j.ctrv.2020.101980] [PMID: 32065879]

[19] Raza A, Sood GK. Hepatocellular carcinoma review: Current treatment, and evidence-based medicine. World J Gastroenterol 2014; 20(15): 4115-27. [http://dx.doi.org/10.3748/wjg.v20.i15.4115] [PMID: 24764650]

[20] Cuestas ML, Oubiña JR, Mathet VL. Hepatocellular carcinoma: overcoming challenges in disease management. Clinical Gastroenterology and Hepatology 2015; 4(3): 252-61.

[21] Gish RG. Hepatocellular carcinoma: overcoming challenges in disease management. Clin Gastroenterol Hepatol 2006; 4(3): 252-61. [http://dx.doi.org/10.1016/j.cgh.2006.01.001] [PMID: 16527686]

[22] Chen F, Zhao X. Prostate cancer: current treatment and prevention strategies. Iran Red Crescent Med J 2013; 15(4): 279-84. [http://dx.doi.org/10.5812/ircmj.6499] [PMID: 24082997]

[23] Harris R, Lohr KN. Screening for prostate cancer: an update of the evidence for the U.S. Preventive Services Task Force. Ann Intern Med 2002; 137(11): 917-29. [http://dx.doi.org/10.7326/0003-4819-137-11-200212030-00014] [PMID: 12458993]

[24] Frame I, Cant S. Current challenges in prostate cancer: an interview with Prostate Cancer UK. BMC

Med 2015; 13(1): 166.
[http://dx.doi.org/10.1186/s12916-015-0411-7] [PMID: 26205142]

[25] Kansagra A, Dahiya S, Litzow M. Continuing challenges and current issues in acute lymphoblastic leukemia. Leuk Lymphoma 2018; 59(3): 526-41.
[http://dx.doi.org/10.1080/10428194.2017.1335397] [PMID: 28604239]

[26] Orthaber K, Pristovnik M, Skok K, Perić B, Maver U. Skin cancer and its treatment: novel treatment approaches with emphasis on nanotechnology. J Nanomater 2017; 2017: 1-20.
[http://dx.doi.org/10.1155/2017/2606271]

[27] Allahverdiyev AM, Parlar E, Dinparvar S, Bagirova M, Abamor EŞ. Current aspects in treatment of breast cancer based of nanodrug delivery systems and future prospects. Artif Cells Nanomed Biotechnol 2018; 46(sup3): S755-62.
[http://dx.doi.org/10.1080/21691401.2018.1511573]

[28] Alqahtani A, Khan Z, Alloghbi A, Said Ahmed TS, Ashraf M, Hammouda DM. Hepatocellular carcinoma: molecular mechanisms and targeted therapies. Medicina (Kaunas) 2019; 55(9): 526.
[http://dx.doi.org/10.3390/medicina55090526] [PMID: 31450841]

[29] Samarasam I. Esophageal cancer in India: Current status and future perspectives. Int J Adv Med Health Res 2017; 4(1): 5-10.
[http://dx.doi.org/10.4103/IJAMR.IJAMR_19_17]

[30] Wang F, Lv H, Zhao B, *et al.* Iron and leukemia: new insights for future treatments. J Exp Clin Cancer Res 2019; 38(1): 406.
[http://dx.doi.org/10.1186/s13046-019-1397-3] [PMID: 31519186]

SUBJECT INDEX

A

B

Neeraj Mishra, Ashish Garg and Neeraj Upmanyu (Eds.)

C

D

K

L

M

N

O

P

R

S

T

V

W

Z

Made in the USA
Las Vegas, NV
15 November 2026

dbea1b3d-6a2f-4ae6-8326-0c3fd0398d26R01